Promoting and sustaining ... *e*

The List of Veterinary Nurses Incorporating The Register of Veterinary Nurses 2010

Revised to 8 Feb 2010

Royal College of Veterinary Surgeons
Belgravia House, 62-64 Horseferry Road, London SW1P 2AF

Telephones:

College: 020 7222 2001
Veterinary Nursing: 020 7202 0788
Library and Information Service: 020 7222 2021
Fax: 020 7222 2004
Email: vetnursing@rcvs.org.uk
Website: www.rcvs.org.uk

ISBN:978-0-902183-16-2
ISSN:1757-0891

Contents

Section 1 **7**

Membership of Veterinary Nurses Council and Sub-Committees
RCVS Contact Information
RCVS Trust Information

Section 2 **15**

Register of Small Animal Veterinary Nurses
Register of Equine Veterinary Nurses

Section 3 **209**

List of Small Animal Veterinary Nurses
List of Equine Veterinary Nurses

Section 4 **273**

Veterinary Nurses and the Veterinary Surgeons Act 1966

Section 5 **281**

Holders of the Diploma in Advanced Veterinary Nursing (Surgical)
Holders of the Diploma in Advanced Veterinary Nursing (Medical)

The VN Register and List

This publication is divided into two sections, to reflect the opening of the Register for Veterinary Nurses on 1 September 2007.

Those joining the Register are entitled to call themselves Registered Veterinary Nurses and use the postnominals RVN. These are listed in the first part of this publication.

RVNs are directly accountable for their professional practice. They demonstrate their commitment to professionalism to both the public and their employers by keeping their skills and knowledge up to date through mandatory Continuing Professional Development (an average of 45 hours over three years), and following the *Guide to Professional Conduct for Veterinary Nurses.*

All veterinary nurses who listed on or after 1 January 2003 were automatically transferred to the Register when it opened: the old List has closed to new entrants. Those listing before this date can transfer if they choose and many have already done so. Otherwise, they remain on the unregulated List, which forms the second part of this publication.

Both the Register and unregulated List are further subdivided into sections for small animal and equine VNs.

For more information about the Register, visit www.rcvs.org.uk/vnregister.

The List of Veterinary Nurses is now closed for the entry of names of new entrants to the profession.

Your personal data and the RCVS

The RCVS holds information relating to veterinary nurses for the purposes of maintaining the List of Veterinary Nurses, of which the Register is a subsection. The VN List and Register will be published each year and contains the following information:-

Name (and any change of name since registration)
The address specified for the Register/List
Telephone number (where known)
Date of listing
Reference number

This information is available upon request in hard copy or electronic format and certain details are also published on RCVSonline (www.rcvs.org.uk).

Information not made available to the public

Additional information requested from nurses includes date of birth (required, but will not be disclosed except in extreme circumstances), additional addresses and other contact information, for example, email, mobile phone and practice details. This information will not be available generally to the public and will not be disclosed without permission.

Updating your details

Nurses should inform the RCVS of any changes in the details of their registration/listing, including change of name, address or status, in writing and within 28 days of any such change. These changes can be modified in the following ways:

- Fill in the online form at www.rcvs.org.uk
- By fax to 020 7222 2004
- To request a form or for further information, contact the Registration Department on 020 7202 0707

Only changes of address may be notified by email and this must be from an email address previously recorded with the RCVS. Email changes should be sent to membership@rcvs.org.uk.

Electronic use of information

Some of the public information from the Register/List is made available on the RCVS website or in electronic format to third parties (within and outside the EU). The information on the RCVS website includes the name, location (but not full address), date of registration and reference number of each veterinary nurse. The information published in the Register/List of those veterinary nurses who have not recorded their objections to their data being used in this manner is occasionally passed onto third parties in accordance with the provisions of the Data Protection Act. Veterinary nurses' objections are recorded on their registration forms and are also reviewed and confirmed when data checks are undertaken. Veterinary nurses who do not wish their Register/List information to be passed on in this manner should contact the Registration Department. The RCVS will never pass on personal data that is not required to be held as part of the Register/List. Individuals may make a request for any personal information held about them under the Data Protection Act.

Section 1

Membership of Veterinary Nurses Council and Sub-Committees

RCVS Contact Information

RCVS Trust Information

MEMBERSHIP OF VETERINARY NURSES COUNCIL AND SUB-COMMITTEES 2009-2010

MEMBERS OF THE VETERINARY NURSES COUNCIL

RCVS Council Members are shown in bold

Symbols: # indicates Chairman + indicates Vice-Chairman

Secretary: Annette Amato

Birbeck A L	Hughes A L	Orpet H
Branscombe E #	Jeffery A K	Swindlehurst P A
Creighton D E +	Kissick K E	Thompson J
Glysen L	**Molyneux J R +**	Torrington H
Goldie C A	**Nute P J**	Yates J M
Hooker R K		

+ Chair, LANTRA Industry Group (House C)

Non-Voting Observers

BVNA

BSAVA

Non-RCVS Council Members

Rev A L BIRBECK MBE MA FRSA	[Appointee 2005-2013]
Ms E A BRANSCOMBE DipAVN(Surgical) RVN	[Elected 2006-2011]
Mrs D E CREIGHTON DipAVN(Surgical) RVN	[Elected 2004-2012]
Mrs L GLYSEN RVN	[Elected 2009-2013]
Mr R K HOOKER BVMS MRCVS	[Appointee 2005-2013]
Mr C J HOUSE BVetMed MRCVS	[LANTRA Nominee]
Mr A L HUGHES BVSc MRCVS	[Appointee 2005-2011]
Mrs K E KISSICK RVN	[Elected 2008-2012]
Mrs A JEFFERY DipAVN(Surgical) RVN	[Elected 2002-2013]
Ms H A ORPET DipAVN(Surgical) RVN	[Elected 2006-2010]
Mrs P A SWINDLEHURST	[Appointee 2008-2012]
Ms J A THOMPSON RVN	[Elected 2007-2011]
Mrs H TORRINGTONBVMS CertSAO MRCVS	[Appointee 2008-2011]
Mrs J M YATES DipAVN(Surgical) RVN	[Elected 2006-2010]

Regular Non-Voting Observers (BSAVA +BVNA)

Awarding Body Board

(Reporting to Veterinary Nurses Council)
Secretary: Annette Amato

Member of RCVS Council and the Veterinary Nurses Council (Chairman)
Nurse member of the Veterinary Nurses Council
RCVS Head of Veterinary Nursing (Awarding Body Manager)
Awarding Body Quality Assurance Manager
Examinations and Higher Education Quality Manager
Sector Skills Council (LANTRA) representative
VN Chief Scrutineer
VN HE Educators (2) (representing university provision)
VN FE Educator (representing VRQ provision)
Centre Representative (representing approved NVQ centres)
Industry representatives from veterinary nursing, and the relevant disciplines of veterinary practice, normally to be recruited via representative organisations

RCVS Awarding Body Examinations Sub-Committee

(Reporting to the Awarding Body Board)
Secretary: Ben Myring

Chairman of the Awarding Body Board (Chairman)
Examinations and Higher Education Quality Manager
RCVS Head of Veterinary Nursing (Awarding Body Manager)
Principal Examiners
Equine Examiner Representative
Small Animal Examiner Representative
Course Provider Members of the Awarding Body Board
Chief Scrutineer

Veterinary Nursing Continuing Education Sub-Committee

Secretary: Annette Amato

Member of RCVS Veterinary Nurses Council (Chairman)
Member of RCVS Veterinary Nurses Council
Lay Member of RCVS Veterinary Nurses Council
DipAVN Senior Examiner
DipAVN Programme Providers
VN CPD providers
RCVS Head of Veterinary Nursing (Awarding Body Manager)
Examinations and Higher Education Quality Manager

ROYAL COLLEGE OF VETERINARY SURGEONS CONTACT INFORMATION

Royal College of Veterinary Surgeons (RCVS)
Belgravia House
62-64 Horseferry Road
London
SW1P 2AF

Switchboard Telephone Number:	**020 7222 2001**
College General Fax Number:	**020 7222 2004**

Principal Staff at the Veterinary Nursing Department

General email - vetnursing@rcvs.org.uk

Head of Department
Elizabeth Earle BA RN TD 020 72020732
(l.earle@rcvs.org.uk)

Deputy Head of Department and Committee Secretary
Annette Amato BSc(Hons) 020 7202 0713 (a.amato@rcvs.org.uk)

Careers advice and student registration
Amy Woods BSc(Hons) 020 7202 0711 (a.woods@rcvs.org.uk)

Examinations and assessment (candidates)
Ben Myring BA(Hons) 020 7202 0738 (b.myring@rcvs.org.uk)

Examiner and examination centre support
Victoria Hedges RVN 020 7202 0782 (v.hedges@rcvs.org.uk)

Centre and course provider approval
Christine James BA(Hons) 020 7202 0711 (c.james@rcvs.org.uk)

Award certificates and listing qualification
Jennifer Orme BA(Hons) 020 7202 0756 (j.orme@rcvs.org.uk)

Awarding Body Quality Assurance Manager
Julie Dugmore RVN 020 7202 0775 (j.dugmore@rcvs.org.uk)

Registration Department
Veterinary Nurses Register/List -
Dorothy Brereton 020 7202 0706 (d.brereton@rcvs.org.uk)

Principal Staff of the College

President's/Registrar's Office	**registrar@rcvs.org.uk**
Secretary/Registrar:	Jane C Hern MA 020 7202 0716 registrar@rcvs.org.uk
Manager, Executive Office:	Lesley Evans 020 7202 0716 l.evans@rcvs.org.uk
Special Projects Consultant:	John Collins BSc(Eng) ACGI 020 7202 0708 j.collins@rcvs.org.uk
Professional Conduct	**profcon@rcvs.org.uk**
Head of Professional Conduct/ Assistant Registrar:	Gordon Hockey MRPharmS, Barrister 020 7202 0718 g.hockey@rcvs.org.uk
Corporate Services	**admin@rcvs.org.uk**
Head of Corporate Services:	Richard Holford PGDCCI(OPEN) 020 7202 0754 r.holford@rcvs.org.uk
Education	**education@rcvs.org.uk**
Head of Education:	Freda Andrews BA(Hons) PGCE 020 7202 0702 f.andrews@rcvs.org.uk
Communications	**communications@rcvs.org.uk**
Head of Communications:	Lizzie Lockett BA(Hons) Oxon 020 7202 0725 l.lockett@rcvs.org.uk
Finance	**finance@rcvs.org.uk**
Head of Finance:	Corrie McCann BSc ACA 020 7202 0724 c.mccann@rcvs.org.uk

Facilities	**facilitiesteam@rcvs.org.uk**
Head of Facilities:	Martyn Webster 020 7202 0765 m.webster@rcvs.org.uk
Registration	**membership@rcvs.org.uk**
Head of Registration:	Christine Fraser BA(Hons) Solicitor 020 7202 0758 c.fraser@rcvs.org.uk
RCVS Trust	**info@rcvstrust.org.uk**
Director:	Cherry Bushell 020 7202 0714 c.bushell@rcvstrust.org.uk
Librarian:	Clare Boulton 020 7202 0721 c.boulton@rcvs.org.uk

RCVS Trust for Veterinary Nurses

The RCVS Trust can support your professional development and practice in two key ways :

1. For information to support your degree or diploma studies, look no further than the **RCVS Trust Library**. The Library holds a large collection of books and journals, which are available on loan. You can also access hundreds of full text electronic journals via your own computer, either at work or home. We offer free Library membership to Registered and Listed Veterinary Nurses.

Check out the website at www.rcvslibrary.org.uk where you can search the Library catalogue, order documents and see the full range of services on offer, or contact us:

RCVS Trust Library
Belgravia House
62-64 Horseferry Road
London SW1P 2AF
Telephone: 020 7202 0752
Fax: 020 7202 0751
Email: library@rcvstrust.org.uk

2. Every year we offer **RCVS Trust Awards** such as travel scholarships or research grants to support your professional development. Past grants awarded to Listed and Registered Veterinary Nurses include:

Name	Project	Award
Sarah Collins, Bristol	IVECCS Congress and AVECCT Examination fee	£1,000
Emma Wilder, Peak Veterinary Practice	Advanced Diploma in Practical Aspect of Companion Animal Behaviour and Training	£2,000

Our grants rounds are advertised in the veterinary press and on our website www.rcvstrust.org.uk so do look out for them.

We always encourage veterinary nurses to get involved in our fundraising activities; either by doing a solo or group sponsored event, joining National Pet Month activities or adopting or buying a book in our listings. We provide resources, advice and PR support to all our eventers, so don't be shy, give us a call if you'd like to get involved.

Call us on 020 7202 0743 to find out more or go to www.rcvstrust.org.uk.

Section 2

Register of Small Animal Veterinary Nurses
Register of Equine Veterinary Nurses

Register of Small Animal Veterinary Nurses 2010

Notes:

1. The current Schedule 3 of the Veterinary Surgeons Act 1966 permits those Veterinary Nurses whose names are on the Register (incorporated as part of the List) of Veterinary Nurses, maintained by the Royal College of Veterinary Surgeons, to carry out any medical treatment or minor surgery (not involving entry into a body cavity) to an animal providing the guidance given in Section 4 of this List, incorporating the Register of Veterinary Nurses, is complied with.
2. The first date after a veterinary nurse's name is the date of initial qualification. The date in brackets (if any) is the date of the last restoration to the Register or List, should a nurse's name have lapsed/been removed from the Register or List at any time. These dates are not intended to indicate the periods for which a name has been on the Register or List. Should information be required as to the full period or total periods a name has been on the Register or List, a request should be made to the Registration Department.
3. Small Animal Veterinary Nurses whose names are on the Register are entitled to use the postnominal letters "RVN" whilst their name is maintained on the Register.

A

ABBEY Jennifer 03/10/2008 Barrow Hill Veterinary Hospital Maidstone Road ASHFORD Kent TN24 8TY w 6437989

ABBITT Gemma Louise 15/07/2005 37 Whitstable Road Faversham Kent ME13 8BG **Tel:** (01795) 535972 w 6293559

ABBOSH Nadine 19/08/1994 5 Buller Mews Bury Lancashire BL8 2BU **Tel:** (0411) 391 329 w 602393X

ABBOTT Christine Ann (nee French) 04/08/1981 (06/06/2002) Briar House Veterinary Surgery 13-15 St Peters Road Broadstairs Kent CT10 2AG **Tel:** (01843) 863395 w 6044381

Claire Michelle 23/12/2008 Woodcote Two Mile Ash Road Horsham West Sussex RH13 0LA **Tel:** 01403730516 w 6429673

ABBOTT Louise Clare (see DAVEY, Mrs)

Phillippa Rachel 21/08/2003 123 South Street Elgin Morayshire IV30 1JB **Tel:** (01343) 542255 w 6276355

ABBOTTS Zoe 10/09/1999 55 Avon Road DEVIZES Wiltshire SN10 1PS w 6185022

ABD'EE Rachel 30/11/2005 4 Battersea Park Road Battersea London SW8 4AA **Tel:** (020) 7627 9256 w 6320256

ABEL Kate Alice 27/03/2008 Diglake House 1 Harridge Lane Scarisbrick Ormskirk Lancashire L40 8HD **Tel:** (01704) 841 527 w 6417199

ABOSCH Katy Louise 12/02/2008 1 Village Mews Wilsden BRADFORD West Yorkshire BD15 0DG **Tel:** (01535) 274563 w 6403834

ABRAHAM Katie Joy 26/07/2004 45 Station Road Little Sutton Ellesmere Port CH66 1NU **Tel:** (0151) 339 2605 w 6302062

Tracy Louise 18/08/2008 36 Danforth Drive Framlingham Woodbridge Suffolk IP13 9HH w 6398180

ABRAHAMS Suzanne 13/09/1999 11 Watermens Square High Street Penge LONDON SE20 7EL w 6185418

ABRAHAMSON Elizabeth 10/09/1999 (07/07/2008) 29 Landseer Gardens SOUTH SHIELDS Tyne and Wear NE34 8HS **Tel:** (0191) 423 1660 w 6138361

ABSON Kirsty Dawn 02/09/2008 10 Watercroft ROCHDALE Lancashire OL11 5PH **Tel:** 01706649148 w 6434436

ACEVEDO-ASHMORE Laura Ann (see ASHMORE, Miss)

ACKERMAN Nicola Anne (nee Lakeman) 28/10/2002 The Veterinary Hospital Colwill Road Estover Plymouth Devon PL6 8RP **Tel:** (01752) 702646 w 6273473

ACKERS Sara Miriam 11/11/2009 Parciau Farm Griffiths Crossing Caernarfon Gwynedd LL55 1TS **Tel:** (01286) 675 038 w 6390458

ACLAND Paula Suzanne 25/04/2005 (06/03/2007) 48 Albert Road St Philips Bristol BS2 0XA **Tel:** (0117) 972 4567 w 6245016

ADAMS Adena Claire 07/05/2009 4 Baden Gardens BASINGSTOKE Hampshire RG23 8BE **Tel:** 01256336938 w 6441883

Alice Elizabeth DipAVN(Medical) (nee Hendry) 10/02/2004 5 Lancaster Road HITCHIN

Hertfordshire SG5 1PE **Tel:** (01462) 612233 w 6285067

Claire Rachel Emily 25/01/2010 Dollars Grove Farm East End North Crawley NEWPORT PAGNELL Buckinghamshire MK16 9HW **Tel:** (01234) 391091 w 6497763

Corrina (nee Belcher) 27/02/2006 Mullacott Veterinary Hospital Bickenbridge Farm Ilfracombe Devon EX34 8NZ **Tel:** (01271) 866770 w 6330123

Elizabeth Katherine Anne 30/01/2009 22 Lampton Close Wool Wareham Dorset BH20 6EW **Tel:** 01929463100 w 6417617

Jayne Louise 13/04/2004 30 Devoke Close Huntingdon Cambridgeshire PE29 6XE w 6287399

ADAMS Julii (see ELLIOTT, Mrs)

Kailee Michele 17/08/2009 Petersfield Veterinary Centre 16-18 St Peters Road Petersfield Hampshire GU31 4AA **Tel:** (01730) 266 431 w 6374431

Kirstie Olivia (nee Hay) 22/02/2007 Birch Heath Road Tarporley Cheshire CW6 9UU **Tel:** (01829) 733777 w 6292800

Louisa Charlotte 06/10/2006 South Moor Vets Derby Road Kingsbridge Devon TQ7 1JL **Tel:** (01548) 852766 w 6320267

Marion (nee Gillow) 22/04/2003 Honeysuckle Cottage 7 The Cross Ilminster Somerset TA19 0EH **Tel:** (07951) 770884 w 6285144

ADAMS Samantha Jaine (see CALDER, Mrs)

Sharon Michelle 16/09/2008 64 Leighton Avenue SWINDON Wiltshire SN3 2HT w 6247062

Sharon Vanessa (nee Newell) 29/07/1974 44 Oakleigh Park Drive Leigh-on-Sea Essex SS9 1RP **Tel:** (01702) 712631 w 6044472

Wendy Elsie Irene (nee Carter) 04/11/1992 (22/08/2006) 12 The Holt Mollington Banbury Oxfordshire OX17 1BE **Tel:** (01327) 262992 w 6012065

ADAMSON Dawn (see HYND, Mrs)

ADAMSON Jaime Sara 10/01/2007 Cobham Veterinary Centre Byfleet Road Cobham Surrey KT11 1DS **Tel:** (01932) 868786 w 6378039

Joanne 09/07/2004 2 High Street Bushey Watford WD23 3DN **Tel:** (020) 8950 2002 w 6369602

Sarah Louise (nee Leavens) 11/09/1998 Garston Veterinary Group Garston House Portway Frome Somerset BA11 1PZ **Tel:** (01373) 451115 w 613105X

ADDISON Gemma (nee Hulson, nee Addison) 28/02/2005 1 Kirby Road Waterbeach CAMBRIDGE CB25 9LX w 6288477

Hayley Ann (nee Corner) 15/11/2001 Oakwood Veterinary Surgery Harper Lane Radlett Hertfordshire WD7 7HY **Tel:** (01923) 853573 w 6251308

ADDISON Joanna Kathryn (see BEEVERS, Mrs)

Marian (nee Davies) 04/02/1992 'Woodside' 48 Third Avenue Gwersyllt Wrexham LL11 4EF **Tel:** (01978) 720325 w 6075740

Stacey Dawn 19/04/2006 67 Bretch Hill BANBURY Oxfordshire OX16 0LE **Tel:** (01295) 254954 w 6342311

ADKINS Amy Lauren 18/08/2009 Blackthorn House 3 Pond Close Newton Longville Milton Keynes Buckinghamshire MK17 0BY **Tel:** (01908) 376 575 w 6440442

ADRIAN Charlotte Ruth (see PACE, Mrs)

ADSHEAD Samantha Joy 27/02/2002 5 Oakfields Hanbury Burton-on-Trent Staffordshire DE13 8TP **Tel:** (01283) 815 226 w 6185946

AGAR Joanne 04/02/2009 3 Silk Mill Way Alkrington Middleton MANCHESTER M24 1QJ **Tel:** 0161653512 w 6446019

AGNEW Heather Jacqueline 30/05/2007 Kingstown Lisnaskea Enniskillen County Fermanagh BT92 5GX **Tel:** (028) 677 23310 w 6377016

Jennifer Ann 19/03/2007 95 Barry Drive Leicester Forest East Leicester Leicestershire LE9 2HJ **Tel:** (0116) 2390 954 w 6363354

AGNEW Lauren (see REID, Mrs)

AHEARNE Jennifer Marie (nee Penny) 03/02/1995 (16/03/2007) 4 Shortwood Close Budleigh Salterton Devon EX9 6QW **Tel:** (01395) 444249 w 6035355

AIKENHEAD Kyley Ann 29/09/2008 69 Neal Road West Kingsdown Sevenoaks Kent TN15 6DG w 6358745

AIKMAN Alison Claire (nee Boyle) 02/02/1998 4 Raynham Drive Loughborough Leicestershire LE11 4TW **Tel:** (01509) 2831314 w 6097753

AINSLIE Lee Anne 22/02/2007 Stoneburn House Vellore Road Maddiston FALKIRK Stirlingshire FK2 0AR w 6261890

AINSWORTH Michelle Joanne (nee Lowe) 15/12/2004 63 London Road South Poynton Stockport Cheshire SK12 1LA **Tel:** (01625) 859019 w 6321983

AIREY Louise 14/09/2005 110 Chichester Road Cleethorpes South Humberside DN35 0JJ **Tel:** (01472) 697207 w 6319101

AITCHISON Gillian Margaret 12/08/2008 87 Grieveship West STROMNESS Orkney KW16 3BQ w 6346865

Nicola Marie 10/02/2004 78 Shay Lane Ovenden Halifax West Yorkshire HX3 6QU **Tel:** (01422) 354542 w 6288862

AITKEN Dawn Lesley 28/06/2005 6 Mansfield Crescent Hawick TD9 8AQ **Tel:** (01450) 378974 w 6325635

Emma Patricia 04/11/2005 15a Hamlyn Road Glastonbury Somerset BA6 8HS w 6344412

Heather 27/04/2006 6 Rostherne Way SANDBACH Cheshire CW11 1WS **Tel:** (01270) 767286 w 6331124

AJCHINGER Helen Louise 10/04/2008 3 Abingdon Road Wolverhampton West Midlands WV1 2PP **Tel:** 07731757631 w 6406441

ALBRIGHTON Sarah-Jane (see REYNOLDS, Mrs)

ALCOCK Claire (nee Sadler) 02/06/2006 14 Baslow Drive Heald Green CHEADLE Cheshire SK8 3HP **Tel:** (01616) 109 867 w 6325349

ALDER Katie Margaret 21/08/2009 Cornhill House West Challow Wantage Oxfordshire OX12 9TD **Tel:** 01235766271 w 6448384

Rebecca Louise 29/10/2008 24 Norman Drive Stilton Peterborough Cambridgeshire PE7 3RS **Tel:** 01733248160 w 6406166

ALDERMAN Eileen Margaret 20/09/1996 4 Church Terrace London NW4 4JU **Tel:** (0208) 2032090 w 6043082

Gareth Edward 04/12/2003 Greenwood Veterinary Clinic 57 Station Approach South Ruislip Middlesex HA4 6SL **Tel:** (020) 8845 8144 m 6144036

Tracy Maud (formerly Cockshoot) 06/03/2006 60 Charles Street Kettering Northamptonshire NN16 9RL w 6304757

ALDERSON Valerie (see HALL, Mrs)

ALDERTON Christopher James 06/08/2008 67 Arnolds Avenue Hutton Brentwood Essex CM13 1EY **Tel:** (01277) 216 900 m 6406804

ALDERWICK Louise Anne 20/03/2008 17 Hylder Close SWINDON SN2 2SL **Tel:** (01793) 729881 w 6372781

ALDHAM Carrie Ann 15/09/2009 14 Mollison Close Woodley Reading RG5 4XG **Tel:** 0189695329 w 6452080

ALDRED Gemma Louise (nee Healey) 27/02/2006 Oakham Veterinary Hospital Ashwell Road Oakham Rutland LE15 7QH **Tel:** (01572) 722646 w 6296188

ALDRIDGE Faye (nee Sherwood) 04/10/2005 49 Skylark Rise Plymouth Devon PL6 7SN **Tel:** (01752) 695258 w 6301798

Samantha Claire 01/07/2009 10 Cornwall Road Whitehill BORDON Hampshire GU35 9PP **Tel:** 01420476978 w 6378809

ALEXANDER Katherine Amanda 21/07/2008 48 Lytton Road London E11 1JH **Tel:** (0208) 925 1740 w 6375872

Katherine Anne (nee Spence) 06/08/1990 The Grate 52 Mancetter Road Nuneaton Warwickshire CV10 0HN **Tel:** (024) 76397962 w 6061104

Laura 26/08/2008 9 Baltersan Gardens Quarter Hamilton Lanarkshire ML3 7QW **Tel:** 07746733569 w 6379557

ALEXANDER Lynda Anne (see LINEY, Mrs)

Victoria Anne 04/02/1994 Treveth Victoria Davidstow Camelford Cornwall PL32 9XS **Tel:** (01840) 261452 w 6067718

ALGAR Denise Yvonne (see GALER, Mrs)

ALLAN Janet Margaret 18/08/1995 10 Blackwall Halifax HX1 2BE **Tel:** (01422) 354106 w 6039622

Lisa 29/09/2009 Flat 0/1 676 Tollcross Road GLASGOW G32 8TB **Tel:** (0141) 550 2134 w 6459395

Lucy 08/04/2008 7 Turners Close WORCESTER WR4 9YX **Tel:** (07966) 403847 w 6366676

ALLAWAY Jacqueline Kim (see JAYNE, Mrs)

ALLDRED Cassie Ann 14/09/2001 12 Near Meadow Long Eaton Nottingham Nottinghamshire NG10 1PZ **Tel:** (0115) 946 5076 w 6228142

ALLEN Amanda Jayne (see DISNEY, Mrs)

ALLEN Claire Rebecca (formerly Tebble) 24/08/1995 The Veterinary Hospital 4 Bath Road Hungerford Berkshire RG17 0HE **Tel:** (01488) 682193/683999 w 6039112

David Philip 17/07/2008 66 Rivermead Stalham NORWICH Norfolk NR12 9PJ **Tel:** (01692) 581415 m 6377269

ALLEN Deborah (see ROBERTS, Mrs)

Elizabeth Georgina 20/07/2007 57 Weston Avenue LEIGHTON BUZZARD Bedfordshire LU7 4QZ w 6328066

Elizabeth Jane 07/11/2008 8 Beaufort Road REIGATE Surrey RH2 9DJ w 6421874

ALLEN Hannah Victoria (see MYBURGH, Mrs)

ALLEN Jacqueline Mary (see SMITH, Mrs)

Kerri Jane 16/02/2009 197 Bryn Place Llay Wrexham Clwyd LL12 0LT **Tel:** 01978720362 w 6416539

Louise Elizabeth 14/05/2007 Three Cross Veterinary Surgery Welyndale Verwood Road Three Legged Cross WIMBORNE Dorset BH21 6RR **Tel:** (01202) 829436 w 6305857

Naomi 10/04/2007 1 Lansbury Road Rugeley Staffordshire WS15 1PD **Tel:** (01889) 585149 w 6283252

ALLEN Rachel (see WAGER, Mrs)

Sarah Leanne 06/07/2004 12 Webley Rise Moseley Parklands Wolverhampton West Midlands WV10 8UH **Tel:** (01902) 782493 w 6270767

Sarah Louise 16/09/2009 112 Apley Way Witney Oxfordshire OX28 5BQ **Tel:** (01993) 200322 w 6466743

ALLENDEN Caroline 13/05/2003 4 Cranmer Close Morden Surrey SM4 4SU **Tel:** (020) 8330 5454 w 6277158

ALLFREE Reuben David William 18/11/2008 190 Graig Road Godrergraig Swansea West Glamorgan SA9 2NZ **Tel:** (01639) 845606 m 6371505

ALLINSON Debbie Ann 21/11/2007 Milton Lodge Hargill Lane LEYBURN North Yorkshire DL8 5NB w 6379491

ALLISON Claire Lewis (nee Kenyon) 18/10/2005 27 The Paddock Kirton BOSTON Lincolnshire PE20 1LA w 6331531

Megan Claire (nee Miles) 29/09/2004 15 Court Lawns Tylers Green Penn High Wycombe Buckinghamshire HP10 8DH **Tel:** (07979) 545315 w 6283351

ALLSEBROOK Lynne (see DURBER, Mrs)

ALLWOOD Judith Margaret 17/01/2006 Fountain Farm 128 Launceston Road Callington Cornwall PL17 8DS **Tel:** (01752) 254167 w 6332532

Sara Sanchia (nee Fox) 09/10/1978 (22/04/1998) Hykeham Green Lincoln Road North Hykeham Lincoln Lincolnshire LN6 8NH **Tel:** (01522) 683300 w 6077930

ALMOND Alison Claire 11/11/2009 Apartment 10 Glasscutter 45 Petherton Road BRISTOL BS14 9BW **Tel:** 01275839213 w 6461045

Hannah Kate 09/11/2005 16 Stamford Street Newmarket Suffolk CB8 8JB **Tel:** (07929) 758359 w 6347195

ALSOP Nicola Kate (see BROWN, Mrs)

ALVES Isabel Margarida Pratas 31/01/2008 83 Meadow Lane LOUGHBOROUGH Leicestershire LE11 1JU w 6398202

ALVSAKER Kirsty Jane McLeod (see HARRISON, Mrs)

AMBROSE Tracy 10/03/2009 124 Graylands Farm Bungalow Oak Hill Wood Street Village GUILDFORD Surrey GU3 3ES **Tel:** (01483) 236593 w 6377027

AMESBURY Emma Louise (see EAGLAND, Mrs)

AMOS Rebecca Louise 21/09/2009 52 High Street Harpole Northampton NN7 4BS **Tel:** 07754735408 w 6452256

ANDERSON Angela (nee Anderson, formerly Green) 25/01/1994 (29/04/2005) PDSA Kings Road Southwick Sunderland SR5 2LH **Tel:** (0191) 5160637 w 6065801

Catherine Eve 30/03/2001 142 Derby Road Long Eaton Nottingham NG10 4ER **Tel:** (0115) 972 7050 w 6214524

Charmain 11/04/2005 3 Valentia Close Bletchingdon KIDLINGTON Oxfordshire OX5 3DF w 6296100

Cheryl 27/08/2008 175 Portobello High Street EDINBURGH EH15 1EU **Tel:** (0131) 669 3790 w 6408894

Emma Jane (nee Seaney) 16/04/2009 3 The Cedars Fleet Hampshire GU51 3YL **Tel:** (01252) 612150 w 6373793

Jenna Louise 13/02/2009 9 Jodrell Close Horndean WATERLOOVILLE Hampshire PO8 9NH w 6443918

Jennifer 21/05/2007 34 High Street Longstanton Cambridge CB24 3BS **Tel:** (01954) 780027 w 6371516

Jillian (nee McIntosh) 14/08/1987 34 Barkers Butts Lane Coventry West Midlands CV6 1DT **Tel:** (02476) 590298 w 6044632

Kerry Michelle 01/12/2008 26 Couston Drive Dalgety Bay DUNFERMLINE Fife KY11 9NX **Tel:** 01383824157 w 6404131

Kirsty 15/04/2004 86b Meadside Avenue Kilbarchan JOHNSTONE Renfrewshire PA10 2LT w 6291304

Leanne Ellen 29/12/2003 207 Forest Glade Langdon Hills BASILDON Essex SS16 6SX **Tel:** (079680) 15580 w 6290424

Lois Anne 08/04/2005 University of Glasgow Veterinary School Garscube Estate Glasgow G61 1QH **Tel:** (0141) 330 5848 w 6318386

Naomi 15/01/2009 113 The Street Mereworth MAIDSTONE Kent ME18 5LU **Tel:** (01622) 814246 w 6261560

Rachel Ann (nee Jefferson) 04/02/2009 The Gables Veterinary Centre First Lane HESSLE East Yorkshire HU13 9HD **Tel:** (01482) 648942 w 6446030

Sian Jessica Susan (nee Ring) 01/09/1999 71 Cromwell Road CATERHAM Surrey CR3 5JF **Tel:** (01883) 330035 w 6121904

Sophie 02/10/2009 26a Teversham Way Sawston CAMBRIDGE CB22 3DF w 6459505

Sophie Jane 17/08/2005 City Road Veterinary Centre City Road Truro Cornwall TR1 2JL **Tel:** (01872) 273959 w 6282207

Tara 10/07/2009 1 Church Street West Wemyss Kirkcaldy Fife KY1 4SX **Tel:** (01592) 650 629 w 6436878

ANDREW Fiona Mairi 16/03/2009 1 Douglas Crescent Kinross Perthshire KY13 8TJ **Tel:** (01577) 830682 w 6345622

ANDREW Gillian Ruth (see MACINTYRE, Mrs)

Katherine Louise 08/08/2005 Pennard House 5 Eardley Road Sevenoaks Kent TN13 1XY **Tel:** (01732) 452344 w 6311434

ANDREWS Beverley Denise (nee Andrews, formerly Smith) 06/11/2000 34 Dombey Close Higham Rochester Kent ME3 7AE **Tel:** (01474) 824 594 w 6136896

Elaine Angela (nee Comerie) 07/08/1988 465/467 Nottingham Road Chaddesden Derby DE21 6NA **Tel:** (01332) 661554 w 6047983

ANDREWS Elizabeth Kate (see LOCKWOOD, Mrs)

Fiona Margaret 12/05/2004 Springfield Surgery Cranbrook Road Hawkhurst CRANBROOK Kent TN18 5EE **Tel:** (01580) 752187 w 6295209

ANDREWS Gemma Valerie (see BRISTOLL, Mrs)

Hayley Louisa 02/09/2009 2 Valleydene Dibden Purlieu Southampton SO45 4NG **Tel:** 02380845660 w 6452102

Kate (nee Honour) 09/09/2002 9 Hetherington Close Slough Berkshire SL2 2HP **Tel:** (01923) 450662 w 6279512

Linzi Marie 08/01/2008 12 Loxley Close Wellesbourne Warwick Warwickshire CV35 9RU **Tel:** (01472) 313637 w 6381471

Lucy Rebecca 27/11/2008 114 Kingshill Road SWINDON SN1 4LQ **Tel:** 01793528677 w 6402470

Victoria Joyce DipAVN(Surgical) (nee Smith) 06/02/1997 5 Wyvern Close Wellesbourne Warwick Warwickshire CV35 9TA w 6098724

ANGEL Eliza Jane 28/02/2003 Eton Veterinary Clinic 31 London Road Tonbridge Kent TN10 3AB **Tel:** (01732) 352004 w 6280007

ANGELL Lisa Jayne 19/03/2007 35 Pavilion Way Ruislip Middlesex HA4 9JR **Tel:** (0208) 868 6240 w 6373991

ANGELL-PARSONS Emily Carole (nee Taylor) 02/03/2009 84 Rugeley Road Chase Terrace Burntwood Staffordshire WS7 1AA **Tel:** (01543) 300025 w 6345743

ANGWIN Claire Emma (see DODGE, Mrs)

ANSELL Elaine Margaret 24/12/2002 (24/11/2006) Priory Veterinary Surgery 139 Brighton Road Redhill RH1 6PS **Tel:** (01737) 765353 w 6277422

Kay Emma 14/05/2007 10 Valley View SANDHURST Berkshire GU47 8EH w 6381218

Laura (nee Knight) 31/03/2003 26 Churchill Road Gloucester Gloucestershire GL1 5DG **Tel:** (01452) 537542 w 6272384

Melanie Louise 21/03/2006 26 Priory Road Ossett West Yorkshire WF5 8QL **Tel:** (01924) 263624 w 6348328

ANSLOW Deborah Penelope 27/08/2008 15 Simmonds Road Hucclecote GLOUCESTER GL3 3HY **Tel:** 07776420949 w 6388874

ANSONIA Heather Jade 31/03/2008 18 Bailey Avenue ELLESMERE PORT CH65 3BJ **Tel:** (01244) 398008 w 6419399

ANSTISS Michelle (see THOMPSON, Mrs)

APLIN Holly Mary Louise 19/10/2009 4 Trinity Terrace Castle Street AXMINSTER Devon EX13 5NR **Tel:** 07921617231 w 6382505

APPADURAI Lisa 09/02/2009 The Croft Sidwell Lane BENFLEET Essex SS7 1LG **Tel:** 07999868520 w 6439639

APPLEBY Nicola 06/07/2004 19 Twizell Lane West Pelton Stanley County Durham DH9 6SH **Tel:** (0191) 370 0796 w 6297937

APPLETON Rachael Julie 18/10/2005 Northdale Veterinary Surgery 48 Victoria Road Worthing West Sussex BN11 1XE **Tel:** (01903) 202474 w 6346425

APPLETON Sharon (see PEAK, Mrs)

APPLEYARD Kate Mary 24/05/2005 2/2 61 Cartside Street GLASGOW G42 9TL w 6296639

Sarah Louise 29/02/2008 Cruggan Farm Portloe TRURO Cornwall TR2 5PS w 6385651

APPS Belinda Jane (see STONER, Mrs)

APPS Carrie Lian 04/11/2008 4 Tudor Close LEIGH-ON-SEA Essex SS9 5AR **Tel:** 01702510395 w 6431895

ARCHARD Rebecca Emily 21/01/2008 1 Coppernets Iford Lewes East Sussex BN7 3JB **Tel:** 01273478565 w 6407123

ARCHBOLD Georgina Suzanne (see VERNOUM, Mrs)

ARCHER Emma DipAVN(Surgical) (nee Davies) 15/02/2002 1 The Cottage Marsh Lane New Buckenham Norwich Norfolk NR16 2BE **Tel:** (01953) 860232 w 6270129

Jacqueline Deborah 03/09/1996 Brunswick Place Veterinary Clinic Brunswick Place Cranbourne Lane Basingstoke Hampshire RG21 3NN **Tel:** (01256) 473371 w 6041573

Louise Jane 08/02/1999 (01/02/2002) Davies Veterinary Specialists Manor Farm Business Park Higham Gobion Hertfordshire SG5 3HR **Tel:** (01582) 883950 w 6128783

ARCHER Shelley Claire (see HOWELL, Mrs)

Zoe Elizabeth 29/09/2004 38 Lowestoft Road Carlton Colville Lowestoft Suffolk NR33 8JD **Tel:** (01502) 531 999 w 6292305

ARENTS Karen Louise (see WARD, Mrs)

ARIMATSU Charlotte 28/08/1997 (17/04/2003) 40 Cherry Hill New Barnet Barnet Hertfordshire EN5 1BG w 6116847

ARME Amanda Jayne 14/09/2005 Mapperley Vets4Pets Unit B 540 Woodborough Road Mapperley Nottinghamshire NG3 5HB **Tel:** (0115) 960 9200 w 6316351

ARMOUR Nicola Ann 13/07/2007 Flat 24 Lincoln Court 634-658 Eastern Avenue Gants Hill ILFORD Essex IG2 6PR **Tel:** (07708) 383226 w 6349483

ARMSTEAD Christine Jennifer 11/11/2004 Victoria Veterinary Clinic 275 London Road Burgess Hill West Sussex RH15 9QU **Tel:** (01444) 233472 w 6290908

ARMSTRONG Deborah Catherine (nee Lyttle) 22/09/2006 47 Grove Park HILLSBOROUGH County Down BT26 6JF w 6296771

Justine Elizabeth 15/09/1999 (08/05/2003) 36 Eastbury Avenue Rochford Essex SS4 1SF **Tel:** (01702) 334235 w 6184857

Kelly Marie 09/05/2006 24 Old Road Clarkhill CASTLEWELLAN County Down BT31 9BW w 6331135

Sarah Jane DipAVN(Surgical) 16/09/1998 7 Asten Fold SALFORD M6 7JH **Tel:** (07709) 058308 w 6132508

ARNALL Suzanne Angela 11/01/2005 73 Bences Lane CORSHAM Wiltshire SN13 0DR w 6326812

ARNOLD Gillian Samantha (see KERROD, Mrs)

ARNOLD Jenny Christine (see CANE, Mrs)

ARNOLD Karen Jane 10/09/2009 6 Wheatfields Thurston BURY ST. EDMUNDS Suffolk IP31 3TE **Tel:** (01359) 232610 w 6459516

Katie Louise 13/11/2009 49 New Road CHATTERIS Cambridgeshire PE16 6BW **Tel:** 01354691282 w 6456304

Kerry Louise 05/07/2006 14 Box End Road Kempston BEDFORD MK43 8RR **Tel:** (07763) 754686 w 6321400

Rachel Shelagh Elouise 06/05/2009 121 Farley Hill Luton Bedfordshire LU1 5EQ **Tel:** 01582619668 w 6449198

ARNUP Julie Rebecca Sarah Jane 02/03/1999 (06/02/2003) Inside Pets At Home Peninsular Park Road Bugsby Way Charlton London SE7 7TZ **Tel:** (020) 8269 1440 w 6123297

ARROUD Michelle Nydia 20/10/2009 94 Norbreck Road Thornton-Cleveleys Lancashire FY5 1RP **Tel:** (01253) 357380 w 6459538

ARROWSMITH Lisa (see BEESLEY, Mrs)

ARTHUR Bonnie Gee 29/06/2007 Harrietsham Vet Clinic, Unit 9 Roebuck Business Park Ashford Road Harrietsham MAIDSTONE Kent ME17 1AB w 6370878

ARUNDELL Louise 01/09/2008 44 Durham Road Stockton-on-Tees Cleveland TS19 0BS **Tel:** (01642) 611 191 w 6434832

ASH Victoria Louise 26/01/2009 4 The Oaks Kempsey WORCESTER WR5 3PN **Tel:** 01905821292 w 6319475

ASHBURN-SCOTT Katherine Ann 25/11/2008 Beech House Veterinary Clinic 35 Harrington Road Brighton BN1 6RF **Tel:** (01273) 505071 w 6429299

ASHBY-PICKFORD Naomi Jane 28/09/2005 6 Hill View Close Ilton ILMINSTER Somerset TA19 9TB **Tel:** (01460) 55963 w 6333269

ASHCROFT Susan 03/10/2007 58 Northgate Pontefract West Yorkshire WF8 1HJ **Tel:** (01977) 600588 w 6281228

ASHEN Claire Louise 29/08/1996 68 Offington Drive WORTHING West Sussex BN14 9PS **Tel:** (01903) 830664 w 6030357

ASHFIELD Samantha Jane 25/02/2003 Park Veterinary Clinic 343a Jockey Road Sutton Coldfield West Midlands B73 5XD **Tel:** (0121) 354 4949/ 2006 w 6275431

ASHFORD Kerri Elysia Natalie 27/11/2008 207 Daventry Road Coventry West Midlands CV3 5HH **Tel:** (02476) 503000 w 6406375

ASHMAN Leigh 04/09/2003 East Villa Craghead STANLEY County Durham DH9 6DY **Tel:** (01207) 232067 w 6244565

ASHMORE Laura Ann (nee Ashmore, formerly Acevedo-Ashmore) 06/12/2004 C/o Royal College of Veterinary Surgeons 62-64 Horseferry Road LONDON SW1P 2AF **Tel:** (0788) 4436493 w 6272725

ASHTON Catherine Margaret 16/12/2005 17 Lynchets Crescent HOVE East Sussex BN3 8EL **Tel:** (01273) 410363 w 6343598

Claire Michelle 17/08/2005 55 Empire Road TORQUAY TQ1 4LF w 6279501

ASHWORTH Claire Louise 15/02/2008 56 Althorp Drive PENARTH South Glamorgan CF64 5FJ w 6383825

Jacqui Louise 07/04/2006 56 Manchester Road Shaw Oldham Lancashire OL2 7DE **Tel:** (01706) 840936 w 6266906

ASKEW Laura 10/08/2001 Coombefield Veterinary Hospital Coombe Lane Axminster Devon EX13 5AX **Tel:** (01297) 630500 w 6170689

ASKEY Nicola Jayne 28/02/2001 36 Greig Court Heath Hayes CANNOCK Staffordshire WS11 7WN **Tel:** (07890) 461193 w 6140530

ASPEY Wendy Anne 11/07/2005 20 Berkeley Grove LEEDS LS8 3RJ **Tel:** (0113) 225 6671 w 6289060

ATHERTON Rebecca Jane 08/04/2005 5 Fraser Road Gosport Hampshire PO13 0UD **Tel:** (01329) 289887 w 6325646

ATKIN Chloe Louise (nee Harris) 31/03/2003 The Veterinary Centre 2-4 Curzon Street Burton-on-Trent Staffordshire DE14 2DH **Tel:** (01283) 535040 w 6284198

ATKINS Amie Jane (nee Levitt) 23/10/2001 46 Southgate Market Weighton York East Riding of Yorkshire YO43 3BQ **Tel:** (01430) 873219 w 6204041

ATKINS Rachel (see LITHGO, Mrs)

Samantha Jane (nee Lavin) 13/01/1999 88 Black Road Macclesfield Cheshire SK11 7BZ **Tel:** (01625) 610351 w 6133738

ATKINSON Catherine Elizabeth 31/10/2005 The Veterinary Surgery Hallfield Lane WETHERBY West Yorkshire LS22 6JU **Tel:** (01937) 582025 w 6343620

Claire 30/11/2006 (23/02/2009) 15 Rosehip Close Plymouth Devon PL6 7TF **Tel:** (01752) 696448 w 6353696

ATKINSON Denise Elizabeth (see DODGE, Mrs)

Gemma Louise 11/03/2009 82a Damson Lane Solihull West Midlands B92 9JP **Tel:** 01216944342 w 6382483

Lindsay (nee Ross) 10/01/2003 2 George Terrace Bearpark DURHAM DH7 7AQ **Tel:** (0191) 3783059 w 6285683

Louise Joanne 29/01/2007 Pet Care Veterinary Surgery 355 Bexley Road Erith Kent DA8 3EZ **Tel:** (01322) 346173 w 6363156

Naomi Karen 26/08/2008 Woodcote Blanches Pierres Lane St. Martin GUERNSEY GY4 6SA **Tel:** (01481) 238345 w 6408905

Susan Elizabeth (nee Thomas) 18/10/2005 26 Highlander Drive The Humbers Telford Shropshire TF2 8JZ **Tel:** (01952) 677 704 w 6342256

Zoe Louise (nee Roper) 03/12/2003 9 Garthends Lane Hemingbrough North Yorkshire YO8 6QW **Tel:** (01757) 630513 w 6267522

ATTRIDGE Kerrie Louise 31/03/2003 32 Cinnamon Street Wapping London E1W 3NJ w 6273308

ATTWATER Fiona Jane DipAVN(Surgical) 01/02/1996 (12/03/2004) 2 Sevenoaks Road Eastbourne East Sussex BN23 7LZ w 6040208

ATTWELL Sarah-Jane Elizabeth 21/03/2007 Allwell House 41a Church Lane Rode FROME Somerset BA11 6PN **Tel:** (01373) 830189 w 6332246

AULD Lucy Alexandra (nee Cromack) 08/01/2008 22 Church Ponds Castle Hedingham HALSTEAD Essex CO9 3BZ **Tel:** 01787461030 w 6404923

AUSTIN Claire 19/01/2009 21 Bow Street Cudworth Barnsley South Yorkshire S72 8JL **Tel:** (01226) 714 522 w 6402547

Emma 19/03/2007 45 Occupation Lane Sheffield South Yorkshire S12 4PS **Tel:** (0114) 239 0685 w 6376356

Joanne Marie 21/11/2005 (27/01/2010) Bucks Farm Bungalow Cookley HALESWORTH Suffolk IP19 0LX **Tel:** (01986) 784458 w 6312039

Jodie Ann 22/03/2004 Rushbrook Leafield Road Shipton-under-Wychwood CHIPPING NORTON Oxfordshire OX7 6EA **Tel:** (07966) 882 457 w 6287410

Julie 30/10/2008 Archway Veterinary Surgery 21 High Street Highworth SWINDON SN6 7AG **Tel:** (01793) 765335 w 6436306

Lucy Emma (nee Gale) 10/12/2002 Barrow Hill House Maidstone Rd Ashford Kent TN24 8TY **Tel:** (01233) 624687 w 6277840

Mairi Mccrindle 06/01/1993 Macclesfield Veterinary Hospital 26/38 Cumberland Street Macclesfield Cheshire SK10 1BZ **Tel:** (01625) 501500 w 6064648

Nicola Danielle 24/02/2004 (16/01/2009) Hillandale Charleswood Road Whitecroft LYDNEY Gloucestershire GL15 4QH w 6293064

AUSTIN Sarah Jayne (see EDWARDS, Mrs)

AVERY Rachel Louise 10/09/2009 24 Ashdown Road Chandler's Ford EASTLEIGH Hampshire SO53 5QW **Tel:** (02380) 269740 w 6449605

Susan Margaret 02/01/1992 (08/05/2003) 12 Broadway Bower Hinton Martock Somerset TA12 6LP **Tel:** (01935) 822985 w 6044836

AVEYARD Charlotte (see DOBSON, Mrs)

AVIS Kimberley Jayne 08/02/2008 5 Mountain View Helsby Frodsham Cheshire WA6 0BA **Tel:** (01928) 725626 w 6376367

AYDON Debbie 30/10/2007 77 The Meadows Grange Park Northampton Northamptonshire NN4 5BU **Tel:** 01604876752 w 6404967

AYLING Katie-Jane (see AYLING-DITTON, Mrs)

AYLING-DITTON Katie-Jane (nee Ayling) 25/02/2003 Horsepond Veterinary Centre Horsepond Meadow South Molton Devon EX36 4EJ **Tel:** (01769) 572226 w 6280194

AYRE Amy Louise (see REID, Mrs)

AYRES Katherine Anne 29/01/2010 Bredy Veterinary Centre Sea Road North Bridport Dorset DT6 4RR **Tel:** (01308) 456 771 w 6465500

AYRES Samantha Anne (see BRADSHAW, Mrs)

B

BABB Laura Caroline (nee Buckland) 16/04/2008 7 Hornbury Close Minety Malmesbury Wiltshire SN16 9YE w 6385607

BABER Angela Mary 22/08/1973 Derrig's Place Spa Boyle Co Roscommon Ireland w 6000107

BACK Joanne 20/11/2008 12 Holme Lea Watford Hertfordshire WD25 0ND w 6436251

BACON Elizabeth Jean 06/10/2006 26 Selworthy Bristol Avon BS15 9RJ **Tel:** (0117) 947 8707 w 6307133

Katie 27/09/1993 (08/10/1999) Queen Mother Hospital for Small Animals Hawkshead Lane North Mymms Hatfield Hertfordshire AL9 7TA **Tel:** (01707) 666366 w 602836X

BADCOCK Sarah Frances 11/03/2005 36 Flowers Yard CHIPPENHAM Wiltshire SN15 3BN **Tel:** (07796) 998489 w 6298531

BADDILEY Antoinette Rose 16/04/2008 12 Wansum Court St. Nicholas at Wade Birchington Kent CT7 0NS **Tel:** (01843) 840898 w 6406320

BADGER Natasha (nee Rice) 09/04/2008 17 Streatfield EDENBRIDGE Kent TN8 5DF **Tel:** (07810) 430902 w 6406936

BADHAM Susan Alice (see QUIN, Ms)

BADMAN Katherine Claire (nee Harris) 29/09/2000 Blackberry Paddock Garden End Farm Panborough WELLS Somerset BA5 1PN **Tel:** (01934) 710202 w 6203392

BAGGS Elizabeth Winifred 14/04/2008 23 Fenton Road LONDON N17 7JL **Tel:** (020) 8889 5108 w 6346876

BAGSHAW Gail Michelle 17/11/2004 174 Wilmslow Road Handforth WILMSLOW Cheshire SK9 3LF w 6291601

BAGSHAWE Jacqueline (see GOULDING, Mrs)

BAIGENT Lynda Jacqueline 02/09/1997 4 Battersea Park Road Battersea London SW8 4AA **Tel:** (020) 7627 9256 w 6112434

Rosemarie Denise (formerly Reveley) 09/08/1983 5 Grange Road Herne Bay Kent CT6 6NH **Tel:** (01227) 364873 w 6059605

BAILEY Cherie (nee Burt) 04/11/2005 75 Bentley Road DONCASTER South Yorkshire DN5 9SD **Tel:** (01302) 784999 w 6247744

Claudia Marie (nee Gilbert, nee Gilbert) 27/09/2006 50 Deer Valley Road PETERBOROUGH PE2 9SN w 6345666

Georgina Anne 22/01/2010 Oakham Veterinary Hospital Ashwell Road Oakham Rutland LE15 7QH **Tel:** (01572) 722646 w 6463795

BAILEY Karen Louise (see STANIER, Mrs)

Kathryn Ann 31/05/1990 Shearbridge Veterinary Group 2 Legrams Lane Bradford West Yorkshire BD7 1ND **Tel:** (01274) 731299 w 6044927

Lisa Marie 05/09/1994 (18/11/1999) Macclesfield Veterinary Hospital 26/38 Cumberland Street Macclesfield Cheshire SK10 1BZ **Tel:** (01625) 501500 w 6037046

BAILEY Michelle Louise (see SMEATH, Mrs)

Nadia Louise 24/08/1998 The Mill 1 Old Road Leighton Buzzard Bedfordshire LU7 2RB **Tel:** (01582) 872773 w 6128240

Nicole Emma 25/02/2002 56 Johnson Way Ford Arundel West Sussex BN18 0TS **Tel:** (01798) 873718 w 6259624

BAILEY Samantha (see BOYCE, Mrs)

BAILEY Sonya Clare (see ELLETT, Mrs)

BAIN Hazel Marie (see JAFFRAY, Ms)

BAINBRIDGE Kerry (see BALCHIN, Mrs)

BAIRD Melissa 09/11/2009 64b Ballyhanedin Road Claudy LONDONDERRY BT47 4ER **Tel:** 07525845925 w 6322071

BAITS Dreana (see BULMER-THOMPSON, Mrs)

BAKE Michala 07/12/2007 33 Alderley Drive Bredbury STOCKPORT Cheshire SK6 2PN **Tel:** (01614) 305431 w 6342322

BAKER Gemma Louise 22/04/2005 Belle Vue Veterinary Clinics Millards Hill Trudoxhill Frome Somerset BA11 5DW **Tel:** (01373) 836186 w 6321917

BAKER Georgina Elizabeth (see HUNT, Mrs)

Janice Rose (nee Chester) 28/07/1992 26 Manor Road Middle Littleton Evesham Worcestershire WR11 8LL **Tel:** (01386) 832398 w 6008864

Louisa (nee Gamble) 29/07/2005 (13/06/2007) Priors Leaze Veterinary Centre Priors Leaze Lane Nutbourne Chichester West Sussex PO18 8RH **Tel:** (01243) 376 000 w 6299983

Louise Charlotte 08/01/2008 205 Chantrey Crescent Birmingham West Midlands B43 7PE **Tel:** 01213604110 w 6373672

BAKER Natalie Joy (see LOCKEY, Mrs)

Sally Victoria 04/12/2003 55 The Burgage Eccleshall STAFFORD ST21 6DR **Tel:** 01543-277205 w 6271977

Sameena Jane 20/02/2009 1 Rowan Place COLCHESTER CO1 1AJ **Tel:** 01206367515 w 6445953

Sarah Jane 16/04/2007 36 Boston Road Kirton Boston Lincolnshire PE20 1DS **Tel:** (01205) 722696 w 6367545

Sonya Lois 24/11/2009 107 East Barnet Road New Barnet Barnet Hertfordshire EN4 8RF **Tel:** (020) 8440 5742 w 6465599

BAKEWELL Amanda Jane (see HODGES, Mrs)

BAKI Rima Selene 24/04/2009 C/o Royal College of Veterinary Surgeons 62-64 Horseferry Road LONDON SW1P 2AF w 6450089

BALCHIN Kerry (nee Bainbridge) 24/11/2004 5 Chestnut Crescent Barnsley South Yorkshire S70 3NW w 6293570

BALDOCK Sarah Catherine (formerly Huddleston) 26/10/2005 Small Animal Teaching Hospital University of Liverpool Leahurst Campus Chester High Road Neston Merseyside CH64 7TE **Tel:** (0151) 795 6100 w 6333885

BALDWIN Katy Sarah Elizabeth (nee Christofe) 16/03/2001 (12/03/2004) 184 Lord Street Hoddesdon Hertfordshire EN11 8NL w 6214117

BALDWIN Laura Natasha (see HIGGS, Mrs)

BALDWYN Daisy Susannah 06/08/2008 Tolleshunt 4 Kents Lane Ettington Stratford-upon-Avon Warwickshire CV37 7SJ **Tel:** (01789) 740386 w 6389259

BALFOUR Anna Christine 22/03/2004 51 Upper Sneyed Road Essington Wolverhampton WV11 2DS **Tel:** (01902) 731127 w 6286596

BALGOWAN June (nee Russell) 12/02/1996 136 Bonnygate Cupar Fife KY15 4LF **Tel:** (01334) 652273 w 6043683

BALINAS Vicky 11/06/2008 10 Langney Drive ASHFORD Kent TN23 5UF **Tel:** (01233) 331594 w 6414427

BALL Emma Langley 15/02/2005 (13/11/2007) 5 Langdon Gardens STANLEY Durham DH9 8RW **Tel:** (01207) 280 360 w 6325382

BALL Emma Shirley (see HALLAM, Mrs)

Gayle Suzanne (nee Hardy) 22/03/2004 Swale Veterinary Surgery Fairfield Way Gallowfields Trading Estate Richmond North Yorkshire DL10 4TB **Tel:** (01748) 826600/822389 w 6268523

Laura Anne 05/07/2006 16 St. Leonards Road Lanstephan LAUNCESTON Cornwall PL15 8LQ **Tel:** (01566) 772861 w 6321411

Michaela 09/06/2009 15 Greenoak Close Abram WIGAN Lancashire WN2 5XN **Tel:** (01942) 711462 w 6443346

Natalie Sarah 30/11/2009 12 Church View CALNE Wiltshire SN11 0FB **Tel:** (01249) 822048 w 6386795

Nikki 14/05/2007 41B Leverton Street London NW5 2PE **Tel:** (020) 7482 0649 w 6293955

Peggy Susan 30/03/2006 40-46 Mount Pleasant Road Northam Southampton Hampshire SO14 0EG **Tel:** (02380) 222622 w 6322423

Sarah Jane 18/05/2009 Longlands Farm Bank Bridge Tarleton Preston Lancashire PR4 6HJ **Tel:** 01772812430 w 6449594

BALLANTYNE Helen Jennifer 07/12/2005 32 Earsham Drive King's Lynn Norfolk PE30 3UZ **Tel:** (01553) 673213 w 6333852

Lynn Janet (nee Paterson) 06/01/1993 Wood of Coldrain Kinross KY13 0QW **Tel:** (01577) 863381 w 6066452

BALLARD Victoria Louise 25/11/2009 New Close Farm London Road HASSOCKS West Sussex BN6 9ND **Tel:** (01273) 843144 w 6464246

BALLINGALL Tracy Margaret (see JONES, Mrs)

BALMAN Katie Louise 30/09/2008 The Dolls House 101 Pilton Street Barnstaple Devon EX31 1PQ **Tel:** 01271344819 w 6380272

BALSDON Sarah - Jayne 20/11/2002 Garston Veterinary Group Garston House Portway Frome Somerset BA11 1PZ **Tel:** (01373) 451115 w 6261571

BANCROFT Sula Diana 14/01/2008 15 Sutherland Grove London SW18 5PS **Tel:** (0208) 789 2572 w 6400677

BANFIELD Victoria Liann (nee Barnes) 22/02/2007 The Donkey Sanctuary Sidmouth devon EX10 0NU **Tel:** (01395) 578 222 w 6351848

BANGHAM Annabel Dawn 26/04/2000 (19/08/2002) 201 Dundee Lane Ramsbottom Bury Lancashire BL0 9HF w 6043967

BANHAM Emma-Louise (see FORDHAM, Mrs)

BANKS Andrea (see O'ROURKE, Mrs)

BANKS Karen (nee Wilson) 22/07/1993 7 Fairview Garway HEREFORD HR2 8RG **Tel:** (01600) 750425 w 6014969

Sandra Dawn (formerly Ritchie) 30/08/1994 33 Junction Road Kirkwall Orkney KW15 1AG **Tel:** (01856) 873403 w 6029148

Tammy Jane (nee Bradbury) 21/08/2002 The Veterinary Surgery Areley Kings Stourport-on-Severn Worcestershire DY13 0LB **Tel:** (01299) 822052 w 6259129

Zoe Ann 06/06/2008 122 Barrells Down Road Bishop's Stortford Hertfordshire CM23 2SY **Tel:** (01279) 831068 w 6413272

BANNING Sarah Louise (nee Stafford) 01/09/1997 3 Lythwood Drive Brierley Hill West Midlands DY5 3QW w 6098757

BANNISTER Amy Susanne 08/11/2006 Ferlys House Overton Park Road Cheltenham Gloucestershire GL50 3BP **Tel:** (01242) 522 429 w 6382252

Julie Ann 30/07/2002 25 Hallam Street Heaviley Stockport Cheshire SK2 6PT **Tel:** (0161) 285 9506 w 6259701

BARATHY Elizabeth Joy 06/10/2006 Glynswood Veterinary Centre Furnham Road Chard Somerset TA20 1AF **Tel:** (01460) 66111 w 6375036

BARBER Estelle (see ST JOHN-SMITH, Mrs)

BARBER Sarah Amy (see HOLDEN, Mrs)

BARBER Susan Anne (formerly Moore) 07/09/1973 8 The Colts Thorley Park Bishop's Stortford Hertfordshire CM23 4DL **Tel:** (01279) 504272 w 6057109

BARCHAM Laura Anne 15/11/2006 Highcliff Veterinary Practice 93 Cliff Lane Ipswich Suffolk IP3 0PQ **Tel:** (01473) 828846 w 6370889

BARCLAY Christine Anne (nee Gauld) 07/09/1999 63 Coniston Drive Priorslee Telford Shropshire TF2 9QW **Tel:** (01952) 210566 w 6130941

Lana Helen (nee Simpson) 01/04/2003 11 Caledonian Court FALKIRK FK2 7FL **Tel:** (01324) 636196 w 6282328

Philippa Jean 24/08/1999 (13/03/2003) Davies Veterinary Specialists Manor Farm Business Park Higham Gobion Hertfordshire SG5 3HR **Tel:** (01582) 883950 w 6184692

BAREFORD Lisa 19/07/2004 53-55 Maidstone Road Footscray SIDCUP Kent DA14 5HB **Tel:** (020) 8300 8111 w 6287421

BARFIELD Amy Louise (nee Palmer) 12/09/2008 47 New Road Coton-in-the-Elms SWADLINCOTE Derbyshire DE12 8ET w 6434700

BARFOOT Laura Louise 11/03/2005 47 Porter Road BASINGSTOKE Hampshire RG22 4JS w 6328088

BARHAM Laura Catherine 08/01/2008 77 Alpha Road Chingford London E4 6TD w 6255763

BARKER Anne Marie 17/07/2008 9 Samantha Mews Havering-Atte-Bower Romford Essex RM4 1QS **Tel:** (07949) 562963 w 6411336

Charlotte 17/11/2009 31 Nuneham Grove Westcroft Milton Keynes Buckinghamshire MK4 4DH **Tel:** (01908) 506344 w 6466787

Gemma Louise (nee Skates) 07/02/2006 32 Swain Court Northampton Northamptonshire NN3 8HT **Tel:** (01604) 416359 w 6329089

Jennifer Elizabeth 11/11/2008 4 The Close CHELTENHAM Gloucestershire GL53 0PQ **Tel:** (01242) 224636 w 6440266

Jill Rebecca (nee Gardner) 30/07/2002 19 Glenbury Grove REDCAR Cleveland TS10 2TN **Tel:** (01642) 476914 w 6270206

Katharine Mary 09/02/2009 91 Station Road Shepley Huddersfield West Yorkshire HD8 8DS **Tel:** 01484609635 w 6434667

Lindsay Dawn (nee Kinson) 16/12/2005 17 Bentley Way TAMWORTH Staffordshire B79 8LJ **Tel:** (01827) 702402 w 6283186

Lisa Mary (nee Munn) 21/06/2005 81 Buxton Drive Bexhill on Sea East Sussex TN39 4AU **Tel:** (01424) 733936 w 6289764

BARLEY Michelle Angela 20/11/2002 (07/08/2008) 5 Lancaster Crescent St. Eval WADEBRIDGE Cornwall PL27 7TP **Tel:** (01841) 540892 w 6259668

BARLOW Emma Victoria 27/11/2009 Forest Veterinary Clinic 7 Park Road Fordingbridge Hampshire SP6 1EQ **Tel:** (01425) 652221 w 6451497

Heather 14/02/1989 55 Cedar Drive Rosedale Estate Torpoint Cornwall PL11 2QQ **Tel:** (01752) 813870 w 6000275

Janine Suzanne 21/10/1993 (31/10/2005) 209a Bacup Road Rawtenstall Rossendale Lancashire BB4 7PA **Tel:** (01706) 225300 w 6011731

Naomi 21/11/2005 4 Fulmar Crescent Box Moor Hemel Hempstead Herefordshire HP1 1SG **Tel:** (07971) 276421 w 6320278

Victoria Michelle 09/09/2008 Moy Farm Chapel Lane Out Rawcliffe Preston PR3 6TB **Tel:** (01253) 701 098 w 6432852

BARNARD Joanna Elizabeth Emilia (see JAMES, Mrs)

Sarah Jane 20/10/2008 18a Valebridge Road Burgess Hill West Sussex RH15 0QY **Tel:** 01444254829 w 6377038

BARNES Alison 11/06/2003 Abbey Veterinary Group 71 Canal Street PAISLEY Renfrewshire PA1 2HP **Tel:** (01505) 683763 w 6274320

Ann 14/03/2006 (11/01/2010) Woodlands Stables Cock Lane Broxbourne HODDESDON Hertfordshire EN11 8LS w 6320817

Anoushka Jennifer 15/12/2009 17 Sunny Walk Bristol Avon BS15 1ED **Tel:** (07780) 880 134 w 6429717

Jessica Marie 21/07/2008 35 Iffley Road OXFORD OX4 1EA w 6375883

Kathryn 19/12/2006 Chester Gates Referral Hospital Unit F Telford Court Chester Gates Chester Cheshire CH1 6LT **Tel:** (01244) 853 823 w 6354521

BARNES Lindsay Anne (see HAWKINS, Mrs)

Louise 19/09/2006 35 Westfield Avenue Yackenthorpe SHEFFIELD S12 4LJ w 6359724

Melanie Joan Maria 08/09/2009 2 Emmetts Place Abbotskerwell Newton Abbot Devon TQ12 5NP **Tel:** (01626) 361900 w 6466699

Pamela 05/06/2006 82 Perowne Way Sandown Isle of Wight PO36 9DT **Tel:** (01983) 407176 w 6312116

Sarah Louise (nee Henderson) 30/08/2006 Shires Veterinary Practice Eccleshall Road Stone Staffordshire ST15 0HJ **Tel:** (01785) 813955 w 6303723

BARNES Victoria Liann (see BANFIELD, Mrs)

BARNETT Sarah 06/04/2009 31 Bibury Close Nailsea North Somerset BS48 2TQ w 6288048

Wendy Jane DipAVN(Surgical) 22/12/1992 Mylva Marefield Lane Burrough on the Hill Melton Mowbray Leicestershire LE14 2QX **Tel:** (079) 2104 1616 w 6044075

BARNHILL Clare Louise 18/04/2005 Old Street Farm Caatterton Tadcaster North Yorkshire LS27 8AG **Tel:** (01937) 833124 w 6301380

BARON Stephanie 29/07/2005 5 Resbury Close Sawston CAMBRIDGE CB2 4DE **Tel:** (01223) 570297 w 6321851

BARR Caroline Frances 19/04/2005 12 Dryden Avenue PORTSMOUTH PO6 4PP w 6323215

BARRABLE Heather Rosemary 31/08/1994 37 Laburnum Drive Whiddon Valley Barnstaple Devon EX32 8PX **Tel:** (01271) 379870 w 6029013

BARRATT Lyndsay Ann 10/10/2008 7 North Wall Cricklade SWINDON SN6 6DU **Tel:** 01793751403 w 6332543

BARRENETXEA Nicola Alaia (see SHAW, Mrs)

BARRETT Gayle Patricia 06/07/2004 8 Grenville Close Meopham Kent DA13 0PH **Tel:** (0794) 1616123 w 6291832

BARRETT Heather Morag (see PACKHAM, Mrs)

Joanne 18/10/2006 6 Home Mead North Waltham BASINGSTOKE Hampshire RG25 2SY **Tel:** 07770868602 w 6321895

Kelly-Louise 18/10/2006 25 Farnborough Avenue SOUTH CROYDON Surrey CR2 8HF w 6301534

BARRETT Ruth Elizabeth (see FARRELL, Mrs)

Stephanie Lara 22/02/2007 High Street Veterinary Hospital 169-170 High Street Lowestoft Suffolk NR32 1HU **Tel:** (01502) 572141 w 6370900

BARRETT Stephanie Leona (see HEDGES, Mrs)

BARRINGTON-WELLS Michelle Elizabeth 26/03/2002 Griffin Barn Oldberrow Henley-in-Arden West Midlands B95 5NU **Tel:** (01564) 793511 w 6205559

BARRON Claire Frances (see DOCHERTY, Mrs)

Jessica Amy (nee Nash) 09/06/2009 160 Hull Grove Sumners Harlow Essex CM19 5RS **Tel:** 01279422066 w 6411534

BARRON Mary Louise (see WANT, Mrs)

BARROS Patricia Marie Vieira 23/02/2005 Chase Veterinary Group 89-91 Seaside Eastbourne East Sussex BN22 7NL **Tel:** (01323) 639331 w 6316373

BARROW Emily Kate 12/10/2009 5 Woodland Close SOUTHAMPTON SO18 5RD w 6461056

BARROW Tracy Joanne (see IVENS, Mrs)

BARRY Nicola Joanne 01/04/2003 11 Bloomfield Way Sawtry Huntingdon Cambridgeshire PE28 5RH **Tel:** (01487) 831892 w 6282108

Teresa Ann 17/07/2009 51 Townsend Way Northwood Middlesex HA6 1TG **Tel:** 07956557986 w 6414504

BARSBY Kelley Louise 19/03/2007 (18/11/2009) 60 Saracen Way PENRYN Cornwall TR10 8PR w 6282053

BARTELS Kate 12/09/1996 (26/05/2006) 4 Castle Street Bridgwater Somerset TA6 3DB **Tel:** (01278) 422121 w 6035049

BARTER Denise Claire (nee Denise Claire) 26/05/2009 438 Hook Road Chessington Surrey KT9 1NA **Tel:** (020) 8397 1776 w 6285540

BARTHOLOMEW Laura Joanne 03/05/2007 Flat 1 Fromus House Street Farm Road Saxmundham Suffolk IP17 1DU **Tel:** (07799) 807913 w 6357909

BARTHOLOMEW Victoria Louise (see SHEARS, Mrs)

BARTLE Rachael Anne 25/02/2003 (23/06/2009) 25 Dipton Grove Cramlington Northumberland NE23 6DR w 6278896

BARTLETT Jane Louise 31/10/2005 3 Bantocks Road Great Waldingfield Sudbury Suffolk CO10 0RT **Tel:** (01787) 377100 w 6342839

Janet Ruth 10/12/2008 RSPCA Putney Animal Hospital 6 Clarendon Drive London SW15 1AA **Tel:** (0300) 123 0716 w 6367556

Marie Louise 22/12/2009 40 Station Road Horrabridge Yelverton Devon PL20 7SS **Tel:** (01822) 854255 w 6426648

BARTLETT Penny Samantha (see BROWNINGS, Mrs)

BARTLEY Christina Ann Margaret 24/11/2009 Cliffe Veterinary Group 21 Cliffe High Street Lewes East Sussex BN7 2AH **Tel:** (01273) 473232 w 6457635

BARTOLOMEO Helen Rose 15/11/2005 5 Hedgerley Barton on Sea NEW MILTON Hampshire BH25 7TD w 6303657

BARTON Claire Emma 15/09/2009 23 Croft Way HORSHAM West Sussex RH12 2AS **Tel:** (01403) 250986 w 6496036

Lucy Louise 25/03/2002 (06/06/2006) 16 Arthur Street LINCOLN Lincolnshire LN5 7UH w 6267544

BARTON Lydia Frances (see THOMPSETT, Mrs)

Sarah-Gay DipAVN(Surgical) 22/01/1996 Harley Wood Farm Upper Basildon nr Reading Berkshire RG8 8NE **Tel:** (01491) 671 681 w 6035220

BARTRAM Debbie 23/05/2008 Penmellyn Veterinary Group Station Road St. Columb Major Cornwall TR9 6BX **Tel:** (01637) 880307 w 6413470

BARTY Emma Charlotte 24/05/2005 (24/09/2009) Elands Veterinary Clinic Station Road Dunton Green Sevenoaks Kent TN13 2XA **Tel:** (01732) 452333 w 6301391

BAS Dawn Anne 22/01/1996 37 Crispin Crescent Beddington CROYDON Surrey CR0 4UG **Tel:** (020) 8681 3043 w 6026624

BASHFORD Laura Kate 20/09/2005 67 Mayflower Close DARTMOUTH Devon TQ6 9JN w 6321862

BASS Heather 08/04/2005 153 Briery Way HEMEL HEMPSTEAD Hertfordshire HP2 7AN **Tel:** 07776418894 w 6307463

BASSETT Kerry 20/01/2000 New Era Veterinary Hospital Victoria Road St Saviour Jersey JE2 7QG **Tel:** (01534) 730521 w 6185165

BATCHELOR Heather Louise 18/10/2005 63 Careys Way WESTON-SUPER-MARE Avon BS24 7HH w 6326229

Helen Louise 19/02/2001 Noah's Ark Veterinary Surgery 54 High Street South Dunstable Bedfordshire LU6 3HD **Tel:** (01582) 606466 w 6212379

Michelle Louise 23/11/2001 32 Park Street Horbury Wakefield West Yorkshire WF4 6AB **Tel:** 01924-283293 w 6259437

BATEMAN Sarah Louise 25/02/2003 (10/02/2009) 28 Bath Road Harlington Hayes Middlesex UB3 5AH **Tel:** (020) 572 6788 w 6254751

BATES Alice Katherine 21/07/2008 33 Bell Road Warnham HORSHAM West Sussex RH12 3QJ **Tel:** (01403) 267096 w 6375894

Bernadette Elisabeth (nee Witt) 25/02/2003 The Old House Killagurteen Waterville Co.Kerry. Ireland **Tel:** (00) 353 877 746 363 w 6276850

Claire Elizabeth 14/04/2009 Elmhurst Farm Rickney Hailsham East Sussex BN27 1SF **Tel:** 01323765862 w 6440750

Joanne Elizabeth 03/12/2003 Lynton House Burgh Road Orby Skegness Lincolnshire PE24 5HR **Tel:** (029) 20862909 w 6290688

Rebecca Charlotte 27/09/2004 3 Durham Close Bagworth Coalville Leicestershire LE67 1BE **Tel:** (07946) 028878 w 6295231

Tarnia Helen 05/01/2005 15 London Road Shenley Radlett Hertfordshire WD7 9EW **Tel:** (01923) 856740 w 6294406

BATEY Karen 15/05/2008 5 Kilpatrick Court Bourtreehill South IRVINE Ayrshire KA11 1JJ **Tel:** (01294) 230572 w 6404736

BATH Rosalind Ann (nee Collins) 25/02/2003 Bishops Stortford Veterinary Hospital Rye Street Bishop's Stortford Hertfordshire CM23 2HA **Tel:** (01279) 654108 w 6272890

BATISTE Clare Margaret 05/08/1976 Glenfield Route Des Blanches St. Martin Guernsey GY4 6AG **Tel:** (01481) 235418 w 6045206

BATLEY Clair (nee Booth) 06/01/1993 16 Heather Court Salendine Nook HUDDERSFIELD West Yorkshire HD3 3SP w 6064681

BATSON Miriam Leanne 07/02/2008 Kings Cottage Longleat Lane Holcombe Radstock Avon BA3 5DU **Tel:** (01761) 232 157 w 6403702

BATT Jennifer Mary 05/01/2005 The Old School Bickleigh Nr Tiverton Devon EX16 8JJ **Tel:** (01392) 271221 w 6297079

BATTEN Vanessa Christine 15/01/1981 6 Pillars Close Mitchell Newquay Cornwall TR8 5DA **Tel:** (01872) 510913 w 6045217

BATTY Emma Jane 13/05/1999 Hopland Cottage Ricehill Kirton Newark Nottinghamshire NG22 9LX **Tel:** (01623) 861232 w 6112751

BAUGH Rachel (nee Burton) 01/10/1999 (25/01/2007) Harper Adams University College Edgmond NEWPORT Shropshire TF10 8NB w 6185440

BAVERSTOCK Kerrie Laura 10/08/2007 The Granary Holmbush Farm Isaacs Lane HAYWARDS HEATH West Sussex RH16 4RY w 6353707

BAVISTER Melissa (see RIVETT, Mrs)

BAWDEN Louise Elizabeth 15/11/2005 Briarfield Eleanora Drive Douglas ISLE OF MAN IM2 3NN **Tel:** (01624) 621878 w 6350869

BAXENDALE Linda Carol (see BURKE, Mrs)

BAXTER Alison Jane (see JENKINSON, Mrs)

BAXTER Amy 12/11/2009 17 Heol Gelynog Beddau PONTYPRIDD Mid Glamorgan CF38 2SG **Tel:** 01443204776 w 6463773

BAXTER Angela Clare (see HARDING, Mrs)

Jill Christine (nee Walmsley) 01/11/1990 64 Alder Drive Hoghton Preston PR5 0AE **Tel:** (01254) 853229 w 6063054

Laura Jane 26/07/2004 Upper Bailey Fold Cottage Bailey Fold Allerton BRADFORD West Yorkshire BD15 8AA w 6298542

Marie Clare 17/08/2005 5 St. Pauls Avenue London NW2 5SS **Tel:** (07834) 618739 w 6297090

BAYCROFT Claire Louise 26/04/2007 15 Ripon Gardens CHESSINGTON Surrey KT9 2QX **Tel:** (020) 8391 5295 w 6321884

BAYFORD Joanne Frances (nee Cude) 26/08/1997 (27/03/2008) 4 Pinfold Lane Somersham HUNTINGDON Cambridgeshire PE28 3EQ **Tel:** (01487) 740082 w 6038491

BAYLIS Kirsty Marie 04/08/2008 7 Hotchkiss Close Wellesbourne Warwick Warwickshire CV35 9JD **Tel:** (01789) 842844 w 6406331

BAYLISS Emma Claire (nee Tripp) 28/02/2007 20 Galingale Way Portishead Bristol Avon BS20 7LU w 6381372

BAYNAM Jodie (nee Parmenter) 07/06/2005 Bridgnorth Veterinary Centre 52 Whitburn Street Bridgnorth Shropshire WV16 4QP **Tel:** (01746) 711561 w 6288972

BAYNES Emma Louise 15/12/2009 50 Skegness Road Stevenage Hertfordshire SG1 2H **Tel:** 01438237542 w 6466853

BAZLEY Catherine Anne (see NEILL, Mrs)

BAZLEY Helena Elizabeth (nee Swan) 30/05/2003 19 Grasmere Avenue Merton Park London SW19 3DY **Tel:** (020) 8540 8645 w 6277257

BEACH Pauline Barbara 23/02/2005 (26/11/2009) 15 Edgehill Gardens Istead Rise Gravesend Kent DA13 9JU **Tel:** (01474) 833964 w 6292052

BEADEL Gemma Kate 22/09/2000 3 East View Writtle Chelmsford Essex CM1 3NL **Tel:** (01245) 420520 w 6203172

BEADLE Paula June (nee Sullivan) 18/09/2003 9 Tealby Close Gilmorton Nr Lutterworth Leicestershire LE17 5PT **Tel:** (01455) 558013 w 6280425

BEAL Claire Louise 09/05/2005 28 Boughthayes TAVISTOCK Devon PL19 8EF **Tel:** (07875) 484 237 w 6277378

Rebecca Jane 14/03/2008 76 Ouseburn Avenue York North Yorkshire YO26 5NN **Tel:** (01904) 788399 w 6388621

BEALE Charlene Layla 05/06/2009 8 The Fields Lower Caldecote Biggleswade Bedfordshire SG18 9BA **Tel:** (07704) 417955 w 6407871

Samantha Louise 05/10/2009 Pound Place Pound Lane Berwick Polegate Sussex BN26 655 **Tel:** (01323) 871684 w 6489370

BEALES Gemma Jane (see SEXTON, Mrs)

BEALEY Joanna Ruth DipAVN(Surgical) 15/11/2001 Cedar Veterinary Hospital 69 Christchurch Road Ringwood Hampshire BH24 1DH **Tel:** (01425) 473683 w 6267379

BEAN Rachel Francesca 27/08/2003 13 Hillside Avenue Grotton Saddleworth OLDHAM OL4 5SG w 6270338

BEANEY Donella Ann 15/01/1990 (20/01/1999) 309 The Ridge Hastings East Sussex TN34 2RA **Tel:** (01424) 751595 w 6045261

Sarah Louise (nee Thompson) 23/12/2003 4 Railway Street Annfield Plain Stanley Durham DH9 7SS **Tel:** (01207) 237 001 w 6283164

BEARD Amy Victoria 01/04/2003 1-2 Lightwoods Road Smethwick West Midlands B67 5AY **Tel:** (0121) 429 1400 w 6277004

Louise Ann 10/06/2003 Batfree Barn Kiln Lane Leigh Sinton MALVERN Worcestershire WR13 5HH w 6289302

Rebecca 25/02/2004 Cheshire Pet Medical Centre Manor Lane Holmes Chapel Cheshire CW4 8AB **Tel:** (01477) 544554 w 6278170

BEASLEY Christine Margaret 03/01/1978 (01/03/2006) Woodlyn Malt Hill Egham Surrey TW20 9PB **Tel:** (01784) 433280 w 6045283

Debra Ann 22/03/2004 The Wylie Veterinary Centre 196 Hall Lane Upminster Essex RM14 1TD **Tel:** (01708) 251200 w 6292723

Karen Anne 28/03/2008 34 Swinbrook Road Carterton Oxfordshire OX18 1DS **Tel:** (01608) 642547 w 6407079

BEASLEY Victoria Louise (see PERRIS, Mrs)

Victoria Margaret (nee Paley) 06/10/2006 19 Cocked Hat Park Sowerby Thirsk North Yorkshire YO7 3HB **Tel:** (01845) 523 892 w 6293207

BEATTIE Nicola Sarah 31/10/2003 4 Staffa Close Wickford Essex SS12 9GG w 6269546

BEAUCHAMP Rachel Lucy (see SINGLETON, Mrs)

BEAUMONT Mandy 14/01/2008 29 May Terrace Barnsley South Yorkshire S70 6HS **Tel:** (01226) 290806 w 6406463

Nichola Ann 20/09/2006 6 Holyoake Terrace Linthwaite HUDDERSFIELD HD7 5NX w 6355115

Samantha Jayne 16/03/2001 42 Meltham Road Honley Holmfirth West Yorkshire HD9 6HL **Tel:** (01484) 323989 w 6214106

BECK Claire Violet 11/02/2009 14 Ladyfields Loughton Essex IG10 3RR **Tel:** 07789174494 w 6425790

BECKETT Jessica Louise 01/12/2008 341 Tamworth Road Long Eaton NOTTINGHAM NG10 3LU **Tel:** (0115) 9728540 w 6429013

BECKHAM Claire Louise 02/06/2004 Durham Vets4Pets Ltd Priory Road Framwellgate Moor Durham County Durham DH1 5HW **Tel:** (0191) 383 0555 w 6284869

BECKWITH Sophie Kate 06/11/2000 84 Mountbatten Road BRAINTREE Essex CM7 9TP w 6203293

BEDDING Sarah Joanne (see CLEMENS, Mrs)

BEDFORD Cheryl Louise (see PLIMMER, Mrs)

BEDFORD Heather Louise 31/03/2003 Spring Lodge Farm Powers Hall End Witham Essex CM8 2HG **Tel:** (01376) 513247 w 6269359

Henrietta Susan 12/01/1988 (10/01/2001) Jacob Mulderweg 26 2597 BS The Hague The Netherlands w 6060053

BEDINGHAM Kirstie Jan (nee Rodgers, formerly Wright) 11/01/1993 (29/05/2001) 12a Ayston Road Uppingham Oakham Rutland LE15 9RL **Tel:** (01572) 822399 w 6065346

BEDRIKOVS Jennifer Michelle 01/05/2009 61 Grange Road Somersham Huntingdon Cambridgeshire PE28 3JT **Tel:** 07729466646 w 6419652

BEDWELL Cresta Ann (nee Coppock) 24/05/2005 34 Brunswick Street Reading Berkshire RG1 6NZ **Tel:** (0118) 967 9147 w 6263485

BEECH Lindsey Ann (nee Garner) 07/02/2007 Village Veterinary Surgery Liverpool Road Buckley Clwyd CH7 3LX **Tel:** (01244) 548866 w 6365719

BEECHEY Jenny Yolande (see PAYNE, Mrs)

BEEDLE Rachel McCarthy 05/04/2005 11 Castle Close Bromley Kent BR2 0YD **Tel:** (020) 8466 8243 w 6284836

BEER Samantha Jayne 10/09/2009 1 Lanes Farm Cottage Dumbleton EVESHAM Worcestershire WR11 7QN **Tel:** 07876714812 w 6465544

BEESLEY Che (see HOBAN, Mrs)

BEESLEY Lisa (nee Arrowsmith) 07/09/1994 14 Swynnerton Way WIDNES Cheshire WA8 9RX **Tel:** (0151) 424 8305 w 6034588

BEESON Sue Ann 09/12/2002 Glenthorne Veterinary Centre 71 Derby Road Uttoxeter Staffordshire ST14 8EB **Tel:** (01889) 562164 w 6274529

BEEVERS Joanna Kathryn (nee Addison) 07/11/2008 2 Old Hall Cottage Dauby Lane Kexby York North Yorkshire YO41 5LJ w 6344060

BEGGS Jennifer Louise 06/08/2008 (21/01/2010) 10h Jubilee Court BANGOR County Down BT19 1PT w 6351144

BELBIN Heather Louise 21/08/1987 (30/03/2000) Old Honeypots Ellis Farm Close Mayford Surrey GU22 9QN **Tel:** (01483) 724597 w 6045363

Valerie Ann (nee Smith) 03/10/1983 (07/10/1998) 3 Myrtle Close Puncknowle Dorchester Dorset DT2 9EH **Tel:** (01308) 898094 w 6060982

BELCHER Clare Louisa 23/12/2003 115 Morley Hill Enfield Middlesex EN2 0BQ **Tel:** (0208) 3639875 w 6279710

BELCHER Corrina (see ADAMS, Mrs)

Karen Louisa (nee Howson) 14/01/1999 (13/02/2002) Forest Lodge Veterinary Centre Station Road Forest Row East Sussex RH18 5DW **Tel:** (01342) 824452 w 6132814

BELDING Samantha (nee Madeley) 25/06/2004 RSPCA Barnes Hill Weoley Castle Birmingham B29 5UP **Tel:** (0300) 123 8652 w 6291843

BELFIELD-SMITH Clare 29/12/2008 61 Childs Way Sheringham Norfolk NR26 8TX **Tel:** 01263822868 w 6439749

BELL Alison (nee Haigh) 03/08/1992 1 Glendene Court New Hey Road Outlane HUDDERSFIELD HD3 3UP w 6007838

Alison Rosemary 04/02/1999 (23/10/2000) 37 Longleat Close Banbury Oxfordshire OX16 9TG **Tel:** (01295) 278742 w 6041008

Anne Gertrude Cora 04/08/1987 8 Carndreen Road Castlederg County Tyrone BT81 7UD **Tel:** (028) 816 79599 w 6045385

Caroline Lucy 30/11/2006 171 Manchester New Road Middleton Manchester M24 1DE **Tel:** (0161) 643 3097 w 6373881

BELL Claire Brownlee (see GARRETT, Mrs)

Gillian 13/04/1989 12 The Crescent Mathern Chepstow Gwent NP16 6JN **Tel:** (0208) 5318517 w 6045396

Jessica Ann 04/01/2006 Stable Cottage Cold Ashby Road Thornby NORTHAMPTON NN6 8SH w 6351617

Joanna Amy 21/05/2007 Tower Wood Veterinary Group 27 Tinshill Road Leeds Yorkshire LS16 7DR **Tel:** (0113) 267 8419 w 6382263

Karen Laura 28/02/2005 6 Horsbrugh Avenue Kilsyth Glasgow G65 9BZ **Tel:** (01236) 824931 w 6285914

Katie Ann 24/10/2008 35 High Street Tattershall LINCOLN LN4 4NP **Tel:** (07979) 641465 w 6431609

Lesley Ann 12/05/2006 70 Portland Street Troon Ayrshire KA10 6QU **Tel:** (01292) 311988 w 6306330

Lindsay Anne (formerly Bell) 20/09/2006 13 Moorfield Square Southfields Northampton Northamptonshire NN3 5BD **Tel:** (01604) 491960 w 6343631

Louise 15/10/1999 5 Foxdale Court Murton SEAHAM County Durham SR7 9GY w 6122249

BELL Nicola Jane (see WARD, Mrs)

Samantha 13/08/2008 56 Ormonds Close Bradley Stoke BRISTOL BS32 0DX **Tel:** (01454) 853748 w 6366709

Samantha Elizabeth (nee Gray) 26/10/2000 62 Burton Road Cottingham North Humberside HU16 5EB **Tel:** (01482) 842 858 w 6203964

Shirley Olivia 08/07/2003 8 clover Road Flitwick Bedford Bedfordshire MK45 1PQ w 6273726

Tara Sinead 24/09/1997 (12/02/2003) 27 Wilton Manor Rathnew Co Wicklow Ireland **Tel:** (01) 2303896 w 6019388

Victoria Louise 07/08/2008 11 The Holloway Compton Wolverhampton West Midlands WV6 8LH **Tel:** ((01902)) 657 235 w 6412040

BELLAS Jane Louise (nee Goodwin) 18/08/1988 (08/05/2002) Westmorland Veterinary Group Riverside Business Park Natland Road Kendal Cumbria LA9 7SX **Tel:** (01539) 722692 w 6051479

Lisa 13/05/2003 38 Kings Road Fairfield Buxton Derbyshire SK17 7NF **Tel:** (01298) 79018 w 6272956

BELLE Jacqueline Michele 12/01/1987 228 Sellincourt Road London SW17 9SB w 604540X

BELTON Gemma Elizabeth 19/07/2006 20 Kilnwood Close Nottingham Nottinghamshire NG3 7AZ **Tel:** (0115) 9112187 w 6317660

Melanie Denise 22/02/2007 9 Jubilee Close Haywards Heath West Sussex RH16 3PJ **Tel:** (01444) 414 126 w 6349516

BENNETT Alice Victoria Margaret 27/02/2007 Brynteg Farm Litchard Hill Bridgend Mid Glamorgan CF35 6HB **Tel:** (07793) 411865 w 6346722

Carol Susan 31/03/2003 15 Saunders Place Fairford Leys Aylesbury Buckinghamshire HP19 7FE **Tel:** (07733) 086629 w 6283681

Catherine Jane 21/01/2008 3 Ivel Close BEDFORD MK41 7EJ **Tel:** (01234) 360631 w 6301435

BENNETT Dawn Agnes (see DUNN, Mrs)

Emma Frances 08/08/2002 31 Park Hill Tiverton Devon EX16 6RW **Tel:** (01884) 255336 w 6274243

Fiona 07/05/2009 28 Hogarth Avenue GOREBRIDGE Midlothian EH23 4AT **Tel:** 07824662101 w 6345644

Hayley Joanne 28/01/2009 100 Nursery Lane South Wootton King's Lynn Norfolk PE30 3NB **Tel:** (01553) 675 856 w 6402492

Jacqueline Louise 24/11/2008 Church Cottage Maynards Green Heathfield East Sussex TN21 0DJ **Tel:** 01435813859 w 6433567

Joanna Louise 21/03/2006 Southfield Veterinary Centre South Walks DORCHESTER Dorset DT1 1DU **Tel:** (01305) 262913 w 6344984

Joanne 17/11/2000 Walton Cottage 5 Foundry Street North HALIFAX West Yorkshire HX3 6RE **Tel:** (01422) 374361 w 6205680

Katherine Anne 27/02/2006 Aston Road Haddenham Buckinghamshire HP17 8AF w 6326240

Kimberley 19/12/2007 Fishery Lodge Noake Mill Lane Water End HEMEL HEMPSTEAD Hertfordshire HP1 3BB **Tel:** 07921147295 w 6401205

Laura Louise 02/03/2009 10 Holly Drive Chingford LONDON E4 7NG **Tel:** 07736934138 w 6373683

Lisa Anne 06/10/2009 2 Broadway Bebington Wirral Merseyside CH63 5NH **Tel:** (0151) 608 7822 w 6460979

Rosemary Karen (formerly Farmer) 01/11/1984 (31/05/2000) 46 Peascroft Long Crendon Aylesbury Buckinghamshire HP18 9AU **Tel:** (01844) 201 034 w 605009X

BENNETT Ruth Ann (see LAMBERT, Mrs)

Samantha Louise 26/08/2008 The Vale Veterinary Group Areley Common STOURPORT-ON-SEVERN Worcestershire DY13 0LB w 6423887

Sarah 13/12/2001 3 Watsons Green Fields Dudley West Midlands DY2 7LW **Tel:** (01384) 561789 w 6261703

Tracy 04/03/1999 55 Park Lane Pinhoe Exeter Devon EX4 9HP **Tel:** (01392) 468365 w 6035344

BENNEY Claire Louise (see HAWKEN, Mrs)

BENNEY Helen Jane (see NORTH, Mrs)

BENNEY Julie Kay (see NESBITT, Mrs)

BENSON Charlotte Margaret 19/02/2009 Dundas Veterinary Group 99 Dundas Street Edinburgh EH3 6SD **Tel:** (0131) 557 1819 w 6492725

Tania Jane (nee Heath) 17/08/2005 23 Bulleid Place ASHFORD Kent TN24 0PW w 6291689

BENSTEAD Sally Jane (nee Gynn) 06/03/2003 Little Briar 17 Lyons Hall Road Bocking Essex CM7 9SG **Tel:** (01376) 345395 w 6278423

BENSTON Shevaun Anne (see CARDIER, Mrs)

BENTLEY Emma Ann 29/08/2000 234b Oxlow Lane Dagenham Essex RM10 7YX w 6204096

Joanne Claire (nee Wilkinson) 03/09/1996 171 Wordsworth Road Horfield Bristol Avon BS7 0EQ **Tel:** (011) 7904 3713 w 6036698

BENTLEY Joy Susann (see FORTIS, Mrs)

Victoria Louisa 26/10/2006 65 Worting Road Basingstoke Hampshire RG21 8YX **Tel:** (01256) 465409 w 6287542

BENTON Emma Margaret 15/02/2008 33 Lymington Avenue Yateley Hampshire GU46 6HA **Tel:** (01252) 861077 w 6300236

BERESFORD Catherine Anne 30/10/2003 20 Albert Road Colne Lancashire BB8 0AA **Tel:** (01282) 863892 w 6280865

BERNI Rhia 26/10/2005 53 Gwar-y-Caeau Pen-y-Cae Port Talbot West Glamorgan SA13 2UR **Tel:** (01639) 882986 w 6330673

BERRY Alix Petra 20/11/2007 Jackson Hill Farm Jackson Hill Queensbury BRADFORD West Yorkshire BD13 2LA **Tel:** (01274) 883916 w 6345875

Carol Lynn (nee Cooper) 05/08/1987 (15/03/2007) 20/22 Campbell Street Belper Derbyshire DE56 1AP **Tel:** (01773) 822 591 w 6076653

Claire Louise 21/05/2007 Mullacott Veterinary Hospital Bickenbridge Farm Ilfracombe Devon EX34 8NZ **Tel:** (01271) 866770 w 6366214

Coleen Ann 04/06/2009 46 Newbury Road Ipswich Suffolk IP4 5EX **Tel:** 01473423764 w 6408883

Lynne Marie 30/10/2003 Wayside Farm Station Road Ansford Castle Cary Somerset BA7 7PA **Tel:** (01963) 350764 w 6287179

BERTONI Lara Andrea 01/04/2003 17 West Street Tadley Hampshire RG26 3ST **Tel:** (01189) 813668 w 6332763

BEST Gemma Louise 10/02/2004 Milehouse Clinic 28 Outland Road Milehouse Plymouth Devon PL2 3DF **Tel:** (01752) 567567 w 6272604

Jennifer Claire 15/11/2006 19 Ryecroft Strensall YORK YO32 5AG **Tel:** (01904) 492656 w 6349681

Jennifer Grace 19/02/2008 18 Honeysuckle Gardens ANDOVER Hampshire SP10 3DD w 6378820

BESTBIER Megan Lucy (nee McCarthy) 19/01/2000 Mill House Veterinary Surgery & Hospital 20 Tennyson Avenue King's Lynn Norfolk PE30 2QG **Tel:** (01553) 771457 w 6121675

BETTERIDGE Jennifer Joanne (nee Smith) 12/07/2004 Pet Doctors Veterinary Clinics 63 Regents Park Road Southampton SO15 8PF **Tel:** (023) 8078 0385 w 6307419

BETTERTON Sally 25/11/1988 (08/07/2008) Harwell Chelveston Road Raunds WELLINGBOROUGH Northamptonshire NN9 6DA **Tel:** (01933) 311260 w 6045556

BETTS Stacey Sarah 19/02/2008 River View Southbourne Grove WICKFORD Essex SS12 0JT w 6357326

BEVAN Hayley Lynne (see OYLER, Mrs)

BEVAN Jodi Laura (see BEVAN-GORE, Mrs)

BEVAN Rebecca Louise DipAVN(Surgical) 03/02/2000 25 The Hedges St. Georges WESTON-SUPER-MARE Avon BS22 7BU **Tel:** (01934) 513800 w 6140541

Sharon Louise 09/08/1990 (03/04/2002) Apple Cottage 415 Jennett Tree Lane Callow End WORCESTER WR2 4UA **Tel:** (01905) 831074 w 6000129

BEVAN-GORE Jodi Laura (nee Bevan) 21/11/2005 3 The Octagon Bulwark CHEPSTOW Gwent NP16 5QJ **Tel:** (01291) 622630 w 6262649

BEVANS Katherine Jane (nee Bust) 04/11/2005 Strickland Farm The Turnpike Halam NEWARK Nottinghamshire NG22 8AE **Tel:** (07900) 853925 w 6333302

BEVERIDGE Daniel Scott 06/03/2008 67 Belgrave Road Keighley West Yorkshire BD21 2HL **Tel:** (07989) 663651 m 6376851

BEVERLEY Rachel Christine 27/10/2008 Park Farm Broad Oak Lane Mobberley KNUTSFORD Cheshire WA16 6JP **Tel:** (01565) 872622 w 6343642

BEVINGTON Jodie Louise 23/05/2008 3 Church View Audlem CREWE CW3 0HN **Tel:** (01270) 812058 w 6374860

BEVINS Sophie Victoria 17/01/2007 (10/02/2009) 61 Tylers Close GODSTONE Surrey RH9 8AW w 6372330

BEVIS Kirsten 19/03/2007 Fulford House Torbay Road Castle Cary Somerset BA7 7DT **Tel:** (01963) 350307 w 6350451

BEYER Sally Jane 13/07/2004 63 Norwich Road Wroxham Norwich Norfolk NR12 8RX **Tel:** (01603) 783 920 w 6298982

BIBBY Nina Lynn 07/02/2005 22 Cinnamon Hill Drive South Walton-le-Dale PRESTON PR5 4QL **Tel:** (01772) 815496 w 6281822

BICHARD Katherine (nee Shannon, formerly Brown) 27/07/1987 8 1/2 Little Street Alderney GUERNSEY GY9 3TT **Tel:** (01481) 822459 w 6078242

BICKFORD Rebecca Joyce (nee Congdon) 29/11/1999 Rose Cottage 13 Dopps Terrace REDRUTH Cornwall TR15 2EP **Tel:** (01209) 210413 w 6186397

BICKLE Jemma Louise (nee Browes) 14/10/2008 2 Proudfoot Way Aylsham NORWICH NR11 6WE w 6434425

BIDDLE Michelle 10/02/2005 29 Southgate Close Goosewell Plymouth Devon PL9 9QL **Tel:** (01752) 408004 w 6298553

BIGGS Helen Joy (see FULLEYLOVE, Mrs)

BIGGS Nicola-Jayne (see JOHNSON, Mrs)

BIGGS Samantha (nee Fletcher) 27/02/2009 10 Larkspur Croft BOSTON Lincolnshire PE21 8EF **Tel:** 01205357554 w 6436284

BIGMORE Donna 08/01/2009 Framlingham College (att: Mark Lavery) College Road Framlingham WOODBRIDGE Suffolk IP13 9EY w 6534074

Helen Elizabeth 17/01/2007 21 Winston Road Churchdown Gloucester Gloucestershire GL3 2QZ **Tel:** (01452) 713843 w 6373243

BILLETT Jennifer Rachel 05/08/2003 C/o Royal College of Veterinary Surgeons 62-64 Horseferry Road LONDON SW1P 2AF w 6278610

BILLINGSLEY Paula Marie 21/03/2007 11 Wembley Road THORNTON-CLEVELEYS Lancashire FY5 4JN **Tel:** (01253) 859119 w 6323226

BILLINGTON Catherine Mary (see MARSHALL, Mrs)

BILLINGTON Melissa Nina (see TAYLOR, Mrs)

BINDER Deborah Louise (see BIRCHER, Mrs)

BINDLOSS Penelope Jane 14/01/1982 173 Warrandyte Road Ringwood North Victoria 3134 Australia **Tel:** (0061) 3 98762111 w 6045603

BINGE Helen Mary 23/01/2009 Petrosa 4 The Cloud Wotton-under-Edge Gloucestershire GL12 7HG **Tel:** (01453) 542092 w 6441949

BINGGELI Lilian 15/04/2008 15 Askham Croft YORK YO24 3FD w 6510259

BINGHAM Alma (nee Rowlands) 14/03/2006 Tyn Ffynnon Llaneilian Amlwch Gwynedd LL68 9NN **Tel:** (077) 250 45198 w 6343202

BINGHAM Heather Louise (see BLADES, Mrs)

Rachael 20/03/2001 (08/05/2003) Copeland Veterinary Surgeons Myton Park Ingleby Barwick Stockton-on-Tees Cleveland TS17 0WA **Tel:** (01642) 760999 w 6204558

BIRCH Jacqui Danielle 22/08/2008 49 Tickfield Avenue SOUTHEND-ON-SEA SS2 6LL w 6433479

Nicola DipAVN(Surgical), DipAVN(Medical) (nee Dixon) 12/01/1990 10 West Croft Much Hoole Preston PR4 4QP **Tel:** (01772) 616771 w 6074521

BIRCHALL Victoria 19/01/2000 Inside Pets at Home Middlebrook Retail Park Middlebrook Bolton Lancashire BL6 6JA **Tel:** (01204) 469478 w 6190588

BIRCHER Deborah Louise (nee Crosier, formerly Binder) 04/09/1996 38 Edinburgh Gardens Braintree Essex CM7 9LH **Tel:** (01245) 473238 w 6099003

Nicola Louise 13/04/2004 3 Sawbridge Close Ellistown Leicestershire LE67 1DH w 6296903

BIRD Claire Karen (nee Scholey) 10/08/1984 Trellyn Abercastle Haverfordwest Dyfed SA62 5HJ **Tel:** (01348) 837762 w 6045614

Leanne Louise 18/01/1999 Bridge Veterinary Centre Commercial Street Pontllanfraith Blackwood Gwent NP12 2JG **Tel:** (01495) 226272 w 6039473

Lisa Jayne (nee Goodall) 31/03/2003 Reaseheath College Nantwich Cheshire CW5 6DF w 6279303

Lucy Kate 30/06/2003 (17/08/2007) 39 New Street Weedon Northamptonshire NN7 4QS **Tel:** (01327) 342232 w 6280986

Marie Louise (nee Rilstone) 25/03/2002 (27/08/2009) New Priory Veterinary Practice The Deneway London Rd Brighton East Sussex BN1 8QR **Tel:** (01273) 540430 w 6262957

Michelle Louise 16/08/2007 Flat 5 Barley House Great Easthall Way SITTINGBOURNE Kent ME10 3TF w 6385200

BIRD Selena Jane (see BURROUGHS, Mrs)

Vanessa Michelle 02/08/2000 Iowna Cottage Colliston ARBROATH Angus DD11 3RP w 6142673

BIRKIN Sarah Jayne 27/11/2008 8 Cygnet Close Filey North Yorkshire YO14 0BJ **Tel:** ((01723)) 516 924 w 6407189

BISBY Emily Charlotte 26/10/2009 Barnsley Vets4Pets Limited 161 Wilthorpe Road Barnsley South Yorkshire S75 1JQ **Tel:** (01226) 289000 w 6460924

BISHOP Alexandra (see BROWN, Miss)

BISHOP Denise Ann 05/11/2008 12 Concorde Drive BRISTOL BS10 6PZ **Tel:** (07967) 362353 w 6426483

Helen Joanne 08/11/2006 (24/11/2009) 28 Marlborough Street Walsall West Midlands WS3 2HZ **Tel:** (07542) 377123 w 6276190

BISHOP Jacqueline Mary (see SMITH, Mrs)

BISHOP Katy (see HEN-BOISEN, Mrs)

Rebecca Ann 24/11/2008 55 Westray Drive Hinckley Leicestershire LE10 0TL **Tel:** 07828581088 w 6440948

BISP Dawn 17/07/2003 22 Leamington Grove Ormesby Middlesbrough Cleveland TS3 0PH **Tel:** (01642) 310757 w 6265267

BLABER Rachel Margaret (see JONES, Mrs)

BLACHFORD Sarah Gillian Mary 26/11/2009 7 Minster Road BROMLEY BR1 4DY w 6440453

BLACK Abigail Anna 03/05/2005 12 Cromwell Court Eynesbury ST. NEOTS Cambridgeshire PE19 2NZ **Tel:** (01480) 407593 w 6274331

Joanne 23/10/2009 74 Lomond Crescent Alexandria Dunbartonshire G83 0RL **Tel:** (01389) 755527 w 6405187

Laura Anne (nee Munro) 08/01/1993 Penguin House Castle Riggs DUNFERMLINE Fife KY11 8SG **Tel:** (01383) 620064 w 6065175

Michelle 22/09/2006 10/3 Royston Mains Gardens Edinburgh Midlothian EH5 1NL **Tel:** (0131) 551 5113 w 6356633

BLACKBOURN Sarah Jane 09/09/1992 (23/03/2000) 1 Rivers Street Place Julian Road Bath BA1 2RS **Tel:** (01225) 313995 w 6005852

BLACKBURN Katherine Jane 05/10/2001 (17/04/2003) 16 Kingsley Gardens Totton SOUTHAMPTON SO40 8ET w 6132676

BLACKBURN Lorna Mary (see LARNDER, Mrs)

Marie 17/11/2004 20 Albert Road Colne Lancashire BB8 0AA **Tel:** (01282) 863892 w 6299917

Penelope Lisa 12/06/1989 4 Quantock Drive Worcester Park Surrey KT4 8JN **Tel:** (020) 8337 8810 w 6045705

Tina Michelle 22/12/2004 The Willows 1 Templegate Walk Leeds West Yorkshire LS15 0EU **Tel:** (0113) 2640116 w 6325030

BLACKBURN Tracy Ann (see OLIVER, Mrs)

BLACKER Helen Margaret 26/04/2007 6 Sherbrooke Close Kirkbymoorside YORK YO62 6LJ **Tel:** (01751) 430600 w 6353718

BLACKERY Katie Louise (nee Havelin) 21/06/2005 94 Skiddaw Close Great Notley BRAINTREE Essex CM77 7UR w 6322082

BLACKETT Beverley (see MALLABAR, Mrs)

BLACKETT Dianne Lorraine Theresa (see SEARLE, Mrs)

BLACKMAN Sharon Patricia (see FILMER, Mrs)

BLACKMORE Charlotte Sara Louise (see RYDZ, Mrs)

BLACKSHAW Emma Catherine Louise (nee Cheshire) 20/04/2005 Pet Doctors Veterinary Clinics 3 Parklands Road Chichester West Sussex PO19 3DP **Tel:** (01243) 782880 w 6325679

BLADES Heather Louise (nee Bingham) 04/02/2002 24 Askam Avenue PONTEFRACT West Yorkshire WF8 2PN w 6269227

BLAGG Helen Mary (nee Williamson) 30/07/1986 (18/11/1999) Woodleigh Broomheath Lane Tarvin Chester CH3 8HD **Tel:** (01829) 740698 w 6010975

BLAIR Hayley Joy 01/06/2007 26 Elford Grove Marston Green BIRMINGHAM B37 7RN w 6376697

BLAKE Jennifer Louise 24/05/2006 3 Layton Lane SHAFTESBURY Dorset SP7 8EY **Tel:** (07966) 513 260 w 6278863

BLAKEMORE Katie Angela 02/11/2004 (10/02/2009) 46 Latebrook Close STOKE-ON-TRENT Staffordshire ST6 5NL w 6257963

BLAKESLEY Melanie Jane (see O'SULLIVAN, Mrs)

BLAKEWAY Laura Dawn 31/10/2008 8 Beeches Grove Bayston Hill SHREWSBURY SY3 0PH w 6388632

BLAKEY Nicola 22/09/1995 33 Keith Close Benwell Newcastle upon Tyne NE4 8HG **Tel:** (0191) 273 1055 w 6037964

BLAMIRES Helen (formerly Skipsey) 28/08/1998 (01/03/2007) Wychwood Cottage West Street Mayfield East Sussex TN20 6DR **Tel:** (07773) 048387 w 6122271

BLANCHARD Joanne Kim 05/07/2006 135 Goldfinch Road POOLE Dorset BH17 7TB **Tel:** (01202) 699905 w 6321422

Katherine Anne 18/10/2006 122 San Diego Road GOSPORT Hampshire PO12 4QT w 6343653

Sarah 28/09/1999 (25/04/2002) 66 Crockfords Road NEWMARKET Suffolk CB8 9BG **Tel:** (01638) 751000 w 6186100

BLANEY Nicola 11/06/2003 Donnington Grove Veterinary Surgery Oxford Road NEWBURY Berkshire RG14 2JB **Tel:** (01635) 47170 w 6261538

BLASDALE Rebekah 26/10/2000 Dunkirk Road Dunkirk Nottingham NG7 2PH **Tel:** (01159) 785787 w 6204602

BLEACH Sarah Louise 06/08/2008 27 Warwick Road Banbury Oxfordshire OX16 2AB **Tel:** 01295266462 w 6413558

BLEAKLEY Jayne 05/09/2000 8 South Mead West Camel Yeovil Somerset BA22 7QQ **Tel:** (01935) 850016 w 615258X

BLEASBY Dawn Marie 09/03/1999 (25/10/2000) 784 Foundry Lane Leeds LS14 6BN **Tel:** (0113) 260 5335 w 6036574

BLENKIRON Rebecca 17/01/2006 The Old School Back Lane Skerne DRIFFIELD North Humberside YO25 9HP w 6332554

BLEZARD Margaret Elizabeth 05/08/1970 29 Moorfield Edgeworth Turton Bolton BL7 0DH **Tel:** (01204) 852908 w 6045807

BLIGHT Kerry-Lianne 06/10/2009 7 Buchans Lawn Broadfield Crawley West Sussex RH11 9NZ w 6436768

BLOCK Emma Louise 12/02/2009 74 Westward Ho Leiston Suffolk IP16 4HU **Tel:** (01728) 832710 w 6352695

BLOOMFIELD Kate 16/01/1989 (21/06/2005) 10 Cutliffe Place Bedford Bedfordshire MK40 4DF **Tel:** (01234) 340797 w 6000209

BLOOR Claire Louise 13/05/2003 6 Lawnwood Avenue Chorley Lancashire PR7 2NF **Tel:** (01257) 411070 w 6287608

Kirsty Joanne 06/08/2007 Hillcrest Animal Health Ltd Water Street Chorley Lancashire PR7 1EX **Tel:** (01257) 262448 w 6371538

BLOOR Samantha Jayne (see GALLAGHER, Mrs)

Sarah Alma 30/10/2008 15 Chilworth Close Crewe Cheshire CW2 6UN **Tel:** 01270664327 w 6442004

BLOWER Nina Rachael (see TUDOR, Mrs)

BLOWES Amy Victoria 17/07/2003 Tregarn Higher Reen PERRANPORTH Cornwall TR6 0AJ w 6268193

BLOWING Kimberley Ann 08/01/2009 15 Hopton Road Thame Oxfordshire OX9 3TS **Tel:** 01844213119 w 6375905

BLOXHAM Lisa 16/08/1995 (19/03/2009) 34 St Georges Avenue Wolstanton Newcastle Staffordshire ST5 8DH **Tel:** (01782) 620683 w 6034963

BLUETT Lisa Jane 28/08/1998 39 Wendover House Chenies Way Watford Hertfordshire WD18 6UW w 611249X

BLUNDELL Frances Anne 15/01/1999 (29/01/2003) Davies Veterinary Specialists Manor Farm Business Park Higham Gobion Hertfordshire SG5 3HR **Tel:** (01582) 883950 w 6138714

Sharon 21/08/1990 (18/05/2005) Inside Pets at Home Unit 1 Didsbury Road STOCKPORT Cheshire SK4 2LQ **Tel:** (0161) 475 5720 w 6045840

BLUNT Natasha Joanne 10/01/2003 53 Queenswood Ave Boothville Northampton Northamptonshire NN3 6JT **Tel:** (01604) 452 517 w 6282570

BLYTH Elizabeth Ann 04/09/1995 (26/02/2001) Brook House Veterinary Hospital 12 Landguard Road Southampton Hampshire SO15 5DJ **Tel:** (02380) 228570 w 6031419

BLYTHE Judith 23/12/1992 Tyn-Y-Celyn Cefn Canol Rhydycroesau Powys SY10 7JG **Tel:** (01691) 654105 w 6044086

BLYTH-TANCOCK Jody Marie (nee Turner) 02/11/2004 16 MacPherson Robertson Way Mildenhall Bury St. Edmunds Suffolk IP28 7RS **Tel:** (01638) 716 883 w 6323545

BOAG Rebecca Louise Ramsey (see WINTER, Mrs)

BOAN Ian 28/05/2008 Blackness Veterinary Surgery 82 Brook Street Dundee Tayside DD1 5BP **Tel:** (01382) 225422 m 6374453

BOARD Virginia Marie Elizabeth 17/11/2004 615 Wells Road Whitchurch Bristol BS14 9BE **Tel:** (01275) 832410 w 6303338

BOARDMAN Catherine 04/04/2006 18 Holmroyd Avenue Cross Hills KEIGHLEY West Yorkshire BD20 7LH **Tel:** (01535) 634360 w 6344071

Melissa Ann 09/09/2008 50 Haydon Street STOKE-ON-TRENT ST4 6JE **Tel:** (01782) 621852 w 6275134

Tracey Ellen (nee Gatward) 02/07/1991 (30/11/2000) Forest Veterinary Centre Eastwick Lodge Harlow Essex CM20 2QT **Tel:** (01279) 437433 w 6045851

BOASE Kirsty Jane 03/05/2007 2c Hales Road CHELTENHAM Gloucestershire GL52 6SE **Tel:** (07796) 318 466 w 6391162

BOAST Clare Louise 04/06/2009 2 Bletchley Close Eldene SWINDON Wiltshire SN3 6BY **Tel:** (01793) 340032 w 6415362

BOBELDIJK Victoria Elizabeth 19/02/2008 10 Enville Way Highwoods COLCHESTER Essex CO4 9UF **Tel:** (01206) 845731 w 6374508

BODDIE Donna Katrina 31/01/2000 26 Rushetts Road Langley Green Crawley West Sussex RH11 7ND w 6191281

BODE Dawn Catherine (nee Layen) 11/11/2004 22 Barley Close Burton-on-Trent Staffordshire DE14 2SX w 6271790

BOGUE Alison Margaret 30/01/2009 Greenstead Auchengray Carnwath LANARK ML11 8LW **Tel:** 01501785535 w 6379458

BOICE Lucy Amanda 16/07/2007 Ark House Veterinary Surgery 22 Hockliffe Street LEIGHTON BUZZARD Bedfordshire LU7 1HJ **Tel:** (01525) 373329 w 6370559

BOL Joanne Elizabeth 16/06/2006 105 Segrave Road Plymouth Devon PL2 3EP **Tel:** (01752) 561 741 w 6333280

BOLDERO Fiona Jane 02/09/1999 (29/11/2001) Grove House Holt Road Fakenham Norfolk NR21 8JG **Tel:** (01328) 862137 w 6149238

BOLTON Abigail 07/05/2009 44 Alma Place CLITHEROE Lancashire BB7 2LF **Tel:** 07845272661 w 6297959

Louisa Jane 27/12/2001 4 Barber End Shefford Bedfordshire SG17 5TB **Tel:** 01462811233 w 6268556

Sarah Elizabeth (nee Mogford) 16/08/2006 16 Campbell Drive Windsor Quay CARDIFF CF11 7QE w 6337537

BONAFIA Harriet Elizabeth (nee Brody) 04/04/2006 Swanspool Veterinary Clinic 1 London Road Wellingborough Northamptonshire NN8 2BT **Tel:** (01933) 222145 w 6324293

BOND Hollie Jane 07/12/2006 Waterdene Veterinary Practice 4 Timber Hill Road Caterham Surrey CR3 6LD **Tel:** (01883) 345277 w 6354092

Joanna 01/05/2008 Milehouse Clinic 28 Outland Road Milehouse Plymouth Devon PL2 3DF **Tel:** (01752) 567567 w 6307397

Joanna Gwen 21/11/2008 11 Bishops Way Andover Hampshire SP10 3EH **Tel:** 01264355418 w 6410775

BOND Katrina Laura (see VENABLES, Mrs)

Lisa Jane (nee Hill) 15/04/2004 5 Slaidburn Close Hawkley Hall Wigan Lancashire WN3 5PX **Tel:** (01257) 426110 w 6293163

Nicola 21/03/2007 Mayfield Avenue Walkden Worsley Manchester M28 3JF **Tel:** (0161) 799 5557 w 6358756

Sally Ann (nee Wood, nee Eastwood) 04/09/1997 34 Richmond Drive North Hykeham LINCOLN LN6 8QY w 602748X

BONE Alison Louise 29/05/2003 11 Bell Court Merlin Road Farnbrough Hampshire GU14 7HR w 6285903

BONIFACE Amanda Jane 21/04/2005 41 Spencerfield Road INVERKEITHING Fife KY11 1PJ **Tel:** (01383) 417064 w 6318397

BONNER Sarah 26/10/2006 6 Lincoln Avenue St. Ives Cambridgeshire PE27 3YF **Tel:** (01480) 497 293 w 6375564

BONNICI Angharad Sarah 14/09/2004 1a The Village Manmoel Blackwood Gwent NP12 0RJ **Tel:** (014795) 371 645 w 6290974

BONSALL Lindsay Anne (see COTTERILL, Mrs)

BONSOR Katie Louise 05/07/2006 10 Hogarth Close BEDWORTH Warwickshire CV12 8TL **Tel:** (024) 76490180 w 6321433

BOON Elizabeth Sarah 06/08/2008 177 Manor Road Cogges Witney Oxfordshire w 6386113

BOOTH Charlotte Elizabeth 22/03/2004 Runnymede Hill Veterinary Hospital Tite Hill Egham Surrey TW20 0NB **Tel:** (01784) 436 367 w 6284935

BOOTH Clair (see BATLEY, Mrs)

Jennifer Helen 05/07/2006 Heightside House Sabden Road Padiham BURNLEY Lancashire BB12 9AD **Tel:** (01282) 775983 w 6321444

Joanne 04/02/2002 The Veterinary Centre Market Street Rugeley Staffordshire WS15 2JH **Tel:** (01889) 582023 w 6260053

Rachel Ann 26/01/1999 (25/10/2000) Donaldson & Partners Miry Lane Thongsbridge HOLMFIRTH HD9 7RY **Tel:** (01484) 684189 w 6135032

Sarah Louise (formerly Puttock) 21/09/1999 211 Elm Drive Hove East Sussex BN3 7JD **Tel:** (01273) 382664 w 6185352

BORLAND Lee-Anne Elizabeth 06/03/2006 Alphavet Veterinary Centre 62 Muirs Kinross KY13 8AU **Tel:** (01577) 863328 w 6281536

Samantha Louise (nee Nash) 11/11/2004 228 Painswick Road Gloucester Gloucestershire GL4 4PH **Tel:** (01452) 529480 w 6273066

BORNMAN Inge 21/03/2007 C/o Braam Botes RMAS Camberley Surrey GU15 4PQ w 6452377

BORRETT Amy 17/09/2009 14a Ryall Road POOLE Dorset BH17 9FA **Tel:** 01202603678 w 6384881

BORRINI Laura 06/05/2008 38 Queens Road Crosby Liverpool Merseyside L23 5TR **Tel:** (0151) 9240600 w 6419927

BORRMANN Melanie Ann (see MACE, Mrs)

BOSWELL Victoria Louise DipAVN(Surgical) (nee Monaghan) 04/12/2003 Fairview House King Street Maidford TOWCESTER Northamptonshire NN12 8HQ **Tel:** (01327) 860952 w 6298113

BOTHWELL Janice Joyce 25/11/2008 Smithston Farm Patna Ayr Ayrshire KA6 7EZ **Tel:** 07845098497 w 6411666

BOUCHARD Louisa Ann 21/04/2004 New Road Cottage La Neuve Route St Peter Jersey JE37 7AU w 6284561

BOUCHER Fiona Ann (nee Hall) 15/12/2003 55 Farnham Road DURHAM DH1 5LL **Tel:** (0191) 3757997 w 6286178

BOUCHER Suzanne Elizabeth (see CAVE, Mrs)

BOUGHEY Barbara Mary (see JAQUES, Miss)

BOUGHTON Clare Louise (see MOORE, Mrs)

BOULTON Katy Victoria 30/06/2003 51 Sycamore Crescent Port Talbot West Glamorgan SA12 8PL **Tel:** (01639) 680744 w 6258051

BOUNDS Anne Louise (nee Richards) 22/08/1990 (08/05/2006) Hollybush Veterinary Group Tenbury Road Cleobury Mortimer Kidderminster Worcestershire DY14 8RB **Tel:** (01299) 271967 w 6059616

BOURN Hannah Louise 09/11/2005 4 Campion Way WITHAM Essex CM8 2XD **Tel:** (01376) 515890 w 6328110

BOURNE Hazel Anne (see SHEPPARD, Mrs)

BOURNE Helen Louise 05/10/2004 204 Bushbury Road Fallings Park Wolverhampton WV10 0NB **Tel:** (01902) 731127 w 6298564

BOVENIZER Susan Sarah 07/12/2005 Friars Moor Veterinary Clinic Ltd Friars Moor Manston Road STURMINSTER NEWTON Dorset DT10 1BH **Tel:** (01258) 472314 w 6278995

BOWATER Helen Ruth (see PLAYFOOT, Mrs)

BOWCOTT Amy DipAVN(Surgical) (nee Tildesley) 24/09/2002 57 Sudeley Dosthill TAMWORTH Staffordshire B77 1JU w 6269997

BOWDEN Carole (see MARTIN, Miss)

BOWDEN Sally Jane 07/08/1990 1975 North Eyre Road Horrellville RD5 Rangiora Canterbury 7475 New Zealand **Tel:** (0064) 3313 2807 w 6046028

BOWDITCH Sally-Ann 04/10/2005 Martock Veterinary Centre Stapleton Road Martock Somerset TA12 6HH **Tel:** (01935) 825199 w 6332862

BOWEN Gemma Louise 04/01/2006 40 Burgess Green Close St. Annes Park BRISTOL BS4 4DG w 6326823

Kate Louise 31/03/2003 40 Thistledown Grove Hampton Dene Hereford HR1 1AZ **Tel:** (01432) 268135 w 6269458

Kathryn Michelle 29/01/2001 The Old Coach House Gunhouse Lane Bowbridge Stroud Gloucestershire GL5 2DB **Tel:** (01453) 766343 w 613455X

BOWEN Rebecca Lucy (see WILLIAMS, Mrs)

BOWEN Sarah Jane (see MAINWARING, Mrs)

BOWERMAN Michelle Catherine (see HODGES, Mrs)

BOWERS Alice Caroline (see BUGG, Mrs)

BOWERS Fiona Jane (see MANN, Mrs)

BOWERS Lynne Helen 31/08/2000 Myerscough College Bilsborrow Preston Lancashire PR3 0RY **Tel:** (01995) 642222 w 6202930

BOWES Vera Elizabeth 30/05/2007 Sandyford Veterinary Hospital 2B Lambs Cross Sandyford Dublin 18 Ireland **Tel:** (00353) 876 459 172 w 6299433

Victoria Louise 31/03/2003 Warwickshire College Moreton Morrell Warwick Warwickshire CV35 9BL **Tel:** (01926) 318000 w 6282834

BOWEY Michelle Claire 28/08/1998 49 Endless Street Salisbury Wiltshire SP1 3UH **Tel:** (01722) 333 291 w 6107752

BOWIE Lisa 08/06/2009 146 Fairview Crescent Danestone ABERDEEN AB22 8ZT **Tel:** 07717001920 w 6408135

BOWKER Catherine Louise (see BROOMFIELD, Mrs)

BOWLER Jemma Kate 20/11/2008 Greenways Prospect Park Great Holland FRINTON-ON-SEA Essex CO13 0HR **Tel:** (01255) 678715 w 6313689

BOWMAN Verity Jane DipAVN(Surgical) 07/05/1976 P.O. Box 3863 Bulawayo Zimbabwe **Tel:** (++) 263 9 287215 w 6046061

BOWN Tina (see EVANS, Mrs)

BOWRON Stacy Jane (see BURLEIGH, Mrs)

BOWSHER Louise Anne 10/12/2009 45 Lewis Lane Cirencester Gloucestershire GL7 1EA **Tel:** (01285) 653151 w 6438341

BOX Verity Lee (see WILLMOTT, Miss)

BOXALL Marie (see JONES, Mrs)

BOYCE Janine (nee Lupetti) 15/11/2001 16 Lynden Close Holyport Maidenhead Berkshire SL6 2LB **Tel:** (01753) 869983 w 6261824

Samantha (nee Bailey) 29/07/2005 108 Summerfield Road Tamworth Staffordshire B77 3PJ **Tel:** (01827) 57531 w 6274397

BOYD Helen Louise (nee Merritt) 13/08/2004 (02/11/2009) 5 Barry Place Derry Hill Calne Wiltshire SN11 9NX **Tel:** (01249) 822161 w 6285584

Jennifer Anne (nee Wilsher) 17/01/2000 4 Bishops Court Kingswells ABERDEEN AB15 8SQ **Tel:** (01224) 745854 w 6133647

Jennifer Vera Anne 05/03/2009 104 Gateside Manor BALLYCLARE County Antrim BT39 9GA **Tel:** 07724929002 w 6354026

BOYD Lesley-Ann Elizabeth (see LYONS, Mrs)

Margaret Deirdre 05/10/2001 Hillcrest Animal Health Ltd Water Street Chorley Lancashire PR7 1EX **Tel:** (01257) 262448 w 6229594

Victoria Mary 14/03/2008 Eastcott Veterinary Hospital 59 Bath Road Swindon Wiltshire SN1 4AU **Tel:** (01793) 528341 w 6366247

BOYLAN Dinah 18/09/2000 9 Silverdale Terrace Greetland Halifax West Yorkshire HX4 8NQ **Tel:** (01422) 379010 w 6204855

BOYLE Alison Claire (see AIKMAN, Mrs)

BOYLE Kelly (see REED, Mrs)

BOYLE Rhona Agnes 22/11/2001 3 Shakespeare Road Bexleyheath Kent DA7 4SF **Tel:** (0208) 2981613 w 6269073

BOYNTON Beverley Jayne (nee Dixon) 23/10/2001 (30/05/2008) Lark Rise Thornborough BEDALE North Yorkshire DL8 2RE **Tel:** (07731) 946830 w 6268248

BRACEY Kathryn Mandy (see MINCHER, Mrs)

BRADBURN Rosemary Patricia (formerly Brapburn) 06/06/2008 18 Davidson Place Newtown St. Boswells Melrose Roxburghshire TD6 0QJ **Tel:** (07784) 320 003 w 6405132

BRADBURY Kathryn Ruth Lynne 04/11/2005 Lime Trees Veterinary Clinic Tean Road Cheadle Stoke-on-Trent ST10 1TW **Tel:** (01538) 752117 w 6343268

Nicola Mary 21/03/2007 The Veterinary Cat Clinic 38 Blackford Avenue Edinburgh EH9 2PP **Tel:** (0131) 466 7110 w 6381229

BRADBURY Tammy Jane (see BANKS, Mrs)

BRADDON Cathy Amanda 23/08/1999 11 Springfield Chase Long Stratton Norwich Norfolk NR15 2WQ **Tel:** (01508) 532589 w 6184978

BRADFORD Charlotte Louise May (see SAMPSON, Mrs)

BRADFORD Joanne 06/08/1991 (22/04/2002) Northumberland Business Park West CRAMLINGTON Northumberland NE23 7RH **Tel:** (0191) 250 3800 w 6046108

BRADFORD Sarah Marjorie (see LUNDSTROM, Mrs)

BRADFORD-CREMER Dreana (see BULMER-THOMPSON, Mrs)

BRADLEY Julie Ann (see WILSON, Mrs)

BRADLEY Laura Jane 21/03/2006 22 Limes Road DUDLEY West Midlands DY1 4AQ **Tel:** (07817) 176545 w 6343015

Lorraine Adele 27/01/1995 (14/08/2007) 1 Chapel Lane Crick Northamptonshire NN6 7TW w 603185X

Louise Sarah 24/02/2004 16 Marlowe Road NORTHWICH Cheshire CW9 7GA **Tel:** (01606) 40046 w 6290292

Sarah Louise (nee Stimpson) 27/08/1996 34 Granville Road Northchurch Berkhampstead Herefordshire HP4 3RN **Tel:** (01442) 870 967 w 6100382

BRADSHAW Katie 09/03/2009 Penhill House Penhill Lane Brixham Devon TQ5 0EY **Tel:** (01803) 850022 w 6421258

Samantha Anne (nee Ayres) 16/12/1998 21 Peterborough Road Wansford PETERBOROUGH PE8 6JN **Tel:** (01780) 781255 w 6141454

BRADY Janine Ann (nee Lackey) 29/12/2003 The Veterinary Surgery Hallfield Lane WETHERBY West Yorkshire LS22 6JU **Tel:** (01937) 582025 w 6279182

Maria Angela 18/10/1996 4 Talbot Park Bangor Co Down BT19 1PH **Tel:** (0289) 1471824 w 6036177

Rachel Anne 06/10/2006 Boness Veterinary Enterprises Ltd 125 Bedford Road Barton le Clay Bedford Bedfordshire MK45 4LP **Tel:** (01582) 612604 w 6294131

BRAGG Caroline Francesca (see O'CONNELL, Mrs)

BRAGG Celia Marie (see PITTS, Mrs)

BRAIME Annmarie 18/03/2008 3 The Willows Quarter Mile Lane Marsh Green EXETER EX5 2EU **Tel:** (07985) 723225 w 6403185

BRAITHWAITE Jennifer Dawn (nee Curtis) 06/04/2009 7 Brierley Road Shafton Barnsley South Yorkshire S72 8QQ **Tel:** 01226717192 w 6344126

BRAMHAM Allison Paula 24/01/1989 30 Belle Vue Road Romford ESSEX RM5 3AY **Tel:** (01708) 728292 w 6046130

BRAND Maria Jayne (nee Russell) 06/03/2006 103 Ashgate Road EASTBOURNE East Sussex BN23 7ER **Tel:** (01323) 740986 w 6332884

BRANDEL Veronica Louise 17/07/2008 62 The Mariners Llanelli Dyfed SA15 2PP **Tel:** 07876274563 w 6384804

BRANDRETH Rebecca Elizabeth (see SADLER, Mrs)

BRANSCOMBE Elizabeth Ann DipAVN(Surgical) 01/12/1986 Davies Veterinary Specialists Manor Farm Business Park Higham Gobion Hertfordshire SG5 3HR **Tel:** (01582) 883950 w 604620X

BRANTON Jenny Louise 21/07/2008 George Veterinary Group George Veterinary Group Hospital 18-20 High Street MALMESBURY Wiltshire SN16 9AU **Tel:** (01992) 424957 w 6377049

BRAPBURN Rosemary Patricia (see BRADBURN, Miss)

BRASSELEUR-EDWARDS Vania Katia 07/11/2008 25 Waypost Court Northampton Northamptonshire NN3 8LN **Tel:** 07748021437 w 6400303

BRATLEY Helen Louise 02/10/2009 Hideaway Cottage Dacre Lane Dacre HARROGATE North Yorkshire HG3 4AG w 6463927

BRAY Angela Louise 07/12/2006 13 Denmark Road Aylestone LEICESTER LE2 8AB w 6370493

BRAZIER Laura Susan 20/11/2009 62 Trench Road Trench TELFORD Shropshire TF2 6PF **Tel:** 07533264912 w 6459670

BREACHER Yvette Sonia 15/12/2004 9 Scizdons Climb GODALMING Surrey GU7 1NL w 6285188

BRECKELL Helen (see GAUCHWIN, Mrs)

BREE Tracey Helen (nee Goudge) 10/01/2007 4 Dorminack Close Whitemoor ST. AUSTELL Cornwall PL26 7WU **Tel:** (01726) 828008 w 6278500

BREEZE Donna Louise 21/07/2008 76 Kenninghall Road East Harling NORWICH NR16 2QD **Tel:** (01953) 718409 w 6375916

BREINGAN Julie Ann 28/08/1996 13 Nightingale Close Mildenhall Bury St. Edmunds Suffolk IP28 7HQ **Tel:** (01638) 510154 w 6097800

BRENNAN Carolyn Lois 14/11/1990 (07/07/2004) Meadowcroft New Road Rotherfield CROWBOROUGH East Sussex TN6 3JT **Tel:** (07980) 207956 w 6046276

Gemma Tracy 10/05/2007 9 Foundry Road Yapton Arundel West Sussex BN18 0HE **Tel:** (01243) 551 513 w 6353729

Natasha Elizabeth 10/07/2009 1 Teal Lane WELLINGBOROUGH Northamptonshire NN8 4TT **Tel:** (01933) 271869 w 6374002

BRENNAND Kerry Louise DipAVN(Surgical) 31/08/1999 (01/03/2002) Baldrand House Bowerham Road Lancaster LA1 3AJ **Tel:** (01524) 32696 w 6185627

BRENSON Joanne Elisabeth 30/07/2004 14 Ambleside Avenue Beckenham Kent BR3 3RW **Tel:** (020) 8402 7005 w 6300401

BRERETON Alison 13/01/2009 670-672 Muller Road Eastville Bristol BS5 6XB **Tel:** (0117) 951 9048 w 6328902

BRESLIN Victoria Claire 03/05/2007 Willett House Veterinary Surgeons 138 Kingston Road Staines Middlesex TW18 1BL **Tel:** (01784) 452048 w 6365653

BRETT Nichola (see JOHNSON, Mrs)

BRETTON Nicola Jayne (see WARREN, Mrs)

BREW Nicola Joanne (nee Houghton-Kennedy) 10/07/2003 (24/08/2009) 64 Eastbourne Road SOUTHPORT Merseyside PR8 4DU **Tel:** (01704) 560439 w 6274199

BREWER Emma Louise (nee Fazackarley) 21/06/2002 5 Hampton Close WATERLOOVILLE Hampshire PO7 8JJ **Tel:** (07793) 816121 w 6204569

BREWER Joanne (see HARPER, Mrs)

Julie Ann DipAVN(Surgical) (nee Ryal) 22/11/1990 (14/07/1999) Eastfield Veterinary Clinic Ltd Station Road North Thoresby GRIMSBY Lincolnshire DN36 5QU **Tel:** (01472) 840209 w 6060097

Louise Anne 24/02/2004 13 Albert Road BRAINTREE Essex CM7 3JQ **Tel:** (01376) 320947 w 6288763

Vicky Jayne 20/03/2008 20 Alfred Close CHATHAM Kent ME4 5EE **Tel:** (01634) 830263 w 6365675

BREWSTER Helen 22/10/2004 4 New Road EVESHAM Worcestershire WR11 2NG **Tel:** (01386) 761416 w 6319255

Joanne Marie 21/04/2008 76 Beresford Road LONDON E17 4LW **Tel:** (020) 8531 5371 w 6330156

BRIANT Anna Louise 31/10/2005 2 Robertson Road Preston Park Brighton East Sussex BN1 5NL **Tel:** (01273) 566595 w 6354532

BRICE Emma Louise (nee Kemp) 24/12/2002 Morella House Overland Ash CANTERBURY Kent CT3 2LF **Tel:** (01227) 720039 w 6284770

BRICK Sarah 27/09/1999 7 Seaview Estate Netley Abbey Southampton SO31 5BP w 6138419

BRICKLES Michaela Ann (nee Thompson) 27/04/2005 92 Rydal Avenue Freckleton PRESTON PR4 1DJ **Tel:** (01772) 635629 w 6323523

BRIDGE Helen Louise (nee Gillatt) 25/02/2003 18 Oaklands Avenue Heanor Derbyshire DE75 7BB **Tel:** (01773) 714034 w 6272736

Kelly Marie 11/04/2008 26 Bennetts Road North Keresley End COVENTRY CV7 8LA **Tel:** (02476) 338819 w 6403383

BRIDGEMAN Jemima Jane 18/12/2008 Flat 1 St. Marys Priory Fernham FARINGDON Oxfordshire SN7 7PP w 6366720

BRIDGER Lucy Anne 10/02/2004 Highcroft Veterinary Group 25 London Road Hailsham East Sussex BN27 3BN **Tel:** (01323) 841666 w 6290017

BRIDGES Linda Marie 01/11/1984 (30/07/1986) Moray Coast Veterinary Group West Road Greshop Estate Forres Morayshire IV36 2GW **Tel:** (01309) 672243 w 6092711

Rebecca Louise 31/10/2008 Flat 1 Holland House 70 Belmont Road HEREFORD HR2 7JW **Tel:** 07749745058 w 6436746

BRIDLE Justine Sarah 19/09/2006 (07/03/2008) Grove Lodge Veterinary Group Ltd 18 Upper Brighton Road Worthing West Sussex BN14 9DL **Tel:** (01903) 234866 w 6287971

BRIDLE Katie Elizabeth (see HARTNOLL, Mrs)

BRIEG Julia Alice Rose (see BRIGG, Miss)

BRIERLEY Tracey 29/06/2007 119 Fakenham Road Great Ryburgh Fakenham Norfolk NR21 7AQ **Tel:** (01328) 829 598 w 6377599

BRIGG Julia Alice Rose (formerly Brieg) 04/06/2008 24 Etheldene Road Cashes Green Stroud Gloucestershire GL5 4RS **Tel:** (07833) 913109 w 6352706

BRIGGS Lyndsey Alicia 07/09/1998 The Blue Cross Animal Hospital Nelson Street Grimsby South Humberside DN32 7SH **Tel:** (01472) 343278 w 6131526

Nicholas Matthew 04/11/2008 70 Morley Road Romford Essex RM6 6XA **Tel:** 07841873875 m 6440937

Sally Elizabeth 10/02/2004 25 Curlew Avenue Eckington SHEFFIELD S21 4HR w 6291150

BRIGHT Deborah Louise 29/05/2003 (03/03/2006) 465/467 Nottingham Road Chaddesden Derby DE21 6NA **Tel:** (01332) 661554 w 6273440

Gillian Roberta (nee Finney) 06/10/2006 2 Midway Exmouth Devon EX8 2PF **Tel:** (01395) 225 386 w 6294417

BRIGHTLEY Fiona Mary 07/01/1992 (16/01/2001) Dovecotewells Farmhouse Glencaple Dumfries Dumfriesshire DG1 4RH **Tel:** (01387) 770097 w 6046312

BRIND Laura 27/03/2009 36 Savoy Court Station Road HARROW Middlesex HA2 6BU **Tel:** (07739) 826189 w 6403669

BRINDLEY Dawn Veronica 23/02/2005 Afon Veterinary Centre Lletty Nedd Pen Y Dre Neath West Glamorgan SA11 3HH **Tel:** (01639) 642739 w 6329870

BRISBOURNE Annette Louisa (nee Jones) 02/08/1988 (22/02/2005) Walford and North Shropshire College Walford Baschurch Shrewsbury Shropshire SY4 2HR w 6054130

BRISTOLL Gemma Valerie (nee Andrews) 12/05/2009 23 The Hayes West Heath Northfield Birmingham West Midlands B31 3QG w 6377280

BRISTOW Michelle Louise (nee Smith) 04/12/1997 (29/01/2008) 14 Sandhurst Road BEXLEY Kent DA5 1DD **Tel:** (020) 8304 8762 w 6118356

BRITLAND Jenny Elizabeth 02/06/2004 Springfield Veterinary Group 39 Moorgate Road Rotherham South Yorkshire S60 2AD **Tel:** (01709) 377241 w 6270745

BRITTEN Amanda Jessie Mary 15/12/2004 191 Broad Street DAGENHAM Essex RM10 9XA **Tel:** (0208) 595 5818 w 6275079

BRITTLE Samantha 04/11/2005 124 School Lane Bushbury Wolverhampton WV10 8HZ **Tel:** (01902) 780451 w 6276454

BRITTON Amie Judith (nee Wilson) 22/09/1999 (28/04/2009) Michael Gibb Veterinary Clinic 88 Shirehampton Road Bristol BS9 2DR **Tel:** (01179) 683706 w 6185814

Kate Elizabeth 04/03/1994 9 Rhyne View Nailsea North Somerset BS48 2FY w 6027821

BROAD Emma Claire 31/08/1999 (09/04/2009) 5 Meadow Way FARINGDON Oxfordshire SN7 7UL w 6129324

Kay Marie (nee Wilkinson) 01/04/2003 (01/06/2009) 11 Langold Drive Norton Doncaster DN6 9GE **Tel:** (01302) 701651 w 6264288

Lisa Caroline 05/07/2006 Parrock Street Veterinary Surgery 144 Parrock Street Gravesend Kent DA12 1EY **Tel:** (01474) 352793 w 6288037

Nichola Rachael 14/09/2009 8 Farnborough Close Maidstone Kent ME16 8UE w 6465511

BROADBENT Lisa Victoria 17/01/2008 9 Albany Court Stantonbury MILTON KEYNES MK14 6DN **Tel:** (01908) 322042 w 6377610

Samantha Jayne (nee Falshaw) 11/11/1999 8 Oakleigh Close Sharlston Common Wakefield West Yorkshire WF4 1ER **Tel:** (01924) 860 149 w 6185979

BROADBRIDGE Nikki Annette 10/10/2008 12 Hartsworth Close Plaistow LONDON E13 0TD **Tel:** 02084727192 w 6423964

BROADHEAD Maree Louise 10/10/2005 Upper Stream Head Farm Black Dyke Lane Thornton Bradford West Yorkshire BD13 3RR **Tel:** (01274) 835116 w 6288565

BROADHURST Lyndsay Joanne (nee Foster) 29/08/2008 14 Granary Halt Rayne Braintree Essex CM77 6AB **Tel:** 07834976997 w 6404890

BROCKBANK Joanne (see CONNOLLY, Mrs)

BROCKS Abigail Victoria 14/01/2008 Clifton Veterinary Surgery Anstey Lane Alton Hampshire GU34 2RH **Tel:** (01420) 82163 w 6404032

BRODRICK Hayley Joanna 16/10/2007 3 Fairway NEWARK Nottinghamshire NG24 4RG **Tel:** (07825) 214267 w 6385596

BRODY Harriet Elizabeth (see BONAFIA, Mrs)

BROMELL Elizabeth Anne (see ROTHEN, Mrs)

BROMFIELD Rachel Sarah 27/04/2006 4 Helnoweth Gardens Gulual Penzance Cornwall TR18 3DT **Tel:** (01736) 350663 w 6323897

BROMLEY Caroline Mary 08/09/2009 North Farm Eaton Mascott Cross Houses SHREWSBURY SY5 6HF **Tel:** (01743) 761031 w 6490745

BROOK Sarah Louise (see TACK, Mrs)

Stacy Marie (nee Lloyd) 26/08/1999 (27/02/2003) 38 Norwood Road MARCH Cambridgeshire PE15 8QF **Tel:** (01354) 660331 w 6185825

BROOKES Jayne Louise 03/10/2007 4 Sandringham Close Whaplode SPALDING Lincolnshire PE12 6UP **Tel:** (07860) 245 390 w 6378534

BROOKES Maxine Helen (see WELLS, Mrs)

BROOKS Andrea (see PIKETT, Mrs)

BROOKS Kirsty Jessica (nee Govey) 23/01/2008 24 Pittmans Field Harlow Essex CM20 3LA **Tel:** 01279868453 w 6325756

BROOKS Laura (see HAYES, Mrs)

Lisa Anne (nee Maskell) 24/08/1995 (10/11/2009) Coastway Veterinary Group Unit 4E, Freshfield Business Park Freshfield Way Brighton East Sussex BN2 0BZ **Tel:** (01273) 692257 w 6034828

Sandra Louise 24/08/1998 Moorland Veterinary Centre St. Lukes House Vicarage Road Leek Staffordshire ST13 6AS w 6112467

Tracy 08/09/1998 (31/01/2006) 2 The Cottages Long Common East Ruston NORWICH NR12 9LA w 6132483

BROOKS Vanessa Joy (see BROOKS - OKE, Mrs)

BROOKS - OKE Vanessa Joy (nee Brooks) 20/01/1998 9 Load Lane Westonzoyland Bridgewater Somerset TA7 0LW **Tel:** (01278) 691041 w 6113573

BROOMER Melanie Anne 30/05/2007 Ash Spinney Bayford Lane Bayford Hertford Hertfordshire SG13 8PR **Tel:** (01992) 511359 w 6383770

BROOMFIELD Catherine Louise (nee Bowker) 19/01/1996 41 Ellwood Road Stockport Cheshire SK1 4BE **Tel:** (0161) 355 0514 w 6041937

BROPHY Sarah Margaret 16/02/2009 61 The Pastures Hatfield Hertfordshire AL10 8PF **Tel:** 01707881469 w 6408927

BROUGH Kay 23/08/1991 (03/04/2002) PDSA PAH Tuxford Close Wolverhampton WV10 0JQ **Tel:** (01902) 459555 w 6075423

BROUGHTON Emma Louise (see BROUGHTON-BEGLEY, Mrs)

BROUGHTON Melanie Jane 27/10/2008 25 London Road King's Lynn Norfolk PE30 5QA **Tel:** (01553) 773168 w 6434293

BROUGHTON-BEGLEY Emma Louise (nee Broughton) 07/02/2006 The Westover Veterinary Centre 40 Yarmouth Road North Walsham Norfolk NR28 9AT **Tel:** (01692) 403202 w 6279556

BROWELL Sharon Michelle 08/01/2008 45 Willowbank Avenue Blackpool Lancashire FY4 3NE **Tel:** (01253) 315526 w 6411006

BROWES Jemma Louise (see BICKLE, Mrs)

BROWN Alexandra (nee Brown, formerly Bishop) 30/01/2001 38 Streamside Mangotsfield Bristol BS16 9EA **Tel:** (0117) 908 9509 w 6204745

BROWN Alexandra Elizabeth (see CLIFTON, Miss)

Alyson Ceri Sharon 17/01/2007 608 Veterinary Group 608 Warwick Road Solihull West Midlands B91 1AA **Tel:** (0121) 705 3044 w 6382285

Anna Elizabeth 21/07/2008 11 High Street Ridgmont Bedford Bedfordshire MK43 0TS **Tel:** (01525) 28863 w 6417606

Audrey Ashton 07/09/1994 (31/03/2006) Ayrton Veterinary Centre Burnhouse Industrial Estate Whitburn West Lothian EH47 0LQ **Tel:** (01501) 744736 w 6032547

Carol (nee England) 17/08/1995 (29/01/2002) 1 School View Polmont FALKIRK FK2 0JW **Tel:** (01324) 718768 w 6043810

Carol Ann 05/08/1980 (14/09/1999) 87 Dugdale Hill Lane Potters Bar Hertfordshire EN6 2DR **Tel:** (01707) 654790 w 6046480

Celia Louise (formerly Rusden) 26/07/1988 (26/01/2004) Bosmarric Old Portreath Road REDRUTH Cornwall TR15 3TQ w 6060075

Claire (nee Buckley) 16/10/1999 79 Mill Lane Wednesfield WOLVERHAMPTON WV11 1DQ **Tel:** (01902) 561378 w 6186265

Elizabeth (nee Chalmers) 28/02/2005 7 Brook Meadow Wirral Merseyside CH61 4YS **Tel:** (0151) 6485619 w 6328913

Elizabeth Jane 04/10/2001 The Veterinary Surgery Inns Park Valley Truckle Camelford

Cornwall PL32 9RX **Tel:** (01840) 212229 w 6229462

Elizabeth Mary 15/07/2005 Camlas Veterinary Practice Waterloo Place Salop Road Welshpool Powys SY21 7HE **Tel:** (01938) 553124 w 6293581

Fiona Jill 02/07/2009 32 Old Auchans View Dundonald Kilmarnock Ayrshire KA2 9EX **Tel:** (01563) 850875 w 6440310

Gillian (nee Brown) 16/01/1996 Kingdom Veterinary Clinic North Street Glenrothes Fife KY7 5NA **Tel:** (01592) 753231 w 6034442

Jennifer Ann 20/02/2009 7 Blandford Road Whitley READING Berkshire RG2 8RA **Tel:** 07815566197 w 6440926

Julianne 07/08/2008 Anrich Veterinary Hospital Caroline Street Wigan Lancashire WN3 4EL **Tel:** (0871) 223 2040 w 6520566

Julie Ann 29/01/2007 17 Tyrells Way Great Baddow Chelmsford Essex CM2 7DP **Tel:** (01245) 474 932 w 6348350

BROWN Kate Samantha (see KING, Mrs)

BROWN Katherine (see BICHARD, Mrs)

Katie Elizabeth 01/02/2010 96 Pound Street Bitterne Village SOUTHAMPTON SO18 6BP **Tel:** (02380) 436953 w 6232586

BROWN Kelly Dawn (see NASTALY, Mrs)

Kelly Louise 21/03/2007 18 Charles Close Gedling NOTTINGHAM NG4 4EH **Tel:** (01158) 400991 w 6344973

Kirsten Fiona 07/12/2007 137 The Oval Clarkston Glasgow Lanarkshire G76 8LX **Tel:** (0141) 633 1259 w 6377621

BROWN Laura Marilyn (see CUNDY, Mrs)

BROWN Lisa Jane (see WILSON, Mrs)

Louise Helen 25/01/1999 (25/01/1999) Cornerstone Veterinary Centre Northwood Park Road Bushbury Wolverhampton WV10 8ET **Tel:** (01902) 397227 w 6108199

BROWN Michelle (see WALKER, Mrs)

BROWN Nicola Gail (see WARING, Mrs)

Nicola Kate (nee Alsop) 17/01/2000 9 Calvados Park Kingsteignton Newton Abbot Devon TQ12 3EE **Tel:** (01626) 351669 w 6191171

Patricia Ann (formerly Willey) 11/05/1972 (01/11/2007) 26 Farthingstone Road Litchborough TOWCESTER Northamptonshire NN12 8JE **Tel:** (01327) 831175 w 6063859

Rosemary Anne 20/07/1993 11 Warren Road Prestatyn Clwyd LL19 7HP **Tel:** (01745) 855877 w 6014991

Samantha 27/08/1999 38 Randalls Drive Hutton BRENTWOOD Essex CM13 1NN **Tel:** (01277) 219179 w 615282X

Samantha Claire (nee Farr) 28/07/1992 Cobweb Barn Eastfield Road Blackford Wedmore Somerset BS28 4NH **Tel:** (01934) 712 820 w 6050114

Serena Joyce 07/02/2007 Capontree Veterinary Centre Greenhill Brampton Cumbria CA8 1SU **Tel:** (01697) 72318 w 6379469

Sharon Jayne (nee Swann) 21/11/1991 11 Balfour Street ST. HELENS Merseyside WA10 4BQ w 6068802

Shona Lindsay 24/02/2009 Morvich House Golf Course Road BLAIRGOWRIE Perthshire PH10 6LJ w 6443830

Sian Julie (nee Nicholas) 30/04/1990 10 Royal Terrace SOUTHEND-ON-SEA SS1 1DY **Tel:** (01702) 348062 w 6057663

Stuart Craig 21/07/2009 353 Haselbury Road Edmonton London N9 9AL **Tel:** 07957488519 m 6325668

Vicky 06/05/2008 39 Carnival Close Ilminster Somerset TA19 9DG **Tel:** (01460) 259 081 w 6488963

BROWN Zoe Clare (see LATTER, Mrs)

Zoe Jane 05/09/2008 49 Portland Road Hove East Sussex BN3 5DQ **Tel:** (01273) 720755 w 6402822

BROWN Zoie Marie (see YESIL, Mrs)

BROWNING Hilary Jane 18/10/2005 1-3 Leopold Road Wimbledon London SW19 7BB **Tel:** (020) 8946 9925 w 6409752

Jacqueline (nee Trevethan) 30/10/2003 Clee Veterinary Centre 441-445 Cleethorpe Road Grimsby N.E. Lincs DN31 3BY **Tel:** (01472) 357430 w 6291854

BROWNINGS Penny Samantha (nee Bartlett) 20/03/1996 (24/04/2002) Cliffe Veterinary Group 21 Cliffe High Street Lewes East Sussex BN7 2AH **Tel:** (01273) 473232 w 6037217

BROWNLOW Laura Louise (nee May) 27/02/2006 Park View Veterinary Group 122 Park View Road Welling Kent DA16 1SJ **Tel:** (020) 8303 2864 w 6316439

BRUCE Alexis (see HORNER, Mrs)

Amie Jane 29/04/2009 Morven View Lumphanan BANCHORY Kincardineshire AB31 4QB **Tel:** 01339883262 w 6407937

Jane Louise Sarah Anderson 29/01/1999 (08/10/2003) 5 Altour Gardens SPEAN BRIDGE Inverness-Shire PH34 4HA w 6137233

Laura Jane 15/12/2004 42 Blair Drive Dunfermline Fife KY12 0JZ **Tel:** (01383) 737993 w 6291469

Sarah Louise 21/01/1997 64 Caernarvon Road Eynesbury ST. NEOTS Cambridgeshire PE19 2RN **Tel:** (01480) 403298 w 6097527

BRUDENELL Gemma 26/07/2002 52 Ford Street Kettering Northamptonshire NN16 0SG **Tel:** (01536) 520593 w 6267456

Natalie Anne DipAVN(Medical) 31/03/2003 15 Augustine Road Minster RAMSGATE Kent CT12 4DG **Tel:** (079) 680 234 37 w 6278126

BRUNWIN Nicola Anne 30/10/2009 Underlea House Church Lane Epwell BANBURY Oxfordshire OX15 6LD **Tel:** (01295) 780318 w 6465269

BRUNYEE Donna Michelle 13/04/2004 82 St. Marys Road Bodmin Cornwall PL31 1NN **Tel:** (01208) 76728 w 6291777

BRUTON Loren 10/11/2009 Polson 12 Woodvale Terrace LAUNCESTON Cornwall PL15 9BN **Tel:** 07976245185 w 6492560

BRYAN Allison Jayne (see JONES, Mrs)

BRYAN Emma Jane 30/10/2007 32 Paulls Close Martock Somerset TA12 6DE w 6387169

Stephanie Wheeldon 26/01/1994 (06/01/2005) 1 Mortimer Close Woolavington BRIDGWATER Somerset TA7 8EH w 606669X

BRYANT Claire Frances (see LOWERISON, Mrs)

BRYANT Gemma 16/06/2004 Gemini White Lane Ash Green Surrey GU12 6HN **Tel:** (01252) 325117 w 6291095

BRYANT Laura Jayne Parry (see INGRAM, Mrs)

Ruth Mary 30/04/2009 April Rise Crosshill Brandesburton Driffield North Humberside YO25 8RB **Tel:** 01964542325 w 6429057

BRYCE Alexa Kirsty 24/11/2008 Hyndhope Hill Cottage Ettrick Valley Selkirk Selkirkshire TD7 5HW **Tel:** (01750) 52213 w 6412403

Jacqueline Sandra 28/08/1980 Ford Farm Dunsford Exeter Devon EX6 7AZ **Tel:** (01392) 811254 w 6088705

BRYCELAND Lesley Anne 05/10/2001 Smithy House East Kilbride Road Rutherglen Glasgow G73 5QU **Tel:** (0141) 634 3183 w 6229605

BRYNING Kirstie 25/02/2003 Tay Veterinary Centre 260 Clepington Road Dundee DD3 8DY **Tel:** (01382) 884411 w 6281118

BRZENCZEK Paula Lisa (nee Wake) 22/12/2004 1 Oakdale Place Pontnewynydd Pontypool Gwent NP4 6PR w 6274309

BUCHAN Elaine Margaret 11/09/2003 4 Kinaldie Cottage Kinellar Aberdeen AB21 0TA **Tel:** (01224) 790945 w 6272626

BUCHANAN Donna Michelle 11/02/2009 67 Laurel Drive East Kilbride Glasgow Lanarkshire G75 9JG **Tel:** 01355520662 w 6436867

Rosemary 04/08/1988 (18/07/2001) Shore Veterinary Centre Ltd 116 Shore Street Gourock Renfrewshire PA19 1QZ **Tel:** (01475) 637312 w 6046651

BUCHELE Kayleigh Jane 15/02/2008 Clarendon House Veterinary Group Ltd Bexfields Farm Galleywood Road Chelmsford Essex CM2 8BY **Tel:** (01245) 353741 w 6383132

BUCKERIDGE Claire Paula 20/09/2005 21 Carrol Grove CHELTENHAM Gloucestershire GL51 0PP **Tel:** (01242) 518388 w 6320839

BUCKINGHAM Sandra Ann 16/06/2004 1 Miles Close Wolverton Rd Blakefields Milton Keynes MK14 5AD **Tel:** 01908-614281 w 6269557

Sian Kadi 06/05/2009 10 Southfield Close Hillingdon Middlesex UB8 3JJ **Tel:** (07979) 624 213 w 6296111

BUCKLAND Laura Caroline (see BABB, Mrs)

BUCKLER Katie Lauren 15/01/2008 104 Coburg Road Dorchester Dorset DT1 2HR **Tel:** (01305) 268 856 w 6402514

BUCKLEY Claire (see BROWN, Mrs)

BUCKLEY Jennifer Claire 17/07/2008 24 Fir Grove Whitehill Bordon Hampshire GU35 9ED **Tel:** (01420) 478077 w 6418189

Louise Anne 31/01/2002 211 Gilmerton Road EDINBURGH EH16 5UD w 6263111

BUCKLEY-REEVES Rebecca Grace 09/11/2005 10 Shortlands Lane Pelsall Walsall West Midlands WS3 4AG w 6246578

BUDD Catherine 26/10/2006 69 Hillsboro Road Bognor Regis West Sussex PO21 2DY **Tel:** (01243) 822 462 w 6368667

Gemma Rachel 10/03/2008 The Veterinary Hospital 118 Victoria Drive Bognor Regis West Sussex PO21 2EJ **Tel:** (01243) 841111 w 6418178

BUGG Alice Caroline (nee Sheriff, nee Bowers) 23/08/1995 103 Carter Street Fordham Ely Cambridgeshire CB7 5JU **Tel:** (01638) 721954 w 6030641

Naomi Dawn 17/07/2008 92 Vicarage Crescent REDDITCH Worcestershire B97 4RR **Tel:** (01527) 451293 w 6349967

BUGLER Karen Michelle 10/10/2000 Badgers Green Waterloo Road Corfe Mullen Wimborne Dorset BH21 3SN **Tel:** (01202) 695960 w 6202490

BULL Heather Susan 15/11/2001 150 Kingston Road Epsom Surrey KT17 2ET **Tel:** (020) 8393 6049 w 6267357

Samantha Jayne 19/01/1998 Hollyoaks Forest Road Nomansland SALISBURY SP5 2BW w 6110889

Shirley Florence Adams 26/01/1989 (11/10/2000) The Surgery Derwent Drive Hayes Middlesex UB4 8DU **Tel:** (020) 8573 0070 w 6046709

Stefanie Ellen 17/07/2008 2 Coldharbour bungalows Plummer Lane TENTERDEN Kent TN30 6TU **Tel:** (07825) 665 493 w 6350319

BULLEN Emma Clare (nee Freeman) 03/08/2001 19 Frant Court Frant TUNBRIDGE WELLS Kent TN3 9DW **Tel:** (01892) 750441 w 6202908

BULLING Catherine 16/01/2009 Orchard View 2 Mill Street CREDITON Devon EX17 3AA **Tel:** 07852472513 w 6535801

BULLOCK Lucy Jane (see DANIELS, Mrs)

BULLOCK Michelle Joanne Merrishaw 21/07/2008 23 Penman Close St. Albans Hertfordshire AL2 3DJ **Tel:** (01727) 810061 w 6375927

Stacey (nee Eltringham) 14/09/2004 Hadrian Veterinary Group Dene Avenue Hexham Northumberland NE46 1HJ **Tel:** (01434) 602703 w 6282768

BULMER-THOMPSON Dreana (formerly Bradford-Cremer, nee Baits) 18/01/1999 (06/01/2010) 68 Northumbrian Way North Shields Tyne and Wear NE29 6XQ **Tel:** (077986) 697261 w 6129663

BULPITT Emma Jayne 15/09/2008 Beech House Veterinary Centre 64 West End Road SOUTHAMPTON SO18 6TG w 6401161

BUNDY Leanne 27/01/2009 30 Pembroke Close Tonteg Pontypridd Mid Glamorgan CF38 1HD **Tel:** 07814461048 w 6439650

BUNGAY Denise Margaret (see PRISK, Mrs)

BUNN Deborah Jane 11/03/2008 St Kitts House High Street Hartley Wintney HOOK Hampshire RG27 8NS **Tel:** (01252) 844044 w 6415527

Katherine Rose 05/01/2005 Uplands Way Vets Ltd Uplands Way DISS Norfolk IP22 4DF **Tel:** (01379) 642865 w 6326625

BUNSTON Lisa Michelle (nee Westlake) 14/12/2006 39 Garland Close EXETER Devon EX4 2NT w 6339264

BUNTING Annabel 13/07/2007 Buntings Nest Kelvedon Road Inworth Colchester Essex CO5 9SN **Tel:** (01376) 571059 w 6349362

Carol 10/10/1990 (27/01/2003) Sileby Hall Cossington Road Sileby Loughborough Leicestershire LE12 7RS **Tel:** (01509) 812445/6 w 6046742

Rosemary Clare 15/11/2005 22 Elmwood Avenue COLCHESTER CO2 9HT w 6342014

BURBIDGE Cecily Ann 07/01/2008 995 8th Conc Road W Puslinch Ontario RR #3 NOB 2JO Canada **Tel:** (Canada) 9056599339 w 6534085

Chloe Louise 01/08/2008 25 Cambridge Road ROCHESTER Kent ME2 3HW **Tel:** 01634718205 w 6401040

Katie Jane 08/06/2006 164 Nuncargate Road Kirkby-in-Ashfield NOTTINGHAM NG17 9EF **Tel:** (01623) 404712 w 6333291

Rachel Karen 20/08/1990 187 High Street STREET Somerset BA16 0NE **Tel:** (01458) 442398 w 6046764

BURCH Stephanie Anne 08/10/2008 104 The Chantrys FARNHAM Surrey GU9 7AN **Tel:** 07748648852 w 6342025

BURCHILL Alison Mariecia (see MCCRICKARD, Mrs)

BURDELL Carley Ellen 16/10/2007 40 Leybourne Avenue Bournemouth Dorset BH10 6HF **Tel:** 07870913026 w 6383858

BURDEN Gemma Louise 27/04/2006 39 Warland Way Corfe Mullen WIMBORNE Dorset BH21 3TH **Tel:** (01202) 699 048 w 6328132

Susan 30/01/1997 (20/11/2001) 7 Spinner Green Easthampstead Bracknell Berkshire RG12 7ED **Tel:** (01344) 489912 w 6039994

BURDETT Claire Jane 21/03/2007 Astonlee Veterinary Surgery Tickford Street Newport Pagnell Buckinghamshire MK16 9BA **Tel:** (01908) 611637 w 6370922

BURDGE Eleanor Margaret (nee Pointon) 15/01/2008 Beaconsfield Farm Harptree Hill West Harptree BRISTOL BS40 6EH w 6389809

BURDOCK Nicole Frances 31/12/2003 Alder House 3 Red House Paddock Tallington Lincolnshire PE9 4RG w 6290644

BURFOOT Rebecca Catherine 20/11/2009 70 Hatch Road Stratton St. Margaret SWINDON SN3 4XY **Tel:** 07852988630 w 6463905

BURGE Felicity Rose 07/08/2001 34 New Dover Road Canterbury Kent CT1 3DT **Tel:** (01227) 765522 w 6113529

BURGESS Christina Valerie 05/10/2009 Curdlands Farmhouse Harthill Road Burwardsley CHESTER CH3 9NU **Tel:** (07905) 927 112 w 6465610

Claire Louise 12/01/2009 24 Station Road Meopham GRAVESEND Kent DA13 0LX **Tel:** (01474) 813122 w 6409510

Claire Louise Frances 24/09/2008 The Veterinary Hospital 118 Victoria Drive Bognor Regis West Sussex PO21 2EJ **Tel:** (01243) 841111 w 6421797

Nancy Joanne 16/12/2005 8 Streamcross Claverham BRISTOL BS49 4LL w 6307474

BURKE Caroline Louise 16/06/2008 61 Woodhouse Lane SALE Cheshire M33 4JZ **Tel:** (0161) 962 2411 w 6380701

Claire Louise 19/01/2005 Bishopton Veterinary Group Bridgehousegate Pateley Bridge HARROGATE North Yorkshire HG3 5HH **Tel:** (01765) 602396 w 6304746

Julia Ann DipAVN(Surgical), DipAVN(Medical) (nee Grout) 29/07/1993 Davies Veterinary Specialists Manor Farm Business Park Higham Gobion Hertfordshire SG5 3HR **Tel:** (01582) 883950 w 6066598

Laura Anne 19/09/2006 58 Ballylucas Road Downpatrick County Down BT30 8SZ **Tel:** (028) 4485 1618 w 6353740

Linda Carol (nee Baxendale) 21/06/2005 (07/08/2007) Park Veterinary Clinic 51 Bury Old Road Prestwich MANCHESTER M25 0FG **Tel:** (0161) 773 1819 w 6290930

BURKE Samantha Jane (see MCMILLAN, Mrs)

BURKE Shirley (see SIMPSON, Mrs)

BURLEIGH Stacy Jane (nee Bowron) 11/01/1993 (29/04/2002) 38 Uppertown Wolsingham BISHOP AUCKLAND County Durham DL13 3ET **Tel:** (01388) 527895 w 6065222

BURLEY Louise Michelle 04/04/2006 61 Doe Royd Lane Sheffield South Yorkshire S5 8GJ **Tel:** (077) 636 57463 w 6334699

BURLINGHAM Faye 07/02/2006 9 Hydean Way STEVENAGE Hertfordshire SG2 9XH **Tel:** (01438) 369390 w 6354543

BURLS Alice Mara 11/11/2004 (09/09/2008) 37 Springfields Padbury Buckingham Buckinghamshire MK18 2AT **Tel:** (01280) 813766 w 6321730

BURN Caroline (nee Pennock) 06/10/1998 Lowna Hambleton Lane Wass Yorkshire YO61 4BH **Tel:** (01347) 868 334 w 6136750

Virginia 11/11/2009 2 Acorn Square Prudhoe Northumberland NE42 5HD **Tel:** 07742134000 w 6439760

BURNETT Beverley-Anne (nee Haines) 02/10/2001 The John Muir Clinic 103 Redcar Road Marske By Sea Cleveland TS11 6HU **Tel:** (01642) 488777 w 6229242

Janet DipAVN(Surgical) 17/09/1981 Bramley Cottage The Common Winterslow Salisbury SP5 1PJ **Tel:** (01980) 863404 w 6046855

BURNEY Nicola Helen (nee Garbutt) 31/03/2003 (24/11/2008) 7 Bennett Street KIDDERMINSTER Worcestershire DY11 6XU **Tel:** (01562) 510146 w 6267533

BURNS Debbie Ann (see MACDONALD, Mrs)

BURNS Emma Louise 16/06/2004 Oundle Veterinary Surgery 92 South Road Oundle Peterborough PE8 4BP **Tel:** (01832) 273521 w 6289236

Sarah Elizabeth 17/10/2007 Summerhill Veterinary Centre 43 Summerhill Avenue Newport Gwent NP19 8FQ **Tel:** (01633) 255394 w 6351177

BURR Emma-Jane Trixie 11/11/2004 32 Strattondale Street Isle of Dogs London E14 3HG **Tel:** (0207) 987 0825 w 6321928

BURRIDGE Nicola Lynn 10/08/1992 White House Veterinary Clinic 1 Linclare Place St. Neots Huntingdon Cambridgeshire PE19 7AH **Tel:** (01480) 216612 w 600873X

BURRILL Rachel Anne (nee Trickett) 21/01/1999 33 Morshead Crescent Fareham Hampshire PO16 7QR **Tel:** (01329) 663881 w 6129630

BURROUGHS Selena Jane (nee Smith, formerly Bird) 15/08/1990 10 Monmouth Way HONITON Devon EX14 2GY **Tel:** (01404) 41722 w 6010363

BURROW Marie Louise (see COLEMAN, Mrs)

BURROWS Gwladys Sian 29/06/2007 Gable End Parc Mawr Farm Senghenydd Caerphilly Mid Glamorgan CF83 4HH **Tel:** (02920) 832316 w 6380283

Lucy Anne 28/02/2007 21 Rock Park BIRKENHEAD Merseyside CH42 1PJ **Tel:** (01516) 453522 w 6342850

BURT Cherie (see BAILEY, Mrs)

BURT Claire Elizabeth 24/02/2000 Chestnut Veterinary Group 1 Hoe Lane Ware Hertfordshire SG12 9LS **Tel:** (01920) 468874 w 6137142

Hannah Jane 08/04/2008 The Firs Bradford on Tone Taunton Somerset TA4 1EX **Tel:** (01823) 461 769 w 6405704

Morwenna 03/05/2007 Ironmine Cottage Grampound Road TRURO Cornwall TR2 4EW **Tel:** (01726) 883524 w 6358338

Rachel 02/03/2009 55 Yeldham Road LONDON W6 8JF **Tel:** 07923358661 w 6540047

Sarah Deana 04/06/2009 31 Arnhem Avenue Aveley South Ockendon Essex RM15 4AT **Tel:** 01708867668 w 6410874

BURTENSHAW Laura Jane 22/02/2007 Flitterbanks Granary The Drive Maresfield Park Maresfield UCKFIELD East Sussex TN22 3ER w 6372341

BURTON Carolyn Lesley 10/09/2009 Chestnut Veterinary Group 1 Hoe Lane Ware Hertfordshire SG12 9LS **Tel:** (01920) 468874 w 6408938

Faye Louise 21/01/1997 102 Golden Vale Churchdown GLOUCESTER GL3 2LX **Tel:** (01452) 555864 w 6039768

BURTON Joanne Elizabeth (see WYNN, Mrs)

Leanne 03/10/2008 Kerswill House Cornwood Ivybridge Devon PL21 9HT **Tel:** (01752) 892390 w 6394352

Leeann 06/06/2003 (15/05/2007) 16 Manse Place Inverkeithing Fife KY11 1AZ **Tel:** (01383) 722818 w 6287531

BURTON Lisa Anne (see EDEN, Mrs)

Pamela Bernice 05/08/1970 4698 Wallaby Drive Victoria British Columbia V9C 4C6 Canada **Tel:** (250) 478 5805 w 6046924

BURTON Rachel (see BAUGH, Mrs)

Sadie May 30/10/2003 Natson Tedburn St Mary Exeter Devon EX6 6ET **Tel:** (01647) 24031 w 6273462

Samantha 14/03/2008 16 Camellia Close Chelmsford Essex CM1 6QZ **Tel:** (01245) 601199 w 6343037

Sarah Helen 22/03/2004 3 Gorringe Close Lower Willingdon Eastbourne East Sussex BN20 9SU w 6295264

Victoria Marian 06/08/2008 80 Elstree Road Hemel Hempstead Hertfordshire HP2 7QP **Tel:** (01442) 216048 w 6378402

BURVILLE Nicola 13/01/2004 290a Queens town Rd Battersea London SW8 4LT **Tel:** (07949) 344745 w 6282471

BUSCOMBE Sarah Lesley (nee Tooley) 26/05/1988 (12/06/2000) Penmellyn Veterinary Group Station Road St. Columb Major Cornwall TR9 6BX **Tel:** (01637) 880307 w 6013499

BUSE Leigh-Anne 28/04/2008 4 Garden Terrace Cullompton Devon EX15 1BN **Tel:** (01884) 34002 w 6366269

BUSH Amy 28/04/2009 132 Footshill Road Bristol Avon BS15 8HE **Tel:** 01179491223 w 6426747

BUSHNELL Victoria Kate 16/10/1998 (25/11/2005) Studley Road Veterinary Surgery 34 Studley Road Luton Bedfordshire LU3 1BB **Tel:** (01582) 723521 w 6121868

BUSSON Amy Elizabeth 04/06/2009 50 Hughes Street SWINDON SN2 2HG **Tel:** (07852) 241162 w 6415307

BUST Katherine Jane (see BEVANS, Mrs)

BUSVINE Gemma Claire 23/03/2007 (09/04/2009) 28 The Maltings Wootton Bassett SWINDON Wiltshire SN4 7EZ w 6370504

BUTCHER Arlene Elizabeth 26/08/2008 17 Elm Drive Cumbernauld GLASGOW G67 3LL **Tel:** (01236) 738734 w 6377412

Clare Louise (nee Cound) 11/03/2005 Bredy Veterinary Centre Sea Road North Bridport Dorset DT6 4RR **Tel:** (01308) 456 771 w 6325701

Deborah Frances 17/07/2008 61 Grange Road Biddulph STOKE-ON-TRENT ST8 7RY **Tel:** 07791500360 w 6381966

BUTCHER Helen Louise (see MOLYNEUX, Mrs)

Kathryn Ann 13/07/2007 38 Clifton Road Ashingdon ROCHFORD Essex SS4 **Tel:** (01702) 540 124 w 6349373

BUTLER Carrie Ann (nee Gilliatt) 31/10/2003 1 Mill Green Road Pinchbeck Spalding Lincolnshire PE11 3PU **Tel:** (01775) 724973 w 6274111

Christopher James 21/11/2005 11 Hillside Terrace Tonypandy Mid Glamorgan CF40 2HJ **Tel:** (01443) 432726 m 6256907

Helen Claire 21/06/2005 Studfall Stone Street Lympne HYTHE Kent CT21 4JP **Tel:** (01303) 266 637 w 6319112

Jane Louise 05/02/1986 7 Cornford Close Portslade Brighton East Sussex BN41 2JE w 604700X

Julia Suzanne (nee Turner) 30/10/2003 Eastfield Veterinary Clinic Ltd Station Road North Thoresby GRIMSBY Lincolnshire DN36 5QU **Tel:** (01472) 840209 w 6287168

Kim Louise 30/10/1998 Walker & Wikeley Veterinary Surgeons Church Street Oakengates Telford Shropshire TF2 6AH **Tel:** (0845) 3004065 w 6137594

Michelle Nathalie Caroline 19/05/2008 6 Lawn Road Tonbridge Kent TN9 2SU **Tel:** (01732) 366164 w 6337768

Sarah Anne 30/10/2003 12 Roy Avenue Beeston Rylands Nottingham NG9 1QG **Tel:** (0115) 925 1197 w 6296485

Sarah Louise 19/07/2006 38 Gascoigne Gardens Woodford Green Essex IG8 9NU **Tel:** (07971) 235484 w 6292470

Sharon Ann 07/11/1975 19 Church Street Southport Merseyside PR9 0QT **Tel:** (01704) 535233 w 6047010

BUTLIN Laura Jane 18/10/2005 155 High Lane East West Hallam Ilkeston Derbyshire DE7 6HY w 6334182

BUTT Katherine Emma 12/11/2009 The Vale Veterinary Centre Station Road Tiverton Devon EX16 4LF **Tel:** (01884) 253355 w 6415296

Katy 06/08/2008 Flat E 10 Parklands Surbiton Surrey KT5 8EA **Tel:** (020) 82410322 w 6385211

Lorna Jean 01/05/2008 Upper Flat Ingram & Partners 1 Barrow Green Road Oxted Surrey RH8 0RA **Tel:** (01883) 723738 w 6394330

BUTTERS Josephine Ann 13/06/2008 80 Cambridge Road STANSTED Essex CM24 8DA **Tel:** 07506672029 w 6408949

Stephanie 25/02/2004 (17/11/2009) 6 Redvers Road BRIGHTON East Sussex BN2 4BG **Tel:** (01273) 380103 w 6292987

BUTTLE Jacqueline Ann 01/10/1982 Mandeville Veterinary Services (Goddard) 131 Carlton Avenue East Wembley Middlesex HA9 8PN **Tel:** (020) 8904 9890 w 6047054

BUXTON Helga Marie 05/07/2006 6 Parkland View Yeadon LEEDS LS19 7DZ w 6344093

BUZZEO Donna Louise 16/07/2008 22 Uplands Road SUDBURY Suffolk CO10 1NX **Tel:** (07791) 305 234 w 6274804

BYE Miranda Marie 24/05/2006 23 Pyms Close Great Barford Bedford Bedfordshire MK44 3HY **Tel:** (01234) 871 157 w 6339000

BYERS Helen Patricia (see GOULD, Mrs)

BYERS Lucy Hannah 20/11/2002 Orchard Veterinary Centre 105 Perry Road Sherwood Nottingham NG5 3AD **Tel:** (0115) 969 3565 w 6279930

BYFIELD Susan Emma 06/05/2009 101 Pool Farm Road Acocks Green BIRMINGHAM B27 7HA w 6388907

BYFORD Lynn Dorothy (nee Thornycroft) 24/09/2002 20 Dunellan Rd Milngavie Nr Glasgow G62 7RE **Tel:** (0141) 956 4258 w 6269788

BYRCH Lucie Ann 31/10/2006 39 Primrose Way Horsford Norwich NR10 3SA **Tel:** (01603) 893 199 w 6380294

BYRNE Charlotte Louise (nee Flett) 08/04/2005 1 Old Oak Close Bolton Lancashire BL2 6SF **Tel:** (01204) 577215 w 6287201

Fionnuala Ann 06/03/2009 15 New Street NEWRY County Down BT35 6JD **Tel:** (028) 3025 2000 w 6386498

Gillian Rose 16/11/2006 Cromlyn House Veterinary Hospital 50 Old Coach Road Hillsborough County Down BT26 6PB **Tel:** (02892) 683711 w 6356358

Joanne Margaret 30/10/2001 34 Meadow Grove Dundalk Co Louth Ireland **Tel:** (00) 353 429336296 w 6205592

BYRNE Lucy Louise (see THORNTON, Mrs)

BYRNES Gemma Louise 14/01/2010 Flat 5, New Plymouth House Dunedin Road Rainham Essex RM13 8LB **Tel:** 07903037507 w 6419718

BYTHEWAY Amy Elizabeth 09/12/2009 3 Sedgley Hall Avenue Dudley West Midlands DY3 3SZ w 6437054

BYWATER Kelly Joanne 14/10/2008 10 Springvale Close Sharlston Common WAKEFIELD West Yorkshire WF4 1TG w 6351188

C

CACICEDO JAROSZYNSKA Irena 08/01/2008 Costa Brava 33 50A ESC DCHA 28034 Madrid Spain **Tel:** 0034917351019 w 6291106

CADBY Michelle Louise 03/08/2006 4 Church Terrace London NW4 4JU **Tel:** (020) 8203 2090 w 6298575

CADDICK Nicola 09/05/2005 85c Haigh Lane Haigh BARNSLEY South Yorkshire S75 4DA w 6289247

CADYWOULD Sarah Dawn 29/06/2007 32 Purcell House 2 Holbrook Close Enfield Middlesex EN1 4UQ **Tel:** (07939) 572459 w 6378204

CAFFERARA Stephanie Jane (see CAFFERATA, Mrs)

CAFFERATA Stephanie Jane (nee Cafferara) 11/04/1973 Manor Farm Cottage 83 Stoke Road Stoke D'Abernon COBHAM Surrey KT11 3PU **Tel:** (01932) 864969 w 608381X

CAIE James David 06/08/2008 4a North Cray Road BEXLEY Kent DA5 3LZ **Tel:** (01322) 336668 m 6306341

CAIN Anne Louise (nee Clarke) 31/01/2000 5 Melrose Crescent Garswood Ashton-in-Makerfield Wigan Lancashire WN4 0SL **Tel:** (01942) 744689 w 6190346

CAINE Emily 29/04/2009 10 Albion Street LEEK Staffordshire ST13 5NL **Tel:** 01538382645 w 6406364

CAIRD Averil Buchanan 21/06/2005 115 High Street Dalkeith Midlothian EH22 1AX **Tel:** (0131) 654 2266 w 6297123

CAIRNEY Karen 03/10/2007 56 Langlee Drive Galashiels Selkirkshire TD1 2EB **Tel:** (01896) 751856 w 6346909

CALCUTT Claire Jane 08/01/1986 (07/01/2002) 1 Easthaven Cottages Whitesmith Lewes East Sussex BN8 6JB **Tel:** (01825) 873094 w 6047112

CALDER Caroline 15/11/2001 33 Hadleigh Court Coxhoe DURHAM DH6 4SJ **Tel:** (0191) 3778196 w 6265586

Katy Leonora 14/12/2006 9 Petershill Gardens Bathgate West Lothian EH48 4DS **Tel:** (01506) 632863 w 6373441

Samantha Jaine (nee Adams) 15/11/2006 2 Southfield Drive Kenilworth Warwickshire CV8 2FR **Tel:** (01926) 852168 w 6352035

CALDICUTT Sarah Leanne 08/08/2005 30 Prior Street HEREFORD HR4 9LB **Tel:** (01432) 267501 w 6297134

CALDWELL Emily Jade 18/02/2009 30 Alandale Road Sompting Lancing West Sussex BN15 0JU **Tel:** 01903753374 w 6421775

CALEY Nicola Jayne 07/06/2005 18 Mallee Crescent Churchtown Southport Merseyside PR9 8NJ **Tel:** (01704) 214 359 w 6320289

CALLAGHAN Louise Rebecca 10/04/2007 23 Cullen Close Yateley Hampshire GU46 6HB **Tel:** (01252) 861 429 w 6385673

CALPEE Alicia Naila Patricia 14/11/2008 31 Irwin Crescent Wakefield West Yorkshire WF1 4RA **Tel:** (01924) 376 754 w 6434249

CALVER Cara Marie (see CALVER-PERKINS, Mrs)

Joanne Mary 15/02/2005 8 Chapel Lane Wickham Market WOODBRIDGE Suffolk IP13 0SD **Tel:** (01728) 747561 w 6319508

CALVER-PERKINS Cara Marie (nee Calver) 02/02/2001 166 Nottingham Road Eastwood Nottingham NG16 3GG **Tel:** (01773) 769298 w 6211862

CALVERT Michelle 12/11/1999 3 Hill Square Cam DURSLEY Gloucestershire GL11 5NJ w 6186375

Rebecca 04/07/2003 Seymour Cottage Veterinary Surgery Weston Road Totnes Devon TQ9 5BT **Tel:** (01803) 866283 w 6259657

CALVO Gillian C (nee Connelly) 25/02/2003 63 Waldemar Road Knightswood GLASGOW G13 3LU **Tel:** (0141) 330 5848 w 6271526

CAMBERS Lorna Ruth 28/08/2009 2 Priors Close Rushden Northamptonshire NN10 9PG **Tel:** (07730) 346483 w 6295242

CAMBRAY Hannah Louise 27/02/2007 Vale Veterinary Group 28 Birmingham Road Kidderminster Worcestershire DY10 2DA **Tel:** (01562) 822692 w 6377863

CAMERON Debbie (nee Hill) 06/02/2002 1-2 Park Street Anlaby Road Hull HU3 2JF **Tel:** (01482) 223688 w 6262462

CAMILLERI Claire Louise (nee Parmenter) 08/03/1999 Barrow Hill House Maidstone Rd Ashford Kent TN24 8TY **Tel:** (01233) 624687 w 6118436

CAMPBELL Amy 29/06/2007 36 Coniston Terrace DUNDEE DD3 0AH w 6372803

Dawn Joyce Agnes (nee Parsons) 09/02/1994 23 Meadow Brook Comber Newtownards County Down BT23 5ED **Tel:** (028) 91873483 w 6068234

Gillian Helen 22/06/2009 7 Inveraray Drive Stenhousemuir Larbert Stirlingshire FK5 4UR **Tel:** (01324) 551314 w 6407926

Hilary 31/03/2003 31 Eskdale Gardens Lowfell Gateshead Tyne and Wear NE9 6NS **Tel:** (0191) 4204672 w 6262011

CAMPBELL Joanne Louise (see WILLIAMS, Mrs)

CAMPBELL Julie Fiona (see WEBSTER, Mrs)

CAMPBELL Lisa Jane (see GUDGIN, Mrs)

Nicola Jean 28/09/2005 33 Bideford Close Farnborough Hampshire GU14 8TL **Tel:** (01252) 371995 w 6349593

Shona 21/03/2007 2 Woodville Road Woodford Bude Cornwall EX23 9JA **Tel:** (01288) 331174 w 6346447

Susan Mary DipAVN(Medical) (nee Hammer) 29/05/2003 Easter Bush Veterinary Centre University of Edinburgh Easter Bush Roslin Midlothian EH25 9RG **Tel:** (0131) 650 7650 w 6277136

Tracy Deborah (nee Marshall) 21/09/1984 16 The Maples Carterton Oxfordshire OX18 3HB **Tel:** (01993) 840880 w 6047203

Victoria Louise 07/02/2007 (09/04/2009) 1 Dakin Close Maidenbower CRAWLEY West Sussex RH10 7LJ **Tel:** (07920) 192648 w 6373276

CAMPBELL-SCARLETT Clare Fiona 14/09/2001 Broadacre Battisborough Cross Holbeton Devon PL8 1JS w 6228164

CAMPHO Victoria Louise 31/10/2005 615 Wells Road Whitchurch Bristol BS14 9BE **Tel:** (01275) 832410 w 6297464

CAMPUZANO Jacqueline Louisa Anne (nee Philips) 04/11/2008 125 Norley Road Cuddington NORTHWICH Cheshire CW8 2TB **Tel:** 07813897702 w 6370614

CANALE Suzi Anna (nee Peak) 02/09/1997 (08/05/2002) 55 Rowan Way WITHAM Essex CM8 2LJ w 6118469

CANE Jenny Christine (nee Arnold) 26/08/1998 (18/11/2005) 12 East Avenue Whetstone LEICESTER LE8 6JG **Tel:** (0116) 286 4133 w 6112536

CANNELL Rachel 30/01/2009 31 Balmoral Close Bedlington Northumberland NE22 5YD **Tel:** 07957981677 w 6445348

CANNING Emily Ann 08/07/2003 343 Earlham Road NORWICH Norfolk NR2 3RQ w 6273638

CANNINGS Sarah Elizabeth 25/02/2003 Manor Farm Veterinary Surgery Green Road Codford Warminster Wiltshire BA12 0NW **Tel:** (01985) 850752 w 6257941

CANNON Catherine Jane 28/09/2005 123 Broadclyst Gardens Thorpe Bay SOUTHEND-ON-SEA SS1 3QY w 6316736

Yvonne June 03/02/1995 (18/07/2007) 23 Plough Close Daventry Northamptonshire NN11 0NX **Tel:** (01327) 301616 w 602959X

CANTILLION Lucy 08/11/2006 Hall Farm Church Lane Roydon King's Lynn Norfolk PE32 1AR **Tel:** (01485) 600022 w 6343048

CAPELL Sarah Elizabeth 10/10/2007 Eastcott Veterinary Hospital 59 Bath Road Swindon Wiltshire SN1 4AU **Tel:** (01793) 528341 w 6401447

CAPON Lisa Nicole 01/04/2008 48 Avondown Road Durrington SALISBURY SP4 8ET w 6510248

CARBONI Joanna 03/07/2009 1 Mount View Southdown BATH BA2 1JX **Tel:** 07875567135 w 6443720

CARD Sharon Paulette 15/04/2004 8 Roberts Way Highweek Newton Abbot Devon TQ13 1SA **Tel:** (01626) 206989 w 6288268

CARDIER Shevaun Anne (nee Benston) 22/04/2002 20 Enchelmaier Street Dayboro Queensland 4521 Australia **Tel:** (00617) 3425 2702 w 6262055

CARE Emma Louise 04/02/2009 45 Meadow Walk Epsom Surrey KT17 2EF **Tel:** 02083933758 w 6429981

CAREY Charlotte 10/02/2004 C/o Royal College of Veterinary Surgeons 62-64 Horseferry Road LONDON SW1P 2AF w 6267181

Emma Louise 23/09/2002 10 Orchid Close Donnington Wood TELFORD Shropshire TF2 7RN w 6270371

CARLISLE Nicola Stacey 06/03/2006 Lite Ltd 23 Fletcher Street STOCKPORT Cheshire SK1 1DY **Tel:** (0161) 480 4801 w 6272340

CARLTON Kelly Louise Yvonne 20/09/1999 39 Lancaster Road Carnforth Lancashire LA5 9LD **Tel:** (01524) 720002 w 6184868

Stacy Louise 18/11/2009 16 Brighton Grove Leeds West Yorkshire LS13 4BP **Tel:** (0113) 2554836 w 6452751

CARLYON-SMITH Celia Betsy 04/10/1993 5 Ely Court Wroughton SWINDON SN4 9JP **Tel:** (01793) 815057 w 6064874

CARNE Hayley Victoria 26/07/2004 Queen Mother Hospital for Small Animals Hawkshead Lane North Mymms Hatfield Hertfordshire AL9 7TA **Tel:** (01707) 666366 w 6284407

CARNELL Heidi Luise 15/01/2008 179 Appleby Street Cheshunt Waltham Cross Hertfordshire EN7 6QX **Tel:** 07890914497 w 6378831

CARPENTER Gillian Mary 23/12/2003 12 Woodsford Lane Moreton DORCHESTER Dorset DT2 8AY **Tel:** (01305) 851631 w 6280667

Katie Terri 14/02/2008 2 Penhale Cottages Penhale Fraddon St. Columb Cornwall TR9 6NA **Tel:** (07894) 438 943 w 6327373

Samantha Anne 05/09/2008 11 Bishops Walk Donnington Wood TELFORD Shropshire TF2 7HP **Tel:** 01952603697 w 6356248

CARR Crystal Francesca Edith Coles 09/07/2008 3 Wood End Farm Cottages Redbourn Road Hemel Hempstead Hertfordshire HP2 7HP **Tel:** (07725) 750687 w 6396046

Geraldine Martina 21/08/2009 Cartoor Moycullen County Galway Ireland **Tel:** (091) 579009 w 6564324

Kerry 02/11/2004 58 Ashley Close Ashdown Manor Killingworth Newcastle upon Tyne NE12 6GD w 6277103

CARRINGTON Andrea (see PIKETT, Mrs)

CARRINGTON Elizabeth Ann 22/10/2003 Medway City Veterinary Centre George Summers Close Strood Rochester Kent ME2 4FF **Tel:** (01634) 718078 w 6230760

CARROLL Judith 11/05/2004 44 Kinnegoe Road Loughgall ARMAGH BT61 8LR w 6304009

Michelle Ann 05/06/2008 96 Wandle Road MORDEN Surrey SM4 6AE **Tel:** (0208) 715 1971 w 6405451

Nicola Linda 10/09/2009 22 Colebrook Gardens Loughton Essex IG10 2HS w 6446888

Terence James 10/04/2003 9 Devizes Avenue BEDFORD MK41 8QT **Tel:** (01582) 652935 m 6281690

CARTER Claire Elizabeth 02/09/2008 55 St. Marks Avenue Northfleet GRAVESEND Kent DA11 9LN w 6424052

Clare-Marie 05/09/2008 35 Essex Way Purdis Farm IPSWICH IP3 8SN w 6437714

CARTER Helen Rosemary (see FIELD, Mrs)

Nichola Suzanne Shirley 29/08/2000 11 Seafield Avenue Scarborough North Yorkshire YO11 3QF **Tel:** (01723) 582621 w 6202589

Sarah Ann 10/09/1998 Stone Lion Veterinary Centre 41 High Street Wimbledon London SW19 5AU **Tel:** (020) 8946 4228 w 6128422

Sarah Anne 07/02/2005 18 Derwent Rd Bicester Oxfordshire OX26 2JA **Tel:** (01869) 600649 w 6285782

Sharon Patricia (nee Woodcock) 24/08/1999 (15/10/2001) Melbourne House Veterinary Centre 60 Hednesford Street Cannock Staffordshire WS11 1DJ **Tel:** (01543) 502197 w 6135451

CARTER Wendy Elsie Irene (see ADAMS, Mrs)

CARTER-WALLER Emma (nee Holmes) 13/04/2004 Spring Head Farm Cottage Windmill Lane Cumberworth Huddersfield HD8 8YE **Tel:** (01484) 540475 w 6279831

CARTLIDGE Tracey Anne 14/10/2002 Rushcliffe Veterinary Centre Collington Way West Bridgford Nottinghamshire NG2 7LR **Tel:** (0115) 982 1717 w 6281305

CARTMEL Laura Jane (see WHITE, Mrs)

CARTMILL Laura Christina 15/10/2004 Cedar Grove Veterinary Clinic 132 Upper Knockbreda Road Belfast BT6 9QB **Tel:** (028) 9070 5777 w 6290336

CARTON Katharine Alexandra 26/10/2006 106 Church Lane Crewe Cheshire CW2 8ER **Tel:** (01270) 569 372 w 6374475

CARTWRIGHT Ann-Marie 01/09/1999 (12/03/2008) 20 Brookside Belper Derbyshire DE56 1UR **Tel:** (01773) 823787 w 6129062

Bonnie Marie (nee Mein) 15/10/2004 25 Sutherland Way STAMFORD Lincolnshire PE9 2TB **Tel:** (07963) 971168 w 6378413

Catherine Mary 24/10/1992 (18/05/2005) 10 Stansfield Close Leigh Lancashire WN7 3DU **Tel:** (01942) 674408 w 6012178

Jennifer Clare (nee Cartwright, formerly Lomas) 18/01/2002 6 Briardene Close Linacre Woods Chesterfield Derbyshire S40 4XY w 6267269

Nicola Ruth 18/09/2003 Windy Ridge Meeting Hill Worstead NORTH WALSHAM Norfolk NR28 9LT **Tel:** (01692) 407547 w 6284165

CARTWRIGHT Rachel Louise (see GLENNON, Mr)

CARTY Alison Ruth (nee Yates) 07/06/2005 8 Glebe Road CHELMSFORD Essex CM1 1QG w 6283791

CARVER Donna DipAVN(Surgical) 22/07/1993 (06/12/2000) 48 Blacket Place Edinburgh Midlothian EH9 1RJ **Tel:** (07909) 721640 w 6015077

Zoe Margaret 22/03/2004 232 Kentfield Lodge London Road PETWORTH West Sussex GU28 9NE **Tel:** (01428) 708155 w 6254619

CASE Nicola Jayne 06/08/2008 33 Waggoners Way Bugbrooke Northampton Northamptonshire NN7 3QT **Tel:** (01604) 832388 w 6420070

Victoria Jane 14/02/2008 Flat 1 12 Thornhill Road SOUTHAMPTON SO16 7AS **Tel:** (02380) 704 092 w 6346931

CASEY Louise Nicola 15/02/2005 Flat 17, Florence Mansions Vivian Avenue LONDON NW4 3UY **Tel:** (020) 8444 2644 w 6299466

CASS Samantha Lucy 29/06/2007 12 Norman Road GRIMSBY South Humberside DN34 4AT **Tel:** 07743407780 w 6376862

CASSELS Elizabeth Jayne 27/04/2009 28 Hillgate Street Terrington St. Clement King's Lynn Norfolk PE34 4NS **Tel:** (01553) 771 457 w 6405044

CASSIDY Victoria Jane 07/12/2006 Pine Grove Veterinary Clinic & Referral Centre 51 Dukes Ride Crowthorne Berkshire RG45 6NE **Tel:** (01344) 774314 w 6316747

CASTELL Laura Jane 07/12/2006 17 Ringwood Road FERNDOWN Dorset BH22 9AA **Tel:** (01202) 581591 w 6357920

CASTLE Emma Louise 13/04/2004 22 Longley Lane Lowerhouses Huddersfield West Yorkshire HD4 6PS **Tel:** (01484) 307741 w 6267786

CATER Gemma Clare (see SIER, Mrs)

CATHCART Lindsay Charlotte (see FLOYD, Mrs)

CATION Louise Anne 25/08/2008 Equipet Veterinary Hospital 24 Nicol Street Kirkcaldy Fife KY1 1NY **Tel:** (01592) 641333 w 6404824

CATT Zoe Jill 17/11/2004 Chimneys Hailsham Road Heathfield East Sussex TN21 8AD **Tel:** (01435) 864422 w 6284858

CAUKWELL Joanne Louise 20/12/2007 52 Grovehill Road Beverley North Humberside HU17 0ED **Tel:** (07833) 793406 w 6382296

CAUSER Nicola Anne (see LAWES, Mrs)

CAVE Clare Louise 29/08/2000 The Park Veterinary Group 519 Saffron Lane Leicester Leicestershire LE2 6UL **Tel:** (0116) 283 1314 w 6203766

Mary-Anne Jubilee 28/01/2009 Regency House Bow Street Langport Somerset TA10 9PS **Tel:** (01458) 250459 w 6438451

Suzanne Elizabeth (nee Boucher) 04/08/1981 Archway Veterinary Practice Ltd Dragon Street Petersfield Hampshire GU31 4JJ **Tel:** (01730) 262101 w 6045997

CAYZER Nicola Elizabeth (see FRITH, Mrs)

CENEY Hayley Louise 30/05/2008 87 Heanor Road Smalley Ilkeston Derbyshire DE7 6DX **Tel:** (01773) 717780 w 6398290

CHACKSFIELD Michelle Jane (see WARD, Ms)

CHADWICK Louise 13/07/2007 10 Regent Close Eaton Socon ST. NEOTS Cambridgeshire PE19 8DT **Tel:** (07731) 845201 w 6347404

CHADWICK Nicola Jane (see CLARK, Mrs)

Victoria (nee Hartley) 21/08/2003 (24/11/2008) 38 Sunningdale RETFORD Nottinghamshire DN22 7NH **Tel:** (01777) 869917 w 6276608

CHALCRAFT Victoria Jean (nee Christie) 25/08/1995 (13/01/2000) Wilbury Veterinary Surgery 20 Wilbury Avenue Hove East Sussex BN3 6HR **Tel:** (01273) 737924 w 6038607

CHALKLEY Nicola Joy 31/05/2001 Piper Garth Marton HULL HU11 5DA **Tel:** (01964) 564867 w 6219749

CHALLICE Louise (nee Whittingham) 06/08/1991 (22/08/2006) 8a Mill Street Torrington Devon EX38 8AL **Tel:** (01805) 623971 w 6075434

CHALLIS Emma Jane 26/08/1994 15 Kingsland Road Shepton Mallet Somerset BA4 5SF **Tel:** (01749) 346 104 w 602799X

Katherine Jane DipAVN(Surgical) 23/01/1997 1 Merton Hall Farm Cottage Madingley Road Cambridge Cambridgeshire CB3 0EP w 6040649

CHALMERS Carol Marie 17/09/2009 Ardene House Veterinary Hospital Kingswells Aberdeen AB15 8PJ **Tel:** (01224) 740700 w 6463784

CHALMERS Elizabeth (see BROWN, Mrs)

CHAMBERLAIN Claire 18/10/2006 16 Northenden Road Gatley Cheadle Cheshire SK8 4DN **Tel:** (0161) 428 5655 w 6365697

Hannah Louise 15/02/2002 22 Foxes Close Hertford Hertfordshire SG13 7UA **Tel:** (01920) 466018 w 6270690

CHAMBERS Andrea Alison Victoria 17/01/1996 Joel Veterinary Clinic Joel Street Farm Joel Street Pinner Middlesex HA5 2PD **Tel:** (020) 8868 3311 w 6043286

Anna Jayne 21/07/2008 257 Kings Acre Road HEREFORD HR4 0SR **Tel:** (01432) 350678 w 6407024

Claire Louise 03/06/2008 93 Brockenhurst Drive Sunderland Tyne and Wear SR4 9NS **Tel:** (0191) 534 6827 w 6398213

Holly Dawn 21/03/2006 The Flat Croft Veterinary Centre 122 Banbury Road Brackley Northamptonshire NN13 6BH **Tel:** (01280) 701544 w 6355126

CHAMBERS Nicole Leeann (see LEE, Mrs)

Sara Jane 08/09/1998 19 Pine Grove SHERINGHAM Norfolk NR26 8QG w 6132472

CHAMPNESS Sarah Elizabeth 05/04/2005 Ashworth Veterinary Group 60 Bridge Road Cove Farnborough Hampshire GU14 0HP **Tel:** (01252) 542121 w 6298586

CHANCELLOR Karen Joanne (nee Perry) 22/02/2007 Hillcroft 50A Hall Street Dudley West Midlands DY2 7BT **Tel:** (01384) 252509 w 6343895

CHANDLER Christine Judith 31/10/2006 (20/01/2010) Stockhurst Cottage Gibbs Brook Lane OXTED Surrey RH8 9PG w 6343675

Elanor Jane 09/05/2005 Hillcroft 50A Hall Street Dudley West Midlands DY2 7BT **Tel:** (01384) 252509 w 6302557

Jennifer Ann (nee Sayers) 26/01/1994 (29/06/1999) Hart House 5 Rodwell Crowborough

East Sussex TN6 2DQ **Tel:** (01276) 855883 w 6067230

Sharon DipAVN(Surgical), DipAVN(Medical) 21/08/1984 3 Whitwell Farm Cottages Whitwell Way Coton Cambridge CB3 7PW **Tel:** (01954) 211787 w 604751X

CHANEY Emma Ernestine 10/01/2007 3 Lindridge Close Redditch Worcestershire B98 0QJ **Tel:** (01527) 526 180 w 6366093

CHANNON Caroline May (see CROSS, Mrs)

CHAPLIN Helen Judith DipAVN(Surgical) 10/09/1999 53 York Road SUDBURY Suffolk CO10 1NF w 6137459

CHAPMAN Angela Jane (formerly Chapman, formerly Lampard) 23/12/2003 20 Besbury Park Minchinhampton STROUD Gloucestershire GL6 9EN w 6289258

Clare 04/08/2008 48 Plough Lane Wallington Surrey SM6 8LN **Tel:** (07967) 351389 w 6414647

CHAPMAN Hannah Louise (see TRYE, Mrs)

Hannah Lucy 04/05/2006 Valentine House Kirton Holme BOSTON Lincolnshire PE20 1SY **Tel:** (01205) 290749 w 6323237

Kara Marie DipAVN(Medical) 22/03/2004 65 Cambridge Street Normanton West Yorkshire WF6 1ES w 6289269

Kirsty Elizabeth 03/03/2008 22 Tamar Grove Western Downs STAFFORD ST17 9SL w 6348361

Nadine 03/09/1992 2 The Cottage Poors End Grainthorpe LOUTH Lincolnshire LN11 7JB **Tel:** (01472) 840082 w 600742X

Rebecca Elizabeth Violet 30/12/2009 Coldwell Farm Lanivet Bodmin Cornwall PL30 5JB **Tel:** 01208832661 w 6442059

CHAPMAN-GREEN Caroline Helen Louise Elizabeh (nee Green) 25/01/1994 (23/08/2002) 6 Chapel Hill St. Erth HAYLE Cornwall TR27 6HL **Tel:** (01736) 755893 w 6065867

CHAPPELL Claire 20/11/2007 60 Hope Street Barnsley South Yorkshire S75 2AY **Tel:** (01226) 291767 w 6384826

Elisabeth Sientje 22/03/2004 8 Townsend Chancellor Park CHELMSFORD CM2 6GB **Tel:** (01245) 466147 w 6286035

Emily Jane 10/04/2008 Avonbank Cottage, Blackston Road Avonbridge Falkirk Stirlingshire FK1 2LB **Tel:** (01324) 861 351 w 6404802

Heidi Marie 09/02/1995 Beaufort Cottage Equine Hospital Cotton End Road Exning Newmarket Suffolk CB8 7NN **Tel:** (01638) 577 754 w 6033562

Louise 28/02/2007 24 Cottam Road High Green SHEFFIELD S35 4PJ **Tel:** (01924) 462365 w 6346942

CHAPPLE-HYAM Alexandra Mae 27/04/2005 Flat 1, 79 Fountain Road Birmingham West Midlands B17 8NP w 6323248

CHARD Mandy Jane 16/09/2008 25 Hallsland Crawley Down Crawley West Sussex RH10 4XZ **Tel:** (01342) 712968 w 6408245

CHARLES Lisa 14/11/2000 Beechwood Veterinary Group Ltd 132 Austhorpe Road Leeds LS15 8EJ **Tel:** (01132) 645422 w 6203359

Tracy (formerly Crocombe) 06/09/2000 2 Aspen Park Road Weston Super Mare Somerset BS22 8AU **Tel:** (01934) 645874 w 6149307

CHARLESWORTH Clare 30/10/2003 11 Skelton Drive Sheffield South Yorkshire S13 7QS **Tel:** (0114) 244 0085 w 6285243

Linda Anne DipAVN(Surgical) 14/01/2000 10 Canney Close Chiseldon Nr Swindon Wiltshire SN4 0PF **Tel:** (01793) 740414 w 6191160

CHARLTON Alison 27/03/2009 Pine Grove Veterinary Clinic & Referral Centre 51 Dukes Ride Crowthorne Berkshire RG45 6NE **Tel:** (01344) 774314 w 6441993

CHARLTON Donna Marie (see JOHNSON, Mrs)

Kelly Louise 31/03/2003 (29/04/2005) 67 Meadrow Godalming Surrey GU7 3HS **Tel:** (01483) 421102 w 6280535

CHARLTON Melanie (see SCOTT, Mrs)

CHASTON Emma Elizabeth 16/09/2008 24 Albert Road South Woodford London E18 1LE **Tel:** (0208) 539 3538 w 6297475

CHATWIN Melody Rachel 10/02/2004 (09/04/2009) 129 Queenswood Drive LEEDS LS6 3LR **Tel:** 07793463013 w 6265520

CHAWNER Lisa Elaine (nee Haldron) 11/05/2004 16 Sir John Pascoe Way NORTHAMPTON NN5 6PQ w 6288873

CHEDZOY Claire Danielle 10/02/2005 Stowey Farm House Fivehead Taunton Somerset TA3 6PR **Tel:** (01460) 281811 w 6299939

CHEESEMAN Jenna Marie 28/09/2009 4 Treegarth Square NOTTINGHAM NG5 5QZ **Tel:** 07879261556 w 6490613

CHEESMAN Carly 11/11/2004 205 Rake Lane WALLASEY Merseyside CH45 5DQ w 6323919

Faye Louise 27/12/2007 Priory Lodge Veterinary Group 31 Pembury Road TONBRIDGE Kent TN9 2JB **Tel:** (01732) 353668 w 6374035

CHEETHAM Nina Susanna 17/02/2009 3 Woodlands Lane Storrington PULBOROUGH West Sussex RH20 3HG **Tel:** 01903743383 w 6433490

CHELL Judith Elizabeth (see PARRY, Mrs)

CHENYLLE-PROCTOR Tina Louise 28/08/1991 (16/11/1998) 10 Valley Gardens WHITLEY BAY Tyne and Wear NE25 9AP **Tel:** (0191) 2096635 w 6061206

CHERRY Helen Louise 12/12/2008 254 Low Lane Horsforth LEEDS LS18 5DN w 6443962

CHESHIRE Emma Catherine Louise (see BLACKSHAW, Ms)

CHESHIRE Jane Elizabeth 01/01/2008 40 Willmore Grove Kings Norton BIRMINGHAM B38 9RE w 6389864

CHESTER Janice Rose (see BAKER, Mrs)

CHESTERTON Alexandra Faye 15/09/1997 22 Harbourer Road Hainault Ilford Essex IG6 3TN **Tel:** (0208) 500 0576 w 6117104

CHETWYND Mandy Helen 13/05/2003 Portland House Veterinary Centre 53 Churchgate Retford Nottinghamshire DN22 6PA **Tel:** (01777) 703663 w 6276432

CHEVINS Kay 08/01/2010 19 Swallowdale Road Melton Mowbray Leicestershire LE13 0AU **Tel:** 07931545603 w 6378424

CHILDS Alison Lindsay 27/02/2006 RSPCA Barnes Hill Weoley Castle Birmingham B29 5UP **Tel:** (0300) 123 8652 w 6313381

Katherine Elizabeth 07/11/2008 62 Parkway Wickham Market WOODBRIDGE Suffolk IP13 0SS **Tel:** 01394387514 w 6434205

CHILTON Heather Louise 06/03/2008 8 Bransdale Mews Normanton West Yorkshire WF6 2SZ **Tel:** (01924) 891 744 w 6404175

Kelly Jane 14/03/1990 (05/11/2001) 70 Brinkley Lane Highwoods COLCHESTER Essex CO4 9XE **Tel:** (01206) 842608 w 6047622

CHIMES Sarah 17/01/2006 21 Richmond Crescent Highams Park London E4 9RT w 6293603

CHISHAM Tracey Mary 10/10/2005 88a Christchurch Road Ringwood Hampshire BH24 1DR **Tel:** (01202) 822030 w 6291172

CHISHOLM Charlotte Louise 07/12/2009 Barrow Hill House Maidstone Rd Ashford Kent TN24 8TY **Tel:** (01233) 624687 w 6493121

CHITTENDEN Maria-Teresa (nee Wildish) 01/10/1999 Fern Cottage Veterinary Surgery 233-235 Park Road Sittingbourne Kent ME10 1ER **Tel:** (01795) 476411 w 615274X

CHITTOCK Sarah Jane 03/03/2005 Trevose 82-84 Commercial Road Hayle Cornwall TR27 4DH **Tel:** (01703) 282979 w 6277631

CHIVERS Elaine Ann DipAVN(Surgical) 20/04/2001 (21/06/2006) Flat 1 31 Main Road Hursley WINCHESTER Hampshire SO21 2JW w 6216119

CHOPPING Helen Frances (nee Gould) 26/03/2002 60 Chapel Hill STANSTED Essex CM24 8AQ **Tel:** (01279) 817415 w 6268853

Nicol 12/11/2009 Highcliff Veterinary Practice 93 Cliff Lane Ipswich Suffolk IP3 0PQ **Tel:** (01473) 828846 w 6459527

CHOWDHARY Davina Elizabeth (see OSBORNE, Mrs)

CHRIMES Kathrine Margaret 10/04/2008 15 Field Close NORTHWICH Cheshire CW8 4UG **Tel:** 07738581048 w 6353762

CHRISMAS Diane Tracey 30/10/2001 23 Spencer Road Ryde Isle of Wight PO33 2NU **Tel:** (01983) 562878 w 6260724

CHRISTIAN Lynda Joyce 20/01/1999 Llys Macsen 66 Bryn Cadno Upper Colwyn Bay LL29 6DW **Tel:** (01492) 532833 w 6119247

CHRISTIE Emma Louise (see MILNE, Mrs)

CHRISTIE Victoria Jean (see CHALCRAFT, Mrs)

CHRISTOFE Katy Sarah Elizabeth (see BALDWIN, Mrs)

CHURCH Alison Fiona (nee Sheen) 02/08/1989 12 Hayes Mead Holbury Southampton Hampshire SO45 2JZ **Tel:** (023) 80890058 w 6060585

Karen Anne 30/11/2006 (09/02/2009) Unit 6 Forest Corner Farm Hangersley Hill Hangersley RINGWOOD Hampshire BH24 3JW **Tel:** (01425) 485615 w 6288070

Natasha Samantha 21/07/2008 6b Beckwith Road London SE24 9LG **Tel:** 07833340821 w 6377060

CHURCHES Amanda Jane 04/06/2009 71 West End STREET Somerset BA16 0LQ **Tel:** (01458) 443884 w 6415417

CHYNOWETH Jacqueline Dawn 15/05/2009 7 Charlotte Close Mount Hawke TRURO Cornwall TR4 8TS **Tel:** (01209) 890 876 w 6429629

CIARCIA Lyndsey Margaret May (nee Ross) 05/09/2003 Ivybank Veterinary Clinic 2 Low Green Road Irvine Ayrshire KA12 8RA **Tel:** (01294) 273161 w 6264706

CILIA Natasha Jayne (see HORNSBY, Mrs)

CLAPHAM Lindsay (nee Drinkwater) 07/02/2005 4 Rushmere Close Raunds Northampton Northamptonshire NN9 6TX w 6307364

Louise 23/08/2004 Hillcrest Animal Health Ltd Water Street Chorley Lancashire PR7 1EX **Tel:** (01257) 262448 w 6272681

CLARE Elizabeth Ann Catherine 23/06/2009 31 Oldfield Drive Wouldham Rochester Kent ME1 3GP **Tel:** 01634686824 w 6434953

Emma Louise (formerly Jenkins, nee Clare) 07/12/2005 Copthorne Veterinary Clinic 114 Copthorne Road Shrewsbury Shropshire SY3 8NA **Tel:** (01743) 360614 w 6342641

CLARE Julie Ann (see DAVIS, Mrs)

Sara-Jane Marie (nee O'Sullivan) 13/09/1996 22 Wheatfield Road Cronton Knowlsey Cheshire WA8 5BU w 6026373

CLARK Alanna 20/07/2009 1 Butchers Row Polehampton Close Twyford READING RG10 9TW **Tel:** 07766166954 w 6432808

Alexandra May 29/11/2007 Toft Lodge Veterinary Centre Raskelf Road Easingwold York North Yorkshire YO61 3LA **Tel:** (01347) 821377 w 6401887

CLARK Alison Grace (see WILLIAMS, Mrs)

Alison Jane 03/09/1998 73 Cawood Drive Skirlaugh Hull HU11 5ER **Tel:** (01964) 562111 w 613527X

Anne-Maire Jane 17/01/2008 59 Berlin Road Hastings East Sussex TN35 5JD **Tel:** (01424) 422 265 w 6396310

Catherine Laura 04/06/2009 140 Rickerscote Road Stafford Staffordshire ST17 4HE **Tel:** 01785603205 w 6407893

Eleanor Louise 14/09/2004 Kohimarama Veterinary Clinic 325 Kohimarama Road Kohimarama 1071 AUCKLAND New Zealand **Tel:** (+61) 210360046 w 6319519

Elizabeth 29/08/1990 21 Haymore Street Middlesbrough Cleveland TS5 6JD **Tel:** 01642850812 w 6047688

Emma Louise 13/07/2007 71 Purbrook Gardens Waterlooville Hampshire PO7 5LE **Tel:** (07941) 076560 w 6347437

Helen Hodge 13/05/2003 19 Swan Crescent GOREBRIDGE Midlothian EH23 4UL **Tel:** (01875) 821717 w 6283901

Katherine Louise 21/11/2005 18 The Avenue Coxhoe DURHAM DH6 4AD **Tel:** (0191) 3771 893 w 6339011

Kelly Ann Maurine 04/06/2009 26 Tabor Avenue Braintree Essex CM7 2SX **Tel:** 01376552716 w 6410852

CLARK Lorraine (see WEBB, Mrs)

CLARK Lucy Ann (see JONES, Mrs)

Nicola Jane (nee Chadwick) 19/04/2005 Madeira Lodge Main Road Tallington Stamford Lincolnshire PE9 4RP **Tel:** (01780) 740137 w 6293966

Rosalind Janet 18/09/2003 25 Barley Close Little Eaton Derby Derbyshire DE21 5DJ **Tel:** (01332) 833 931 w 6252375

Ruth Margaret 06/02/2002 9 Tatton Close LEEK Staffordshire ST13 8NS **Tel:** (01538) 382330 w 6268149

CLARK Sallyanne (see FAIRS, Mrs)

Sarah Ann 31/03/2008 1 Bridge Court Hoole Lane Chester Cheshire CH2 3DW **Tel:** (07841) 526325 w 6403471

Sarah Jane 16/01/1996 The Veterinary Clinic School Way Okehampton Devon EX20 1EU **Tel:** (01837) 52148 w 6042420

Tessa Lorraine 19/09/2008 57 Stanley Grove London SW8 3PD **Tel:** (020) 7627 0682 w 6385640

Victoria Constance Alexan 28/08/1998 4 Everest Court Balderton Newark Nottinghamshire NG24 3PZ **Tel:** (01636) 701 725 w 6132789

Victoria Samantha (nee Clark, formerly Lyons) 27/08/1996 (16/04/2003) C/O 61 School Road Ashford Middlesex TW15 2BT **Tel:** (01784) 211845 w 6029884

CLARKE Ami Hannah 24/09/2009 26 Brampton Road MELTON MOWBRAY Leicestershire LE13 0NA **Tel:** 01664854168 w 6464345

CLARKE Anne Louise (see CAIN, Mrs)

Charmaine Dionne Sabrina 09/09/2008 51 Pinner Park Avenue Harrow Middlesex HA2 6JY **Tel:** 02084201165 w 6378556

Helen Elizabeth (nee Walker) 05/02/1999 Chapel House Veterinary Practice Ltd Hady Hill Chesterfield Derbyshire S41 0DZ **Tel:** (01246) 222 232 w 613375X

Helena Mary 17/04/1999 (26/10/2000) 165 Union Street DUNSTABLE Bedfordshire LU6 1HA w 613447X

Jennifer Kay 06/08/2008 9 Almsford Drive York North Yorkshire YO26 5NR w 6377423

Julie Ann 23/12/2003 39 Summerfield Road SOLIHULL West Midlands B92 8QB **Tel:** (0121) 742 3745 w 6279688

Kaylee Ann 10/03/2009 Parkside Veterinary Centre 61 Ruskin Road Carshalton Surrey SM5 3DD **Tel:** (020) 8395 8222 w 6437505

CLARKE Laura Anne (see COOPER, Mrs)

Lesley Frances 14/10/2008 32 Magherabeg Road DROMORE County Down BT25 1RS **Tel:** (028) 92699675 w 6328143

Michelle (nee Cook) 02/08/1988 Coco Markus House Nelson street Grimsby North East Lincolnshire DN32 7SH **Tel:** (01472) 343278 w 6047702

Michelle Louise 04/03/2009 39 Rathbone Close Rugby Warwickshire CV21 4EP **Tel:** 01788334750 w 6413547

Philippa Dawn 03/12/2003 30 Baxters Walk Malvern Worcestershire WR14 2DY w 6280887

Sarah Louise 18/11/2009 64 Sermon Drive Swanley Kent BR8 7HT **Tel:** (01322) 409778 w 6340353

Sarah Louise May (nee Roberts) 21/05/2009 19 Rosedale Road Bentley DONCASTER South Yorkshire DN5 0JP **Tel:** 07894211299 w 6400215

Sharna Louise (nee Clarke, formerly Jordan) 25/02/2000 (28/03/2008) 3 Keir Road WEDNESBURY West Midlands WS10 0HL **Tel:** (0121) 531 0425 w 6191050

Trudy Celeste 15/07/2005 12b Chilton Way Dover Kent CT17 0QA **Tel:** (01304) 826806 w 6322434

Wayne Anthony 11/03/2008 125 Storforth Lane Hasland CHESTERFIELD Derbyshire S41 0PZ **Tel:** (01246) 233834 m 6406232

CLARKSON Louise Carol (nee Foan) 06/06/2003 (24/04/2006) 23 Worlebury Hill Road Weston-super-Mare Avon BS22 9SQ **Tel:** (01934) 625 773 w 6274540

CLAY Donna Marie (nee Parden) 24/01/2000 C/o Royal College of Veterinary Surgeons 62-64 Horseferry Road LONDON SW1P 2AF w 6190907

Marie Louise 04/02/2009 14 Beverley Crescent Grimsby South Humberside DN32 9SX **Tel:** 01472344679 w 6423909

Sarah Katie 31/03/2008 53 Selborne Close PETERSFIELD Hampshire GU32 2JB **Tel:** (07885) 693785 w 6330695

CLAYTON Amanda Jane (see SMITH, Mrs)

CLAYTON Keri Eileen Margaret 12/12/2008 Rosemount Tachbrook Road LEAMINGTON SPA Warwickshire CV31 3DD **Tel:** 07793003893 w 6350462

CLAYTON-HART Joanne Clare 13/05/2003 23 Amberwood Close Calmore SOUTHAMPTON SO40 2ST **Tel:** (07773) 529481 (work) w 6286981

CLEAR Melanie Sara 24/09/2001 63 Pine Way Cheriton Folkstone Kent CT19 4QL **Tel:** (01303) 274099 w 6228549

CLEAVER Allyson 25/02/2003 Swanspool Veterinary Clinic 1 London Road Wellingborough Northamptonshire NN8 2BT **Tel:** (01933) 222145 w 6279754

CLEMENS Sarah Joanne (nee Bedding) 22/03/2004 Crossroads Veterinary Centre 54 West Wycombe Road High Wycombe Buckinghamshire HP11 2LP **Tel:** (01494) 459095 w 6287432

CLEMENT Selina Kimberley 20/11/2008 9 Deacon Road Kingston upon Thames Surrey KT2 6LT w 6436196

CLEMENTS Jane (nee Clements, formerly Pulford) 23/01/2003 (23/01/2006) Prospect Cottage

Brains Green BLAKENEY Gloucestershire GL15 4AJ w 6281701

Katrina Louise 21/05/2009 The Veterinary Centre James Street Louth Lincolnshire LN11 0JW **Tel:** (01507) 602828 w 6434601

CLIFFORD Claire Louise (see NASH, Mrs)

CLIFFORDE Emma Louise 20/11/2000 C/o Royal College of Veterinary Surgeons 62-64 Horseferry Road LONDON SW1P 2AF w 6205812

CLIFT Clare 16/10/2000 Riverside Beaufort EBBW VALE Gwent NP23 5NT **Tel:** (01495) 305465 w 6203260

CLIFTON Alexandra Elizabeth (formerly Brown) 01/09/1997 (18/02/2008) 1 Hagg Bush Cottage Hagg Bush Lane Burn Selby YO8 8LE **Tel:** (01757) 270018 w 6115694

CLINCH Gemma Louise 13/02/2009 11 Bluebell Close Burghclere Down ANDOVER Hampshire SP10 3XE **Tel:** (075005) 56697 w 6420103

CLOSE Samantha Leigh 13/03/2008 41 Quantock Close Bristol Avon BS30 8UT **Tel:** (0117) 9611175 w 6418629

Sarah Danielle 09/07/2007 119 Avocet Way Langford Village BICESTER Oxfordshire OX26 6YW **Tel:** (07841) 869670 w 6352486

CLOUGH Claire Louise (see HOBSON, Mrs)

CLOUT Suzanne Maria (see KIRBY, Mrs)

CLOWES Helen Charlotte 06/06/2008 11 Claydon Crescent NEWCASTLE Staffordshire ST5 4JR w 6378567

Sarah Louise (nee Cooper) 23/08/1995 (27/07/1999) 29 Sycamore Road RADSTOCK Somerset BA3 3NL w 6031281

CLUE Joanna Elizabeth (formerly Rhodes) 11/01/2005 The Veterinary Surgery Higher Trenant Wadebridge Cornwall PL27 6HB **Tel:** (01208) 813258 w 6317748

COATES Stephanie Ann 03/06/2003 35 Roker Park Road Roker Sunderland SR6 9PL **Tel:** (0191) 516 0056 w 6275871

COATSWORTH Michelle Jane (nee Tipping) 17/11/2003 1 Clock Row Norton Malton North Yorkshire YO17 9BE w 6291645

COBB Lucy Ann (see EDE, Mrs)

COBB Lynsey 05/01/2005 4 Radcliffe Way Bracknell Berkshire RG42 1FR **Tel:** (01344) 457894 w 6277950

COBHAM Louise Christine 07/08/2008 81 Quentin Road London SE13 5DG **Tel:** (0208) 3186144 w 6402701

COBURN Sarah Amanda 22/02/2007 Cheadle Hulme Veterinary Hospital 2-4 Queens Road Cheadle Hulme Cheshire SK8 5LU **Tel:** (0161) 485 8444 w 6371560

COCHRANE Nicola 19/03/2007 4 The Wynd Biggar Lanarkshire ML12 6BU **Tel:** (01899) 221169 w 6373386

COCKBURN Cheryl Anne DipAVN(Surgical) 25/09/1996 131 Craigielea Road Renfrew PA4 8EW **Tel:** (0141) 587 0653 w 609640X

Gail Michelle 22/08/2008 12 Lena Avenue Whitley Bay Tyne and Wear NE25 8TF **Tel:** (0191) 252 9876 w 6434491

Nichola Jane 13/10/2000 3 Bedwellty Pits Tredegar Gwent NP22 4BW w 6202809

COCKERILL Sandra 03/03/2009 53 Durrington Road Bournemouth Dorset BH7 6PY **Tel:** (01202) 426434 w 6434315

COCKLIN Michelle (nee Long) 22/08/1997 (06/09/2007) 337 St. Helens Road LEIGH Lancashire WN7 3PQ **Tel:** (01942) 679797 w 6116213

COCKSHOOT Tracy Maud (see ALDERMAN, Mrs)

CODD Victoria Marie 16/08/2007 Orwell Veterinary Group Hartree Way Grange Farm Kesgrave Ipswich Suffolk IP5 2BZ **Tel:** (01473) 333677 w 6376378

COE Anna Marie 11/10/2004 (18/02/2008) 8 Allysum Walk BILLERICAY Essex CM12 0SR w 6292085

Helen Lucy (nee Parker) 21/01/1998 The Old Appleyard 124 Poolbrook Road Malvern Worcestershire WR14 3JF **Tel:** (01684) 576139 w 6101728

COFFEY Sarah Louise 08/08/2005 Thameswood Veterinary Clinics Ltd 62-64 Purton Road Swindon SN2 2LZ **Tel:** (01793) 526780 w 6282845

COFFEY Vanessa Louise (see CUNNINGHAM, Mrs)

COGBILL Deborah Ann 28/11/2008 59 Sunnyside Road BRIDGEND Mid Glamorgan CF31 4AF **Tel:** (01656) 652751 w 6260240

COGGLES Venetia Ann 31/08/1993 41 Eastwood Rise Leigh-on-Sea Essex SS9 5BT w 602684X

COKER Amy Louise 05/01/2009 E C Straiton & Partners Llp The Veterinary Hospital Cannock Road Penkridge STAFFORD ST19 5RY w 6440354

COLBERT Carly 06/03/2008 35 Newbury Avenue Great Coates Grimsby South Humberside DN37 9NQ **Tel:** (01472) 315765 w 6415197

Craig Nigel 15/04/2008 5 Barnett Grove CONGLETON Cheshire CW12 4WF m 6339022

COLBORNE Hannah Louise (nee Woodward) 19/09/2008 129 Montgomery Close Stewartby Bedford Bedfordshire MK43 9LP **Tel:** (07920) 770144 w 6420829

COLBURN Katrina Petra 07/02/2007 New Priory Veterinary Practice The Deneway London Rd Brighton East Sussex BN1 8QR **Tel:** (01273) 540430 w 6371571

COLE Gemma Rose 21/08/2009 112 John Newton Court WELLING Kent DA16 2AG **Tel:** 02082989405 w 6434458

Jennie Patricia 29/07/2005 23 Whitley Road WHITLEY BAY Tyne and Wear NE26 2EW w 6321939

Nicola 13/04/2004 Wingrave Veterinary Surgery 84 Mulgrave Road Sutton Surrey SM2 6LZ **Tel:** (020) 8642 9100 w 6287443

Rebecca Dawn 22/12/2004 8 Batterby Green Hempton FAKENHAM Norfolk NR21 7LY **Tel:** (01328) 855 434 w 6307155

Selina Dawn 07/07/2008 Arbury Road Veterinary Surgery 32 Arbury Road Cambridge CB4 2JE **Tel:** (01223) 361911 w 6366104

Wendy Lynne (nee Duke) 30/11/2006 3 The Maltings Roydon Road Stanstead Abbots

Hertfordshire SG12 8HG **Tel:** (01920) 877200 w 6291524

COLEMAN Caroline Naomi 18/09/2007 93 Beechcroft Road Longlevens Gloucester Gloucestershire GL2 9HE w 6370944

Danielle Louise 30/07/2004 7 Morris Gardens Ampthill BEDFORD MK45 2RU w 6299950

COLEMAN Emma Louise (see MCLEAN, Mrs)

Gemma Louise 07/07/2008 5 The Longthorns Frome Somerset BA11 4FD **Tel:** (07794) 432180 w 6376389

COLEMAN Karen Jane (see HUNTER, Mrs)

COLEMAN Katie Louise (see WILL, Mrs)

Katy Elizabeth (nee Johnson) 19/07/2004 Barnsley Vets4Pets Limited 161 Wilthorpe Road Barnsley South Yorkshire S75 1JQ **Tel:** (01226) 289000 w 6286739

Lindy 06/03/2006 75 Gateside Avenue Cambuslang GLASGOW G72 7YF **Tel:** (0141) 6410344 w 6346953

Marie Louise (nee Burrow) 04/03/2008 The Green Veterinary Surgery Skelton Penrith Cumbria CA11 9SQ **Tel:** (01768) 484258 w 6417034

Miranda Lee 16/06/2006 53-55 Maidstone Road Footscray SIDCUP Kent DA14 5HB **Tel:** (020) 8300 8111 w 6270635

Victoria Louise (nee Wheeler) 21/11/2005 27 Sycamore Avenue Woodford Halse Daventry Northamptonshire NN11 3ST **Tel:** 07985641957 w 6332675

COLERIDGE SIMPSON Rebecca Louise (see TAYLOR, Mrs)

COLES Geraldine Elaine DipAVN(Surgical) 21/01/1997 458 Havering Road ROMFORD Essex RM1 4HR w 6107854

Kate Anna 20/10/2008 86 Washford Farm Road ASHFORD Kent TN23 5YD **Tel:** 01233330917 w 6342036

Laura Claire 17/09/2007 4 Beaufort East London Road Bath BA1 6QD **Tel:** (01225) 312061 w 6357931

Linda Sally 15/01/1981 Boness Veterinary Enterprises Ltd 125 Bedford Road Barton le Clay Bedford Bedfordshire MK45 4LP **Tel:** (01582) 612604 w 6000344

COLESHILL Rebecca 21/08/2003 34 Warwick Close Chippenham Wiltshire SN14 0YD **Tel:** (01249) 446 232 w 6280392

COLFER Melanie Yvonne 02/06/2004 6 Mayoral Terrace Haverfordwest Dyfed SA61 2PH **Tel:** (07739) 490908 w 6285474

COLING Sharon Jane (nee Powell) 17/02/2000 (10/12/2009) Avonvale Veterinary Centres Ltd 88 Coventry Street Southam Warwickshire CV47 0EA **Tel:** (01926) 812826 w 6033110

COLLETT Ruth (formerly O'Grady) 22/02/1999 76 Acacia Road Falmouth Cornwall TR11 2LA w 6138532

COLLEY Janet Ann 07/02/2007 565 Green Lane Goodmayes Ilford Essex IG3 9RJ **Tel:** (020) 8590 0181 w 6301072

Ruth Anne 13/08/2003 38 Burns Way Wath Upon Dearne Rotherham South Yorkshire S63 6ED **Tel:** (01709) 878372 w 6281206

COLLIDGE Stephanie Ruth 10/02/2004 Flat 4 117 Parkway LONDON NW1 7PS **Tel:** (07899) 904 166 w 6297992

COLLIER Jill Irene 06/08/2007 Chestnut Cottage Astrop Road Kings Sutton Banbury Oxfordshire OX17 3PS **Tel:** (01295) 812040 w 6366115

Kimberley Anne 14/09/2004 4c Stoneybank Terrace Musselburgh Midlothian EH21 6NL **Tel:** (0131) 440 0654 w 6290028

Lisa 16/08/2006 12 Shincliffe Avenue Sunderland Tyne and Wear SR5 5UB **Tel:** (0191) 5499 854 w 6346469

COLLINS Alison (nee Mann) 11/11/1999 (13/04/2006) Merlin Veterinary Group Easter Langlee Melrose Road Galashiels Selkirkshire TD1 2UH **Tel:** (01896) 753759 w 6148868

Anna Mary 24/09/2009 32 Elsdon Road Gosforth NEWCASTLE UPON TYNE NE3 1HY **Tel:** 07776268868 w 6465027

Haley Karen (nee Hornsby) 05/10/2004 The Veterinary Practice Millennium Way Braintree Essex CM7 3GX **Tel:** (01376) 325511 w 6267005

Janice Valerie 26/08/1998 Deep Well Cottage 44 Lynch Hill Kensworth DUNSTABLE Bedfordshire LU6 3QY w 6134254

Joanne Lesley 27/11/1996 19 Audnam Wordsley Stourbridge West Midlands DY8 4AJ **Tel:** (01384) 372849 w 6097946

Josephine Mary 31/10/2006 32 Richards Close Tonedale WELLINGTON Somerset TA21 0BE w 6375047

Julie Anne 23/08/2005 83a Emmanuel Road HASTINGS East Sussex TN34 3LE w 6299477

Lisa Jayne (nee Stead, formerly Daw) 24/08/1998 64 Elgar Crescent Pensnett Brierley Hill West Midlands DY5 4JJ **Tel:** (01384) 346452 w 6098768

Naima Melissa 18/05/2009 Ground Floor Flat 5 Station Approach East Hassocks West Sussex BN6 8HN **Tel:** 01273842477 w 6435811

Rachael Mary 24/11/2004 8 North Hyde Road HAYES Middlesex UB3 4ND w 6314657

COLLINS Rosalind Ann (see BATH, Mrs)

Sarah Michelle DipAVN(Medical) (nee Klyn) 15/08/1995 (02/02/2000) University of Bristol Intensive Care Unit Dept of Clinical Veterinary Science Langford House Bristol BS40 5DU w 6036789

Sharon Louise 24/05/2005 Avon Lodge Veterinary Group 21 Stratford Road Salisbury SP1 3JN **Tel:** (01722) 412211 w 6290941

COLLINSON Lucy Hannah Elizabeth (see TOMLIN, Mrs)

COLPMAN Georgina Mary 03/06/2008 Higher Mount Farm Kebs Road Todmorden Lancashire OL14 8SD **Tel:** (01706) 813 946 w 6388654

COLSTON Storm Louise 02/10/2009 Thornbury House Hollins Lane Hawarden DEESIDE Clwyd CH5 3JX **Tel:** (01244) 533874 w 6493308

COLVILL Lisa Marie 07/02/2007 The Elms Church Lane Abridge ROMFORD RM4 1AD w 6355137

COLVILLE Susan Joan 28/09/2005 (04/02/2009) 54 Norfolk Place Chafford Hundred GRAYS Essex RM16 6DE **Tel:** (01375) 482901 w 6280480

COLVIN Melanie Ann 26/01/2000 Pet Care Veterinary Surgery 355 Bexley Road Erith Kent DA8 3EZ **Tel:** (01322) 346173 w 6145743

COLWELL Frances Clare (see EASTERBROOK, Mrs)

COMAN Claire Joanne 25/09/2009 5 Honey Close NORWICH NR1 4LJ **Tel:** 01603433668 w 6461023

COMBAY Sarah Jane (see COMBOY, Mrs)

COMBER Anna Elizabeth (see SPECHT, Mrs)

COMBOY Sarah Jane (nee Newall, formerly Combay) 04/09/1998 Willows Veterinary Group 70 High Street Winsford Cheshire CW7 2AP **Tel:** (01606) 592714 w 613383X

COMERIE Elaine Angela (see ANDREWS, Mrs)

COMPTON Carole Louise 13/10/2009 25 Kemble Green East Newton Aycliffe County Durham DL5 5AS **Tel:** (01325) 617568 w 6367688

CONCAH Kathryn 15/12/2004 Coco Markus House Nelson street Grimsby North East Lincolnshire DN32 7SH **Tel:** (01472) 343278 w 6311456

CONDON Olive Maria 04/06/2003 91 Onslow Gardens WALLINGTON Surrey SM6 9PX w 6254993

CONGDON Rebecca Joyce (see BICKFORD, Mrs)

CONLON Lisa Tammy 01/10/2008 97 Bankton Park East Livingston West Lothian EH54 9BN **Tel:** (01506) 430047 w 6373397

CONN Alison (nee Sedgwick) 22/08/1997 16a Harrow Gardens Warlingham Surrey CR6 9ES **Tel:** (01883) 372432 w 6118855

CONNELLY Gillian C (see CALVO, Mrs)

Liza Hart 22/12/2009 6 Lorne Terrace LOCHGILPHEAD Argyll PA31 8LS **Tel:** (01546) 603083 w 6491427

CONNERTY Harriet Jane 03/10/2007 Oundle Veterinary Surgery 92 South Road Oundle Peterborough PE8 4BP **Tel:** (01832) 273521 w 6368799

CONNOLLY Joanne (nee Brockbank) 22/11/2001 Wesham House Farm Fleetwood Road Wesham Preston Lancashire PR4 3HD **Tel:** (01772) 671654 w 6268644

CONNOR Dannielle 08/08/2005 20 Beeston Close South Oxhey Watford Hertfordshire WD19 6LF **Tel:** (0208) 421 0344 w 6283021

Davina Gillian 31/03/2003 (03/03/2006) 88 Chamberlain Street St. Helens Merseyside WA10 4NN **Tel:** (01772) 744229 w 6269766

CONSTABLE Samantha Dawn 05/07/2006 Sutton Farm Veterinary Surgery Tilstock Crescent Sutton Farm Shrewsbury Shropshire SY2 6HW **Tel:** (01743) 352274 w 6330167

Sharon Jane 02/02/1987 27 The Street Gillingham Beccles Suffolk NR34 0LH **Tel:** (01502) 710703 w 6048014

CONSTANT Rachael Yvette 23/07/2008 9 Ullswater Close Biggleswade Bedfordshire SG18 8LX **Tel:** 01767317986 w 6371824

CONVERY Natalie Anne 13/07/2007 3 Bacon Street Guiseley LEEDS LS20 9LH **Tel:** (07813) 267749 w 6347448

CONWAY Emer Colette 12/07/2006 Glascarn Lane Ratqath Co Meath Ireland Ireland **Tel:** (003531) 825 7429 w 6258194

Norma 27/07/1979 (12/12/2005) The Old Cider House Westdown Farm Sandy Bay Exmouth Devon EX8 5BU **Tel:** (01395) 275116 w 6048036

Una Mary 09/06/2009 6 Shanroy Park Pomeroy Dungannon County Tyrone BT70 2RP w 6443434

COOK Anne Monica 05/08/1976 1 Uphill Grove Mill Hill LONDON NW7 4NH w 6085566

COOK Annika Maria (see GROOMBRIDGE, Mrs)

COOK Bethan Sian (see SPENCER, Mrs)

Charlotte Jane 24/11/2008 1 Barden Cottages The Green Leigh Tonbridge Kent TN11 8QN w 6408960

Claire Louise 02/04/2009 46 Courtney Park Road Langdon Hills BASILDON Essex SS16 6RE w 6386520

Denise Deborah 19/02/2001 M Y F Training Hippodrome House Station Road ALDERSHOT Hampshire GU11 1LZ w 6212401

COOK Donna-Marie (see MAYNARD, Mrs)

COOK Hannah Elizabeth (see DAVIES, Mrs)

Kathryn 14/01/2008 Station Farm London Road Six Mile Bottom Newmarket Suffolk CB8 0UH **Tel:** (01638) 572012 w 6400446

Kerry Elizabeth 08/09/2009 The Lodge Ross Road Gorsley Ross-On-Wye Herefordshire HR9 7SP **Tel:** (01989) 720137 w 6466941

Kimberley Louise 15/07/2009 Clifton Villa Green Lane Staines Middlesex TW18 3LT **Tel:** (01784) 461788 w 6383143

COOK Michelle (see CLARKE, Mrs)

Michelle Sally 27/09/2000 Bredy Veterinary Centre Sea Road North Bridport Dorset DT6 4RR **Tel:** (01308) 456 771 w 6141476

Rachael Melanie 07/12/2005 45 Lewis Lane Cirencester Gloucestershire GL7 1EA **Tel:** (01285) 653151 w 6332257

Rachel Louise 05/07/2006 132 Brookfield Road Grimsby South Humberside DN33 3JL **Tel:** (01472) 598984 w 6322203

Rosanna Jane 09/07/2007 70 Back Lane Okeford Fitzpaine BLANDFORD FORUM Dorset DT11 0RP **Tel:** (01258) 861 557 w 6352497

Samantha Jane 06/07/2004 Riverside Veterinary Surgery 2 Scotter Road Eastleigh Hampshire SO50 6AJ **Tel:** (023) 8062 0607 w 6301259

Samantha Jane 06/08/2007 31 Stromness Place Southend-on-Sea Essex SS2 4JH **Tel:** (01702) 610434 w 6358767

Samantha Jane 03/12/2003 The Dragon Veterinary Clinic 496 Hornsey Road London N19 4EF **Tel:** (020) 7272 3354 w 6278951

COOKE Amanda 24/01/1997 11 Hawarden Road Caterham Surrey CR3 5QT **Tel:** (01883) 343258 w 6076846

COOKE Anna Marie (see STRINGER, Mrs)

Collette 04/01/2008 1 Ffordd Aeron Coedpoeth WREXHAM Clwyd LL11 3NY **Tel:** 07745150947 w 6392119

COOKE Emma Jane (see LIGHT, Mrs)

Gemma Louise 24/11/2009 155 Den Lane Springhead Oldham OL4 4RE w 6466160

Jenny Caryl Mary (nee Irvine) 05/04/2005 (18/02/2008) 155a Movilla Road Newtownards Co Down BT23 8RL **Tel:** (028) 9181 9147 w 6291216

COOKE Sarah Jane Louise (see LANSLEY, Mrs)

Valerie Ann 21/03/2006 3 Dunbar Street Hopeman ELGIN Morayshire IV30 5TD w 6348658

COOKNELL Rebecca Louise 25/09/2009 18 Horsham Close Banbury Oxon OX16 1XR **Tel:** (01295) 266108 w 6489480

COOKSLEY Emma 31/10/2005 27 Burgess Green Close St. Annes Park BRISTOL BS4 4DG w 6326306

COOKSON Andrea 11/11/2008 3 Ash Road Winwick Warrington Cheshire WA2 8NQ **Tel:** 01925653216 w 6413349

COOMBES Nichola Anne 13/04/2004 Royal Veterinary College Hawkshead Campus Hawkshead Lane North Mymms Hatfield Hertfordshire AL9 7TA **Tel:** (01707) 666665 w 6290952

COOMBS Rachel Anne 16/12/2005 1 Cheviot Way Oldland Common BRISTOL BS30 8QB w 6326317

COOPER Bernadette (see SIMS, Ms)

COOPER Carly Natasha 16/10/2007 84 MacDonald Avenue Hornchurch Essex RM11 2NE **Tel:** (01708) 475184 w 6386806

COOPER Carol Lynn (see BERRY, Mrs)

COOPER Cathryn Lesley (see JENNINGS, Mrs)

Charlene Barbara 10/09/2009 23 Captains Close Sutton Valence Maidstone Kent ME17 3BA **Tel:** (01622) 840298 w 6402745

Claire Elizabeth 02/02/1994 51 New Laithe Hill HUDDERSFIELD HD4 6RF **Tel:** (01484) 534623 w 6067387

Claire Louise 04/11/2005 Flat 4 513 Old Chester Road Rockferry BIRKENHEAD Merseyside CH42 4NG w 6332807

COOPER Danielle Louise (see URWIN, Mrs)

Emma Louise (nee Miss Hodson) 25/02/2004 80 Toad Hall Crescent Chattenden ROCHESTER Kent ME3 8PA w 6255477

Holly 28/09/2007 148 Newchapel Road Kidsgrove Stoke-on-Trent Staffordshire ST7 4RT **Tel:** (01782) 773099 w 6376873

Janet Linda 04/01/2006 22 Kings Avenue SUNBURY-ON-THAMES Middlesex TW16 7QE **Tel:** (01932) 761146 w 6344104

Julie Ann 25/06/2009 3 The Villas Foxt Road Foxt Stoke-on-Trent Staffordshire ST10 2HJ **Tel:** (01538) 266730 w 6433457

Laura Anne (nee Clarke) 18/01/1993 (12/07/2007) 40 Portesham Way Canford Heath Poole Dorset BH17 9HB **Tel:** (01202) 694606 w 6065426

Lisa (nee Frost) 24/08/1999 26 Hillview Bicknacre Chelmsford Essex CM3 4XD **Tel:** (01245) 227242 w 6185253

Lucy Jane 15/09/2009 47a Winchester Road Chandlers Ford Eastleigh Hampshire SO53 2GF **Tel:** (023) 8025 2543 w 6303668

Marta Elizabeth 29/06/2007 21 Stafford Street Aberdeen Aberdeenshire AB25 3UN w 6313326

COOPER Nadine Anne (see FLETCHER, Mrs)

Natasha Jayne 23/07/2001 Severn Veterinary Centre Berkeley House Berkeley Way Worcester Worcestershire WR4 9UP **Tel:** (01905) 756156 w 6040933

Rebecca Mary 24/05/2006 125 Victoria Road NORTHWICH Cheshire CW9 5RQ **Tel:** (01606) 330 136 w 6304394

Samantha Marika 13/03/2009 22 The Wickets MAIDENHEAD Berkshire SL6 6TT **Tel:** 01628630132 w 6435404

COOPER Sarah Louise (see CLOWES, Mrs)

COPELAND Barbara Anne (see JONES, Mrs)

COPLEY Emma 05/08/2003 47 Denhale Avenue Flanshaw Wakefield West Yorkshire WF2 9EG **Tel:** (0113) 2525818 w 6204360

COPPING Helen Louise 10/04/2007 63 Esk Avenue Whitehaven Cumbria CA28 8AL **Tel:** (01946) 696071 w 6346964

COPPOCK Cresta Ann (see BEDWELL, Mrs)

CORBETT Lesley Jayne (see LATHAM, Mrs)

CORBETT Michelle Patricia (nee Trigg) 29/01/1999 (27/05/2008) 21 Watch Elm Close Bradley Stoke BRISTOL BS32 8AL **Tel:** (0117) 9073206 w 6133603

Terri-Ann Coral (nee Young) 13/08/2002 (21/01/2009) Crossways Ruthin Road Coedpoeth WREXHAM Clwyd LL11 3US w 6270492

CORBIN Emma Jane 29/10/2004 Mainstone Veterinary Clinic Mainstone Romsey Hampshire SO51 6BA **Tel:** (01794) 513157 w 6254377

CORCORAN Maria May (nee Tyson) 10/12/2007 Orwell Veterinary Group Hartree Way Grange Farm Kesgrave Ipswich Suffolk IP5 2BZ **Tel:** (01473) 333677 w 6398169

Victoria Louise 22/08/2008 14 Farnborough Court Middleton St. George DARLINGTON County Durham DL2 1UH **Tel:** (01325) 335835 w 6409609

CORDER Katie Louise 16/06/2004 52 Shaftesbury Drive Maidstone Kent ME16 0JR **Tel:** (01622) 670470 w 6285221

CORFMAT Julie 13/07/2004 5 Bob Amor Close Faversham Kent ME13 8BW **Tel:** (07951) 094 434 w 6296133

CORKER Michelle Catherine 30/10/2007 20 Wayside Court Brimington CHESTERFIELD Derbyshire S43 1BS **Tel:** (01246) 235604 w 6403416

CORMACK Wendy Margaret 06/06/2003 2 East View Dacre Banks HARROGATE North Yorkshire HG3 4EQ w 6274551

CORNELIUS Trudy Irene 24/06/2004 4 Taunton Street BLACKPOOL FY4 3BH w 6284341

CORNER Hayley Ann (see ADDISON, Mrs)

CORNER Stephanie Louise 16/05/2006 Grove Farm Carlton Miniott THIRSK North Yorkshire YO7 4NJ **Tel:** (01845) 523 518 w 6333874

CORNES Kate Lindsey 15/07/2005 1 Newcastle Road Arclid SANDBACH Cheshire CW11 2UE **Tel:** (01477) 500310 w 6327505

CORNWELL Debbie Susan 20/01/1999 23 Wigton Crescent Bristol Avon BS10 6DU w 6137630

CORNWELL Laura Anne (see LANDER, Mrs)

CORREIA Marielsy Matty De Freitas 07/02/2005 (06/03/2009) 132 Sertina House Poynders Gardens London SW4 8PD **Tel:** (0208) 6751590 w 6294153

CORSON Anne Margaret PhD 16/08/1982 Eton Veterinary Clinic 31 London Road Tonbridge Kent TN10 3AB **Tel:** (01732) 352004 w 6010115

CORY Julie DipAVN(Medical) 25/01/1994 9 The Rookery BRANDON Suffolk IP27 0JZ w 6065845

COSGROVE Gemma Kate (nee Robson) 09/05/2005 28 Queens Road Seaton Sluice Tyne and Wear NE26 4DS **Tel:** (0191) 237 1089 w 6322093

Michelle Marie DipAVN(Surgical) (nee Furlong) 09/01/1990 (13/09/1999) 207 Daventry Road Coventry West Midlands CV3 5HH **Tel:** (02476) 503000 w 6050839

COSTELLO Melanie Jane 14/02/2000 P O Box 7733 Ashbourne Derbyshire DE6 9BQ w 6190687

Michael Peter De Lacy 02/03/1992 The Philippa & George Adams Centre 6 Amersham Vale New Cross London SE14 6LD **Tel:** (020) 8691 0577 m 6048251

Noleen Bridget 11/09/1986 The Flat 30-32 Newland Road Worthing West Sussex BN11 1JR w 6092890

COSTELLOE Lucy Ann 30/09/1983 (02/12/1999) 6 Westleigh Avenue LEICESTER LE3 0HG w 6048262

Samantha Rachel Joyce 09/07/2007 Warrenside Cottage The Warren Caversham READING RG4 7TQ **Tel:** (0118) 947 3508 w 6352519

COSTER Lauren Dawn 20/11/2009 53A Church Road ALDERSHOT Hampshire GU11 3PR **Tel:** 07791788047 w 6465434

COTTERILL Lindsay Anne (nee Bonsall) 19/03/2007 Alfreton Park Veterinary Hospital 216 King Street Alfreton Derbyshire DE55 7DF **Tel:** (01773) 832218 w 6375454

COTTLE Sarah 17/08/2005 45 Stanhope Drive Horsforth Leeds West Yorkshire LS18 4ES **Tel:** (0113) 2819663 w 6326053

COTTRELL Carol Yvonne 30/10/1990 7 Falkland Road Southport Merseyside PR8 6LG **Tel:** (01704) 501779 w 6048295

Jane DipAVN(Surgical) (nee Wilkinson) 06/08/1990 Donnington Grove Veterinary Surgery Oxford Road NEWBURY Berkshire RG14 2JB **Tel:** (01635) 47170 w 6063826

COULBORN Lisa Marie (nee Fildes) 22/08/2000 4 Est Bank Road Holcombe Brook Ramsbottom Bury Lancashire BL0 9RA w 6202358

COULTER Alison Ruth 10/03/2009 Flat 2 17 Buckhurst Road BEXHILL-ON-SEA East Sussex TN40 1QF w 6255950

COULTHARD Claire Elaine 11/03/2005 7 Howley Close Irlam Manchester M44 6RY w 6307815

COULTRUP Sarah Ruth (see FOWLER, Mrs)

COUND Clare Louise (see BUTCHER, Mrs)

COUPE Charlotte Ellen Louise (see GUYMER, Miss)

COURT Jennifer Mary 23/02/2005 14 Burlington Road New Malden Surrey KT3 4NY **Tel:** (020) 8942 2202 w 6318826

COURTNADGE Ruth 13/04/2004 Treig Kendoon Dalry St Johns Town of Dalry CASTLE DOUGLAS Kirkcudbrightshire DG7 3UB w 6289665

COUSINS Amanda Jayne 03/05/2005 123 Heathcote Road Whitnash Leamington Spa Warwickshire CV31 2LX **Tel:** (01926) 337790 w 6319266

COUTTS Pauline Jane 11/02/1998 16 Kellands Avenue Inverurie Aberdeenshire AB51 3YJ **Tel:** (01467) 622466 w 6107876

COVE Vivien Jean (nee Salt) 29/07/1977 134-136 Osmaston Road Derby Derbyshire DE1 2RF **Tel:** (01332) 345119 w 6048331

COWAN Jennifer Anne 06/08/2007 27 Seaview Terrace Edinburgh Midlothian EH15 2HD **Tel:** (0131) 669 5333 w 6373650

COWAP Deborah Jayne (see RODEN, Mrs)

COWARD Kirsty Louise (nee Howard) 12/07/2004 Capstone Sandley GILLINGHAM Dorset SP8 5DZ **Tel:** (01747) 825297 w 6302568

COWDEN Jane Alexandra (see HARDING, Mrs)

COWDEROY Mandy Colleen 30/07/1973 3 Sayerland Road Polegate East Sussex BN26 6NU **Tel:** (01323) 731450 w 6000297

COWIN Deborah Wilhelmina (see WILLIAMS, Mrs)

COWLEY Jane (see PARREN, Mrs)

COWLING Dawn Alison (see VOSE, Mrs)

COWNE Sarah Elizabeth 07/02/2006 23 Henbury House Gardens Sturminster Marshall WIMBORNE Dorset BH21 3TZ w 6330332

COX Andrew Martin 02/06/2006 Stone Lion Veterinary Centre 41 High Street Wimbledon London SW19 5AU **Tel:** (020) 8946 4228 m 6292525

Donna Alison DipAVN(Surgical) 08/10/1992 (17/08/2001) Hillocks Farm Stanton Ashbourne Derbyshire DE6 9DZ w 6006481

Emma Victoria 15/05/2009 55 Great Meadow Way AYLESBURY Buckinghamshire HP19 7GF **Tel:** 01844212000 w 6400237

Helen Louise 04/09/1997 (25/05/2005) Tremain Veterinary Practice Ltd 1 Farm Mill Lane WITNEY Oxfordshire OX28 4BJ **Tel:** (01993) 703146 w 6117192

Julia Louise 02/06/2004 Flat 6, South Mount High Road Whetstone LONDON N20 0PJ **Tel:** (020) 8908 0822 w 6290050

Julia Mary (nee Thomason) 29/07/1974 100 Heather Road Binley Woods Coventry West Midlands CV3 2DB **Tel:** (024) 7654 0036 w 6000377

COX Laura Catherine (see SMITH, Mrs)

Leila Alexandra 31/03/2003 13 All Saints Avenue Westbrook Margate Kent CT9 5QW **Tel:** (01843) 295662 w 6268358

COX Lisa Ann (see MANSFIELD, Mrs)

Michelle Elizabeth 06/02/2009 The Swallows Brockley Way Claverham BRISTOL BS49 4PT **Tel:** 01934834718 w 6419938

Samantha Jane 04/06/2009 56 Furze Lane Godalming Surrey GU7 3NP **Tel:** 07826928462 w 6418101

Stephanie Ruth 18/10/2006 Blacklands Cottage Cottles Lane Woodbury Exeter Devon EX5 1EE **Tel:** (01395) 233534 w 6347591

COX Suzanne Denise (see WOOD, Mrs)

Tracy Clare 13/03/2008 2 Langlands Stoke-sub-Hamdon Somerset TA14 6QA **Tel:** 07791269311 w 6400457

COXON Alison Kathleen Nancy 29/08/1997 (25/04/2002) Rainsbrook Veterinary Group 12 Upper Grove Street Leamington Spa Warwickshire CV32 5AN **Tel:** (01926) 422592 w 6038695

Zillah May (nee West) 10/02/2004 Hannam House Lamberts Lane Midhurst West Sussex GU29 9EA **Tel:** (01730) 816833 w 6292096

COYLE Victoria Elizabeth 09/02/2009 29 Basil Way South Shields Tyne and Wear NE34 8UA **Tel:** 07534996747 w 6426395

COZENS Susan Lilian (see NEWHAM, Ms)

CRABB Janice Elizabeth 15/11/2001 1 Chichester Close Ilfracombe Devon EX34 8PW **Tel:** (01271) 866 513 w 6262638

Kerrie Jacqueline Tugela 13/06/2008 376a High Street Aldershot Hampshire GU12 4NA **Tel:** (01252) 331638 w 6416363

CRADDOCK Alison Marie 14/01/2000 Melbourne House Veterinary Centre 60 Hednesford Street Cannock Staffordshire WS11 1DJ **Tel:** (01543) 502197 w 613607X

CRAIG Julie (nee Devine) 24/11/1998 (19/06/2008) 50 Niven Road INVERKEITHING Fife KY11 1EE **Tel:** (01383) 419110 w 6132326

Louise Elizabeth 29/06/2007 19 Stroan Road Dervock BALLYMONEY County Antrim BT53 8BZ **Tel:** (028) 207 42265 w 6326856

Suzanne 30/10/2003 (09/03/2009) 29 Lawrie Terrace LOANHEAD Midlothian EH20 9AR **Tel:** (0131) 448 1645 w 6282306

CRAIK Jillian Elizabeth 14/05/2007 Smithy House East Kilbride Road Rutherglen Glasgow G73 5QU **Tel:** (0141) 634 3183 w 6377632

Kim Alyson 08/06/2006 357-359 Anniesland Road GLASGOW G13 1XT **Tel:** (0141) 959 6100 w 6324458

CRANE Frances Elizabeth 28/02/2005 15 Nelson Road EXETER EX4 1BG **Tel:** (01392) 439975 w 6293361

CRANE Joanna Margaret (see TUCKER, Mrs)

CRANGLE Julia Elizabeth (see HENWOOD, Mrs)

CRAVEN Jane Matilda Margaret (see LAMONT, Mrs)

CRAVEN Jessica Amy 10/11/2009 Amery Veterinary Group Amery Hill Alton Hampshire GU34 1HS **Tel:** (01420) 82384 w 6431840

CRAWFORD Amanda Claire 19/04/2006 Westway Veterinary Centre 426-428 West Road Newcastle upon Tyne NE5 2ER **Tel:** (0191) 274 7910 w 6348372

CRAWFORD Jennifer Lorna (see CRAWFORD-ALLEN, Mrs)

Michelle Elizabeth 19/01/2000 Walnut Cottage West Street Thorne DONCASTER South Yorkshire DN8 5QU w 6116100

CRAWFORD-ALLEN Jennifer Lorna (nee Crawford) 29/12/1983 (26/10/2000) Cedar Grove Veterinary Clinic 132 Upper Knockbreda Road Belfast BT6 9QB **Tel:** (028) 9070 5777 w 6000457

CRAWLEY Harriet Loveday 01/09/2008 111 Market Street Musselburgh East Lothian EH21 6PZ **Tel:** (0131) 665 2124 w 6377434

CREIGHTON Dorothy Elizabeth DipAVN(Surgical) (nee Green) 14/09/1992 Sebright House Boreham Road Great Leighs Chelmsford Essex CM3 1PR **Tel:** (01245) 362 451 w 6006663

CRESSWELL Michelle (formerly Cresswell, formerly Isaacs) 17/07/2003 26 Desford Road Liverpool Merseyside L19 3RD **Tel:** 01514273844 w 6286607

CREWDSON Heather Frances 10/09/2009 South Lakes Veterinary Centre Victoria Road Ulverston Cumbria LA12 0BY **Tel:** (01229) 582900 w 6456315

CREWE Kerry Ann (see JACKSON, Mrs)

CRICHTON Victoria Louise 16/08/2006 14 Beattie Rise Hedge End SOUTHAMPTON Hampshire SO30 2RF w 6334171

CRISP Kirsten Louise 03/12/2003 (26/02/2009) 84 Kitchener Crescent Poole Dorset BH17 7HX **Tel:** (01425) 473683 w 6278401

CRITCHLEY Angela Margaret 05/06/2006 92 Acorn Way Woodthorpe YORK YO24 2RP **Tel:** (01904) 703353 w 6356666

CROCKETT Ann Mary 19/01/1998 8 Empress Avenue Woodford Green Essex IG8 9EA **Tel:** (020) 8558 5918 w 6107898

Gemma Louise 07/02/2007 14 Parsons Lawn North Shoeburyness Essex SS3 8BN **Tel:** (01702) 584 687 w 6299488

CROCOMBE Tracy (see CHARLES, Miss)

CROFT Angela Marie 23/09/2002 Forest Veterinary Centre 32 Waltham Road Woodford Green Essex IG8 8EB **Tel:** (020) 8505 4078 w 6272769

Sharon 04/10/2005 183 Cross Flatts Grove LEEDS LS11 7BR w 6346975

CROFTON Claire Louise 16/08/2006 7 Perry Street Gardens Chislehurst Kent BR7 6PT **Tel:** (07736) 111153 w 6351210

CROFTS Helen Felicity (nee Weaver) 05/04/2006 Oathall Veterinary Group 30 Oathall Road Haywards Heath West Sussex RH16 3EQ **Tel:** (01444) 440224 w 6331289

Helen Mary (nee Howell) 14/01/1988 20 Pentrebane Street Grangetown Cardiff CF11 7LL **Tel:** (029) 20252071 w 6000956

Jodie Ann 21/11/2005 14 Shortbrook Way Westfield Sheffield South Yorkshire S20 8LB w 6352728

Kimberley 22/12/1992 Drove Veterinary Hospital 252 Croft Road Swindon Wiltshire SN1 4RW **Tel:** (01793) 522483 w 6044177

CROLL Tina Marie 23/01/2008 66 Milner Road CATERHAM Surrey CR3 6JR w 6403009

CROMACK Lucy Alexandra (see AULD, Mrs)

CROMBIE Elaine (see MURRAY, Mrs)

CROMPTON Holli Louise Beale 29/04/2009 25 Ryall Road POOLE Dorset BH17 9FA **Tel:** 07710956801 w 6409565

Stacey Ann 07/02/2005 1 Whitley Avenue Latchford WARRINGTON WA4 1UN **Tel:** (01925) 658951 w 6327615

CROOK Samantha Patricia 29/08/2008 25 Cereleton Park Charlton Marshall Blandford Forum Dorset DT11 9PL **Tel:** 01258458926 w 6425713

Sarah Rachel DipAVN(Medical) 23/12/2003 Davies Veterinary Specialists Manor Farm Business Park Higham Gobion Hertfordshire SG5 3HR **Tel:** (01582) 883950 w 6278786

CROOKS Nicola Jayne 26/03/2008 2 Cherry Tree Close Romiley Stockport Cheshire SK6 4HD **Tel:** 07766410181 w 6406870

CROOM Charlotte Elizabeth 01/05/2009 1 Bitchams Mead Bere Regis Wareham Dorset BH20 7ND **Tel:** 01929471905 w 6443907

CROOME Yvonne Margaret (see GIRDWOOD, Mrs)

CROOSE Vanessa Margaret 27/02/2008 Grove Farm Huntington Kington Herefordshire HR5 3PJ **Tel:** (07960) 690 449 w 6410115

CROSIER Deborah Louise (see BIRCHER, Mrs)

CROSS Caroline May (nee Channon, formerly Stone) 15/01/1990 Seadown Veterinary Hospital Frost Lane Hythe Southampton Hampshire SO45 3NG **Tel:** (023) 8084 2237 w 6047520

Danielle Marie 02/09/2008 The Animal Hospital Stinchcombe Dursley Gloucestershire GL11 6AJ **Tel:** (01453) 542092 w 6421698

CROSS Elaine Marie (see CROSS-JOHNSON, Mrs)

Gail Susan (nee Roberts) 10/04/2003 L.I.T.E. Ltd 3a Church Street St. Helens Merseyside WA10 1BA **Tel:** (01744) 24062 w 6275002

Louise Claire 23/01/1995 (27/02/2002) Lite Ltd Training Agency 3a Church Street ST. HELENS Merseyside WA10 1BA **Tel:** (01744) 24062 w 6030754

Nicola Jane 09/04/2009 67 Garden Street HYDE Cheshire SK14 4AU **Tel:** (07809) 208408 w 6343686

CROSS-JOHNSON Elaine Marie (nee Cross) 04/08/2008 The Flat Garage Creslow Aylesbury Buckinghamshire HP22 4EH **Tel:** (01296) 715 660 w 6411622

CROSSLEY Angela Dawn (see JONAS, Mrs)

CROSSLEY Kathryn 06/08/2008 1 The Flat Town Head Farm Newbiggin PENRITH Cumbria CA11 0HT **Tel:** (01768) 487020 w 6417045

CROSSMAN Rebecca Elizabeth Jane (nee Esser) 13/08/2003 6 Fountain Mews Kelross Road Highbury London N5 2QH **Tel:** (020) 7272 3354 w 6287256

CROSSTHWAITE Helen Elizabeth (see ROONEY, Mrs)

CROUCH Andrea Jane 18/06/2008 9 Huntingdon Road Southend-on-Sea Essex SS1 2XU **Tel:** (01702) 464 808 w 6403636

Heather Jane 27/11/2009 54 Old Chapel Road Swanley Kent BR8 8LJ **Tel:** (01322) 662838 w 6406045

Kirsty Alexandra (nee Moir) 11/02/2009 79 Robertson Road DUNFERMLINE Fife KY12 0AR **Tel:** 01383726031 w 6429310

CROUCHER Louise Elaine 17/03/2009 Berry House Veterinary Practice 41 Nightingale Road HITCHIN Hertfordshire SG5 1RE **Tel:** (01462) 451 500 w 6413371

Natalie Isabelle (nee Haggett) 05/04/2005 (04/04/2008) 92 Willow Close St. Georges WESTON-SUPER-MARE Avon BS22 7SF w 6307870

CROUCHER Tristan Mark (see REID-CROUCHER, Mr)

CROW Aimee Lynda Marie 18/01/2008 Ash Croft Veterinary Surgery 169 St. Neots Road Hardwick CAMBRIDGE CB23 7QJ w 6353773

Rebecca Leann 12/05/2004 Hykeham Green Lincoln Road North Hykeham Lincoln Lincolnshire LN6 8NH **Tel:** (01522) 683300 w 6296144

CROWE Lisa (nee Mansfield) 23/07/1993 19 Hill Top Way Stanton Bury St. Edmunds IP31 2EB **Tel:** (01359) 252 368 w 6015317

CROWELL Stacey Michelle 19/03/2007 7 Berries Avenue Bude Cornwall EX23 8QE **Tel:** 01288354632 w 6378072

CROWLEY Clair Elizabeth 22/02/2007 Maindee House Veterinary Surgeon Mount Pleasant Road Pontnewydd Cwmbran Gwent NP44 1AN **Tel:** (01633) 483208 w 6349351

Ita Carmel 11/08/1989 Flat 2 Westergate 20 Corfton Road LONDON W5 2HT w 6048546

CROWSON Claire Rebecca 24/11/2009 76 Rosewood Close TAMWORTH Staffordshire B77 3PD **Tel:** (01827) 61118 w 6490536

CROWTHER Charlotte Anne 20/11/2002 218 Huddersfield Road Shelley Huddersfield HD8 3LH w 6280018

CRUICKSHANK Claire 02/06/2008 283 Lee Crescent North Bridge of Don Aberdeen Aberdeenshire AB22 8GF **Tel:** (01224) 820170 w 6379480

CRUM Lee-Ann 06/03/2006 (06/08/2009) 22 Orchard Street Baillieston GLASGOW G69 7XA w 6283857

CRUMP Jessica Jane (nee Wilson) 03/02/1999 The Cheshire Pet Medical Centre Ltd Manor Lane

Holmes Chapel Crewe Cheshire CW4 8AB **Tel:** (01477) 544 554 w 6116712

Louise Jane 10/10/2005 38 Clyde Street Hilton Derby Derbyshire DE65 5ND **Tel:** (01283) 732662 w 6320982

Rosie Scott 11/11/2009 Elm Cottage Brockham Green Brockham BETCHWORTH Surrey RH3 7JS **Tel:** (01737) 842293 w 6496179

CRUNDWELL Sophie Gabrielle 24/09/2008 Cobblers Yard Farmhouse Leggs Lane Langton Green Tunbridge Wells Kent TN3 0RQ **Tel:** (01892) 520 296 w 6390150

CRUTCHLEY Mandy Nicola (see LEWIS, Mrs)

CRUZ David Richard 24/02/2004 Garland Cottage 22 Church Street SOUTH BRENT Devon TQ10 9BE m 6286618

CUBLEY Zoe Anne 27/03/2008 11 Anchor Way Pill Bristol Avon BS20 0JY **Tel:** (01275) 371544 w 6414449

CUDE Joanne Frances (see BAYFORD, Mrs)

CULLEN Jasmine Therese 14/01/2008 30 Medway Drive WELLINGBOROUGH Northamptonshire NN8 5XT **Tel:** (01933) 392935 w 6397861

CULLEN Josephine (see JONES, Mrs)

Louise 07/02/2006 20 Fen Avenue FAREHAM Hampshire PO16 0TD **Tel:** (01329) 288845 w 6353784

CULLEN Louise N G (see GLYSEN, Mrs)

Teresa Jane 18/10/2006 Manor Veterinary Centre 113-119 Kent Road Halesowen West Midlands B62 8PB **Tel:** (0121) 422 5411 w 6355148

CULLEY Deborah Jane 30/04/1975 39 Westbury Lane Newport Pagnell Buckinghamshire MK16 8PN **Tel:** (01908) 614509 w 6048568

CULLUM-HANSHAW Kathryn Sarah DipAVN(Surgical) (nee Hanshaw) 02/09/1988 2 Sibleys Terrace School Road Terrington St John PE14 7SH **Tel:** (01945) 880 624 w 6052257

CULSHAW Natalie 05/04/2005 39 Broughton Road WALLASEY Merseyside CH44 4DT **Tel:** (07944) 364035 w 6284572

CULVER Amy Elizabeth 12/09/2008 22 Highland Drive LOUGHBOROUGH Leicestershire LE11 2HU w 6425779

Olivia Jane 30/11/2006 15 Springfield Grove Bristol Avon BS6 7XG **Tel:** (0117) 942 7661 w 6367589

CUMBERBEACH Nicola Lyn 09/09/2004 45 Liberty Hall Road ADDLESTONE Surrey KT15 1SS **Tel:** (01932) 842 406 w 6313700

CUMBRIDGE Nicola Susan 05/12/2007 18 Pound Road CHATTERIS Cambridgeshire PE16 6RL w 6398257

CUMMINGS Kate Alison (nee Hersey, formerly Haynes) 26/08/1997 Jilmar Biltur Road Ipplepen Newton Abbot Devon TQ12 5QL **Tel:** (01803) 812565 w 6108596

Melanie (nee Dick) 07/08/1989 (03/03/2006) 41 Beckingthorpe Drive Bottesford Nottingham NG13 0DN **Tel:** (01949) 842916 w 6049164

CUMMINS Wendy Jane DipAVN(Surgical), DipAVN (Medical) 28/01/1992 Prospect Veterinary Centre 1 Wakefield Road Sowerby Bridge West Yorkshire HX6 2AP **Tel:** (01422) 833960 w 6048615

CUMNER Charlotte Ann 13/11/2007 Green Pastures Veterinary Centre Green Pastures Moor Lane Weston-super-Mare Somerset BS24 7LA **Tel:** (01934) 622022 w 6387279

CUNDY Laura Marilyn (nee Brown) 28/08/1998 (10/11/2009) 3 Chipperfield Drive BRISTOL BS15 4DP **Tel:** (0117) 967 4688 w 6112514

CUNLIFFE Gemma Irene (see MACALISTER, Mrs)

CUNLIFFE Samantha Jayne 17/09/2007 PDSA 7 Warwick Road Old Trafford Manchester M16 0JW **Tel:** (0161) 862 9530 w 6376884

CUNNINGHAM Jacqueline Margaret (see RIDDELL, Mrs)

CUNNINGHAM Vanessa Louise (nee Coffey) 15/05/1990 47 Caledonian Road Stamford Lincolnshire PE9 2TG **Tel:** (01780) 765473 w 6047848

CUPPENS Philippiene Francisca Adrianna 14/12/2006 Veterinary Health Centre 11 Market Place Wymondham Norfolk NR18 0AS **Tel:** (01953) 600066 w 6340507

CURETON Julie 09/03/2001 Riversdale 1 Finsbury Avenue YORK YO23 1LW **Tel:** (07719) 253473 w 6213919

CURNOW Sarah Louise 04/12/2003 The Veterinary Centre Drump Road Redruth Cornwall TR15 1PS **Tel:** (01209) 214737 w 6277532

Tanya Cara 24/05/2006 22 Courtland Drive Queensferry Deeside Clwyd CH5 1UQ **Tel:** (01244) 810090 w 6347602

CURRAGH Lindsay Dawn 19/08/2008 8 Knock Green Belfast County Antrim BT5 6GJ **Tel:** 07849139902 w 6351232

CURRAN Jemma Lorraine 11/01/2005 (07/02/2007) 12 Station Avenue North Fencehouses Houghton Le Spring Tyne and Wear DH4 6HS w 6317176

Ruth Ann 08/01/2008 80 Bishops Court Road Downpatrick County Down BT30 7PD **Tel:** (028) 44841574 w 6366280

CURRIE Joanna Kathryn 21/07/2008 Flat 1 196 Worple Road Wimbledon LONDON SW20 8PN w 6378237

CURRY Adele Louise 18/10/2006 41 Byram Park Road Byram Knottingley West Yorkshire WF11 9EA w 6351595

CURRY Sharon (see JENKINSON, Mrs)

CURTIN Frances Louise 10/11/2008 7 St. Helens Place Armadale BATHGATE West Lothian EH48 3EX **Tel:** (01501) 739581 w 6408729

CURTIS Jennifer Dawn (see BRAITHWAITE, Mrs)

CURTIS Laura 11/04/2005 43 Vandyck Avenue Keynsham BRISTOL BS31 2UH **Tel:** (0117) 9861995 w 6301468

Sharon Louise 01/09/2008 32 Chilcompton Road Midsomer Norton RADSTOCK BA3 2PQ w 6436339

CUSACK Clare Joanna 14/09/2009 2A Acacia Road HAMPTON Middlesex TW12 3DS **Tel:** 07738364209 w 6346161

CUTLER Bonnie (nee Williams) 15/04/2009 30 School Road BRIERLEY HILL West Midlands DY5 1BE **Tel:** (01384) 361075 w 6386894

CUTLER Victoria (see MILNE, Mrs)

CUTMORE Heather Ann 06/02/2009 18 Galeborough Avenue Woodford Green Essex IG8 9PL **Tel:** 02085279654 w 6371582

D

DACUNHA Keeley Jane 11/05/2004 Donaldson & Partners Miry Lane Thongsbridge HOLMFIRTH HD9 7RY **Tel:** (01484) 684189 w 6284660

DAGGER Sarah Harcourt (nee Wilsdon) 24/01/1997 (03/06/2003) 35 Thestfield Drive Staverton TROWBRIDGE Wiltshire BA14 8TT **Tel:** (01225) 774486 w 6027366

DAGLISH Katie Anne 19/03/2007 18 Field Street Shepshed Loughborough Leicestershire LE12 9AL **Tel:** (01509) 503850 w 6374046

DAKEYNE Georgina Katie 17/02/2009 1 Village Street Petersfield Hampshire GU32 2AH **Tel:** 07929636819 w 6447152

DALBY Anna Jane 01/03/2000 Daws Cottage Loxbeare Tiverton Devon EX16 9RH **Tel:** (01884) 881332 w 6190742

DALE Rebecca Alison (nee Richardson) 30/11/2006 71 Simmance Way Amesbury Salisbury Wiltshire SP4 7TB **Tel:** (01980) 626 598 w 6375190

D'ALELIO Nadia 21/03/2007 9 London Road Yaxley Peterborough Cambridgeshire PE7 3NG **Tel:** (01733) 243 078 w 6375718

DALLOW Mary Josephine (nee Nugent) 25/04/1975 (12/12/2005) Windward Jacob Ladder Lane Claines Worcester WR3 7RT **Tel:** (01905) 455 538 w 6075263

DALLY Louise (nee May) 09/04/1998 Tredower Farm St. Minver WADEBRIDGE Cornwall PL27 6RG **Tel:** (01208) 813018 w 6131118

DALY Kelly Alexandra 06/08/2007 57 Manorbier Crescent Rumney Cardiff South Glamorgan CF3 3NE **Tel:** (029) 2079 9322 w 6359130

Leigh Crawford (nee Stone) 01/03/2001 (08/02/2005) 5 Ardgay Road BONNYBRIDGE Stirlingshire FK4 2FL **Tel:** (01236) 630648 w 6132825

Nicola Diane (nee Drayner) 23/07/1993 33 Main Street Denton NORTHAMPTON NN7 1DQ **Tel:** (01604) 891825 w 6005411

DAMANT Hayley marie (see EADE, Mrs)

DANDO Melanie Kate 11/05/2004 24 Abbeydale Road South Sheffield South Yorkshire S7 2QN **Tel:** (0114) 2363391 w 6290523

DANIEL Maya Kristina Nadine (see YATES, Mrs)

Nerys Angharad 14/01/2008 Church Lane Llanbadarn Fawr Aberystwyth Dyfed SY23 3QU **Tel:** (01970) 612526 w 6377643

DANIELL Joanne Elizabeth (see MASON, Mrs)

DANIELLS Claire Elizabeth 23/10/2001 Lyndale Moorend Grove Cheltenham Gloucestershire GL53 0EX **Tel:** (01242) 517199 w 6259228

DANIELS Laura Jane 27/01/2009 14 Kestrel Close Congleton Cheshire CW12 3FA **Tel:** 07821755400 w 6442026

Lois DipAVN(Surgical) 22/01/1985 Norton Radstock College Ellsbridge House Bath Road Keynsham Bristol BS31 1TL **Tel:** (01179) 863898 w 6048728

Lucy Jane (nee Bullock) 01/04/2003 2 Dyas Road Kingstanding Birmingham B44 8SF **Tel:** (0121) 377 7215 w 6280931

Rosanna Clare 14/05/2007 Pinewood Veterinary Practice 23 Crown Street Chorley Lancashire PR7 1DX **Tel:** (01257) 276517 w 6377654

DANN Nichola Louise (see HATCH, Mrs)

DARBY Lynn DipAVN(Surgical) (nee Jones) 09/11/1988 (03/06/2003) University of Glasgow Veterinary School Garscube Estate Glasgow G61 1QH **Tel:** (0141) 330 5848 w 6054210

DARBY Victoria Anne (see PHEYSEY, Mrs)

DARBYSHIRE Emma Jane (see ROBY, Mrs)

DARLING Emma Louise (nee Havercroft) 01/09/1997 126 Linton Woods Lane Linton on Ouse York North Yorkshire YO30 2TF **Tel:** (01347) 848880 w 6117680

Fiona Menzies 08/06/2006 10 Glenbrook Road Balerno Midlothian EH14 7BE **Tel:** (0131) 449 3751 w 6324469

DARLOW Gemma-Chantel Patricia 17/04/2008 13 Gladstone Road MARGATE Kent CT9 5ST **Tel:** 07969906734 w 6410159

DARNELL Georgina Jayne 30/12/2008 Chase Veterinary Group 103-105 London Road St. Leonards-on-Sea East Sussex TN37 6AT **Tel:** (01424) 424870 w 6425658

DAVEY Hayley Claire 27/01/2010 Flat 2 New Era Veterinary Hospital Victoria Road St. Saviour JERSEY JE2 7QG **Tel:** 07700332286 w 6580043

Laura Rachel 12/02/2009 Salathiel Grove Road Cranleigh Surrey GU6 7LH **Tel:** 07843005861 w 6374651

Louise Clare (nee Abbott) 10/10/2005 3 Orchard Close Burringham Scunthorpe South Humberside DN17 3UT **Tel:** (01724) 783500 w 6331927

Marie DipAVN(Surgical) 21/01/1999 (26/10/2000) 171 Worthing Road Rustington Littlehampton West Sussex BN16 3PR **Tel:** (01903) 785 235 w 6117261

Tamzin 14/05/2003 21 Ventonlace Grampound Road Truro Cornwall TR2 4TA **Tel:** (01726) 883046 w 6285859

DAVIDSON Anna Katherine 24/11/2004 (17/09/2008) Mayhew Animal Home Trenmar Gardens LONDON NW10 6BJ **Tel:** (020) 8969 7110 w 6261945

Jane 28/02/2005 The Garden Flat 21 Muswell Road LONDON N10 2BJ w 6289830

Karen Jayne (nee Wood) 28/08/1991 6 Oxford Road Wakefield West Yorkshire WF1 3LB **Tel:** (01924) 376813 w 6064171

Pauline Anne 28/06/2005 59 Mile End Place Inverness Inverness-Shire IV3 8JH **Tel:** (01463) 238878 w 6316769

DAVIES Bethan Helen 07/02/2006 28 Buckfield Road Leominster Herefordshire HR6 8SF **Tel:** (01568) 611066 w 6350297

Carly Jane 24/05/2005 49 Summerhill Avenue NEWPORT Gwent NP19 8FQ w 6319695

Carrie Ann (nee Keoghane) 27/09/1999 The Croeso Veterinary Hospital Ltd 111 Whitchurch Road Cardiff CF14 3JQ **Tel:** (029) 2061 9899 w 6149191

DAVIES Claire Louise (see GRIFFITHS, Mrs)

DAVIES Emma (see ARCHER, Mrs)

Gaynor Elizabeth 07/01/1986 (04/04/2007) Willow Pool Toll Bar Cross CHULMLEIGH Devon EX18 7AF w 6048808

Gemma 13/07/2004 85 Walden Close Ouston Chester le Street County Durham DH2 1TG **Tel:** (0191) 3701511 w 6296661

Gemma Frances 24/05/2002 27 Bulkeley Street Stockport Cheshire SK3 9HD **Tel:** (0161) 4776680 w 6205581

Hannah Elizabeth (nee Cook) 11/05/2004 49 Wentworth Way Doddington Park LINCOLN LN6 0WE **Tel:** (07970) 782790 w 6290325

Janine Marie 27/04/2006 (19/06/2008) 114 Riesling Drive LIVERPOOL L33 1SH **Tel:** (0151) 548 0121 w 6346733

Jennifer Annette 10/02/2005 Hartlepool Vets4pets Ltd Unit 2, Belle Vue Neighbourhood Hartlepool Cleveland TS25 1QF **Tel:** (01429) 224555 w 6318408

Kathryn Ann 29/06/2007 (03/02/2009) Lowesmoor House Veterinary Centre 18 Rainbow Hill Worcester WR3 8LX **Tel:** (01905) 723361 w 6293229

Kelly (nee Russ) 24/12/2002 PDSA PAH Tuxford Close Wolverhampton WV10 0JQ **Tel:** (01902) 459555 w 6283945

Laura Leigh 22/05/2009 Flat 2 Lletty Nedd Pen Y Dre Neath West Glamorgan SA11 3HH **Tel:** (01639) 642739 w 6418211

Lauren Elizabeth 12/12/2005 (08/07/2008) 7 Graig Park Avenue NEWPORT Gwent NP20 6GZ **Tel:** (01633) 770101 w 6263232

Leanne (nee Richardson) 08/01/2008 1 Hillside Abercych BONCATH Dyfed SA37 0HD **Tel:** (07890) 503094 w 6411897

Linda 26/08/1999 (08/02/2005) 61 Ratcliffe Drive Stoke Gifford Bristol Avon BS34 8TX **Tel:** (07761) 737215 w 6135123

Lisa Michelle 03/01/2008 Ty Newydd Llanwddyn Oswestry Shropshire SY10 0LZ **Tel:** (01691) 870 659 w 6390381

Louise Marie (nee Walters) 23/02/2005 Unit A1 Priestley Road Wardley Business Park Worsley Manchester M28 2LY **Tel:** (0161) 794 4999 w 6296892

DAVIES Marian (see ADDISON, Mrs)

DAVIES Michelle Joanne (see TAYLOR, Mrs)

DAVIES Nicola (see HOPKINS, Mrs)

Nicola Joanne 12/02/2009 102 Parc y Fro Creigiau Cardiff South Glamorgan CF15 9SB **Tel:** 02920892706 w 6415153

Rachael Louise (nee Foster) 10/10/2008 58 Northgate Pontefract West Yorkshire WF8 1HJ **Tel:** (01977) 600588 w 6276014

Rebecca Megan 17/01/2006 Blaven 5 Drybourne Avenue Shildon County Durham DL4 1HZ **Tel:** (01388) 772734 w 6324491

DAVIES Rosemary Ann (see HUGHES, Mrs)

Samantha Jane 18/10/2005 60 Cinder Road DUDLEY West Midlands DY3 2RJ w 6332565

Sara Elizabeth 01/09/1997 Inglebury Wesley Hill Machen Caerphilly Mid Glamorgan CF83 8QH **Tel:** (01633) 440 892 w 6099036

Tammy 10/12/2002 (18/03/2009) Afallon Maesycrugiau PENCADER Carmarthenshire SA39 9DN **Tel:** (01570) 480746 w 6277554

Tracey Louise (nee Mawer) 28/08/1997 8 Lilac Drive Penyffordd Chester CH4 0GF **Tel:** (01244) 545725 w 6116290

Victoria Clare 19/03/2007 34 Tyisha Road Llanelli Dyfed SA15 1RW **Tel:** (01554) 774817 w 6330706

DAVIS Amanda Carol 08/09/2005 22 Parkside Road Pinhoe EXETER EX1 3TN **Tel:** (01392) 469328 w 6305263

Andrea 29/12/2003 Christchurch Veterinary Surgery 49 Christchurch Street Ipswich Suffolk IP4 2DF **Tel:** (01473) 255789 w 6293097

Catherine Anne 03/05/2007 1 Kings Road High Wycombe Buckinghamshire HP11 1SA **Tel:** (078) 869 42491 w 6376400

Claire Joanne 18/10/2005 (18/11/2009) 2 Sunshine Terrace TAVISTOCK Devon PL19 0HT **Tel:** (07766) 770475 w 6323270

Constance 21/09/1976 (16/03/2004) 15 Cissbury Road Ferring Worthing West Sussex BN12 6QJ **Tel:** (01903) 507354 w 6048841

Craig Anthoney 10/08/2007 47 Ibstock Close Redditch Worcestershire B98 0PH **Tel:** 01527525451 m 6376411

Elizabeth Jean 27/12/2007 34 Geltsdale Avenue Carlisle Cumbria CA1 2RL **Tel:** 07932522868 w 6401139

Helen Elizabeth 26/10/2005 Davies Veterinary Specialists Manor Farm Business Park Higham Gobion Hertfordshire SG5 3HR **Tel:** (01582) 883950 w 6288576

DAVIS Hellen Paula (see JORDAN, Mrs)

Julie Ann (nee Clare) 31/08/1999 Guide Dogs, Tollgate House Banbury Road Bishops Tachbrook Leamington Spa Warwickshire CV33 9QJ **Tel:** (01926) 651226 w 6117115

DAVIS June Ann (see ROGERS, Mrs)

Katrina Louise 07/02/2007 Leadon Vale Veterinary Centre Lower Road Trading Estate Ledbury Herefordshire HR8 2DJ **Tel:** (01531) 632276 w 6349527

Kay Helen 29/01/2010 Birchcroft Churchill Avenue Hatfield DONCASTER South Yorkshire DN7 6LU **Tel:** 07703492431 w 6466479

Kelly Louise 28/02/2005 Abbotsbury St. Marys Road Meare Glastonbury Somerset BA6 9SS **Tel:** (01458) 860 289 w 6297508

DAVIS Lianne (see TIFFNEY, Mrs)

DAVIS Samantha Rebecca (see POSNER, Mrs)

Sara Louise 22/12/2004 (25/02/2009) Rouken Glen Veterinary Surgery East Lodge Rouken Glen Road Giffnock Glasgow G46 6UG w 6260251

Sarah Jane 19/07/2004 13 Brook End LONGHOPE Gloucestershire GL17 0QT w 6267764

Tracy Louise 06/08/2008 Teignview Veterinary Group Hospital Hill Dawlish Devon EX7 9NS **Tel:** (01626) 862020 w 6321191

DAVISON Amanda Jane (see ELLIS, Mrs)

DAVISON Emma 30/10/2007 70A Devon Drive Brimington CHESTERFIELD Derbyshire S43 1DY **Tel:** (01246) 209625 w 6403438

Karen Louise 13/07/2007 3 Briton Close South Croydon Surrey CR2 0JH **Tel:** (07720) 328330 w 6347459

Pauline Elizabeth 09/04/2009 219 Killinchy Road Comber Newtownards County Down BT23 6AB **Tel:** (028) 97541334 w 6253112

DAVISON-WHITE Nicola 15/02/2005 Oakwood Redford Hamsterley Forest BISHOP AUCKLAND County Durham DL13 3NL **Tel:** (07939) 435 790 w 6307826

DAVY Rebecca Emma 26/03/2008 3 Ralph Cottages Ford Manor Road Dormansland Surrey RH7 6NZ **Tel:** (01342) 835071 w 6410269

DAW Emma Melinda 27/11/2000 Flat 2 Fairfield House New Town UCKFIELD East Sussex TN22 5DG w 6204338

DAW Lisa Jayne (see COLLINS, Mrs)

DAWES Sharon 27/07/1992 8 Cranwell Close Shenley Brook End Milton Keynes Buckinghamshire MK5 7BU **Tel:** (01908) 506776 w 6050602

DAWSON Kim Jennifer Rachel 04/02/2002 34 Garlondes East Harling NORWICH NR16 2NR w 6257270

Kim Louisa 06/12/2004 1 Woodlands Place Banchory Kincardineshire AB31 5ZP **Tel:** (01330) 823830 w 6289841

Louise Victoria 02/06/2004 11 Jackson Way Quinton Birmingham B32 1BS **Tel:** (0121) 4221068 w 6290710

DAY Amanda Jane (nee Lock) 23/02/2005 35 St. Johns Road WINCHESTER Hampshire SO23 0HQ **Tel:** (01962) 620477 w 6317253

DAY Angela (see PORTER, Mrs)

Kelly Anne 11/07/2005 158 Chingford Mount Road Chingford London E4 9BS **Tel:** (020) 8529 0111 w 6305527

DAY Nicola Anne (see JOHNSON, Mrs)

Sarah Louise 13/04/2004 The Old Barn Quemerford Gate Cherhill Calne Wiltshire SN11 8UL w 6283802

Tara Louise 05/04/2005 Moorland Veterinary Centre St. Lukes House Vicarage Road Leek Staffordshire ST13 6AS **Tel:** (01538) 382129 w 6317429

Victoria Louise 02/11/2004 28 Lower Church Road COWES Isle of Wight PO31 8JG w 6297684

DAYKIN Stephanie Jane 01/12/2008 70 North Park Fakenham Norfolk NR21 9RQ **Tel:** 01328856325 w 6443753

DE LA COUR Georgia Elisabeth 07/04/2003 New Era Veterinary Hospital Victoria Road St Saviour Jersey JE2 7QG **Tel:** (01534) 730521 w 6269117

DEACON Jessica Fay (nee Smith) 16/09/2008 4 Mitre Pitch WOTTON-UNDER-EDGE Gloucestershire GL12 7JP **Tel:** 01453520374 w 6437945

Kathleen Teresa 27/09/2004 Flat 2, Sileby Hall Cossington Road Sileby Loughborough Leicestershire LE12 7RS **Tel:** (0116) 2693711 w 6323281

DEAKIN Patricia Anne (nee Evans) 30/05/2007 2 Black & White Cottages Pulford Drive Eccleston CHESTER CH4 9JH w 6383165

DEAMER Camilla 04/03/2009 242 Ladyshot HARLOW Essex CM20 3EU **Tel:** 01279302953 w 6428980

DEAN Carrie Kendra 20/11/2009 9 Eastfield Avenue Scartho GRIMSBY South Humberside DN33 2PD **Tel:** 01472581758 w 6449539

Cassandra Lillian 04/02/2009 The Veterinary Hospital Cannock Road Penkridge Stafford ST19 5RY **Tel:** (01785) 712235 w 6444116

Donna Therese 28/04/2008 137 Bottleacre Lane Loughborough Leicestershire LE11 1JF **Tel:** (01509) 214057 w 6404956

Lesley Fiona (nee Saunders) 16/04/1999 (31/10/2005) Brook Farm Harleston Road Rushall DISS Norfolk IP21 4RT **Tel:** (01379) 853306 w 6137572

DEANE Caroline Sophie (see REEDER, Mrs)

DEANE Helen Lorraine 11/07/2005 19 Fernhurst Crescent BRIGHTON BN1 8FA w 6301479

DEAR Emily Jane 15/04/2009 48 Guest Road Eastleigh Hampshire SO50 6AQ **Tel:** 07894076851 w 6438209

DEBBAGE Nikki Marie 16/08/2007 15 Uplands Road North Carlton Colville LOWESTOFT Suffolk NR33 8AZ **Tel:** (01502) 569 404 w 6328935

DEBNAM Alison Clare (see ROBINSON, Mrs)

DECRUZ Karen Ann (nee Honey) 22/08/1994 (11/09/2006) 106 Bridge Lane FRODSHAM Cheshire WA6 7HZ w 6024922

DEDMAN Janet Lois (see HARRIS, Mrs)

DEEGAN Vera Catherine (see ROGERS, Mrs)

DEER Laura Susan 21/06/2002 (11/08/2006) Ark Veterinary Centre 14 Church Lane Lexden Colchester Essex CO3 4AF **Tel:** (01206) 572410 w 6269249

DEFRIES Claire Ilana Natalie DipAVN(Medical) 30/10/2001 77 New Road Croxley Green Rickmansworth Hertfordshire WD3 3EN **Tel:** (01923) 772388 w 6267159

DEGNAN Laura 06/09/2007 214 Bath Road Kettering Northamptonshire NN16 9LZ **Tel:** (01536) 525124 w 6323292

DELESTINNE Linde Peggy Ive 21/02/2008 Grote Molenweg 81A Herent 3020 Belgium **Tel:** (0032) 162 03151 w 6503131

DELL Janet 03/02/1997 (13/03/2003) 71 Larkholme Parade Fleetwood Lancashire FY7 8QY **Tel:** (01253) 779042 w 6098688

DELLOU Sarra Jean Nadwa 11/11/2009 2 The Gallops Roke Bere Regis WAREHAM Dorset BH20 7JN **Tel:** 07854422704 w 6489293

DELOOZE Leanne (nee Hipperson) 13/04/2004 14 Barrymore Avenue Warrington Cheshire WA4 1RT **Tel:** (01925) 491937 w 6300456

DEMETRIOU Jessica Rachel 13/11/2006 Rosemullion Veterinary Practice Isaac House Angel Centre Tyacke Road Helston Cornwall TR13 8RR **Tel:** (01326) 572596 w 6296672

DENBY Claire Louise 24/04/2009 1 Drysdale Close Firhouse Road West Tallaght Dublin 24 Ireland **Tel:** (00353) 87 6729300 w 6549606

DENCH Sara Pamela 17/01/2008 2 The Green Thurlby Bourne Lincolnshire PE10 0EB **Tel:** (01778) 420 462 w 6398301

DENHOLM Stephanie Louise 07/12/2005 34 Moray Park Terrace Culloden INVERNESS IV2 7RW **Tel:** (01463) 798060 w 6317187

DENISE CLAIRE Barter (see BARTER, Miss)

DENMAN Nicola Michelle 30/10/2003 Pilgrims St. James Road FLEET Hampshire GU51 3YX w 6282955

DENNESS Daniel John 05/04/2005 (26/01/2007) 9 Oak Farm Gardens Headcorn Ashford Kent TN27 9TZ **Tel:** (01662) 891894 m 6292998

DENNEY Georgina Louise 19/04/2005 Beacons Veterinary Centre Ashfield Place Llanfaes Brecon Powys LD3 8EG **Tel:** (01874) 622464 w 6292778

DENNING Joanne Catherine 24/11/2004 White House Bartlow Road Ashdon SAFFRON WALDEN Essex CB10 2HY **Tel:** (01799) 584 355 w 6319123

DENNINGTON Sandra Christine (nee Dennington, formerly Dennington-Crane) 25/01/1988 (21/07/1999) 30 Eastbury Close Bowers Brook Widnes Cheshire WA8 9WW **Tel:** (0151) 420 7718 w 6014368

DENNINGTON-CRANE Sandra Christine (see DENNINGTON, Miss)

DENNIS Georgina Brenda (see HILLS, Mrs)

DENNIS Natalie Chantal 21/03/2007 1 Queens Court Doncaster South Yorkshire DN5 9QE **Tel:** (01302) 787 023 w 6346986

DENNISON Michele Marie 06/12/2004 Dean Cottage Dean Bottom South Darenth Dartford Kent DA4 9JX **Tel:** (07980) 33 95 73 w 6284495

DENT Alana 09/05/2008 34 Marjoram Place Conniburrow Milton Keynes Buckinghamshire MK14 7AQ **Tel:** (01908) 610982 w 6418134

Emma Louise 07/02/2008 30 Arnold Close Castle Gresley Swadlincote Derbyshire DE11 9HF **Tel:** (01283) 213707 w 6323974

Jillian Renee 13/08/1964 17 Ancton Way Elmer Sands Bognor Regis West Sussex PO22 6JW **Tel:** (01243) 585666 w 6049095

Tamasina Louise 04/01/2006 36 Boston Road Kirton Boston Lincolnshire PE20 1DS **Tel:** (01205) 722696 w 6251033

DENTICE Laura Ellen 16/04/2008 Stanton Hall Stanton Morpeth Northumberland NE65 8PR **Tel:** 01670772641 w 6402789

DENTON Rebecca Clare (see SWINDELLS, Mrs)

DERNIE Michelle Elizabeth 11/12/2009 259 Bilton Road Rugby Warwickshire CV22 7EQ **Tel:** (01788) 812650 w 6432896

DERRIMAN Emma Jennifer 22/10/2008 56 Ladies Mile Road Patcham BRIGHTON BN1 8QF **Tel:** (01273) 727433 w 6400435

DERRY Marie Linda 08/01/2008 12 Christchurch Road Hucknall Nottingham Nottinghamshire NG15 6SA **Tel:** 01159636735 w 6400017

Stephanie Jayne (formerly Stephanie Jayne) 28/04/2006 1-5 Hugh Street London SW1V 1QQ **Tel:** (020) 7932 2370 w 6299499

DERWENT Rebecca Eloise 29/09/2009 15 Ash Close Bitterne Southampton SO19 5SD **Tel:** 07821423869 w 6492648

DESODT Lee Marylyn Phyllis 27/10/2009 25/6 South Clerk Street EDINBURGH EH8 9JD **Tel:** 07516959163 w 6379579

DEVANEY Jane 19/01/2001 415 Woodchurch Road Prenton Wirral Merseyside CH42 8PF **Tel:** (0151) 201 8606 w 6204283

DEVINE Fiona 14/09/2009 4 Benedict Place 17 St. Marys Road Netley Abbey SOUTHAMPTON SO31 5HQ **Tel:** (02380) 455141 w 6492307

DEVINE Julie (see CRAIG, Mrs)

DEVLIN Julie (see HENSTEAD, Mrs)

DEVONSHIRE Alison Jane (nee Hall) 15/11/2001 Orwell Veterinary Group Hartree Way Grange Farm Kesgrave Ipswich Suffolk IP5 2BZ **Tel:** (01473) 333677 w 6261901

DEWAR Aileen Margaret Jane 27/03/2009 4 Braeside Place Reddingmuirhead Falkirk Stirlingshire FK2 0DD **Tel:** 07841484106 w 6377456

DEYA BERNAT Maria Christina 01/09/2008 Camino la Villalonga N.7 07100 Soller Mallorca Spain **Tel:** 07872171732 w 6400061

DE-ZILLE Angela Jade 18/01/1988 58 Union Road Deal Kent CT14 6AR **Tel:** (01304) 375571 w 6062196

DI MATTEO Maria Adelina 04/10/2005 23 Highertown Highertown Truro Cornwall TR1 3QE **Tel:** (01872) 273408 w 6339055

DI SALVO Jacqueline Carol Anne 30/10/2003 8 Boughton Drive RUSHDEN Northamptonshire NN10 9HX **Tel:** (01933) 358079 w 6285177

DIACK Louise Dorothy (see MISKELLY, Mrs)

DIAS-JAYASINGHE Abigail Jayne 05/07/2006 88 Crouch House Road EDENBRIDGE Kent TN8 5EP **Tel:** (01732) 300651 w 6321543

DIBB Charlotte Joanne (see HORSLEY, Mrs)

DICK Lynsey Michelle 30/10/2003 133d Rannoch Rd Letham Perth PH1 2DQ **Tel:** (01738) 449173 w 6282427

DICK Melanie (see CUMMINGS, Mrs)

DICKENS Kelly 29/08/2000 7 Minster Road Minster on Sea Sheerness Kent ME12 3JD **Tel:** (01795) 662578 w 6203436

Laura Maureen 06/11/2008 Diamond Farm Wisbech Road Tipps End Welney Wisbech Cambridgeshire PE14 9SQ w 6418145

Michelle 25/03/2009 6 Ridge Lane Oldbury Nuneaton Warwickshire CV10 0RB **Tel:** 07852135523 w 6405033

DICKENSON Laura Elizabeth 19/05/2009 48 Waverley Road KENILWORTH Warwickshire CV8 1JN **Tel:** (01926) 859374 w 6374519

DICKINSON Allison (nee Gore) 24/04/1981 (05/11/2004) Barn Lodge Veterinary Hospital 54A Southport Road Ormskirk Lancashire L39 1LX **Tel:** (01695) 572837 w 6049186

Judith Emily 12/09/1997 (01/03/2002) 27 Woodside View Bolton on Dearne ROTHERHAM South Yorkshire S63 8GZ w 6115821

DICKINSON Susan Elizabeth (see JONES, Mrs)

DICKSON Amy Alice 07/04/2009 44 Red Cat Lane Burscough Ormskirk Lancashire L40 0RD **Tel:** (01704) 893613 w 6389347

Laura 04/05/2006 19 Linnhe Avenue Glasgow Lanarkshire G44 3NY **Tel:** (07884) 247755 w 6349692

Sara Ann Louise 11/07/2005 (15/06/2007) 18 Makbrar Place DUMFRIES DG1 4BD **Tel:** (01387) 265077 w 6298630

DIGBY Claire Michelle 23/01/2003 37 Oval Road South DAGENHAM Essex RM10 9DP **Tel:** (020) 8596 0753 w 6260262

DIGBY Lisa Marie (see FIELD, Mrs)

DILLON Emma Louise 11/05/2009 17 Hollands Way Kegworth DERBY DE74 2GQ **Tel:** 07837029144 w 6417474

DINGLE Helen Louise (see HARRIS, Mrs)

DINGLE Katie Jane DipAVN(Surgical) (nee Richardson) 24/01/1995 The Veterinary Surgery Higher Trenant Wadebridge Cornwall PL27 6HB **Tel:** (01208) 813258 w 6033766

DINNELL Tracy Jane (nee Dinnell, formerly Henderson) 26/08/1997 16c Niddrie Mill Crescent EDINBURGH EH15 3ET w 6108224

DIPPLE Emily (see DYCHE, Mrs)

DIPPLE Nichola Jane 14/03/2006 9 Lyecroft Avenue Birmingham West Midlands B37 6SZ **Tel:** (0121) 603 2597 w 6346491

DISNEY Amanda Jayne (nee Allen) 23/09/1987 (28/10/2002) 4 Hastings Close Fleckney Leicester Leicestershire LE8 8UG **Tel:** (01162) 404061 w 6049233

DISTON Maxine Ann 14/09/2009 42 St. Philips Drive EVESHAM Worcestershire WR11 2RJ **Tel:** (01386) 765712 w 6271405

DIVALL Grant Adam 17/08/2005 Pet Doctors Veterinary Clinics Brooklyn Road Seaford East Sussex BN25 2DU **Tel:** (01323) 894568 m 6281481

DIX Gemma (see IRWIN-PORTER, Mrs)

DIXON Beverley Jayne (see BOYNTON, Mrs)

Catherine Amy 16/07/2007 P D S A Woolfall Heath Avenue Liverpool Merseyside L36 3YD **Tel:** (0151) 480 2288 w 6357040

Claire Louise 01/09/1999 29 Sopwith Crescent Merley Wimborne Dorset BH21 1SH **Tel:** (01202) 883089 w 6149158

Gemma 30/10/2003 15 Merlin Court Waterstone Park Stone Kent DA9 9TB w 6292734

Jacqueline 12/05/2004 2 Greenside Drive Lostock Green NORTHWICH Cheshire CW9 7SR w 6287113

Jayne Elizabeth 01/09/1995 Beechwood Veterinary Group 335 Chapeltown Road Leeds West Yorkshire LS7 3LL **Tel:** (0113) 262 1189 w 6039542

Kathryn Joy (nee Rundle) 26/02/2000 16 Reddington Road Plymouth Devon PL3 6PS **Tel:** (07813) 753968 w 6190357

Kay 02/09/2009 66 St. Ives Place Murton Seaham County Durham SR7 9LD **Tel:** 07921909675 w 6437560

Laura Jane 13/07/2004 38 Forester Close Seaton Carew HARTLEPOOL Cleveland TS25 1JE w 6292536

DIXON Nicola (see BIRCH, Mrs)

Roxanne Jayne 24/03/2009 5 Naburn Place Leeds West Yorkshire LS14 2DB **Tel:** (0113) 2645422 w 6443676

DIXON Tanzi Louise (see RIDGE, Mrs)

DOBBS Amanda Jayne 10/12/2009 58 The Parkway Cottingham North Humberside HU16 5HB **Tel:** 01482847363 w 6447163

DOBSON Anna Louise 08/01/2008 T/A Bonham Veterinary Centre 19 Central Street Ramsbottom Bury Lancashire BL0 9AF **Tel:** (01706) 827787 w 6280062

Cally Frances 22/04/2008 74 Brookfield Road Grimsby South Humberside DN33 3JL **Tel:** (01472) 593970 w 6415186

Charlotte (nee Aveyard) 20/09/1996 Abbey House Veterinary Hospital Commercial Street Morley Leeds West Yorkshire LS27 8AG **Tel:** (0113) 252 5818 w 6039575

Cheryl May 21/05/2009 AbbeyVET 60 Cross Street London N1 2BA **Tel:** (020) 7226 8555 w 6400248

Kerry-Ann 10/09/2009 Quaint Cottage Greenbottom Truro Cornwall TR4 8QJ **Tel:** (01872) 561477 w 6425768

Sharon Louise 06/09/1995 9 Lambton Terrace New Penshaw Houghton le Spring Tyne and Wear DH4 7PL **Tel:** (0191) 3858353 w 6036097

Sharon Terri 06/08/2007 32 Lemon Grove Whitehill Bordon Hampshire GU35 9BE **Tel:** (01420) 472912 w 6356215

DOCHERTY Claire Frances (nee Barron) 02/03/2001 Chestnut House Veterinary Centre Sutton Grange Saltshouse Road Hull HU8 9HL **Tel:** (01482) 787366 w 6213567

Denise Heather 21/03/2003 St Clair Veterinary Group 2 Pottery Street Kirkcaldy Fife KY1 3ET **Tel:** (01592) 599500 w 6282284

Lynn 02/10/1990 (12/04/2002) 3 Coopers Close CHIGWELL Essex IG7 6EX w 6049244

Steven Thomas 10/12/2002 77 Westgate Driffield North Humberside YO25 6TA m 6268666

DODD Carli Ann (nee Gibson, formerly Dood) 02/02/2001 4 Squarehouse Barns Tattenhall Lane Tattenhall CHESTER CH3 9NH **Tel:** (07712) 764476 w 6211873

Lindsey Anne 09/07/2007 18 St. Johns Road Rowley Park STAFFORD ST17 9AS w 6352530

Victoria (nee Ion) 25/02/2003 Langford Veterinary Services Ltd Langford House Bristol North Somerset BS40 5DU **Tel:** (01934) 852422 w 6279523

DODGE Claire Emma (nee Angwin) 05/09/2000 The Veterinary Surgery Harleigh Road Bodmin Cornwall PL31 1AQ **Tel:** (01208) 72323 w 6203381

Denise Elizabeth (nee Atkinson) 16/09/1981 53 Cedar Drive Keynsham Bristol BS31 2TX **Tel:** (01179) 864306 w 6049266

DODSON Emma 23/02/2009 54 Dunvegan Avenue KIRKCALDY Fife KY2 5TG **Tel:** 01592201625 w 6438242

DOHERTY Maura (see MONTAGUE, Mrs)

DOLAN Amanda 13/01/2000 73 Ravensby Park Gardens Carnoustie Angus DD7 7NY **Tel:** (01241) 858600 w 6190390

DOLBEAR Elaine Rachel 16/08/2006 456-458 Hagley Road West Oldbury West Midlands B68 0DL **Tel:** (0121) 422 2902 w 6436053

DOLLEY Emma Rose 15/02/2005 252 Miller Way Thornbury Plymouth PL6 8UQ **Tel:** (01752) 786 153 w 6293119

DOLPHIN Kylie Sarah 09/04/2009 3 Auclum Close Burghfield Common READING RG7 3DY **Tel:** 01189832916 w 6407585

DONAGHY Lesley Ann 11/11/2004 Pinewood Veterinary Practice 23 Crown Street Chorley Lancashire PR7 1DX **Tel:** (01257) 276517 w 6296155

DONALD Alison Sarah (nee Donald, formerly Varney) 21/08/1998 88 Lechmere Avenue Woodford Green IG8 8QG **Tel:** (0208) 5512274 w 6130850

Emma Victoria 28/02/2007 10 Coral Avenue Liverpool Merseyside L36 2PZ **Tel:** (0151) 290 0195 w 6385233

DONALD Sarah Louise (see THOMAS, Mrs)

DONALDSON Janette Boyd (see YOUNG, Mrs)

DONNAI Maria 09/09/1996 (15/10/2001) 136-138 County Road South Hull HU5 5NA **Tel:** (01482) 505333 w 6041700

DONNELLY Claire Amanda Elaine 28/06/2005 9 Segarsdean Terrace HADDINGTON East Lothian EH41 4RJ **Tel:** (07956) 897054 w 6297156

Lisa Marie 12/01/2009 Glenabo Fermoy Co Cork Ireland **Tel:** 00353863446159 w 6282680

DONOVAN Michelle Rowena Simone DipAVN(Medical) 23/09/1999 Lanwades Park Kentford Newmarket Suffolk CB8 7UU **Tel:** (01638) 552700 w 6185000

DOOD Carli Ann (see DODD, Mrs)

DOOLAN Alyson Margaret (nee Robertson) 19/01/2000 Shore Veterinary Centre Ltd 116 Shore Street Gourock Renfrewshire PA19 1QZ **Tel:** (01475) 637312 w 603943X

DORAN Kate Maria 21/07/2008 19 Keedonwood Road BROMLEY BR1 4QJ **Tel:** (07834) 600488 w 6345897

Rachelle Mary 21/08/2008 26 Hargill Drive Washington Tyne and Wear NE38 9EY **Tel:** (0191) 4178225 w 6416528

DORES Charlotte Ruby 27/05/2009 8 Brannel Green St. Stephen ST. AUSTELL Cornwall PL26 7DG w 6411996

DOREY-PHILLIPS Claire Louise 15/12/2004 36 Ridgewood Gardens Cimla Neath West Glamorgan SA11 3QF w 6299961

DORNEY Caroline Pietruszka 07/07/2009 13 Collingwood Terrace Whitley Bay Tyne and Wear NE26 2NP **Tel:** 07908134621 w 6374189

DORRICOTT Katherine Mary (nee Thompson) 10/04/2003 17 St. Nicholas Road Wallasey Wirral Cheshire CH45 8NG **Tel:** (0151) 6396295 w 6271988

DORRIES Katie Maria 04/12/2003 (21/01/2009) 13 North Street DOVER Kent CT17 9QX **Tel:** (01304) 208236 w 6283593

DORSETT Emma Jane (see DORSETT-WHEELEY, Mrs)

DORSETT-WHEELEY Emma Jane (nee Dorsett) 04/12/2007 2 Church Cottage Winston Stowmarket Suffolk IP14 6LG **Tel:** (01728) 861303 w 6353234

DORWARD Beth Sophie (nee Osborn) 15/01/1998 Crossways House Tattersett Road Syderstone Kings Lynn Norfolk PE31 8TJ **Tel:** (01485) 578 123 w 6118312

DOUGHTY Lucy Catherine 22/08/1995 1 Church Piece Cottages Queens Street Farthinghoe Brackley Northamptonshire NN13 5NY **Tel:** (01295) 712799 w 6036224

DOUGLAS Nicola Helen 10/09/1997 (19/02/2001) PDSA Kings Road Southwick Sunderland SR5 2LH **Tel:** (0191) 516 0636 w 6076176

DOUSE Katherine Elizabeth 14/09/2004 (28/07/2008) Wickham Green Farm Crookwood Potterne Devizes Wiltshire SN10 5QS **Tel:** (01380) 840429 w 6296683

DOVE Helen Jane (nee Duffin) 24/01/2005 Long Howe End Farm Witherslack GRANGE-OVER-SANDS Cumbria LA11 6RH **Tel:** (015395) 52316 w 6316538

DOVER Janet Elizabeth (see TATE, Mrs)

DOWD Sarah Jane 16/09/1998 20 Latham Lane Kitt Green Orrell Wigan Lancashire WN5 0JQ **Tel:** (01942) 212996 w 6115843

DOWLER Lucy Alexandra 26/10/2005 14 Eliot Close Long Eaton NOTTINGHAM NG10 3LS w 6344137

DOWLEY Lisa Maria (nee Munnery, formerly Herst) 27/08/1997 Manor Veterinary Clinic Shearway Business Park Shearway Road Folkestone Kent CT19 4RH **Tel:** (01303) 273203 w 6029589

DOWLING Christine 30/10/2003 1 Starlight Farm Close Verwood Dorset BH31 7BS **Tel:** (01202) 814 067 w 6280645

DOWNES Andrea Jane 25/02/2000 (19/04/2005) 8 Bramerton Lodge Bramerton Norwich Norfolk NR14 7ZQ **Tel:** (07717) 280335 w 6190269

DOWNIE Hannah 31/10/2003 16 Gustory Road Crantock Newquay Cornwall TR8 5RG **Tel:** (01637) 830053 w 6269612

DOWNS Katherine 21/06/2005 7 Marl Park Scoriton Nr BUCKFASTLEIGH Devon TQ11 0HZ **Tel:** (01364) 631050 w 6274408

DOWNSBOROUGH Kay 29/12/1983 (31/07/2006) 18 Woodlands Mount Halifax West Yorkshire HX3 6HR **Tel:** (01422) 321 890 w 604938X

DOYLE Hillis Alexandra 06/02/2008 58 Ravenswood Drive Caskieberran Glenrothes Fife KY6 2NZ **Tel:** (01592) 560606 w 6295715

DRAIN Wendy Marie 24/11/2009 Petkind Veterinary Centre 14 Commonwealth House Montreal Road Tilbury Essex RM18 7QX **Tel:** (01375) 840979 w 6417111

DRAKE Claire Louise 30/11/2009 Prospect House Frome Road Bradford-on-Avon Wiltshire BA15 1LA **Tel:** (01225) 862656 w 6492252

DRAYNER Nicola Diane (see DALY, Mrs)

DREW Owen William 14/03/2006 12 Marlborough Road Colliers Wood LONDON SW19 2HG **Tel:** (020) 8543 2528 m 6345435

DREWITT Claudia Hannah 17/01/2006 174 Pine Road BOURNEMOUTH BH9 1ND w 6318837

DREYER Marie Frances 03/06/2003 (18/02/2009) 102 Nutley Lane REIGATE Surrey RH2 9HA **Tel:** (01737) 246665 w 6286629

DRING Kathryn Sarah (nee Grundy) 06/02/1997 Wood Farmhouse Broadgate Weston SPALDING Lincolnshire PE12 6JA w 6117636

DRINKWATER Lindsay (see CLAPHAM, Mrs)

DRISCOLL Jennifer Louise 21/07/2008 57 Herongate Road London E12 5EH **Tel:** (0208) 9896978 w 6375971

Kirsty Louise 23/04/2008 73 Cherry Way Hatfield Hertfordshire AL10 8LG **Tel:** (01707) 891038 w 6413008

Louise Marie (nee Levitt) 27/05/2003 Bruton Veterinary Surgery 25 High Street Bruton Somerset BA10 0AH **Tel:** (01749) 813291 w 6278918

DRIVER Abigail Beth (see MASSEY, Mrs)

DRUCE Kelly Louise 28/02/2001 Black Horse Inn Harrow Road WEMBLEY Middlesex HA0 2QP w 6144273

DRUMMOND Juliet Christina DipAVN(Medical) 31/01/1997 (07/11/2000) 24 Abbeydale Road South Sheffield South Yorkshire S7 2QN **Tel:** (0114) 2363391 w 610764X

Suzanne 01/07/2008 38 Purcell Road Luton Bedfordshire LU4 0RD **Tel:** (01582) 709952 w 6359141

DRURY Judith 21/01/1999 (16/05/2003) 1 Alder Close Forest Town Mansfield Nottinghamshire NG19 0NQ **Tel:** (01623) 468887 w 6138598

Vicky Christine 12/06/2009 Pilgrim Veterinary Surgery Fydell Street Boston Lincolnshire PE21 8LE **Tel:** (01205) 366872 w 6417573

DRURY-GORHAM Sarah Louise (nee Edwards) 02/06/2004 Coastway Veterinary Group Unit 4E, Freshfield Business Park Freshfield Way Brighton East Sussex BN2 0BZ **Tel:** (01273) 692257 w 6274364

DRYLAND Hayley Louise 22/03/2004 2 Waterside Terrace Ninn Lane Great Chart Ashford Kent TN23 3DD **Tel:** (01233) 638377 w 6293658

D'SOUZA Anna Marie 10/06/2009 112 Marlborough Hill Harrow Middlesex HA1 1UA **Tel:** 02088610119 w 6407904

DU HEAUME Julie Rose 31/10/2008 Les Eturs Veterinary Centre Rue des Eturs Castel Guernsey GY5 7DT **Tel:** (01481) 257708 w 6419388

DUDDY Jody Katy 27/02/2007 3 Fairfield Cottages Leatherhead Road Bookham LEATHERHEAD Surrey KT23 4RA **Tel:** (01372) 456247 w 6351243

DUDLEY Amanda Jane 21/03/2007 57-59 Broadleys Clay Cross Chesterfield Derbyshire S45 9JN **Tel:** (01246) 862266 w 6374541

DUFF Amanda Louise 11/08/2009 312 Cowley Mansions Mortlake High Street London SW14 8SL **Tel:** (07957) 159 136 w 6437010

Angela 15/02/2005 (22/02/2008) The Beach Appartment The Promenade STONEHAVEN Kincardineshire AB39 2RD **Tel:** (01567) 763656 w 6291326

Claire 02/04/2009 10 Kippielaw Gardens Easthouses Dalkeith Midlothian EH22 4JA **Tel:** (0131) 6604247 w 6346997

Claire Louise 12/07/2006 Veterinary Hospital Fyfield Barrow Walnut Tree Local Centre Milton Keynes Buckinghamshire MK7 7AN **Tel:** (01908) 397777 w 6354609

Helen Elizabeth 26/01/2009 116 Glenhugh Road Cullybackey Ballymena County Antrim BT42 1EJ **Tel:** 07732361943 w 6433468

DUFF Sarah Maria (see ORR, Mrs)

DUFFELL Emily Jayne 08/01/2008 White Cross Vets 1238 London Road Alvaston Derby DE24 8QP w 6400721

Sophie Claire 15/12/2009 144 Melton Road Stanton-on-the-Wolds Keyworth NOTTINGHAM NG12 5BQ w 6457712

DUFFILL Teri 29/08/2000 18 Parkhead Avenue Edinburgh EH11 4SG **Tel:** (0131) 539 9816 w 6205086

DUFFIN Helen Jane (see DOVE, Mrs)

DUFFY Amanda Mary 08/04/2008 4 Altananam Park BALLYCASTLE County Antrim BT54 6EE **Tel:** (028) 20768868 w 6322456

Lorraine Eunice 19/01/1998 (29/01/2008) 1 Jubilee Cottages Arley NORTHWICH Cheshire CW9 6LZ w 6115876

DUGGAN Deirdre Mary 23/11/2001 Kealnagower House Kenmare Co Kerry Ireland **Tel:** 064-41202 w 6259239

Shenade Lucinda DipAVN(Surgical) (nee Moore) 16/07/2002 21 The Anchorage Killyleagh County Down BT30 9UH **Tel:** (028) 4482 1303 w 6268985

DUGMORE Julie Maureen 13/08/1987 (12/12/2002) 123 Weggs Farm Road Duston Northampton Northamptonshire NN5 6HF **Tel:** (01604) 584304 w 6049732

DUHIG Emma Elizabeth 21/07/2008 2 Elmfield Court Wickham Street Welling Kent DA16 3DF **Tel:** 07903584770 w 6377071

DUKE Wendy Lynne (see COLE, Mrs)

DUMELOW Melanie Rachel (see PATTEN, Mrs)

DUMELOW Michelle Louise 24/07/2003 9 Carnforth Close Stapleford NOTTINGHAM NG9 7EZ w 6280315

DUNBAR-UNCLES Katherine Wendy 30/07/2009 Drove Veterinary Hospital 252 Croft Road Swindon Wiltshire SN1 4RW **Tel:** (01793) 522483 w 6431642

DUNCAN Hayley Louise (see DUNCAN LANE, Mrs)

DUNCAN Jennifer Ann 27/11/2009 2 Place Farm Court Rowhedge Road COLCHESTER Essex CO2 8ER **Tel:** (01206) 510191 w 6491361

Rachel Anne 17/09/2009 Croft of Cultalonie Farm Kirkmichael Blairgowrie Perthshire PH10 7NA **Tel:** 01250881253 w 6412029

DUNCAN LANE Hayley Louise (nee Duncan) 13/05/2003 84 Chapel Lane Coppull Chorley Lancashire PR7 4PN **Tel:** (01257) 795614 w 6275563

DUNCAN-BROWN Lucy Elizabeth (nee Ince) 18/10/2005 Wangfield House Wangfield Lane Curdridge Southampton Hampshire SO32 2DA **Tel:** (01489) 786520 w 6328979

DUNHAM Amber Frances 21/11/2005 77 High Street Purton Swindon Wiltshire SN5 4AB **Tel:** (01793) 771869 w 6353058

DUNKLEY Zoe Louise 27/02/2006 Orchard Veterinary Centre 21 Church Street Oldbury West Midlands B69 3AF **Tel:** (0121) 544 8951 w 6287080

DUNKS Lucy Caroline 18/08/2009 25 Lugano Close Waterlooville Hampshire PO7 6AT **Tel:** 07596638085 w 6447141

DUNLOP Karen 04/02/2008 21a Coldharbour Lane Bushey Hertfordshire WD23 4NP **Tel:** (07736) 037 018 w 6383869

DUNMALL Hannah 11/03/2008 17 Ansell Road Dorking Surrey RH4 1QN **Tel:** (01306) 640509 w 6376422

DUNN Cheryn Anne 23/08/2004 Waterdene Veterinary Practice 4 Timber Hill Road Caterham Surrey CR3 6LD **Tel:** (01883) 345277 w 6373606

Dawn Agnes (nee Bennett) 06/08/1980 (05/11/2004) 24 Dove Street Stewkley Leighton Buzzard Bedfordshire LU7 0HT w 6000515

DUNN Hayley (see MOOTIEN, Ms)

DUNN Helen Marjorie (see LASHLEY, Mrs)

Michelle June (nee Parton) 24/11/2004 27 Ferguson Street Wolverhampton West Midlands WV11 2JU **Tel:** (01902) 651541 w 6287597

DUNNACHIE Fiona 29/08/2000 Drummond House 49 Main Street Callander Perthshire FK17 8DX **Tel:** (01877) 330383 w 6202314

DUNNE Hayley Jane 24/02/2004 9 Crescent Road Wokingham Berkshire RG40 2DB **Tel:** (0118) 979 3200 w 6276751

DUNNETT Emma-Clare Louise 07/02/2006 The Village Animal Hospital CVS (UK) Ltd Guards Avenue Coulsdon Road Caterham Surrey CR3 5ZD **Tel:** (01883) 348483 w 6344786

DUNNING Claire Pamela 08/04/2005 Burnham House Veterinary Surgery 33-35 Castle Street Dover Kent CT16 1PT **Tel:** (01304) 206989 w 6301501

DUNTHORNE Michael John 07/02/2006 27 Bamber Place NEWCASTLE Staffordshire ST5 7PG **Tel:** (01782) 852840 m 6328946

DUNWORTH Sharon Louise 20/05/2002 (06/04/2009) 29 The Park Redbourn ST. ALBANS Hertfordshire AL3 7LR w 6261681

DURAN Stephanie 11/07/2005 88-92 Merton High Street Merton London SW19 1BD **Tel:** (020) 8254 1400 w 6299543

DURBER Lynne (nee Allsebrook) 23/02/1987 2 Crescent Grove Hartshill Stoke-on-Trent ST4 6EN **Tel:** (01782) 613863 w 6049506

DURICKI Natalie Tracy 22/06/2009 70 Strangers Lane Canterbury Kent CT1 3XG **Tel:** (01227) 450 432 w 6440244

DUROSE Sarah Christina 24/01/2005 20 Forfar Road Southmuir Kirriemuir DD8 5BY **Tel:** (01575) 572643 w 6317682

DURSTON Tamsin 30/06/2003 88-92 Merton High Street Merton London SW19 1BD **Tel:** (020) 8254 1400 w 6267907

DUTTON Abigail Beth (see MASSEY, Mrs)

DUTTON Sally Elizabeth (formerly Dutton) 28/02/2005 2 Freestone Road Southsea Hampshire PO5 3NA **Tel:** (07780) 541026 w 6299972

DWORAK Katarzyna Maria 15/10/2008 70 Oldfield Circus Northolt Middlesex UB5 4RU **Tel:** 02084235330 w 6386135

DWYER Julie 07/02/2005 77 Renville Rd Broadgreen Liverpool L14 3LN **Tel:** (0151) 281 7867 w 6285320

DYCHE Emily (nee Dipple) 20/04/2005 5 Hawthorne Crescent BURNTWOOD Staffordshire WS7 4RZ w 6302645

DYDE Rebecca Jayne 21/08/1985 Paws Veterinary Health Centre Edward Street Nuneaton Warwickshire CV11 5RP **Tel:** (024) 7638 4064 w 6049539

DYER Claire Serena 15/11/2001 Duddery Cottage The Duddery Wickhambrook Newmarket Suffolk CB8 8UN **Tel:** (01440) 821295 w 6270910

Nicola Louise 29/12/2003 Cliffe Veterinary Group 21 Cliffe High Street Lewes East Sussex BN7 2AH **Tel:** (01273) 473232 w 6280370

Penny 22/02/2007 Prince Bishop Veterinary Hospital 1 Plantation Street Leadgate Consett County Durham DH8 7PP **Tel:** (01207) 590340 w 6285364

Rachel Elizabeth DipAVN(Medical) 24/09/2001 25 West Glade Farnborough Hampshire GU14 0JE **Tel:** (01252) 523135 w 6228637

DZIUBA Louise 24/01/2000 Gamston Veterinary Centre Unit B, Gamston District Centre Gamston Nottingham NG2 6PS **Tel:** (0115) 981 6262 w 6191347

E

EADE Abigail Charlotte 10/02/1997 (02/11/2009) The Veterinary Hospital 118 Victoria Drive Bognor Regis West Sussex PO21 2EJ **Tel:** (01243) 841111 w 6100666

Hayley Marie (formerly Damant, nee Damant) 04/11/1999 7 Chingford Avenue Clacton-on-Sea Essex CO15 4US w 6185869

EADIE Julia Marie 18/10/2006 9 Cosham Road Peel Hall Wythenshawe MANCHESTER M22 5AL **Tel:** (0161) 442 9462 w 6291656

EAGLAND Emma Louise (nee Amesbury) 11/09/2003 Stable Cottage Lower Norton Lane Kewstoke WESTON-SUPER-MARE Avon BS22 9YR w 6286321

EARLE Tracey Ann 17/01/1996 (06/08/2002) 19 Southern Close TORQUAY TQ2 8QJ **Tel:** (01626) 867038 w 6031055

EARNSHAW Nicola Jane (nee Yates) 21/08/1995 3 Turner Avenue Lostock Hall PRESTON PR5 5LW **Tel:** (01772) 626002 w 6024161

EASOM June 04/11/1980 Hollywell Farm High Road South Wingfield ALFRETON Derbyshire DE55 7LX w 6049572

EASON Lorraine 15/11/2001 7 Mayors Place TENTERDEN Kent TN30 6JX **Tel:** (0788) 440 0993 w 6264167

EAST Tracey Louise (nee Medland) 14/11/1990 5 Mudgley Cross Road Mudgley Nr Wedmore Somerset BS28 2XW **Tel:** (01934) 710520 w 6056648

EASTERBROOK Frances Clare (nee Colwell) 26/07/1993 (19/04/2002) Milehouse Clinic 28 Outland Road Milehouse Plymouth Devon PL2 3DF **Tel:** (01752) 567567 w 6015088

EASTHAM Julie Ann 15/04/2004 Cromwell Veterinary Hospital 36-36a St. Johns Street HUNTINGDON Cambridgeshire PE29 3DG **Tel:** (01480) 52601/52222 w 6293372

EASTMAN Laura Teri Ann 14/11/2008 16 The Croft Cocking Midhurst West Sussex GU29 0HQ **Tel:** 01730817490 w 6416770

EASTMENT Rebecca Gemma 12/03/2008 21 Haverhill Crescent Nottingham Nottinghamshire NG5 5AW **Tel:** (0115) 9550 359 w 6396332

EASTWICK Annette Tracy (nee Strevens) 27/01/1999 154 High Street Ramsgate Kent CT11 9TT **Tel:** (01843) 591899 w 6121595

EASTWOOD Caroline Helen 29/06/2007 85 Alpine Drive Wardle Rochdale Lancashire OL12 9NY w 6384837

Jacqueline Louise (nee Freestone) 17/01/1996 15 Bakers Way Morton BOURNE Lincolnshire PE10 0XW w 6040445

Nicola Jane (formerly Whitehead) 22/01/1985 (18/05/2004) The Old Stores Lowthorpe Southrey Lincoln Lincolnshire LN3 5TD w 6063644

EASTWOOD Sally Ann (see BOND, Mrs)

EATON Katy Jane 02/03/2007 416 Myers Grove Lane Sheffield South Yorkshire S6 5LA **Tel:** (0114) 234 3934 w 6383154

EBBRELL Sandra 04/07/2008 23 Daneswell Drive Moreton Wirral Merseyside CH46 1QD **Tel:** (0151) 677 2411 w 6411886

ECCLES Sarah Jane 09/06/2009 10 Rawthey Gardens Sedbergh Cumbria LA10 5DZ **Tel:** 07725947157 w 6444347

EDDY Lauren Elizabeth 16/09/2008 Glebe House St. Breock Wadebridge Cornwall PL27 7JS **Tel:** 07969208952 w 6410940

EDE Lucy Ann (nee Cobb) 28/08/1998 Inside Pets At Home Burrfields Retail Park Burrfields Road Portsmouth Hampshire PO3 5LZ **Tel:** (023) 9265 0655 w 6117137

Priscilla Louise 17/09/2003 Penmellyn Veterinary Group Station Road St. Columb Major Cornwall TR9 6BX **Tel:** (01637) 880307 w 6258084

EDEN Lisa Anne (nee Burton) 29/06/2007 Grange Farm East Lancashire Road Leigh Lancashire WN7 3SD **Tel:** (01942) 673915 w 6286970

EDES Natasha Louise 31/10/2005 37 Wordsworth Place Horsham West Sussex RH12 5PR **Tel:** (01403) 243009 w 6345908

EDGAR Catherine (formerly Johnstone) 19/04/2005 Veterinary Health Centre Ltd 4 Greeways Lytham St. Annes Lancashire FY8 3LY **Tel:** (01253) 729309 w 6323358

Christina 04/11/1999 35 Fircroft Avenue Lancing West Sussex BN15 0NW **Tel:** (01903) 763220 w 6185550

EDGAR Gillian Linda (see LANE, Mrs)

Kelly Lorraine 08/09/2009 Newbury Fen Road Pakenham BURY ST. EDMUNDS Suffolk IP31 2LS **Tel:** 07725400797 w 6464917

Vicki 08/09/2009 Westway Veterinary Centre 426-428 West Road Newcastle upon Tyne NE5 2ER **Tel:** (0191) 274 7910 w 6466435

EDGE Emily Jane 28/09/1999 Hill Top Farm Lyme Park Disley Stockport Cheshire SK12 2NS **Tel:** (01625) 858918 w 6145448

EDGE Victoria Ella (see FLUDE, Mrs)

EDMED Rebecca Jane 30/11/2005 1 Myrtle House Lees Road Brabourne Lees ASHFORD Kent TN25 6QE w 6330178

EDWARD Andrea Jane (nee Hodge) 16/09/1999 (18/11/2005) 84 Brook Vale Waterloo LIVERPOOL L22 3YB **Tel:** (0151) 928 7882 w 6184967

EDWARDS Carolyn Elizabeth Margam 16/06/2008 2 Langford Place Gardens Langford BRISTOL BS40 5BS **Tel:** (01934) 861 082 w 6382714

Claire 20/11/2008 71a Congleton Road Biddulph Staffordshire ST8 6EF **Tel:** (01782) 522100 w 6429145

David Richard 02/02/1995 (05/11/2001) 47 Netherley Road Hinckley Leicestershire LE10 0RD **Tel:** (01455) 637615 m 6033507

Dawn 05/10/1998 124 Cheadle Road Cheddleton Leek Staffordshire ST13 7HW **Tel:** (01538) 360222 w 6115887

Elizabeth Grace 07/02/2005 22a Chelsham Road South Croydon Surrey CR2 6HY w 6290534

Gemma Elaine 09/05/2005 Afon Veterinary Centre Lletty Nedd Pen Y Dre Neath West Glamorgan SA11 3HH **Tel:** (01639) 642739 w 6311742

Gemma Louise 22/09/2009 4 Maple Drive Firsdown Salisbury Wiltshire SP5 1SY **Tel:** (01980) 862 832 w 6440475

Helen 11/10/2004 10 Hanover Court Annitsford Cramlington Northumberland NE23 7RX **Tel:** 07946591713 w 6322016

Helen Louise 01/08/1989 Anwell Veterinary Centre 41 Brighton Road Coulsdon Surrey CR5 2BF **Tel:** (020) 8668 6151 w 6049663

Jane Elizabeth 20/01/1998 33 Ramsons Way St Fagans CARDIFF CF5 4QY **Tel:** (02920) 593510 w 6043388

EDWARDS Jayne Margarette (see FARRELL, Mrs)

Jo-Anne Elise 19/03/2007 (23/02/2009) Inside Pets at Home Centre Retail Park Broadway Royton Oldham Lancashire OL2 5HX **Tel:** (0161) 624 7539 w 6363200

Joanne Louise 27/12/2001 Corner Veterinary Clinic 1 Stayton Road Sutton Surrey SM1 1QY **Tel:** (020) 8641 6126 w 6260988

Lisa Jane 12/09/1997 (25/04/2002) 74-76 Chorley New Road Bolton Greater Manchester BL1 4BY **Tel:** (01204) 525066 w 6038764

Nicola Louise (nee Hunter) 29/08/1997 24 Shields Road Sunderland Tyne and Wear SR6 8ND **Tel:** (0191) 548 3371 w 611206X

Nicola Louise (nee Jackson) 09/09/2004 11 Dewhurst Road Cheshunt Hertfordshire EN8 9PG w 6286222

Philippa Jane 29/09/2008 9 Ash Road Ashurst SOUTHAMPTON Hampshire SO40 7AT w 6412865

EDWARDS Rachael Dawn (see MCCOOEY, Mrs)

Sarah Jane 27/02/2006 Willesley Equine Clinic Ltd Byams Farm Willesley Tetbury Gloucestershire GL8 8QU **Tel:** (01666) 880566/ 880501 w 6273979

Sarah Jayne (nee Austin) 29/10/1997 (24/10/ 2000) Damory Veterinary Clinic Damory Lodge Edward Street Blandford Forum Dorset DT11 7QT **Tel:** (01258) 452626 w 6107708

EDWARDS Sarah Louise (see DRURY-GORHAM, Mrs)

Sophie Anne 06/07/2004 Hilltop Cottage Priory Lane Thurgarton Nottinghamshire NG14 7GR **Tel:** (01636) 830681 w 6284396

EDWARDS Susan Dianne (see HOWARTH, Mrs)

Victoria Jane 19/03/2007 74a Front Street East Bedlington Northumberland NE22 5AB w 6355159

EGAN Fiona Helen 15/10/2008 47 Beech Avenue Whitefield Manchester Lancashire M45 7EN **Tel:** 01617963784 w 6392108

EGGINTON Joanne 16/07/2007 25 Elm Tree Avenue Upper Poppleton YORK YO26 6HL w 6352739

EGLIN Samantha Joanne (see HOLLIDAY, Mrs)

EGMORE Louise (see WOODSBY, Mrs)

ELFORD Kelly Marie 02/10/2001 38 Littlegate Road PAIGNTON Devon TQ3 3AZ w 6229264

ELKINS Susan Anne 27/04/2001 (22/04/2003) Calder Veterinary Group/Calder Vets Savile Road Dewsbury West Yorkshire WF12 9LN **Tel:** (01924) 465592 w 6216471

ELLETT Sonya Clare (nee Bailey) 10/08/1992 8 Browns Drive Southgate Swansea SA3 2AE **Tel:** (01792) 234496 w 6008139

ELLIOT Sarah Jane (nee Hubbleday) 01/08/1987 (25/01/2002) 608 Veterinary Group 608 Warwick Road Solihull West Midlands B91 1AA **Tel:** (0121) 705 3044 w 6053432

ELLIOTT Caroline Alice Mary 04/02/2002 38 Speerstown Road Moorfields Ballymena County Antrim BT42 3DD **Tel:** (02825) 891983 w 6262330

Cathryn 10/09/1999 (07/08/2003) 5 Landon Close Walton CHESTERFIELD Derbyshire S42 7LX w 6185330

Julie 26/10/2006 Clare Veterinary Group 75 Ballynure Road Ballyclare County Antrim BT39 9AG **Tel:** (028) 9332 2223 w 6322049

Julii DipAVN(Surgical) (nee Adams) 29/07/1987 (05/08/1999) 11 Forgefields Herne Herne Bay Kent CT6 7TB **Tel:** (01227) 372396 w 6044461

Lisa 03/05/2007 17 Marigold Close Brayton SELBY North Yorkshire YO8 9RF **Tel:** (01757) 709976 w 6325712

Lynda Jacqueline Ann 04/02/2009 100 Crocknamack Road PORTRUSH County Antrim BT56 8JW **Tel:** 07715710372 w 6406573

Melanie 02/10/2009 1 Marlowe Place Houghton-le-Spring Tyne And Wear DH5 8HZ **Tel:** (0191) 5844285 w 6466897

Sarah-Jane 13/07/2007 150 Scalby Road Scarborough North Yorkshire YO12 5QP **Tel:** (078) 4166 5848 w 6349384

ELLIS Amanda Jane (nee Davison) 19/01/1989 PDSA PetAid Hospital Stoneygate Lane Felling Gateshead Tyne & Wear NE10 OLX **Tel:** (0191) 4382881 w 6094344

Carolyn Sara 06/08/2007 Great Kettle Barn Great Asby APPLEBY-IN-WESTMORLAND Cumbria CA16 6EX **Tel:** (078) 450 26000 w 6376895

Christine Suzanne 01/06/2009 Downland Veterinary Group 71 Havant Road Emsworth Hampshire PO10 7NZ **Tel:** (01243) 377141 w 6438385

Deborah Patricia 23/08/1989 25 Battle Road St. Leonards-on-Sea East Sussex TN37 7AA **Tel:** (01424) 428525 w 6049798

Denise Lynn 28/09/2005 Cherry Trees Riffhams Lane Danbury CHELMSFORD CM3 4DS **Tel:** (01245) 222569 w 6345930

ELLIS Jacqueline (see HADDON, Mrs)

Jade Louise 17/03/2009 Southfield Veterinary Centre South Walks DORCHESTER Dorset DT1 1DU **Tel:** (01305) 262913 w 6420092

Joanna Ruth (nee Melling) 06/03/2001 Holly Cottage 24 Fall Lane Hartshead LIVERSEDGE West Yorkshire WF15 8AR **Tel:** (01274) 242744 w 6203821

Kersty Selina 03/01/1992 23 Nelson Road BASILDON Essex SS14 1QQ **Tel:** (07912) 521 601 w 6015565

Lauren Claire 02/06/2004 50 Brooklands Park Laindon BASILDON Essex SS15 6BE **Tel:** (01268) 766314 w 6287751

Nicola Jayne 19/09/2006 51 Boughton Lane Moulton Northampton Northamptonshire NN3 7LE **Tel:** (01604) 462768 w 6365708

Samantha Denise 27/04/2005 12 Collet Walk GILLINGHAM Kent ME8 9QL w 6317352

Stella (nee Garnett) 13/04/2004 156 Middlewich Road Rudheath Northwich Cheshire CW9 7DU w 6282658

ELLISON Anne Elizabeth 01/10/1986 2 Lapwing Wilnecote Tamworth Staffordshire B77 5NW **Tel:** (01827) 283856 w 6049801

ELMER Beverley-Jane 13/08/1993 (07/03/2008) 21 Priors Gardens RUISLIP Middlesex HA4 6UG w 603118X

ELMER Polly Anna (see MILLER, Mrs)

ELMS Sally Lorna 25/02/2003 Laburnum Cottage Peaslake Guildford Surrey GU5 9RR **Tel:** (01306) 730395 w 6255994

ELPHICK Andrea Margaret 20/01/1999 (12/12/2002) 59 Broomwood Gardens Pilgrims Hatch BRENTWOOD Essex CM15 9LH **Tel:** (01277) 211682 w 6133057

ELSDON Jayne Margarette (see FARRELL, Mrs)

ELSON Michelle Dawn 14/09/2005 42 Havelock Road LUTON Bedfordshire LU2 7PR **Tel:** (01582) 481915 w 6273957

Samantha Sarah 26/10/2006 (18/11/2009) 110 Whitland Road Hartcliffe BRISTOL BS13 9QL w 6376444

ELTRINGHAM Stacey (see BULLOCK, Mrs)

ELVIDGE Lindsay Marie 13/04/2004 3 The Rindle Cheadle STOKE-ON-TRENT Staffordshire ST10 1PS w 6296705

ELWOOD Laura Jane 11/07/2005 The Ardmore Veterinary Group 57 Cornard Road Sudbury Suffolk CO10 2XB **Tel:** (01787) 372588 w 6323303

ELY Samantha Elizabeth 09/02/2009 The Castle British Road St. Agnes Cornwall TR5 0TY **Tel:** 01872552242 w 6438319

EMBY Elizabeth Caroline (see MARKS, Mrs)

EMERY Sarah Louise 29/03/2000 Little Orchard Gills Lane Rooksbridge Axbridge Somerset BS26 2TZ **Tel:** 01934750059 w 6185275

EMMOTT Victoria Louise 26/07/2006 58 New Park Road Lee Mill Bridge IVYBRIDGE Devon PL21 9EB w 6328154

ENEVER Lucy Helen Elizabeth 03/05/2007 17 Juniper Bracknell Berkshire RG12 7ZG **Tel:** (01344) 646 679 w 6371835

ENGLAND Carol (see BROWN, Mrs)

ENGLAND Cheryl Anne (see MARR, Mrs)

ENGLISH Jean Eileen (nee Evans) 26/04/2002 2 Perthneidr Cottages Sarnau Llandysul SA44 6QG **Tel:** (01239) 654645 w 6267687

ENOS Francesca 06/12/2004 38 Highwalls Avenue DINAS POWYS Vale of Glamorgan CF64 4AP w 6306187

EPPS Fiona Carmen 17/08/2005 Mews End Cottage 33 Bath Hill Keynsham Bristol Avon BS31 1HQ **Tel:** (01179) 583835 w 6316483

ERRINGTON Gail (see HOPPER, Mrs)

ERSKINE Jennifer Hazel 29/06/2007 2 Lawhead Place Penicuik Midlothian EH26 9JU **Tel:** (01968) 674107 w 6382725

Katie Joan 22/01/2010 13 Byrons Lane MACCLESFIELD Cheshire SK11 7JW w 6498962

ESLER Katie Rose 24/06/2004 3 Blakeney Grove Nailsea North Somerset BS48 4RG **Tel:** (01275) 853671 w 6285232

ESPLEY Clare Louise (nee Smith) 17/02/1998 (22/04/2002) Castle Vets Pet Healthcare Centre 1 Tilehurst Road Reading Berkshire RG1 7TW **Tel:** (0118) 957 4488 w 6129277

ESQUILANT Karen 03/05/2007 12 Sycamore Drive Park Street ST. ALBANS Hertfordshire AL2 2PJ w 6349010

ESSER Rebecca Elizabeth Jane (see CROSSMAN, Mrs)

ETHERINGTON Cheryl Alison 13/11/2006 Mid Sussex Veterinary Clinic More House Farm Ditchling Road Wivelsfield HAYWARDS HEATH West Sussex RH17 7RE w 6367600

ETHERINGTON Claire (see WILSON, Mrs)

EVANS Alison 08/05/2008 1 Lamborough Crescent Clarbeston Road Dyfed SA63 4UZ **Tel:** (01437) 731411 w 6291194

Amy 31/10/2006 33 Beech Road Alresford Hampshire SO24 9JS **Tel:** (01962) 732393 w 6357942

Anneliese Jade 22/08/2008 Chimneys Hailsham Road Heathfield East Sussex TN21 8AD **Tel:** (01435) 864422 w 6436229

EVANS Beverley Ann (see WILLIAMSON, Mrs)

Catherine Louise 20/01/2009 56 Askwith Road Hindley Green Wigan Lancashire WN2 4NS **Tel:** 07917798749 w 6412502

EVANS Cheryl (see ROBERTS, Mrs)

EVANS Elaine Sharon (see WHALE, Mrs)

EVANS Helen Tracy (see PARRISH, Ms)

EVANS Jean Eileen (see ENGLISH, Mrs)

EVANS Linzi Angela (see NUTTALL, Mrs)

Lucy Kate Madeley 16/06/2008 Pembrey Heol y Bryn HARLECH Gwynedd LL46 2TU **Tel:** (01766) 780 999 w 6380734

EVANS Maria Anne (see WYER, Mrs)

Melissa May 05/09/2008 4 Anderson Walk Bury St. Edmunds Suffolk IP32 6QH **Tel:** (01284) 750 987 w 6435382

Meriel Carys 29/08/2000 36 Argyll Avenue Southall Middlesex UB1 3AT **Tel:** (020) 85712210 w 6202985

Nicole 12/05/2004 32 Hedgers Close Ashton Bristol Avon BS3 2SX **Tel:** (01761) 233396 w 6298641

EVANS Patricia Anne (see DEAKIN, Mrs)

Rebecca Linda 17/01/2008 Pet Doctors 125-129 Chertsey Road Woking Surrey GU21 5BP **Tel:** (01483) 769881 w 6344148

Ruth 14/12/2006 Knolton Hall Lodge Oswestry Road Overton WREXHAM Clwyd LL13 0LG w 6375058

Sarah-Jayne 30/11/2006 138 Todmorden Road Bacup Lancashire OL13 9TZ **Tel:** (07980) 078380 w 6330717

Sian Louise 05/10/2004 64 Westbourne Avenue Emsworth Hampshire PO10 7QU **Tel:** (01243) 375860 w 6256874

EVANS Sian Marie Anne (see WILTSHIRE, Mrs)

Tara 27/02/2006 Veterinary Surgery Cinque Ports Street Rye East Sussex TN31 7AN **Tel:** (01797) 222265 w 6344159

Tina (nee Bown) 18/01/1999 (01/03/2006) 172 Seafield Road Southbourne Bournemouth Dorset BH6 5LJ w 6135360

EVANS Victoria Jane (see PEACOCK, Mrs)

Victoria Mary 23/08/2004 230 Foley Road Newent Gloucestershire GL18 1SR **Tel:** (01531) 821 945 w 6278566

EVASON Stephanie Jayne 04/02/2009 9 Victoria Street Rawtenstall ROSSENDALE Lancashire BB4 7PT **Tel:** 01614088810 w 6392097

EVE-RAW Emma Victoria 06/06/2001 27 Bullhead Road BOREHAMWOOD Hertfordshire WD6 1HW **Tel:** (020) 82072861 w 6191468

EVERDEN Amy Louise 24/04/2009 32 Virginia Walk Gravesend Kent DA12 5UL **Tel:** 01474747715 w 6417133

EVERITT Rachel Catherine 01/04/2009 Flat 1 Brookmead Horsham Road Cranleigh Surrey GU6 8DJ **Tel:** 07810118182 w 6402536

EWERS Nicola Jane (nee Watson) 01/04/2003 Edgewood Veterinary Group Chelmsford Road Purleigh Chelmsford Essex CM3 6QR **Tel:** (01621) 828381 w 6267203

EWING Melissa Jane (nee Thompson) 24/06/2004 Park View Veterinary Group 122 Park View Road Welling Kent DA16 1SJ **Tel:** (020) 8303 2864 w 6288224

EWINS Karen Nicola 26/08/1997 100 Greenway Gardens Greenford Middlesex UB6 9TX **Tel:** (0208) 5789098 w 6099127

F

FACER Bridget Sarah 14/09/2004 162 Addison Road Bilton Rugby Warwickshire CV22 7EY **Tel:** (01788) 334 977 w 6289533

FAHY Elisha Marie 20/09/2006 101 The Glebe Church Road Ballina Co Mayo Ireland **Tel:** (0035396) 73512 w 6293383

FAIRBAIRN Christine (nee Wild) 14/01/1982 North Lodge Whitfield Hexham Northumberland NE47 8LR **Tel:** (01434) 345313 w 6063768

FAIRHURST Kristoffer Graham 31/10/2003 5 Cliffe Lane Great Harwood Blackburn Lancashire BB6 7PY **Tel:** (01254) 888457 m 6290072

FAIRLEY Anna 15/02/2005 (03/03/2009) 2 Winchester Avenue York North Yorkshire YO26 4RU **Tel:** (01904) 781632 w 6325734

FAIRS Sallyanne (nee Clark) 25/08/1998 45 The Hill Glapwell Chesterfield Derbyshire S44 5LX **Tel:** (07903) 183877 w 6128728

FALBERG Andrea Jane 14/09/1999 Glan-Yr-Afon West Grove Lane Hundleton Pembroke Dyfed SA71 5RE **Tel:** 01646622995 w 6145823

FALSHAW Samantha Jayne (see BROADBENT, Mrs)

FANE-GLADWIN Helen Victoria 25/08/1999 14 Burlington Road New Malden Surrey KT3 4NY **Tel:** (020) 8942 2202 w 612903X

FARION Tracey 24/05/2005 21 Elliot Place TROWBRIDGE Wiltshire BA14 9TQ **Tel:** (01225) 760732 w 6307485

FARLEY Elizabeth Louise 31/03/2003 36 Boston Road Kirton Boston Lincolnshire PE20 1DS w 6249427

FARMER Abigail 31/08/1999 Bowbridge Surgery Bowbridge Stroud Gloucestershire GL5 2LA **Tel:** (01453) 762350 w 613420X

Katharine Lindsay Mary 15/04/2004 27 Page Close BALDOCK Hertfordshire SG7 6PT w 6272010

Linda Jane 23/02/2005 (30/01/2009) Marlcroft Lindley Hall Farm Fenny Drayton NUNEATON Warwickshire CV13 6BP **Tel:** (024) 76372013 w 6320872

FARMER Rosemary Karen (see BENNETT, Mrs)

FARNELL Dean Stephen 07/02/2006 108 Barrier Point Road Royal Victoria Docks LONDON E16 2SD m 6347030

FARNWORTH Laura Anne (nee Jones) 23/12/2003 38 Adolphus Street Whitburn Sunderland Tyne and Wear SR6 7DJ w 6289401

FARR Linda Patricia (formerly Hill) 02/10/1998 Bodkin Farm Ingleberry Road Shepshed LOUGHBOROUGH Leicestershire LE12 9DE **Tel:** (01509) 504057 w 6140177

FARR Samantha Claire (see BROWN, Mrs)

FARRALL Lynn (nee Robinson) 04/02/2002 65 Field Lane CREWE Cheshire CW2 8ST **Tel:** (01270) 560323 w 6260647

FARRANT Jennifer Susan 06/02/2008 53 Portman Drive Billericay Essex CM12 0PE **Tel:** (01277) 631025 w 6386597

Victoria Clare 02/09/1997 Chimneys Hailsham Road Heathfield East Sussex TN21 8AD **Tel:** (01435) 864422 w 6117002

FARRELL Cristina Ana (nee Manso, nee Manso) 14/09/1998 Chase Veterinary Group 89-91 Seaside Eastbourne East Sussex BN22 7NL **Tel:** (01323) 639331 w 6138259

Hayley Louise 15/11/2006 53 Markland Road Dover Kent CT17 9LY **Tel:** (01304) 225502 w 6379106

Jayne Margarette (formerly Elsdon, formerly Edwards) 30/01/1991 (12/02/2003) Miramar Veterinary Centre 15 Holt Road Sheringham Norfolk NR26 8NA **Tel:** (01263) 822293 w 6049845

Jayne Sarah 15/02/2008 15 Chiswick Close Murdishaw RUNCORN Cheshire WA7 6HQ w 6376906

Ruth Elizabeth (nee Barrett) 31/03/2003 (22/12/2008) 85 Barnes Avenue Dronfield Woodhouse DRONFIELD Derbyshire S18 8YF **Tel:** (01246) 414756 w 6283890

Sarah Jane (nee Roberts) 07/04/2006 65 Queens Park Rise BRIGHTON BN2 9ZF **Tel:** (01273) 382506 w 6337867

FARRICKER Louise Michelle 03/06/2009 82 Wellington Road Ashton-under-Lyne Lancashire OL6 6DP **Tel:** (0161) 330 2514/4839 w 6439529

FARRINGTON Nicola Victoria 22/09/2004 Oak Cottage Bagot Street Abbots Bromley Rugeley Staffordshire WS15 3DB **Tel:** (07815) 424494 w 6296166

FAULKINER Sian Caroline Shackleton 09/09/2009 3 Broadcroft Grove Tingley Wakefield West Yorkshire WF3 1TU **Tel:** 01132380546 w 6449517

FAULKNER Carolina Anne Vega 18/02/2009 39 Penzance Road Romford Essex RM3 9NR **Tel:** 07816276960 w 6449484

Katie Jane 29/09/2008 56 Barnfield Way OXTED Surrey RH8 9QG w 6396343

Lesley Jean 20/01/1998 4 Battersea Park Road Battersea London SW8 4AA **Tel:** (020) 7627 9256 w 6076154

Melissa Jayne 28/08/2008 88 Blackthorn Drive LEICESTER LE4 1BJ **Tel:** 07729197328 w 6413404

Stephanie Ann 08/09/2009 48 Rosehill Road IPSWICH IP3 8ET **Tel:** (01473) 425562 w 6459428

FAVELL Sally-Anne 31/10/2008 65 Ely Road Little Downham Ely Cambridgeshire CB6 2SN **Tel:** (01353) 699 655 w 6435481

FAZACKARLEY Emma Louise (see BREWER, Mrs)

FEAR Nikki Jane 14/03/2006 80 High Street Lytchett Matravers POOLE Dorset BH16 6BJ **Tel:** (01202) 623757 w 6330189

FEARN Gary Stuart 04/11/2008 Croft Cottage Moor Lane Ockbrook DERBY DE72 3SA m 6429112

Lisa Margaret 11/03/2009 1 East Weald Drive Ashford Road TENTERDEN Kent TN30 6LX **Tel:** 07980611147 w 6445117

FEARON Daina Charlotte 24/10/2008 27 Marlborough Way Uttoxeter Staffordshire ST14 7HL **Tel:** (01889) 560737 w 6404142

FEDERICO Renata Rose Mary 07/01/2008 Elizabeth Street Veterinary Clinic 55 Elizabeth Street London SW1W 9PP **Tel:** (020) 7730 9102 w 6502746

FEDRICK Hollie Roxanne 09/09/2009 231 Greystoke Avenue BRISTOL BS10 6BB **Tel:** 07917405531 w 6492571

FEENEY Clare Louise (nee Osborne) 20/09/2005 14 Church End Avenue Runwell Wickford Essex SS11 7JD **Tel:** (01268) 572198 w 6258403

FELGATE Anna Claire 27/08/2003 74 Hillcrest Avenue Dereham Norfolk NR19 1TD w 6268468

FELL Lisa Karen (see LAYE, Mrs)

FELLOWS Mary Christina 25/07/2008 148 Polwhele Road Newquay Cornwall TR7 2TN **Tel:** 07530500313 w 6244279

FELSTEAD Anne Margaret (nee Nelson) 23/12/2003 Letchworth Veterinary Centre Ltd Norton Way North Letchworth Garden City Hertfordshire SG6 1BS **Tel:** (01462) 685882 w 6291876

Christina Kathleen 21/05/2007 5 Ash Way ROYSTON Hertfordshire SG8 7LG **Tel:** (079) 312 32356 w 6321653

Karen Louise 27/08/2003 13 School Rd Ludham gt Yarmouth Norfolk NR29 5QN **Tel:** (01692) 678554 w 6282141

FELTON Karen 21/01/1997 Meadowcroft 5 The Green Flempton Nr Bury St. Edmunds Suffolk IP28 6EL **Tel:** (01284) 728741 w 6099138

FENN Julia Elizabeth 04/02/2009 Queen Mother Hospital for Small Animals Hawkshead Lane North Mymms Hatfield Hertfordshire AL9 7TA **Tel:** (01707) 666366 w 6438352

FENNELL Teresa Jayne (see RIDLEY, Mrs)

FENOULHET Joanna Margaret 30/10/2007 15 Oak Avenue Farndon Newark Nottinghamshire NG24 3TQ **Tel:** 07759192958 w 6401469

FENTON Vivienne Maeve 11/09/1978 Old Church Veterinary Group The Mall Ballyshannon Co Donegal Ireland **Tel:** (00353) 719851559 w 6050205

FEREDAY Emily Catherine Joy 29/08/2008 Mauna Loa Pitt Lane Appledore BIDEFORD Devon EX39 1QB **Tel:** 07815847635 w 6440904

FERGUS Kim Alexandra (nee McGimpsey) 05/10/1993 (08/01/2009) Unit 7 & 8 Brownlow Street Whitchurch Shropshire SY13 1QW **Tel:** (01948) 662424 w 6064772

FERGUSON Carly Ann 02/06/2006 Fammau View The Village Burton Neston Merseyside CH64 5TQ **Tel:** (0151) 336 2231 w 6347041

Lucy Elizabeth 18/09/2007 Mayfield Avenue Walkden Worsley Manchester M28 3JF **Tel:** (0161) 799 5557 w 6297530

FERGUSSON Mhairi 11/06/2008 Woodlea Byre North Berwick East Lothian EH39 5PH **Tel:** (01620) 893304 w 6377467

FERN Nicola Lorraine 01/02/1994 The Cottage Montpellier Court Boarden Barn Exmouth Devon EX8 1TP **Tel:** (01395) 273393 w 6067489

FERNEE Rosanne Mary 09/07/2007 18 Garden Lane ROYSTON Hertfordshire SG8 9EH **Tel:** (01763) 243395 w 6352541

FERRIER Angela (nee Thomson) 27/01/2000 33 Kirkfield East Livingston Village Livingston EH54 9BA w 6141705

FERRIS Clare 03/12/2003 7 Snave Close Litherland Liverpool L21 8QG w 6286640

Sian Kelly 09/07/2007 10 Llys y Fedwen Mornington Meadows CAERPHILLY Mid Glamorgan CF83 3QJ **Tel:** (029) 2088 9186 w 6352552

Tamsin Louise Dixon 29/05/2008 13 Rivendell Weston-super-Mare Avon BS22 7GD **Tel:** (07795) 380794 w 6379117

FERRY Claire Louise 28/04/2006 1-5 Hugh Street London SW1V 1QQ **Tel:** (020) 7932 2370 w 6284451

FIELD Claire Jane (see JERVIS, Mrs)

FIELD Helen Rosemary (nee Carter) 01/02/1999 93 Victoria Road Barking Essex IG11 8PZ **Tel:** (0208) 5144735 w 613439X

Katie Louise 22/10/2004 32 Carisbrooke Drive Weston Downes STAFFORD ST17 9JY w 6320047

Lisa Marie (nee Digby) 10/04/2003 6 Amber Close Teynham Sittingbourne Kent ME9 9TF **Tel:** (01634) 329502 w 6285958

Menna Rachel 06/10/2009 The Willows Muddles Green Chiddingly Lewes East Sussex BN8 6HN **Tel:** (01825) 872681 w 6375069

Sally Anne 20/08/2002 Harddfan Dynant Fach Road Pontyberem Llanelli Dyfed SA15 5LW **Tel:** (01269) 831209 w 6244521

FIELDING Jodie Ann 08/09/1997 (08/06/2009) 1 Holborne Close NEWBURY Berkshire RG14 6ST **Tel:** (01635) 569152 w 6112547

Kerry Louise 23/12/2003 Pines Veterinary Clinic 146a Bath Road Maidenhead Berkshire SL6 4LB **Tel:** (01628) 776699 w 6270250

Rikki 06/08/2008 The Paddock 53 Cherrydown West Basildon Essex SS16 5AW **Tel:** (01268) 533636 w 6321719

FIELDSON Natasha Ann (nee McLean) 03/09/2004 15 Rothbury Drive ASHINGTON Northumberland NE63 8TQ w 6268259

Victoria Ann (nee Savell) 27/01/2005 Wilson Veterinary Group 5-11 Tenters Street BISHOP AUCKLAND County Durham DL14 7AD **Tel:** (01388) 602707 w 6294461

FILDES Lisa Marie (see COULBORN, Mrs)

FILER Stephanie Clare 13/02/2009 5 St. Francis Drive Wick Bristol Avon BS30 5PQ **Tel:** 01179323660 w 6350836

FILLINGHAM Caroline 03/03/1989 (27/01/2010) Foxwood House Butterley Park RIPLEY Derbyshire DE5 3QW w 6050271

FILMER Sharon Patricia (nee Blackman) 23/12/2003 (12/01/2009) Shrubbery Veterinary Centre 65 Perry Street Northfleet Gravesend Kent DA11 8RD **Tel:** (01474) 333141 w 6286343

FINAN Carol Patricia 10/09/1981 156 Dudwell Lane Halifax Yorkshire HX3 0SH **Tel:** (01422) 300429 w 6091671

FINCH Alison Ruth 31/12/2003 59 Goatstown Close Hollywood Drive Dublin 14 Eire Ireland **Tel:** (00) 353 863611016 w 6284902

Amanda Jayne 19/01/1995 (02/12/1999) 204 Bushbury Road Fallings Park Wolverhampton WV10 0NB **Tel:** (01902) 731127 w 6035730

Amy Louise 27/05/2009 35 Peckover Close Rowley Regis West Midlands B65 0AU **Tel:** 01215592359 w 6381823

Danielle Sarah 02/12/2009 18 Butts Park Newton Ferrers Plymouth Devon PL8 1HY **Tel:** (01752) 872608 w 6425647

Joanne Clare 18/10/2006 (29/07/2008) 89 Mayles Road SOUTHSEA Hampshire PO4 8NR **Tel:** (02392) 737096 w 6272164

Sharon Lorraine 04/01/2006 32 Crescent Way HORLEY Surrey RH6 7LL **Tel:** (01293) 435583 w 6305109

FINDLAY Joanne (nee Wilde) 19/08/1994 20 Oakes Lane Brockholes Holmfirth HD9 7AR **Tel:** (01484) 667713 w 6032059

FINDLAY Leana (see THORPE, Mrs)

Maxine Anne 06/08/2008 10 Bankton Glade Livingston West Lothian EH54 9DG **Tel:** (01506) 460670 w 6377478

Sandra 29/08/2000 16 Cuthbert Place Kilmarnock Ayrshire KA3 1DT **Tel:** (079) 217 04827 w 6202523

FINEGAN Gillian Ann Catherine (see SHALA, Mrs)

FINLAYSON Rachel Elizabeth 07/02/2005 Moray Coast Veterinary Group West Road Greshop Estate Forres Morayshire IV36 2GW **Tel:** (01309) 672243 w 6286090

FINNEY Gillian Roberta (see BRIGHT, Mrs)

FINNEY Stephanie 10/07/2009 28 Caverswall Road Stoke-on-Trent Staffordshire ST3 6PE **Tel:** (01782) 599637 w 6400985

FINNIE Jessica Helygen 07/04/2009 3 Blackford Glen Road EDINBURGH EH16 6AD w 6436834

FINZEL Charlotte Violeta 16/09/2009 New Priory Veterinary Practice The Deneway London Rd Brighton East Sussex BN1 8QR **Tel:** (01273) 540430 w 6316549

FIRTH Nicole Amy 31/10/2008 62 Leigh Road Walsall West Midlands WS4 2DS **Tel:** (01922) 428669 w 6410687

FISH Jenna Amanda 12/09/2008 8 Crowhill Godmanchester Huntingdon Cambridgeshire PE29 2LP **Tel:** 01480350921 w 6429640

Karen Louise (nee Hulme) 06/08/1991 66 Church View Longhorsley Morpeth Northumberland NE65 8UQ **Tel:** (01670) 788040 w 6053512

FISHER Amanda Jane 03/09/1990 Molesey Veterinary Centre 4 Park Road East Molesey Surrey KT8 9LE w 6050329

Christine Ann 22/09/2004 44 Mogul Lane Halesowen West Midlands B63 2QW **Tel:** 01384638686 w 6294230

Emily Alexandra 15/04/2008 44 Glossop Road South Croydon Surrey CR2 0PU **Tel:** (0208) 6513305 w 6405429

Hannah Faye 21/07/2008 7 Norman Close Thorpe Willoughby Selby North Yorkshire YO8 9NS **Tel:** (01757) 702554 w 6375993

Leigh Sally 29/01/2009 94 Pithall Road Shard End BIRMINGHAM B34 7PT **Tel:** 01212410695 w 6445293

Victoria Anne 19/08/2008 8 Averon Rise Moorside OLDHAM OL1 4NX **Tel:** (0161) 633 5050 (Work) w 6355170

Victoria Maria 10/05/2007 7 Sandy Way Croydon Surrey CR0 8QT **Tel:** (020) 8777 5530 w 6387180

FISHER Zoe Ellen Crichton (see WALTON, Mrs)

FITZEARLE Gail Erin 01/10/1999 2 Near The Windmill Otten Road Belchamp Otten Sudbury Suffolk CO10 7BH **Tel:** (01787) 278502 w 613594X

FITZER Rachael Ann 29/01/2010 32 Burlish Avenue Olton Solihull BIRMINGHAM B92 8BF **Tel:** (0121) 704 2022 w 6466006

FITZGERALD Denise Ann 01/09/2009 12 Wansford Park BOREHAMWOOD Hertfordshire WD6 2PH **Tel:** (07949) 091560 w 6293020

FITZ-GERALD Lisa Jayne (see HOWE, Mrs)

FITZPATRICK Alexandra Adrienne 06/08/2007 Dandenong Veterinary Hospital 118 Princes Highway Dandenong Victoria 3178 Australia **Tel:** (0061) 3 9792 4787 w 6349472

Colette 17/11/2008 92 Blakemere Close Redditch Worcestershire B98 0LZ **Tel:** 01527502731 w 6413536

FITZROY Susan Carol 11/01/2005 The Freda Powell Centre 1c Eynsham Drive Thamesmead London SE2 9RQ **Tel:** (020) 8311 6695 w 6305538

FLACK Samantha Karen 22/02/2007 Flat 132 Griffin Court Black Eagle Drive Northfleet GRAVESEND Kent DA11 9AP w 6370515

Sarah Therese 10/09/2009 11 Pleasant Drive BILLERICAY Essex CM12 0JL **Tel:** (01277) 632216 w 6466380

Tammy Marie 21/12/2007 23 Blackbird Road Beck Row BURY ST. EDMUNDS Suffolk IP28 8HL **Tel:** (01842) 860189 w 6411424

FLANAGAN Claire Marie (formerly Readman) 28/12/2000 Highgate Veterinary Clinic 173 Highgate Kendal Cumbria LA9 4EN **Tel:** (01539) 721344 w 6205042

Hayley Ann 19/01/1998 207 Daventry Road Coventry West Midlands CV3 5HH **Tel:** (02476) 503000 w 6043617

FLANAGAN Zena Maxine (see MCFADZEAN, Mrs)

FLATMAN Sarah Jayne 27/09/2006 92 Montbelle Road London SE9 3NY **Tel:** (020) 8480 7320 w 6367259

FLEMING Kitty 05/08/2008 Arch Cottage John Beales Hill Pilton Shepton Mallet Somerset BA4 4DB **Tel:** 01749890296 w 6406947

FLEMONS Amy Laura 26/11/2007 68-70 Mill Lane West Hampstead London NW6 1NJ **Tel:** (020) 7794 1777 w 6363211

FLETCHER Amie Sarah 28/02/2005 4 Churchill Avenue ALDERSHOT Hampshire GU12 4JR **Tel:** (01252) 656484 w 6320058

FLETCHER Bryony (see WATKINS, Mrs)

Janine 28/07/1986 125 Malvern Drive North Common Bristol BS30 8UY **Tel:** (01179) 604917 w 6050431

Nadine Anne (nee Cooper) 13/07/1992 16 The Lawn Fakenham Norfolk NR21 8DT **Tel:** (01328) 855809 w 6008842

Ruth Elizabeth 14/11/2008 58 Jessop Street Codnor RIPLEY Derbyshire DE5 9RN w 6425735

FLETCHER Samantha (see BIGGS, Mrs)

FLETCHER Virginia DipAVN(Medical) 09/09/1988 7 Keats Walk Harrogate North Yorkshire HG1 3LN **Tel:** (01423) 566688 w 6051774

FLETT Charlotte Louise (see BYRNE, Mrs)

Rebecca Emily 11/03/1998 (27/03/2007) 21 Kinross Road Sleaford Lincolnshire NG34 8GB w 6130894

Selina Lois Evelyn 23/02/2005 26 Churchfields Kingsley Bordon Hampshire GU35 9PJ **Tel:** (01420) 476 125 w 6313711

FLINT Keri Dawn 06/12/2004 New Priory Veterinary Practice The Deneway London Rd Brighton East Sussex BN1 8QR **Tel:** (01273) 540430 w 6277543

Teresa Ann 13/08/2003 5 Upper Farm Road Oakley Basingstoke Hampshire RG23 7HN **Tel:** (01256) 781604 w 6267610

FLOOK Wendy (see WOOD, Mrs)

FLOYD Amy Louise 30/08/2000 Fivelands Veterinary Centre 98 Alcester Road BIRMINGHAM B13 8EG **Tel:** (0121) 449 3716 w 6204239

Lindsay Charlotte (nee Cathcart) 18/10/2006 The Veterinary Hospital 23 Wellington Street Thame Oxfordshire OX9 3BW **Tel:** (01844) 212000 w 6370933

FLUDE Victoria Ella (formerly Edge, nee Edge) 11/05/2000 Daleside 309-311 Liverpool Road Birkdale Southport Merseyside PR8 3DE **Tel:** (01704) 575606 w 6191369

FLYNN Lucy Jayne (nee Sullivan) 05/04/2005 32 Kelfield Avenue Birmingham West Midlands B17 0QL **Tel:** (0121) 6040663 w 6292921

FOAN Louise Carol (see CLARKSON, Mrs)

FOEKEN Jessica Janna 10/12/2007 8 Harwood Road LONDON SW6 4PH w 6502724

FOGARTY Deborah Fiona (nee Malton) 08/09/1997 Rodbaston College Vet Nurse Department Penkridge Stafford ST19 5PH **Tel:** (01785) 712209 w 6076187

FOGGO Tara (see LYNCH, Mrs)

FOGGON Peter 19/11/2009 Coastway Veterinary Group Unit 4E, Freshfield Business Park Freshfield Way Brighton East Sussex BN2 0BZ **Tel:** (01273) 692257 m 6435888

FOLEY Joanne Margaret 08/01/2008 The Mews Veterinary Centre Preseland Road LIVERPOOL Merseyside L23 5TE **Tel:** (0151) 924 2025 w 6332818

Katie Louise 22/02/2007 3 Pipers Ash RINGWOOD Hampshire BH24 1UF w 6348416

FONTAINE Samantha Joanna DipAVN(Medical) 27/02/2002 1/1 194 Earl Street Glasgow Lanarkshire G14 0BY **Tel:** (01506) 431657 w 6271537

FOORD Natalie (see ROBERTS, Mrs)

FOOTE Shelley Louise (nee Wenban) 14/05/2007 Killivose Cottage St. Allen TRURO Cornwall TR4 9DG **Tel:** (07971) 700 653 w 6374200

FOOTER Christopher Brian 31/10/2003 (16/12/2009) 99 Great Mistley Basildon Essex SS16 4AZ **Tel:** (01268) 458561 m 6272703

FORBES Nicola 22/03/2004 17E Waulking Mill Road CLYDEBANK Dunbartonshire G81 5AJ w 6287234

Rachel Mary (nee Hay) 04/07/2007 45 Tollohill Crescent Aberdeen Aberdeenshire AB12 5EN **Tel:** (07709) 353586 w 6349219

FORD Carly Marie 30/05/2008 15 Gadwell Road Walton Cardiff Tewkesbury Gloucestershire GL20 7RT **Tel:** (01684) 293942 w 6333676

Carol Elizabeth (nee Palmer) 24/02/2000 70 Brinkley Lane Highwoods COLCHESTER Essex CO4 9XE **Tel:** (01206) 842608 w 6118345

Elizabeth Mary 31/10/2008 26 Roberts Road London E17 4LR **Tel:** 02085319735 w 6431675

Gareth 22/08/1997 98 Conway Road Newport Gwent NP19 8NW **Tel:** (07904) 411724 m 6112616

FORD Julia Michelle (see SMITH, Mrs)

FORD Michelle (see SANDERS, Mrs)

Samantha Louise 15/02/2008 129 Bulls Head Lane COVENTRY CV3 1FW **Tel:** (02476) 449172 w 6405649

Terrie 17/08/1981 Flat 1 181 Bow Road Bow London E3 2SJ **Tel:** (0208) 9814995 w 6089458

FORDE Emma Kristina Hazel 22/12/2009 14 Boscaswell Downs Pendeen Penzance Cornwall TR19 7DR **Tel:** (01736) 785674 w 6440068

FORD-FENNAH Stuart James 31/10/2006 Cheetham House The Drove Bridgwater Somerset TA6 4BA **Tel:** (01278) 450080 m 6326350

Victoria Emma 27/04/2006 Lavender House White Street North Curry TAUNTON Somerset TA3 6HL w 6326471

FORDHAM Emma-Louise (nee Banham) 18/09/2003 4 Dowland Close Stanford-le-Hope Essex SS17 8QX **Tel:** (07739) 802972 w 6284913

FORDYCE Hayley (nee Tisdale) 06/10/2006 8 Setter Combe Warfield BRACKNELL Berkshire RG42 2FD w 6281404

FOREMAN Emma Dee (nee Simcock) 14/10/2002 36 Henderson Close HAVERHILL Suffolk CB9 7SU **Tel:** (01440) 704088 w 6273517

Louise Jane 25/06/2004 145 Cobham Road Fetcham Leatherhead Surrey KT22 9HX **Tel:** (01372) 379636 w 6283362

Sadie Marie 27/02/2006 Eastgate Veterinary Clinic 31 Bury Road Thetford Norfolk IP24 3AW **Tel:** (01842) 753991 w 6353806

FORNAI Francesca Daniela 28/09/2009 3 Poundbury Business Centre Poundbury Dorchester Dorset DT1 3WA **Tel:** (01305) 267083 w 6445513

FORREST Jay Lesley 18/10/2005 180 Merthyr Road Whitchurch CARDIFF CF14 1DL **Tel:** (02920) 529446 w 6254894

Jennifer Audrey BSc 10/02/2004 The Annex The Close Church Lane Fringford BICESTER Oxfordshire OX27 8DL **Tel:** (07939) 003171 w 6298025

Julie (nee Walton) 26/08/1997 17 Thorpe Avenue Whitwell Worksop Nottinghamshire S80 4PU **Tel:** (01909) 720031 w 6116632

FORRESTER Kerry Louise 03/05/2007 27 Apedale Road Newcastle-Under-Lyme Staffordshire ST5 6BH **Tel:** (01782) 565372 w 6375080

FORSHAW Kathryn Anne 06/06/2003 The Maisonette 1 Denmark Road Exeter EX1 1SL w 6274573

Kimberley Elizabeth 13/01/2004 5 Woodcote Cottages Pigeonhouse Yard Sutton Scotney Winchester Hampshire SO21 3JU **Tel:** (01962) 760579 w 6287883

FORSTER Stephanie Caroline (see WINTER, Mrs)

FORSYTH Amanda Cameron (see KELSO, Mrs)

FORSYTH June Brenda 06/07/2004 Meadows Veterinary Centre Station Road Oldmeldrum Inverurie Aberdeenshire AB51 0EZ **Tel:** (01651) 872481 w 6292558

Rhona Anne 04/10/2005 25 Lovers Lane Scone PERTH PH2 6RG **Tel:** (01738) 552712 w 6318430

FORTIS Joy Susann (nee Bentley) 26/10/2005 13 Windmill Row Glemsford SUDBURY Suffolk CO10 7QG w 6344995

FOSTER Claire Louise 22/09/2004 Congleton Veterinary Centre West Heath Retail Park Sandbach Road Congleton Cheshire CW12 4NB **Tel:** (01260) 272131 w 6307837

Emma Louise 21/06/2005 379 Bury Road Tonge Fold Bolton Lancashire BL2 6DE **Tel:** (01204) 385856 w 6263122

Jennifer 23/12/2008 8 Duddingston Avenue Kilwinning Ayrshire KA13 6RP **Tel:** (077) 325 18189 w 6440277

Kate 24/01/2008 Bro-Dawel Llanrhydd Ruthin Denbighshire LL15 2UP **Tel:** (01824) 704407 w 6387818

Katherine Elizabeth 07/01/2009 29 Ribble Lane Chatburn Clitheroe Lancashire BB7 4AG **Tel:** 01200440217 w 6441080

FOSTER Lyndsay Joanne (see BROADHURST, Mrs)

Melanie Kim 10/08/2007 40 Arden Road Furness Green CRAWLEY West Sussex RH10 6HS **Tel:** (077) 93738261 w 6284506

FOSTER Rachel Louise (see DAVIES, Mrs)

Sarah 01/10/1982 (22/01/2007) Mole End 3 Underwood Cottages Clyst Hydon CULLOMPTON Devon EX15 2NT **Tel:** (01884) 277958 w 6050646

FOSTER Sarah Ann (see KIRK, Mrs)

FOSTER Sarah Louise (see WALKER, Mrs)

Victoria Helen Lisa 29/06/2007 The White Cottage Hallingbury Place Great Hallingbury Bishop's Stortford Hertfordshire CM22 7UE **Tel:** (01279) 652251 w 6376004

FOTHERGILL Glenys 06/03/2006 Number 2 Townhead Farm Newbiggin Stainton PENRITH Cumbria CA11 0HT **Tel:** (07913) 855 178 w 6344797

FOTHERINGHAM Lynne Christina (see NIMMO, Mrs)

FOULKES Victoria Louise 15/07/2008 15 Maes y Llan Llanfairtalhaiarn ABERGELE Clwyd LL22 8SF **Tel:** (01745) 720 258 w 6410346

FOWLER Catherine Grace 14/03/2006 Caldew Veterinary Hospital Carlisle House Townhead Road Dalston Carlisle Cumbria CA5 7JF **Tel:** (01228) 710208 w 6349703

Celine Danielle 04/06/2009 Bolt House Love Lane West Meon Petersfield Hampshire GU32 1HS w 6407915

Claire Louise 15/05/2009 128 Drysdale Avenue London E4 7PE **Tel:** (0208) 529 4470 w 6440233

Lysbeth Jane (nee Threlfall) 02/09/1998 (12/07/2005) 12 Windermere Road Handforth Wilmslow Cheshire SK9 3NH w 6034602

Nichola Jane Shirley (nee Sadler) 19/03/2007 Oakfield Veterinary Group 2 Margaret Road Atherstone Warwickshire CV9 1EE **Tel:** (01827) 713 149 w 6347316

Sarah Jane 23/03/2006 Galemire Veterinary Hospital Galemire CLEATOR MOOR Cumbria CA25 5QX **Tel:** (01946) 810295 w 6344808

Sarah Ruth (nee Coultrup) 28/08/1997 45 St. Laurence Drive Broxbourne Hertfordshire EN10 6LH **Tel:** (01992) 414381 w 6026839

FOX Angela Marie 30/01/1991 PDSA Kings Road Southwick Sunderland SR5 2LH **Tel:** (0191) 516 0636 w 6050679

Claire Dawn 26/10/2005 Sileby Hall Cossington Road Sileby Loughborough Leicestershire LE12 7RS **Tel:** (01509) 812445/6 w 6346249

Emma Jayne 30/09/2008 22 Reedmace Tamworth Staffordshire B77 1BH **Tel:** 0182760729 w 6433182

Gemma Anne 12/12/2005 45 Middlemoor Road Frimley CAMBERLEY Surrey GU16 8BT **Tel:** (01276) 676274 w 6329650

Gemma Verity Paula (nee Taylor) 09/06/2008 9 Allington Rise Taylors Farm Sherfield-on-Loddon HOOK Hampshire RG27 0ST w 6412491

Geraldine Mary 16/02/2009 17 Brae Court Moy DUNGANNON County Tyrone BT71 7UB **Tel:** 02887789629 w 6404010

Joanna Kim 27/02/2006 5 Carisbrooke Crescent Chandler's Ford EASTLEIGH Hampshire SO53 2LQ **Tel:** (023) 80904262 w 6301523

Julie Ann Marie 07/02/2006 228 Painswick Road Gloucester Gloucestershire GL4 4PH **Tel:** (01452) 529480 w 6260603

Leanne Joan 04/10/2005 72 Endlebury Road Chingford London E4 6QG **Tel:** (020) 8542 5080 w 6290094

Lisa Marie 31/03/2003 (25/06/2008) 10 Hainault Close BENFLEET Essex SS7 2LL w 6279743

Rebecca Louise 19/11/2007 Little Couchman Green Farm Couchman Green Lane Staplehurst Tonbridge Kent TN12 0RT **Tel:** (01580) 891436 w 6411435

Samantha 06/03/2006 Feldon Veterinary Centre 1 Guy Street Leamington Spa Warwickshire CV32 4RX **Tel:** (01926) 423161 w 6343719

FOX Sara Sanchia (see ALLWOOD, Mrs)

Serena 18/04/2008 Flat G Clifton Mansions 54 St. Giles High Street LONDON WC2H 8LH w 6507234

Suzanne Elizabeth 07/02/2007 Oathall Veterinary Group 30 Oathall Road Haywards Heath West Sussex RH16 3EQ **Tel:** (01444) 440224 w 6366159

FOX Victoria Elisabeth (see HEDGES, Mrs)

FOXALL Emma Louise 29/11/2007 9 Woodcroft Close Annitsford CRAMLINGTON Northumberland NE23 7UF w 6377181

FOXLEY Rebecca Jane 22/12/2009 40 Wivelsfield Road Saltdean BRIGHTON BN2 8FQ **Tel:** (07793) 814166 w 6497499

FRADLEY Kerry 03/05/2005 Lemburg Greenhill Lane Riddings Alfreton Derbyshire DE55 4AY **Tel:** (01773) 541070 w 6318276

FRALEY Jennifer Anthea 09/07/2007 3 Kenilworth Drive KIDDERMINSTER Worcestershire DY10 1YD **Tel:** (01562) 60847 w 6352563

FRAMPTON Rosemary 16/08/1977 12 Roberts Street Sneinton Nottingham NG2 4QD **Tel:** (01159) 599030 w 6050704

FRANCE Jane (nee France) 21/01/1999 (21/01/2010) Pennington House Veterinary Centre Newlands Road LEIGH Lancashire WN7 4HA **Tel:** (01942) 673777 w 6129685

FRANCIS Catherine Sian 09/03/2005 St Runwalds Veterinary Surgery 94A Maldon Road Colchester Essex CO3 3AP **Tel:** (01206) 572173 w 6268072

Claire Rachel 25/10/1999 (02/11/2006) 42 Criffel Avenue Streatham Hill LONDON SW2 4BN w 6117432

Jane (nee Walton) 30/07/1987 33 High Street Stalham Norwich NR12 9AH **Tel:** (01692) 580171 w 6063098

Joanna Louise 02/10/2009 100 Maison Dieu Road Dover Kent CT16 1RU **Tel:** (01304) 206989 w 6408168

Nicola Lesley 06/03/2008 46 Wisbech Road Thorney PETERBOROUGH PE6 0SD **Tel:** (01733) 270429 w 6398224

Rachel Suzanne 13/03/2002 Anneth-Lowen 3 Sheilas Court Trewartha Estate Carbis Bay St. Ives Cornwall TR26 2TQ **Tel:** (01736) 794801 w 6255543

Sarah Louise 01/10/2008 Station Farm London Road Six Mile Bottom Newmarket Suffolk CB8 0UH **Tel:** (01638) 572012 w 6434370

FRANKLIN Hayley Anne 10/02/2004 Honeysuckle Veterinary Surgery Tunnel Road Beaminster Dorset DT8 3HB **Tel:** (01308) 862312 w 6285628

Sharon (formerly Franklin) 18/12/2007 Rivendell King William Lane Curry Rivel LANGPORT Somerset TA10 0HB **Tel:** (01458) 253878 w 6382340

FRANKS Joanna Elizabeth 04/03/2008 44 Sibland Road Thornbury BRISTOL BS35 2EP **Tel:** (01454) 417927 w 6378622

FRASER Catherine Amy (nee Rees) 24/11/2004 (11/01/2010) 17 Rossall Drive ASHBY-DE-LA-ZOUCH Leicestershire LE65 2QN w 6319761

Claire Louise 07/08/1990 46 Stirling Crescent Hedge End SOUTHAMPTON SO30 2SB w 6050748

Diann 18/09/2007 Ayrton Veterinary Centre Burnhouse Industrial Estate Whitburn West Lothian EH47 0LQ **Tel:** (01501) 744736 w 6355181

Faye Claire 13/07/2004 Flat 6 38 Coundon Road Coventry West Midlands CV1 4AW **Tel:** (02476) 594 242 w 6305549

Jill Marie 11/09/1998 (18/02/2008) Glen Bridge Farm Todley Hall Road Oakworth KEIGHLEY West Yorkshire BD22 0PX **Tel:** (01274) 580785 w 6133294

FRASER Julie Fiona (see ROBERT, Mrs)

Lisa Marie (nee Gough) 25/08/1998 126 Penn Road Datchett Berkshire SL3 9JE **Tel:** (01753) 594131 w 6134130

Susan Mary 17/01/1984 The Shepton Veterinary Group Allyn Saxon Drive Shepton Mallet Somerset BA4 5QH **Tel:** (01749) 343955 w 6089673

FRATER Dawn (nee Wardle) 24/01/2005 75 Dene View Crescent Sunderland Tyne and Wear SR4 0LP **Tel:** (0191) 534 5478 w 6325888

FRAWLEY Christine 16/09/2004 Animal Hospital 37 Main Road Tallaght Dublin 24 Ireland w 6296716

FRAZER Aimee Lyn 22/04/2008 2 Longdyke Farm Steading Shilbottle ALNWICK Northumberland NE66 2HQ **Tel:** (01665) 581523 w 6402459

FRAZER Claire Louise (see TAYLOR, Mrs)

FREEMAN Dawn 28/01/1999 12 Atkinson Road Maidenbower CRAWLEY West Sussex RH10 7JY **Tel:** 07740345578 w 6017697

Donna Marie 03/10/2007 31 Charnwood Street Coalville Leicestershire LE67 3DH **Tel:** (07850) 897458 w 6374563

FREEMAN Emma Clare (see BULLEN, Mrs)

Katherine Elizabeth 10/08/2007 22 London Road CIRENCESTER Gloucestershire GL7 1AE w 6351826

Melanie Anne 24/09/2001 44 Storth Lane Broadmeadows South Normanton Alfreton Derbyshire DE55 3AA **Tel:** (01773) 511195 w 6228571

FREESTONE Jacqueline Louise (see EASTWOOD, Mrs)

FRENCH Christine Ann (see ABBOTT, Mrs)

FRENCH Lindsay Alexandra 10/05/2007 22 Hogarth Way Bournemouth Dorset BH8 0DX **Tel:** (01202) 394358 w 6359801

Sally Nicola BSc 25/06/2004 93 Sea Place Worthing West Sussex BN12 4BH **Tel:** (01903) 700252 w 6284242

Victoria Grace 24/05/2005 8 The Leas FAVERSHAM Kent ME13 7QE w 6317407

FRESNEAU Kerry Anne 29/01/2007 1 Hawthorn Close Stowupland Stowmarket Suffolk IP14 4DQ **Tel:** (01449) 675 095 w 6366786

FREWIN Henrietta Louise 23/12/2003 Riverside Veterinary Clinic 17 Severnside South Bewdley Worcestershire DY12 2DX **Tel:** (01299) 402960 w 6279402

FREYTAG Jennifer Jane 19/09/2006 16 Dalsholm Place GLASGOW G20 0UH w 6350000

FRIAR Richard William 29/10/1986 Cedarmount Veterinary Clinic 67 Bryansburn Road Bangor County Down BT20 3SD **Tel:** (02891) 271364 m 6050817

FRIEND Michaela Lorraine 04/08/2003 326 Mutton Lane Potters Bar Hertfordshire EN6 2AX **Tel:** (01227) 373510 w 6230320

FRITH Laura Jane 13/02/2009 The Veterinary Hospital 175 Newport Lincoln Lincolnshire LN1 3DZ **Tel:** (01522) 800333 w 6426252

FRITH Laura Kate (see WALTERS, Mrs)

Nicola Elizabeth (formerly Hine, formerly Cayzer) 24/08/1998 240 Sigston Road BEVERLEY North Humberside HU17 9PL w 613156X

FRODSHAM Anne-Marie (nee Sewell) 19/07/2004 12 South Terrace ALDERLEY EDGE Cheshire SK9 7HA w 6291051

FROGLEY Samantha Jane 17/02/2009 1 Gladwish Cottages Headcorn Road Sutton Valence MAIDSTONE Kent ME17 3EL **Tel:** 07903963134 w 6451849

FROST Diana Jean 31/07/1992 13 College Road Thurlton Norwich NR14 6QZ **Tel:** (01508) 548237 w 6008081

Helen Frances (nee Mouzer) 05/10/2004 3 Eastlands Court St Peters Road Rugby Warwickshire CV21 3QP **Tel:** (01788) 575300 w 6275827

Kelly Marie 31/10/2003 17 Hardwick Street Langwith Mansfield Nottinghamshire NG20 9DR w 6287652

FROST Lisa (see COOPER, Mrs)

Lowri Wynne (nee Williams) 21/05/2007 Wern Veterinary Surgery Greenfield Road Ruthin Denbighshire LL15 1EY **Tel:** (01824) 702445 w 6375674

Sarah Marie 23/11/2001 30 Lavender Road Swanwick ALFRETON Derbyshire DE55 1RR w 6274144

FRY Bridget Louise 10/09/1996 (05/05/2005) 10 Pope Crescent Enderby LEICESTER LE19 4QT **Tel:** (01162) 849 456 w 6031066

Nichola Claire 26/01/1998 (13/02/2004) 48 Albert Road St Philips Bristol BS2 0XA **Tel:** (0117) 972 4567 w 6107989

FRYER Charlene Jayne 30/11/2007 3 Frank Street LINCOLN LN5 8AL **Tel:** (07828) 184194 w 6367061

FUIT Nicole 13/11/2006 59 Mornington Blvd Waikiki 6169 Western Australia Australia **Tel:** (00) 618 9592 2947 w 6443544

FULLALOVE Jane Susan 29/10/2004 28 Alderbury Lea Bicknacre Essex CM3 4XQ **Tel:** (01245) 226627 w 6295330

FULLBROOK Megan Jean 30/05/2007 Haven Veterinary Practice 35 Holland Road Clacton-on-Sea Essex CO15 6EH **Tel:** (01255) 422150 w 6334556

FULLEYLOVE Helen Joy (nee Biggs) 02/02/1999 (26/10/2006) 102 Moseley Avenue Coundon Coventry West Midlands CV6 1HQ **Tel:** (02476) 594242 w 6143531

FULLS Judith 14/01/1992 (21/01/2008) Arago Clinica Veterinaria Carrer Cirerer 2 B 07008 Palma De Mallorca Spain **Tel:** (00) 34 971 47 9354 w 6065244

FULTON Elaine 14/01/2008 25 Little Hoddington Upton Grey Basingstoke Hampshire RG25 2RN **Tel:** (01256) 862230 w 6383176

FURBER Georgina Mary 01/09/2009 21 Ledbury Road Hereford HR1 2SY **Tel:** (01432) 356253 w 6489018

FURLONG Michelle Marie (see COSGROVE, Mrs)

FURLOW Joanna Teresa 26/11/2008 51 Sycamore Drive HUNTINGDON Cambridgeshire PE29 7JA **Tel:** 07500141181 w 6434788

FURMSTON Lynda Pauline 23/03/2007 11 Greenshank Close Newton-le-Willows Merseyside WA12 9RT **Tel:** (01925) 221 677 w 6372836

FURNESS Allison Valerie (see LITTLEHALES, Mrs)

FURNISS Emma Elizabeth Sarah 10/03/2009 4 Ancaster Road Leeds West Yorkshire LS16 5HH **Tel:** 07926883003 w 6409400

FURNISS Melissa Louise (see HARRIS, Mrs)

FURNIVAL Kirsty Anne (nee Wright, formerly Hare) 22/08/1997 4 Brambles Courtyard Freemens Way Deal Kent CT14 9WP **Tel:** (01304) 366262 w 6040376

FYSH Emma Marion 12/09/1996 Mill House Veterinary Surgery & Hospital 20 Tennyson Avenue King's Lynn Norfolk PE30 2QG **Tel:** (01553) 771457 w 6099218

G

GADD Gillian Mary 18/01/2002 Castle Vets Pet Healthcare Centre 1 Tilehurst Road Reading Berkshire RG1 7TW **Tel:** (0118) 957 4488 w 6185902

GAIN Andrew David 01/02/2008 3 Park Lane Fareham Hampshire PO16 7JU **Tel:** (01329) 237619 m 6378842

GALDAS Caroline Michelle 06/02/2009 95 Woodhall Avenue BRADFORD West Yorkshire BD3 7BU **Tel:** 07946470142 w 6438572

GALE Heather Elena 29/08/2000 Thorn House Business Centre 30 Ballot Road Irvine Strathclyde KA12 0HW **Tel:** (01294) 278232 w 6138725

GALE Lucy Emma (see AUSTIN, Mrs)

Sian Marie 22/09/2008 April Cottage Old London Road Coldwaltham PULBOROUGH West Sussex RH20 1LF **Tel:** 07814231633 w 6437890

GALER Denise Yvonne (nee Algar) 25/08/1999 (01/12/2006) 48 Schoolfield Glemsford Sudbury Suffolk CO10 7RE w 6116789

GALES Anna 19/10/2007 9, Platinum Court Silver Way Romford Essex RM7 8EB **Tel:** 02085506119 w 6370977

GALLACHER Amy Marie 02/09/2008 30 Bertelin Road STAFFORD ST16 3JJ w 6441861

Jacqueline (nee McCrone) 04/02/1992 (27/10/2003) 79 Langmuirhead Road Kirkintilloch GLASGOW G66 5DJ **Tel:** (0141) 5885977 w 6002148

GALLAGHER Ciara Helen 17/01/2006 116 Station Road Kegworth DERBY DE74 2FR w 6326361

Jane Alison 19/01/2009 45 Yoxall Road Shirley SOLIHULL West Midlands B90 3SD **Tel:** 07846949870 w 6433050

Jeanette Butler 03/08/1972 (21/03/2001) Earlswood Veterinary Hospital 193 Belmont Road Belfast BT4 2AE **Tel:** (028) 9047 1361 w 6000774

Kerrie-Ann DipAVN(Medical) (nee MacDonald) 02/09/1998 Acorn House Veterinary Surgery Linnet Way Bedford MK41 7HN **Tel:** (01234) 261839 w 6132665

Muriel Patricia 20/11/2002 51 Fountain Hill Mell Co Louth Ireland **Tel:** (00) 353 877 985896 w 6279479

Samantha Jayne (nee Bloor) 30/10/2003 Lime Trees Veterinary Clinic Tean Road Cheadle Stoke-on-Trent ST10 1TW **Tel:** (01538) 752117 w 6284814

GALLETLY Kerry Rachel 25/11/2008 18 Butts Bridge Road Hythe Southampton Hampshire SO45 3HF **Tel:** 02380843534 w 6433105

GALLOWAY Karyn Anne 09/07/2008 Alver Veterinary Group 30 Stubbington Green Stubbington Hampshire PO14 2LE **Tel:** (01329) 667551 w 6391921

GALVIN Paula (see WYNNE, Mrs)

GAMBLE Louisa (see BAKER, Mrs)

GAMBLE Rebecca Louise (formerly Hodgson) 07/11/2008 Dog Vane Veterinary Clinic 289 Yarm Road DARLINGTON County Durham DL1 1BA **Tel:** (01325) 469165 w 6436240

GAMMON Rebecca Kate 02/09/2008 14 Eaton Crescent SWANSEA SA1 4QJ **Tel:** 01792470551 w 6408223

GANNAWAY Helen Margaret 31/01/1991 75a Princess Road Urmston MANCHESTER M41 5SQ w 6050908

GAPP Amanda Jayne 06/03/2006 Holly House Veterinary Clinic 101 Market Street Hindley Wigan WN2 3AB **Tel:** (01942) 526222 w 6347074

GARBETT Kim 19/12/2006 Moor Cottage Veterinary Hospital London Road Binfield Bracknell Berkshire RG42 4AA **Tel:** (01344) 450345 w 6363222

GARBO Amy Maria 18/02/2008 Meridian Veterinary Practice Ltd 11 Edith Avenue Peacehaven East Sussex BN10 8JB **Tel:** (01273) 585386 w 6405286

GARBUTT Marie Elizabeth 05/12/2008 62 Edward Road COVENTRY CV6 2GR w 6417144

GARBUTT Nicola Helen (see BURNEY, Mrs)

GARCIA Samara Louise 09/06/2009 Hillcrest Animal Health Ltd Water Street Chorley Lancashire PR7 1EX **Tel:** (01257) 262448 w 6443401

GARDINER Emma Jane 06/10/2006 Southcrest Veterinary Centre 97 Mount Pleasant Redditch Worcestershire B97 4JD **Tel:** (01527) 550111 w 6357051

Jody Future Melissa 10/02/2005 7 Church Road Colmworth BEDFORD MK44 2JX w 6300027

Lindsey 08/09/2009 8 McFadden Crescent Kintore INVERURIE Aberdeenshire AB51 0SD **Tel:** (07973) 678168 w 6453367

Louise Catherine 10/04/2003 Ayrton Veterinary Centre Burnhouse Industrial Estate Whitburn West Lothian EH47 0LQ **Tel:** (01501) 744736 w 6282240

Maria Louise (nee Price) 13/03/2009 Arrowfield Veterinary Group Butt's Meadow Hatton Gardens Kington Herefordshire HR5 3DD **Tel:** (01544) 230567 w 6433424

Sally Deborah 29/08/1995 255 Barnwell Road Cambridge Cambridgeshire CB5 8SL **Tel:** (01223) 243535 w 6039509

GARDNER Jennifer Clare 19/04/2005 1 Gaw Hill View Aughton ORMSKIRK Lancashire L39 3QX w 6323314

GARDNER Jill Rebecca (see BARKER, Mrs)

GARDNER Lindsay (see MACAUSLAND, Mrs)

Sarah Ruth 08/11/2006 49 Askham Lane York North Yorkshire YO24 3HB **Tel:** (01904) 798 896 w 6372352

GARLAND Emma Louise (see JAMESON, Mrs)

GARLIKE Joanna Rachel 17/07/2008 29 Carisbrooke Court Romsey Hampshire SO51 7JQ **Tel:** (01794) 521592 w 6378853

GARNER Hayley Marie 19/03/2007 8 Raby Court Ellesmere Port Merseyside CH65 9DZ **Tel:** (0151) 5122159 w 6375498

James Oliver 04/01/2006 16 East of England Way Orton Northgate Peterborough Cambridgeshire PE2 6HE **Tel:** (01733) 552932 m 6351265

Jennifer Claire 17/09/2007 (02/12/2009) Ashlands Veterinary Centre 119 Leeds Road Ilkley West Yorkshire LS29 8JS **Tel:** (01943) 817000 w 6374585

GARNER Lindsey Ann (see BEECH, Mrs)

GARNETT Emma Jane 01/02/2008 40 Mayfair Close Great Sankey Warrington Cheshire WA5 3PL **Tel:** (01925) 488706 w 6404076

GARNETT Stella (see ELLIS, Mrs)

GARRARD Fiona 16/09/2002 20 Knowsley Court Tudor Grange Kenton Bankfoot Newcastle upon Tyne NE3 2FJ **Tel:** (0191) 2868072 w 6275332

Fiona Jean 06/10/2006 73 Markyate Road Slip End Luton Bedfordshire LU1 4BU **Tel:** (01582) 451 415 w 6357337

GARRATT-BRIDLE Elizabeth Anne 28/10/2008 56 Forgefields Herne Bay Kent CT6 7TF **Tel:** 07952964844 w 6431686

GARRETT Alexandra Jane 22/03/2004 1 Old Eign Hill Hampton Park Hereford Herefordshire HR1 1TU **Tel:** (01432) 357222 w 6292569

Claire Brownlee (nee Bell) 13/04/2004 20 The Spinney Burgess Hill West Sussex RH15 8AG **Tel:** (01444) 870015 w 6287564

Jennifer Alison 13/05/2003 69 Findhorn Place Edinburgh EH9 2PD **Tel:** (0131) 6670050 w 6282295

GARROD Louise Rachael 21/07/2008 38 Beech Way Dickleburgh DISS Norfolk IP21 4NZ **Tel:** (01379) 741261 w 6376015

Rachel Elizabeth Clare DipAVN(Medical) 22/09/1999 Apartment 16 The Nile 24 City Road East MANCHESTER M15 4TA w 6184780

GARROOD Emma Louise 11/05/2009 Chestnut Veterinary Group 1 Hoe Lane Ware Hertfordshire SG12 9LS **Tel:** (01920) 468874 w 6446910

GARTON Rebecca (see HANCOCK, Mrs)

GARTSIDE Susan Julia 03/02/1995 (05/02/2007) 71 Tickford Street Newport Pagnell Buckinghamshire MK16 9AW **Tel:** (01908) 216386 w 6038447

GARVEY Connie Alison (nee Gilchrist) 17/08/1994 (30/10/2000) 1 Sillswood Olney Buckinghamshire MK46 5PL **Tel:** (01243) 711755 w 6026486

GARWOOD Tracy Louise 25/01/1999 North Kent Referrals Warren Road Blue Bell Hill CHATHAM Kent ME5 9RD **Tel:** (01634) 666655 w 613543X

GASCOYNE Heidi 04/08/2008 2 Fern Cottages GLASGOW G13 1NH **Tel:** 01419599194 w 6520555

GASKILL Clair Marie 13/12/2001 85 Garway Liverpool Merseyside L25 5LP **Tel:** (0151) 475 0696 w 6261725

GASKIN Sharon Theresa DipAVN(Surgical) (nee O'Connor) 16/08/1982 (19/07/1999) 82 Wellington Road Ashton-under-Lyne Lancashire OL6 6DP **Tel:** (0161) 330 2514/4839 w 6051016

GATES Chantel Louise 15/07/2008 23 Buckton Road Borehamwood Hertfordshire WD6 4HN **Tel:** (07958) 244 495 w 6415450

Victoria Louise 02/06/2006 Wood Street Veterinary Hospital 74 Wood Street Barnet Hertfordshire EN5 4BW **Tel:** (020) 8449 0074 w 6283384

GATHERER Mary Elizabeth 18/01/1995 4 Milliken Drive Kilbarchan Renfrewshire PA10 2AW **Tel:** (01505) 706253 w 6036009

GATT Gertrude 27/07/1992 24 St. Margaret Street Dunfermline Fife KY12 7PE **Tel:** (01383) 732897 w 6051038

GATWARD Tracey Ellen (see BOARDMAN, Mrs)

GAUCHWIN Helen (nee Breckell) 04/08/1992 21 Norbreck Close Great Sankey Warrington WA5 2SJ **Tel:** (01925) 791755 w 6008853

GAUDIANO Frances Jane 21/08/1998 Yew Tree Veterinary Centre Horsham Road Cranleigh Surrey GU6 8DP **Tel:** (01483) 275665 w 6129823

GAUGHAN Laura 11/08/1989 (28/01/2010) 38 Melbourne Road BUSHEY Hertfordshire WD23 3LN **Tel:** (020) 8387 4246 w 6051049

GAULD Christine Anne (see BARCLAY, Mrs)

GAYLARD Lindsey Marie (formerly Scarsbrook) 27/09/2004 Martock Veterinary Centre Stapleton Road Martock Somerset TA12 6HH **Tel:** (01935) 825199 w 6305219

GAYLOR Donna Elaine (nee Macdonald) 19/09/2006 Easter Bush Veterinary Centre University of Edinburgh Easter Bush Roslin Midlothian EH25 9RG **Tel:** (0131) 650 7650 w 6303734

GAZEY Katie Jean (nee Mold) 22/08/1995 5 The Pines Woodlands Park Bedworth Warwickshire CV12 0NZ **Tel:** (024) 76640536 w 6030073

GEDDES Donna Ann 25/02/2003 116 Calder Place Falkirk Stirlingshire FK1 2QQ **Tel:** (01324) 610852 w 6271559

GEESIN Victoria Emma 29/04/2009 222 West Street Bedminster BRISTOL BS3 3NE **Tel:** 07711292091 w 6340364

GEMMELL Sarah Rosalind 24/11/2009 31 Someries Road Hemel Hempstead Hertfordshire HP1 3PJ w 6466468

GEOGHEGAN Nicola Ann 23/08/2005 Novartis Animal Health Frimley Business Park Frimley

CAMBERLEY Surrey GU16 7SR **Tel:** (01276) 694402 w 6301545

GEORGE Caroline Sally-Jane DipAVN(Surgical) 22/09/1987 Canterbury College New Dover Road CANTERBURY Kent CT1 3AJ w 6051118

Corinne 29/10/2004 14 Shelton Road SHREWSBURY Shropshire SY3 8SS w 6290369

Donna Louise 18/10/2006 63 Lonsdale Avenue Cosham PORTSMOUTH Hampshire PO6 2PU w 6345457

Emily Elizabeth 28/04/2006 (31/01/2008) 13 Belvedere Crescent Bewdley Worcestershire DY12 1JX **Tel:** (01299) 400647 w 6286871

Louise Janette 19/03/2007 Morley Veterinary Centre 31 Bridge Street Taunton Somerset TA1 1TQ **Tel:** (01823) 276959 w 6382362

GERRARD Emma Louise 08/09/2005 Ty Crwban 12 Berllan Deg Llansantffraid Powys SY22 6FF **Tel:** (01691) 670067 w 6346546

June Doreen 15/11/2001 Buchan Veterinary Clinic 29 Finlayson Street Fraserburgh Aberdeenshire AB43 9JQ **Tel:** (01346) 510099 w 6258535

GERRARD Lauren Ann Edith (see WADE, Mrs)

GERRARD Sarah Louise (see JONES, Mrs)

GETHING Victoria Sarah 06/02/2009 63 Camden Road Broadstairs Kent CT10 3DS **Tel:** (01843) 861 644 w 6445535

GETTINS Clare 30/08/2006 50 Tuscan Road Sunderland Tyne and Wear SR3 4NA **Tel:** (01915) 512295 w 6348427

GEYELIN William 19/09/2006 Grove Lodge Veterinary Group Ltd 18 Upper Brighton Road Worthing West Sussex BN14 9DL **Tel:** (01903) 234866 m 6290105

GIBBISON Helen 23/02/2005 George Veterinary Hospital 18-20 High Street Malmesbury Wiltshire SN16 9AU **Tel:** (01666) 823165 w 6300005

GIBBONS Jodie Louise 10/09/2009 Claremont Newent Gloucestershire GL18 1EB **Tel:** 07890715893 w 6429277

Ruth (nee Shepard) 21/05/2007 68 Calico Crescent Carrbrook Stalybridge Cheshire SK15 3FJ **Tel:** (01457) 834 027 w 6373078

GIBBS Lucy Anne 04/07/2007 88 Edale Stoney Delph TAMWORTH Staffordshire B77 4HF **Tel:** (01827) 703 290 w 6352574

GIBSON Amanda Jane (see RAWLINSON, Mrs)

GIBSON Carli Ann (see DODD, Mrs)

GIBSON Caroline 16/07/2002 Flat C 26 Grey Street NEWCASTLE UPON TYNE Tyne & Wear NE1 6AE w 6265949

GIBSON Catherine Louise (see TIDD, Mrs)

Clare 26/04/2007 Kirkton Veterinary Centre Fetteresso Stonehaven Kincardineshire AB39 3UP **Tel:** (01569) 764140 w 6373287

Dawn 17/01/2008 4 Fisherbeck Park Ambleside Cumbria LA22 0JT **Tel:** (015394) 33440 w 6405748

Erin Michelle Jude 10/02/2004 1 Chestnut Ave Corby Northamptonshire NN17 2ER **Tel:** (01536) 394 828 w 6285452

Jean Ann 22/01/1985 Kingfisher Veterinary Practice Tower Hill Road Crewkerne Somerset TA18 8EQ **Tel:** (01460) 77790 w 605113X

Katherine Claire 19/12/2006 Phoenix Veterinary Centre 93 Portsmouth Road Camberley Surrey GU15 1HT **Tel:** (01276) 21225 w 6372858

Kira Jayne 26/08/2003 20 Albert Road Colne Lancashire BB8 0AA **Tel:** (01282) 863892 w 6280854

Rachel (nee Hillaby) 09/02/1999 (09/01/2004) Bollington Veterinary Centre Middlewood House Grimshaw Lane Bollington Macclesfield Cheshire SK10 5JB **Tel:** (01625) 572999 w 6140519

Rebecca Jayne 27/04/2005 11 Ashfield Place Fagley BRADFORD West Yorkshire BD2 3JB w 6327076

Tyrina 17/07/2008 17 Bamborough Court Dudley CRAMLINGTON Northumberland NE23 7HW **Tel:** 07738590031 w 6351276

GIDLEY Rebecca Louise 19/09/2006 58 Elmside EXETER Devon EX4 6LR w 6305296

GIFFARD Kelly-Marie 19/12/2006 7 Griffin Field Stewkley Leighton Buzzard Bedfordshire LU7 0GZ w 6354620

GIFFORD Elizabeth Anne 07/01/2010 52 B Pretoria Avenue London E17 7DR **Tel:** 07724171360 w 6440486

GIFFORD Sarah Kathleen (see SONLEY, Mrs)

GILBERT Clare Elizabeth 21/04/2005 14 Lindford Way Kings Norton Birmingham B38 0BD **Tel:** (0121) 459 0698 w 6284704

GILBERT Claudia Marie (see BAILEY, Mrs)

Jayne Emily Victoria 08/11/2006 The Flat Three Countries Equine Hospital Stratford Bridge Ripple Tewkesbury Gloucestershire GL20 6HE **Tel:** (07810) 481623 w 6301556

Toni Joanne 17/01/1997 (23/02/2000) 19 Weelsby Avenue Grimsby North East Lincolnshire DN32 0AH **Tel:** (01472) 322 166 w 6108279

GILBEY Sophie Lucinda 10/01/2003 Spring Lodge Farm Powers Hall End Witham Essex CM8 2HG **Tel:** (01376) 513247 w 6281492

GILCHRIST Connie Alison (see GARVEY, Mrs)

GILES Emma Louise 26/04/2002 (02/11/2009) Rosebank Cottage The Square Moreton Pinkney DAVENTRY Northamptonshire NN11 3SH w 6274859

Karen Yvonne 13/02/2009 1 Harrogate Close Higher Openshaw Manchester Lancashire M11 1WX **Tel:** (0161) 3302514 w 6407145

Laura Kate 07/06/2005 (28/02/2007) Dobles Cottage Tolland Lydeard St. Lawrence TAUNTON Somerset TA4 3PP **Tel:** 01984667417 w 6325745

Samantha 08/05/2008 9 Jerusalem Lane New Inn Pontypool Gwent NP4 0NR **Tel:** (01495) 752152 w 6391866

GILKES Kerry Anita (see ROBERTS, Mrs)

GILKES Tracy 29/01/1992 (21/07/1999) 4 Smith Street Spratton Northampton NN6 8HW **Tel:** (01604) 820095 w 6051231

GILL Casey Louise 29/12/2008 Flat 61 Buxton Court Thoresby Street LONDON N1 7TL **Tel:** 07789702332 w 6534052

Lisa 20/12/1996 Abbeydale Veterinary Centre 91 Preston New Road Blackburn BB2 6AY **Tel:** (01254) 681811 w 610828X

Lisa Michelle 24/07/2003 56 Thornes Moor Road Thornes Wakefield West Yorkshire WF2 8PX **Tel:** (01924) 374970 w 6267599

GILL Samantha Helen (see THOMPSON, Mrs)

GILL Samantha Louise (see LOVEDAY, Mrs)

Zoe Jane 11/09/2009 The Maltings Fordham Road Newmarket Suffolk CB8 7AA **Tel:** (01638) 662253 w 6465423

GILLARD Helen (see HOLLINGSWORTH, Mrs)

GILLATT Helen Louise (see BRIDGE, Mrs)

GILLESPIE Jeana Louise 28/07/2008 102 Broomside Lane Durham County Durham DH1 2QT **Tel:** 01913830879 w 6402217

Laura 10/03/2008 135 Sandringham Road South Gosforth Newcastle Upon Tyne NE3 1QB w 6403933

GILLETT Judith Frances 17/01/2006 A1 Oaktree Caravan Site Allington Lane West End Southampton Hampshire SO30 3HR **Tel:** 02392262346 w 6334193

GILLIATT Carrie Ann (see BUTLER, Mrs)

GILLOW Marion (see ADAMS, Mrs)

GILMAN Kelly Ann 29/01/2008 Easing Farm Thorncliffe Leek Staffordshire ST13 8UR **Tel:** (01538) 300277 w 6388698

GILMORE Nicole Louise 02/03/2001 58 Oatlands Road Shinfield READING Berkshire RG2 9DN **Tel:** (01189) 883953 w 6213578

GIRDWOOD Yvonne Margaret (nee Croome) 10/01/1991 (26/10/2000) Dragon Veterinary Centre Unit 7, Concord House Concord Washington Tyne and Wear NE37 2AS **Tel:** (0191) 417 6923 w 6048499

GIRLING Claire Louise (see THOMAS, Mrs)

GITTINS Alexander John 26/08/2009 West Bar Veterinary Hospital 19 West Bar Street Banbury Oxfordshire OX16 9SA **Tel:** (01295) 262332/267531 m 6449418

GLAICHOVA Monika 12/09/2008 11 Castle Street Caerleon NEWPORT Gwent NP18 1BR w 6440409

GLASBEY Charlotte Elizabeth 03/12/2008 10 Bridge Street Barford WARWICK CV35 8EH **Tel:** 07971489562 w 6416407

GLASS Corale Ann 03/09/2009 40 Long Close Station Road Lower Stondon HENLOW Bedfordshire SG16 6JS **Tel:** 0788943229 w 6445623

Seante Marie 01/06/2007 16 Hazelbank Terrace Edinburgh Midlothian EH11 1SL **Tel:** (0131) 477 4385 w 6382846

GLASSPOOLE Donna Marie (see GOODWIN, Mrs)

GLAZEBROOK Emma Elizabeth (see RAVEN, Ms)

GLEAVE Emma Louise (see PROUSE, Mrs)

GLEDHILL Joanne 18/10/2006 6d Ryecroft Street OSSETT West Yorkshire WF5 9EL **Tel:** (01924) 261756 w 6359152

GLEESON Laura Kirsten 07/01/2010 24 Venetia Road LONDON W5 4JD **Tel:** 02088405365 w 6492593

GLENDINNING Taryn Elizabeth 13/08/2008 (13/08/2008) South View Kirk Ireton Ashbourne Derbyshire DE6 3JW **Tel:** (01335) 370739 w 6043107

GLENNON Rachel Louise (nee Cartwright) 08/07/2003 (22/09/2008) Wood Bank Brockwell Lane Triangle SOWERBY BRIDGE West Yorkshire HX6 3PQ **Tel:** (01422) 835090 w 6275915

GLENWRIGHT Gail Ann DipAVN(Surgical) (nee Hawkes) 15/08/1990 29 Thornton Crescent Loup Farm Blaydon Tyne and Wear NE21 4BA **Tel:** (0191) 414 0195 w 6052541

GLICKSMAN Rebecca Louise (see MISSEY, Miss)

GLOVER Sarah Patricia 18/10/2005 (20/04/2009) 37 Woodshawe Rise Braunstone LEICESTER LE3 1RL w 6330728

GLYSEN Louise N G (nee Cullen, nee Jackson) 22/07/1993 North Highland College Ormlie Road Thurso Caithness KW14 7EE w 6015102

GOAD Elisabeth Jane 05/02/2009 3 Farriers FORDINGBRIDGE Hampshire SP6 1FE w 6437912

GOANE Amanda Ellen (nee Hibbert) 27/01/1999 32 Stocks Way Shepley West Yorkshire HD8 8DL **Tel:** (01484) 605681 w 6099477

GOATEN Janet Diane (see HIGERTY, Mrs)

GODDARD Andrea Rachel (see ROWLAND, Mrs)

GODDARD Lucy Ann DipAVN(Surgical), DipAVN(Medical) 05/04/1994 64 Elgar Drive Shefford Bedfordshire SG17 5RA w 6034169

GODDERHAM Natasha Jayne (see GOODERHAM, Mrs)

GODFREY Alison Sarah (see YOUNG, Mrs)

GODFREY David 20/05/2003 84 Trent Rd Beston Rylands Nottingam NG9 1LQ **Tel:** (0115) 9254235 m 6282922

Jemma 10/02/2004 18 Holliday Street Berkhamsted Hertfordshire HP4 2EE **Tel:** (01442) 873122 w 6291678

Megan Emily Jean 02/03/2009 Flat 8 Forum House Lemsford Road HATFIELD Hertfordshire AL10 0FG w 6440222

Melanie Jane 02/09/2009 89 Windmill Hill Lane DERBY DE22 3BN **Tel:** 01332343085 w 6495783

Rebecca Victoria 24/04/2009 Cedar Veterinary Hospital 69 Christchurch Road Ringwood Hampshire BH24 1DH **Tel:** (01425) 473683 w 6365730

GODFREY Sian (see HOLMAN, Mrs)

GODSMARK Rachael 08/04/2005 (04/11/2009) 34 Glebe Estate Tilney All Saints KING'S LYNN Norfolk PE34 4SN **Tel:** (01553) 829729 w 6296441

GOLBY Gemma Louise 04/04/2006 De Montfort Veterinary Hospital 44 Merstow Green Evesham

Worcestershire WR11 4BH **Tel:** (01386) 446095 w 6328165

GOLDIE Melanie Anne (nee Turnbull) 17/09/2008 25 Harper Terrace Yeadon Leeds LS19 7RP **Tel:** (01132) 505522 w 6379392

GOLDIE Yvonne Munro (see SHAW, Mrs)

GOLDING Grace Kelly 26/03/2008 203 Firestone House Clayponds Lane Brentford Middlesex TW8 0GW **Tel:** (07776) 237121 w 6382373

Sarah 03/06/2004 St Anne's Veterinary Group 6 St Anne's Road Eastbourne East Sussex BN21 2DJ **Tel:** (01323) 640011 w 6280359

GOLDSMITH Faye (see HINCHLIFFE, Mrs)

GOLLICK Amanda Jane 02/09/2008 Animal Medical Centre Thurnscoe Business Park Thurnscoe Rotherham South Yorkshire S63 0BH **Tel:** (01709) 897354 w 6437538

GOMORY Rita Gabriella 05/04/2005 (04/03/2009) 96 Aspinall Road Brockley LONDON SE4 2EG w 6325074

GOOD Rosemary Christine 04/10/1975 (02/11/2007) 13 The Strand Quainton AYLESBURY Buckinghamshire HP22 4AS **Tel:** (01296) 651565 w 6085169

GOODALL Christina Jane 15/10/2008 1 Sleningford Rise BINGLEY West Yorkshire BD16 2SQ w 6434238

Karen Ann 19/02/2001 Springfield Veterinary Group 451 Richmond Road Sheffield South Yorkshire S13 8LW **Tel:** (0114) 264 8913 w 6212423

Karen Michelle 05/09/2008 7 Kenchurchill Drive Horbury WAKEFIELD West Yorkshire WF4 6JU w 6436526

Leanne Tracey 24/05/2006 5 Morrells Close DIDCOT Oxfordshire OX11 7DJ w 6313722

GOODALL Lisa Jayne (see BIRD, Mrs)

GOODE Susan Elaine (see SUTTON, Mrs)

GOODERHAM Jenny Lesley 10/08/2009 Sunny Banks Deerton Street Teynham Sittingbourne Kent ME9 9LJ **Tel:** 01227765522 w 6410247

GOODERHAM Katie Anne (see SAMSON, Mrs)

Natasha Jayne (nee Langrish, nee Godderham) 11/09/2003 178 Locks Road Locks Heath Southampton Hampshire SO31 6LE **Tel:** (01489) 607001 w 6273506

GOODES Katie Jayne (nee Nolan) 03/09/1998 (09/02/2009) Petersfield Veterinary Centre 16-18 St Peters Road Petersfield Hampshire GU31 4AA **Tel:** (01730) 266 431 w 6118276

GOODEY Melanie 08/07/2003 148 Howitts Gardens Eynesbury ST. NEOTS Cambridgeshire PE19 2NU w 6273693

GOODHEW Charlotte Mary 05/09/2008 Goodacres Burtons Lane Wellington Heath Ledbury Herefordshire HR8 1NF **Tel:** 07845654660 w 6440860

GOODING Naomi Ruth (see STARKEY, Mrs)

GOODLET Karen 24/05/2005 (14/01/2009) 56 Milndavie Crescent Strathblane GLASGOW G63 9DF **Tel:** (01360) 770962 w 6277851

GOODRIDGE Holly Rose Amy 26/05/2009 17 Dover Close Fareham Hampshire PO14 3SU **Tel:** 01329661053 w 6429167

GOODWIN Donna Marie (nee Glasspoole) 28/01/1998 Oakland House Old Station Way Holt Norfolk NR25 6DH **Tel:** (01263) 713200 w 6117512

Ellen Lisa 27/02/2007 100 Falmouth Road Redruth Cornwall TR15 2QP **Tel:** (01209) 203902 w 6357755

GOODWIN Jane Louise (see BELLAS, Mrs)

Ruth Mary 06/10/2006 12 Chesterfield Close Winsford Cheshire CW7 2NS **Tel:** (01606) 593 487 w 6302073

GORDON Jenny (nee Osborne) 04/02/2002 14 Mornington Avenue Rochford Essex SS4 1DN **Tel:** (01263) 758537 w 6268237

Julia 16/05/2000 (07/05/2002) 23 Spalt Close Hutton Brentwood Essex CM13 2UN **Tel:** (01277) 202632 w 6152830

Karen DipAVN(Surgical), DipAVN(Medical) (nee Sharpe) 23/11/1991 Davies Veterinary Specialists Manor Farm Business Park Higham Gobion Hertfordshire SG5 3HR **Tel:** (01582) 883950 w 6004065

Kelly Marie 04/06/2009 167 The Spinney Bar Hill Cambridge Cambridgeshire CB3 8TW **Tel:** 01954789047 w 6407684

Laura Kate 23/09/2009 121 Lower Street Pulborough West Sussex RH20 2BP **Tel:** (01798) 872089 w 6452124

Marie Elaine (nee Stockwell) 30/03/2001 (04/05/2004) No 1 Bramston Way Southfields Laindon Essex SS15 6TP **Tel:** (01268) 564664 w 6214645

GORE Allison (see DICKINSON, Mrs)

GORE Emma Lucy 21/03/2007 Toachim House Veterinary Surgery Toachim House South Road Faversham Kent ME13 7LR **Tel:** (01795) 531313 w 6373694

Sharon Ann 28/09/2005 Anchorage Barn Veterinary Clinic Fakenham Road East Rudham King's Lynn Norfolk PE31 6TA **Tel:** (01485) 528221 w 6353102

GOREY Kirstin Eleanor (nee Ramage) 03/06/2003 175 Portobello High Street Edinburgh EH15 1EU **Tel:** (0131) 669 3790 w 6280579

GORLEY Lesley Ann 20/09/2005 3 Ashtree Farm Cottages L T Broughton Cockermouth Cumbria CA13 0WZ **Tel:** (01900) 829412 w 6291799

GORMAN Emily Clare 28/02/2005 4 Avonside Bantham KINGSBRIDGE Devon TQ7 3AR w 6318441

GORMLEY Claire Elizabeth 16/06/2008 1 Hospital Cottages Madingley Road CAMBRIDGE CB3 0ES w 6400743

GOSDEN Caroline Ann 10/09/1981 (03/02/2003) Glen Rosa The Bostal Castletown Upper Beeding STEYNING West Sussex BN44 3TR **Tel:** (01903) 814239 w 6051515

Sarah Louise 26/04/2007 40 Pertwee Drive Chelmsford Essex CM2 8EA **Tel:** (01245) 472 639 w 6350506

GOSLING Chloe Edwina 12/05/2004 Swallows Barn Mickleton BARNARD CASTLE County Durham DL12 0JW **Tel:** (01833) 641134 w 6278390

GOSS Corinna 27/01/1994 (04/11/1999) Milehouse Clinic 28 Outland Road Milehouse Plymouth Devon PL2 3DF **Tel:** (01752) 567567 w 6066725

GOTTS Claire Louise 14/10/2008 41 Main Road Kesgrave Ipswich Suffolk IP5 1AG **Tel:** 01473623798 w 6419905

GOUDGE Tracey Helen (see BREE, Mrs)

GOUGH Claire Louise (nee Potter) 22/08/1997 (16/07/2003) 40 Southernlea Road BURNHAM-ON-SEA Somerset TA8 2ER w 6116450

GOUGH Lisa Marie (see FRASER, Mrs)

GOUGH Nicola Jayne (nee Nye) 17/08/2005 45 Manor Park Avenue Pontefract West Yorkshire WF8 2PX **Tel:** (01977) 708244 w 6272087

Sarah Elizabeth 31/10/2003 Dubai Falcon Hospital P.O. Box 23919 Dubai United Arab Emirates **Tel:** (00) 44 784 306 4740 w 6293009

GOULD Claire Anne (formerly Scott) 20/03/2001 (09/04/2009) 76 Harwood Drive HOUGHTON LE SPRING Tyne and Wear DH4 5NY w 6204272

Felicity Ellen May 15/09/2009 23 Thornewill Drive Stretton Burton-on-Trent DE13 0HY **Tel:** (01283) 533250 w 6452311

GOULD Helen Frances (see CHOPPING, Mrs)

Helen Patricia (nee Byers) 13/05/2003 The Veterinary Surgery Hollybush Road Bridgnorth Shropshire WV16 4AR **Tel:** (01746) 763 998 w 6280821

Peter James 11/03/2008 19 Sheffield Road Chesterfield Derbyshire S41 7LR **Tel:** (01246) 202590 m 6403427

GOULDEN Harriet Nicole 04/06/2009 8 Sharnbrook Gardens Sharnford Hinckley Leicestershire LE10 3QD **Tel:** (01455) 271662 w 6407838

GOULDING Catherine Tracey DipAVN(Surgical) 29/07/1992 15 Alder Avenue Ashton-in-Makerfield Lancashire WN4 0LS **Tel:** (01942) 202632 w 6051526

Jacqueline (nee Bagshawe, formerly Millington) 13/12/1984 15 Albion Road New Mills High Peak Derbyshire SK22 3EX **Tel:** (01663) 747441 w 6091955

Lana Ruth (nee Norman) 07/08/1991 3 Banks Cottages Mountfield East Sussex TN32 5JZ **Tel:** (01580) 880849 w 6057765

Sarah Patricia 02/07/2009 9 Fourth Avenue Walsall West Midlands WS8 6JQ **Tel:** (01543) 453 324 w 6434887

GOURLEY Helen Louise 31/08/2005 158 Upper Rd Greensland Carrickfergus Co Atrim BT38 8RW **Tel:** 02890-854803 w 6276531

GOVEY Kirsty Jessica (see BROOKS, Mrs)

GOW Angela Melanie 21/09/2009 36 Megson Drive LEE-ON-THE-SOLENT Hampshire PO13 8BA **Tel:** 02392551587 w 6490712

Victoria June 10/10/2008 7 Middlebrook Green MARKET HARBOROUGH Leicestershire LE16 7DW w 6419729

GOWEN Helen (see PETHER, Mrs)

GOWER Louise Ruth Elizabeth 29/02/1996 (10/05/2004) 34 Chisholm Close Southampton Hampshire SO16 8GU **Tel:** (023) 8034 3727 w 6038094

GRACE Louise 14/04/2008 27 Home Mead CHELMSFORD CM2 8SN w 6383187

GRAEF Nikki Jayne 02/11/2004 5 Russel Croft Aston fields Bromsgrove Worcestershire B60 3EF **Tel:** (01527) 576 747 w 6284011

GRAHAM Elizabeth Patricia 10/10/1967 4 The Spires Grove Killinchy Newtownards County Down BT23 6UH w 6051570

Emma Louise 18/10/2006 9 Elizabeth Gardens Dibden Purlieu Southampton Hampshire SO45 4NF **Tel:** (023) 8022 6679 w 6374596

Gillian 06/02/2009 Mid-Corses Parkgate Dumfries Dumfriesshire DG1 3NN **Tel:** (01387) 860 431 w 6440332

GRAHAM Gillian Frances (see MCPHAIL, Mrs)

GRAHAM Jo-Anne (see STEVENS, Mrs)

GRAHAM Mary-Ellen (see STEPHENSON, Mrs)

Myra 26/10/2005 6 Wavell Drive Rosehill Industrial Estate Carlisle CA1 2ST **Tel:** (01228) 521393 w 6339066

Pamela Elizabeth 03/02/2005 (29/02/2008) 133 Ballyutoag Road Belfast County Antrim BT14 8ST **Tel:** (02890) 825 338 w 6267643

Shereen Natalie Jayne 30/05/2008 Willow Veterinary Group 2 Willen Road NEWPORT PAGNELL Buckinghamshire MK16 0DF w 6332268

GRAIN Katherine Rachel 12/12/2007 70 The Crossways Otley West Yorkshire LS21 2AR w 6400281

GRANGE Vanessa Helen (nee Wright) 02/02/1995 Amical Veterinary Centre Ltd 90 High Street March Cambridgeshire PE15 9LQ **Tel:** (01354) 652246 w 603126X

GRANT Claire 24/04/2008 12 Thatcham Court YEOVIL Somerset BA21 3DT **Tel:** 07816121576 w 6420048

Karen Louise 28/08/1998 (23/10/2000) 41 Heritage Drive Carron Falkirk Stirlingshire FK2 8EL **Tel:** (0131) 4421368 w 6130511

Kirsty Sarah (nee MacNaughton, nee Scullard) 22/02/2000 P D S A Veterinary Centre 2b Hutchison Crossway 7 Slateford Road Edinburgh EH14 1RR **Tel:** (0131) 443 6178 w 6191325

Lindsay Anne 29/08/1997 (23/06/2000) 33 Junction Road Kirkwall Orkney KW15 1AG **Tel:** (01856) 873403 w 6032004

Sarah 12/05/2004 33 Silken Court Off Marlborough Road Warwickshire CV11 5NN w 6289346

GRANTHAM Hollie Paula 14/09/2009 Horton Hall Farm Henfield Road Smalldole West Sussex BN5 9XJ **Tel:** (01903) 814146 w 6451486

Sarah Louise 02/03/2007 (22/01/2009) 59 Galloway Crescent BROXBURN West Lothian EH52 6XP **Tel:** (01506) 859695 w 6354642

GRANVILLE Trudie Anne (see VALE, Mrs)

GRAPES Laura Elizabeth 24/04/2009 10 Rectory Lane Poringland Norwich Norfolk NR14 7ST **Tel:** (01508) 494 824 w 6436020

GRAUDINS Hayley Louise 02/03/2007 40 Carnhywell Road Llanelli Dyfed SA14 9EE **Tel:** (01554) 778 767 w 6368821

GRAVENOR Zoe Angela (see LESZCZYNSKI, Mrs)

GRAVER Shelley Susan 21/08/2009 31 Pullman Court Streatham Hill LONDON SW2 4ST **Tel:** 07505559206 w 6447757

GRAVETT Alexandra Beverley 27/08/1999 13 Park Avenue Keymer Hassocks West Sussex BN6 8LT **Tel:** (01273) 845877 w 6142753

Sarah Louise (formerly Hope) 01/02/2008 2 St. Andrews Road Whitehill BORDON Hampshire GU35 9QN **Tel:** (01420) 472737 w 6354675

Terence Richard 02/06/2000 (31/01/2002) 2 St. Andrews Road Whitehill BORDON Hampshire GU35 9QN **Tel:** (01420) 472737 m 6191457

GRAY Amy Jane 14/10/2008 36 Farington Drive Marton-in-Cleveland MIDDLESBROUGH Cleveland TS7 8PH **Tel:** 01642311274 w 6372363

Georgina Jade 09/06/2009 80 Trent Road Shaw OLDHAM OL2 7YL **Tel:** 01706841435 w 6377082

Lisa Allison 09/03/2005 3 Holy Island HEXHAM Northumberland NE46 3QL w 6313733

Lisa Pauline 14/03/2006 Cairnview Balmenach Cromdale Grantown on Spey Moray-shire PH26 3PF **Tel:** (01479) 873326 w 6347096

Lorna Jane Gunn 06/10/2009 Milton of Duthil Carrbridge Inverness-Shire PH23 3NA **Tel:** 01479841413 w 6429728

Nicola Louise Samantha 21/03/2006 The Park Veterinary Group 519 Saffron Lane Leicester Leicestershire LE2 6UL **Tel:** (0116) 283 1314 w 6342058

GRAY Samantha Elizabeth (see BELL, Mrs)

Samantha Jenny 15/06/2009 10 George Street BLAIRGOWRIE Perthshire PH10 6HA **Tel:** 07850100580 w 6382747

Sarah Jane 02/08/1993 3 Kennett Road Moulton Newmarket Suffolk CB8 8QR **Tel:** (01638) 751601 w 6066634

Sophie Louise 12/05/2004 Davies Veterinary Specialists Manor Farm Business Park Higham Gobion Hertfordshire SG5 3HR **Tel:** (01582) 883950 w 6292789

Teresa Doreen 18/04/2005 (18/03/2009) 35 Isca Road EXETER Devon EX2 8BQ w 6321213

Victoria Louise 16/04/2008 Flat 1, 20 Osborne Road BROADSTAIRS Kent CT10 2AE w 6334204

GRAYSTON Rebecca Kim 16/06/2008 3 Copse Close BURY ST. EDMUNDS Suffolk IP33 2TD **Tel:** (01284) 700 118 w 6380756

GREAVES Doreen Molly (see LAWRENCE, Mrs)

GREAVES Jennifer 08/09/2005 73 Eastcroft Road WALLASEY Merseyside CH44 4BW **Tel:** (0151) 6397696 w 6296936

Tammy Jane 18/10/2007 12 Market Garden Close Thurmaston LEICESTER LE4 8NW **Tel:** 07908207268 w 6408201

GREEN Angela (see ANDERSON, Miss)

GREEN Angela Mary 19/02/2001 207 Daventry Road Coventry West Midlands CV3 5HH **Tel:** (02476) 503000 w 6212434

Carla Louise 04/09/1997 Green Cottage 157 High Street Teddington Middlesex TW11 8HH **Tel:** (0208) 977 5350 w 609931X

GREEN Caroline Helen Louise Elizabeh (see CHAPMAN-GREEN, Mrs)

Christine Michelle 01/06/2007 5 Park Cottages Mayles Lane Wickham FAREHAM Hampshire PO17 5NH **Tel:** (01329) 833656 w 6357953

Claire (nee Marlow) 10/01/2007 Anchor House Station Row Shalford Guildford Surrey GU4 8BY **Tel:** (01483) 502057 w 6265696

Clare Marie 01/09/2008 Middlecave House 89 Middlecave Road Malton North Yorkshire YO17 7NQ **Tel:** (01653) 600079 w 6429068

Deborah Kay 02/09/2008 7 Millholme Walk Camberley Surrey GU15 1RY w 6406144

GREEN Dorothy Elizabeth (see CREIGHTON, Mrs)

Eleanor Jayne 24/01/2006 16 Raedwald Drive Bury St. Edmunds Suffolk IP32 7DA **Tel:** (01284) 700169 w 6337779

Elizabeth Ann 30/10/2003 Village Vet Hampstead 11 Belsize Terrace London NW3 4AX **Tel:** (020) 7794 4948 w 6288378

Hannah Christa 07/02/2008 87 Watford Road Cotteridge Birmingham B30 1NP **Tel:** (0121) 459 4333 w 6342586

Jean Ann (nee Whordley) 08/10/1975 17 Union Street Chasetown Lichfield Staffordshire WS7 3XX **Tel:** (01543) 676794 w 6063735

Jenny 13/11/2009 43 Temple End High Wycombe Buckinghamshire HP13 5DN **Tel:** (01494) 522956 w 6453202

Kelly Hannah 02/09/2009 27 Youngs Avenue Balderton Newark NG24 3FG **Tel:** (01636) 701523 w 6452278

Lynsey Roseanna 05/02/2008 Dovehouse Cottage Diss Road Tibenham NORWICH NR16 1PW w 6373716

Marcala Anne 09/06/2009 12 Norwich Crescent Rayleigh Essex SS6 9QR **Tel:** 01268783180 w 6443412

Natalie Marie 05/02/2009 77 Farringdon Way Tadley Hampshire RG26 3UA **Tel:** 01189815181 w 6437461

Nicola 09/10/1998 9 Chancel Way Monkbretton Barnsley S71 2HS **Tel:** (01226) 200476 w 6140202

Nicola (nee Seghini) 21/07/1993 14 Gordon Road Blyth Northumberland NE24 3EL w 606650X

Rachael Dawn 22/02/2007 34 Chenery Drive Norwich Norfolk NR7 8RR **Tel:** (01603) 429 754 w 6377665

Rebecca Jane 04/11/2005 62 Stone Hill ST. NEOTS Cambridgeshire PE19 6AA **Tel:** (07748) 141120 w 6352772

Rebecca Louise 10/05/2007 94 Evelyn Crescent Sunbury on Thames Middlesex TW16 6LZ **Tel:** (01932) 429282 w 6290391

Sarah Heather 12/01/2010 Oakhaven Showley Road Clayton-le-Dale Blackburn Lancashire BB1 9DP **Tel:** (01254) 812444 w 6441817

Stephanie Elizabeth 27/04/2009 36 Talbot Avenue Bristol Avon BS15 1HD **Tel:** 01179608846 w 6438616

Stephanie Jayne 15/11/2001 3 Aston Mead SALISBURY Wiltshire SP1 3HJ **Tel:** (01722) 413 327 w 6258920

GREEN Susan Vanessa (see MCDONALD, Mrs)

GREENAWAY Dawn Pauline (nee Williams) 17/01/1996 The Veterinary Practice Millennium Way Braintree Essex CM7 3GX **Tel:** (01376) 325511 w 6030528

Elona Clare 14/08/1989 (17/04/2001) 70 Brinkley Lane Highwoods COLCHESTER Essex CO4 9XE **Tel:** (01206) 842608 w 6051741

GREENHOUGH Joanna Elizabeth (nee Jiggins) 06/09/1993 Pennywhistle Cottage Nantwich Road Chorley Green Nantwich CW5 8JR **Tel:** (01270) 524 605 w 6026737

GREENSLADE Heather Julie 19/08/1976 (17/01/2002) Newhill Farm Whitnage Uplowman TIVERTON Devon EX16 7EZ **Tel:** (01884) 821699 w 6051796

GREENSMITH Tracy Anne (nee Lawrence) 23/02/2005 (21/01/2008) 6 Mill Lane Barton under Needwood Burton-on-Trent Staffordshire DE13 8HE **Tel:** (01283) 713 378 w 6293746

GREENWOOD Kylie Jane 10/10/2005 Calder Veterinary Group/Calder Vets Savile Road Dewsbury West Yorkshire WF12 9LN **Tel:** (01924) 465592 w 6289357

Matthew James 18/09/2007 The Veterinary Surgery 23 Mill Hill Road PONTEFRACT West Yorkshire WF8 4HR **Tel:** (01977) 702056 m 6351859

GREETHAM Philippa Anne 03/05/2005 (16/01/2009) 7 Netherfield Close ALTON Hampshire GU34 2EP **Tel:** (077813) 700606 w 6300016

GREGORY Joanna 02/03/2007 Avon Lodge Veterinary Group 21 Stratford Road Salisbury SP1 3JN **Tel:** (01722) 412211 w 6357964

Katherine Elizabeth 27/04/2005 Fitzpatrick Referrals Ltd Halfway Lane Eashing Godalming Surrey GU7 2QQ **Tel:** (01483) 423761 w 6324524

Kelly-Marie 18/03/2009 5 Peterhead Amington Tamworth Staffordshire B77 3QS **Tel:** 07515388515 w 6419663

Ruth Louisa 14/03/2006 Wildbore Veterinary Group 5 Newcastle Street Worksop Nottinghamshire S80 2AS **Tel:** (01909) 472059 w 6344170

Stephanie Louise 20/09/2005 20 Burn View BUDE Cornwall EX23 8BZ w 6302205

GREGORY FITZGERALD Helen Lucy 31/08/2005 29 Sunnydale Park OSSETT West Yorkshire WF5 0RJ w 6318936

GREGSON Jamie Eleanor 26/11/2007 90 Spring Terrace Road Stapenhill Burton-upon-Trent Staffordshire DE15 9DX **Tel:** (01283) 568162 w 6376917

Susan June (nee Gregson, nee Hunt) 08/08/2002 Ashcroft Veterinary Surgery 59 Main Street Frodsham Cheshire WA6 7DF **Tel:** (01928) 733228 w 6202336

GRETA Lorraine 05/10/2001 41 Brackendale Elton Chester Cheshire CH2 4PQ **Tel:** (01928) 726112 w 6229682

GRETTON Johanna Michelle 08/09/2005 8 Thurlaston Close Peterborough Cambridgeshire PE3 6LD **Tel:** (01733) 267124 w 6324018

GREY Claire Louise (see ORAM, Mrs)

GRIBBLE Sarah Jane 29/06/2009 Flat 2, Kaber Court Grafton Street LIVERPOOL L8 6RY **Tel:** 07792840974 w 6426241

GRICE Christine Yvonne 10/04/2007 2 Harvard Road Solihull West Midlands B92 8ET w 6240616

GRIERSON Elaine 04/09/1997 8 Blands Row Pilning BRISTOL BS35 4NF w 6115989

GRIEVE Elizabeth Louise 24/02/2004 61 The Rock Helsby Frodsham Cheshire WA6 9AS **Tel:** (0161) 9294388 w 6345402

GRIEVE Kim (see SOUTTAR, Mrs)

Louise 10/11/2009 Flat 1/2 126 Gallowhill Road PAISLEY Renfrewshire PA3 4TY **Tel:** (07738) 096 319 w 6455138

GRIFFIN Joanna Louise 27/05/2009 60 Dart Road Farnborough Hampshire GU14 9PF **Tel:** 01252514730 w 6400644

Julia Claire (nee Wadham-Smith) 05/08/1976 29 Claremont Avenue BOURNEMOUTH BH9 3EZ **Tel:** (01202) 518764 w 6085613

Siobhan Lisa 21/09/2009 Chestnut Veterinary Group 87 Ware Road Hertford Hertfordshire SG13 7EE **Tel:** (01992) 554466 w 6465313

GRIFFITH Helen (nee Turner) 03/12/2003 19 North Farm Road FARNBOROUGH Hampshire GU14 9AD **Tel:** (01276) 608932 w 6290468

Sandra 23/12/2003 160 Morden Road Mitcham Surrey CR4 4DD **Tel:** (020) 8640 0367 w 6292580

GRIFFITHS Caroline Alexandra 05/10/2004 19 Dorothy Crescent Clawes Worcester WR3 7DD **Tel:** (01905) 454 940 w 6286684

Claire Louise (nee Davies) 17/11/2004 4 School Road Cyrnant Neath West Glamorgan South Wales SA10 8NR **Tel:** (01639) 750 856 w 6282801

Emma Louise 14/09/2004 5 Norristhorpe Avenue LIVERSEDGE West Yorkshire WF15 7AD w 6303239

Hayley Sarah 28/01/2008 Abrooks Quarry Road Rock Kidderminster Worcestershire DY14 9SE **Tel:** 01299832602 w 6370537

Kaye 16/12/2009 52 Ridgewalk Way Ward Green Barnsley S70 6TH **Tel:** 01226247119 w 6466721

Kelly Jayne 21/12/2009 397 Turves Green Longbridge Birmingham B31 4DB w 6466666

Kerry Ann 15/06/2009 115 Cann Hall Road Leytonstone London E11 3NJ **Tel:** 07969683058 w 6407673

Megan 03/02/2009 2 Sweethope Farm Cottages Kelso Roxburghshire TD5 7RZ **Tel:** 01573470713 w 6446998

Rhian Elizabeth 15/02/2008 90 Tre Garth Machynlleth Powys SY20 8HY w 6388720

Tracy Leigh Dawn (nee Lemke) 05/09/1994 178 Park Road London N8 8JT **Tel:** (020) 8340 5453 w 6037793

GRIGGS Sarah Louise 27/01/2005 (09/02/2009) 73 Sycamore Road CHALFONT ST. GILES Buckinghamshire HP8 4LG **Tel:** (01494) 872498 w 6316802

GRIMASON Hayley Louise 14/11/2008 Ground Floor Flat 1 Jocelyn Road BUDLEIGH SALTERTON Devon EX9 6SF **Tel:** 07759151828 w 6330739

GRIMBLE Katie Lynn 22/01/2008 118 Bluehouse Road London E4 6HR **Tel:** 02085290573 w 6382384

GRIMES Deborah Ann 11/05/2004 42 Oulston Road Fairfield Stockton-On-Tees Cleveland TS18 4HU **Tel:** (01642) 891568 w 6287344

GRIMMETT Laura Jayne 24/03/2009 34 Westleas Horley Surrey RH6 8AF **Tel:** 07912418696 w 6437263

GRINYER Katie Ann 10/11/2009 St Anne's Veterinary Group 6 St Anne's Road Eastbourne East Sussex BN21 2DJ **Tel:** (01323) 640011 w 6456381

GRIST Eleanor Margaret 14/03/2006 64 West End Road Bitterne Southampton Hampshire SO18 6TG **Tel:** (02380) 447797 w 6349538

GROOMBRIDGE Annika Maria (nee Cook) 30/11/2005 10 Highacres Loders BRIDPORT Dorset DT6 3SE w 6344764

Tracy Jane (nee Limbrick) 27/02/2006 42 Terrace Road Elvington DOVER Kent CT15 4EJ **Tel:** (01304) 831892 w 6332609

GROUT Julia Ann (see BURKE, Mrs)

GROVES Claire Marie Joanne 24/11/2005 70 Brinkley Lane Highwoods COLCHESTER Essex CO4 9XE **Tel:** (01206) 842608 w 6325085

Samantha Jane 24/11/2005 Cogges Veterinary Surgery Cogges Hill Road Witney Oxfordshire OX28 3XY **Tel:** (01993) 772 627 w 6344181

GROVES-HAMBIDGE Nicola Caroline (see WIGHT, Mrs)

GRUNDY Kathryn Sarah (see DRING, Mrs)

GRYCUK Catriona Mackinnon 01/06/2007 198 Upper Craigour EDINBURGH EH17 7SH **Tel:** (0131) 6644899 w 6349197

GUDGE Christopher Martyn 06/08/2008 47 Coulsons Road Bristol Avon BS14 0NN **Tel:** (01275) 830360 m 6353817

GUDGEON Deberah Kathleen 28/02/2001 (30/03/2004) Wood Green Animal Shelter 601 Lordship Lane London N22 5LG **Tel:** (08701) 904440 w 6186155

Sarah Leanne 11/08/2009 21 Blackberry Lane Potterne Devizes Wiltshire SN10 5NZ **Tel:** 07724241551 w 6368832

GUDGIN Lisa Jane (nee Campbell) 28/08/1998 Jennayr 7 Elizabeth Road Daventry Northamptonshire NN11 9DP **Tel:** (01327) 872216 w 6117068

Nicola Jane 29/12/1992 56 Glebe Crescent New Bilton Rugby Warwickshire CV21 2HQ w 6066270

GUEST Leanne 04/07/2007 6 Dudley Crescent Halifax West Yorkshire HX2 8LE **Tel:** (01422) 241 924 w 6387829

GUILD Hannah (see POLLOCK, Mrs)

GUINAN Diane Elizabeth DipAVN(Surgical) 06/02/1986 2 Hillcrest Cottages Hermongers Lane Ellens Green Rudgwick West Sussex RH12 3AH **Tel:** (07930) 899590 w 6051956

GUITE Laura Jennifer 13/11/2006 32 Penarth Road Manchester Lancashire M22 4AR **Tel:** (0161) 998 4414 w 6358349

GULLIVER Kerry Louise (nee Spiller) 18/01/2002 40 Rookery Crescent Cliffe ROCHESTER Kent ME3 7RH w 6270800

GUNN Emma Joanne 24/11/2009 2 Garnetts Takeley BISHOP'S STORTFORD Hertfordshire CM22 6RJ **Tel:** (01279) 871266 w 6456359

Kerry Marie 14/11/2008 (Gunn) Bardnaclavan Janetstown Thurso Caithness KW14 7XF **Tel:** 01862894223 w 6408806

Michelle Amy 05/01/2005 59 Albemarle Road TAUNTON Somerset TA1 1BD **Tel:** (07967) 120051 w 6297552

GUNNER Megan Nessa 19/03/2007 (21/05/2009) Golden Valley Veterinary Hospital Nailsea Park Nailsea North Somerset BS48 1BD **Tel:** (01275) 852140 w 6356688

Natalie Joanne 20/11/2009 8 Andrews Close HEREFORD HR1 2JX **Tel:** (01432) 357 222 w 6457657

GUNSMAN Rebecca Louise (see MILLS, Mrs)

GUNTER Marie Louise 01/02/2010 Pet Doctors Veterinary Clinics Brooklyn Road Seaford East Sussex BN25 2DU **Tel:** (01323) 894568 w 6489843

GURDEN Julie Frances 29/07/2005 88 Prospect Avenue STANFORD-LE-HOPE Essex SS17 0NJ **Tel:** (01375) 678190 w 6303349

GURNETT Eleanor Jane 27/02/2006 Pennard House 5 Eardley Road Sevenoaks Kent TN13 1XY **Tel:** (01732) 452344 w 6307848

GURNEY Angela Clare 30/11/2005 Shrubbery Veterinary Centre 65 Perry Street Northfleet Gravesend Kent DA11 8RD **Tel:** (01474) 333141 w 6297266

Victoria Rosanne 26/04/2007 12 West End Lane Potton Sandy Bedfordshire SG19 2RD **Tel:** (01767) 260069 w 6375509

GUTHRIE Emma Catherine (see HIRST, Mrs)

Nicola Sadie 11/08/2008 150 Kingston Road Epsom Surrey KT17 2ET **Tel:** (020) 8393 6049 w 6403823

GUY Alison Claire 11/02/2008 Folly Gardens Veterinary Clinic No 1 Folly Gardens Barton Road Tewkesbury Gloucestershire GL20 5QP **Tel:** (01684) 292244 w 6403361

Deborah Kathleen 22/03/2004 Rosemont Charlton Shaftesbury Dorset SP7 0EN w 6246204

GUYAN Nina Jayne 17/01/2006 Grove Lodge Veterinary Group Ltd 18 Upper Brighton Road Worthing West Sussex BN14 9DL **Tel:** (01903) 234866 w 6331509

GUYMER Charlotte Ellen Louise (formerly Coupe) 23/02/2005 (20/10/2008) 33 Andrew Crescent WATERLOOVILLE Hampshire PO7 6BE **Tel:** (07861) 762821 w 6319541

GWYNNE Kirsty 02/02/2001 Braeriach Hope Mansell Ross-on-Wye Herefordshire HR9 5TL **Tel:** (01989) 750890 w 6211906

GYNN Sally Jane (see BENSTEAD, Mrs)

H

HADDON Jacqueline (nee Ellis) 03/02/1997 530 Etruria Road Basford Newcastle Staffordshire ST5 0SX w 6039906

HADDRELL Georgina Faye 03/06/2004 136 Woodend Road Frampton Cotterell South Gloucestershire BS36 2HX **Tel:** (0117) 9569038 w 6295341

Jessica Bethryn 17/08/2009 12 Sheringham Avenue London N14 4UE **Tel:** (0208) 360 6781 w 6406452

HADINGHAM Nicola Jayne 09/09/1996 Deben Valley Equine Veterinary Clinic Birds Lane Framsden Stowmarket Suffolk IP14 6HR **Tel:** (01728) 685123 w 6099375

HADLAND Emma Jane 24/06/2004 15 Lady Bailey Park Winterbourne Whitechurch Blandford Dorset DT11 0HJ **Tel:** (01258) 880467 w 6288114

HADWEN Catherine Cheryl 24/01/1997 Midcliffe Farm Hartington Buxton Derbyshire SK17 0AZ **Tel:** (01629) 650187 w 6098236

HADWIN Celia Anne 19/12/2006 High Aulthurstside Farm Woodland BROUGHTON-IN-FURNESS Cumbria LA20 6AE **Tel:** (01229) 716382 w 6322236

HAGGER Abigail Jemima 09/04/2009 23 Church Lane Deal Kent CT14 9QG **Tel:** (01304) 365660 w 6354653

HAGGETT Natalie Isabelle (see CROUCHER, Mrs)

HAIGH Alison (see BELL, Mrs)

HAIGH Kerry Louise 31/10/2005 331 Yew Tree Road Withington Manchester M20 3FP **Tel:** (0161) 445 2282 w 6230210

HAINE Lisa Rosamund 28/09/2005 13 Poplar Farm Close Milton-under-Wychwood CHIPPING NORTON Oxfordshire OX7 6LX **Tel:** (01993) 830078 w 6321961

HAINES Beverley-Anne (see BURNETT, Mrs)

HAINEY Sarah Morgan (nee West) 06/10/2006 Hykeham Green Lincoln Road North Hykeham Lincoln Lincolnshire LN6 8NH **Tel:** (01522) 683300 w 6345589

HALDRON Lisa Elaine (see CHAWNER, Mrs)

HALE Victoria Jane 06/11/2000 22 Ashley Walk LONDON NW7 1DU w 6202325

HALES Michelle Linda (see RICHMOND, Mrs)

HALEWOOD Gemma Louise 19/09/2006 4 Timon Avenue BOOTLE Merseyside L20 9DZ **Tel:** (0151) 286 2647 w 6304768

HALEY Michelle 02/03/2009 8 Greenwood Fold BRADFORD West Yorkshire BD4 6EZ **Tel:** 07900317601 w 6423920

Samantha 24/04/2008 2 Ashfield Gardens Falmouth Cornwall TR11 2TZ **Tel:** (01326) 317805 w 6415472

HALL Alison Jane (see DEVONSHIRE, Mrs)

HALL Catherine Dawn 30/05/2007 Windwhistle Cottage Kings Lane Woodlands WIMBORNE Dorset BH21 8LZ **Tel:** (01202) 824 234 w 6276740

Claire Louise 11/11/2009 61 Colebrook Road Shirley Solihull West Midlands B90 2JZ **Tel:** (0121) 745 6161 w 6447471

Emily Katherine 24/12/2002 5 Cullcott Close Yoxford SAXMUNDHAM Suffolk IP17 3GZ w 6279171

Evadne Madelaine 15/02/1999 Church Cottage Victory Road North Tamerton Holsworthy Devon EX22 6RY **Tel:** (01409) 271383 w 6139693

HALL Fiona Ann (see BOUCHER, Mrs)

Gemma Kathleen 11/03/2009 159 Thimblemill Road SMETHWICK West Midlands B67 6LR **Tel:** 01215339327 w 6333357

Georgina Hannah (nee Sall) 04/01/2006 Blackcraig Croft Methlick ELLON Aberdeenshire AB41 7HN w 6333456

HALL Jane (see TAYLOR, Mrs)

Jill (nee Townson) 30/06/2003 (11/03/2008) 9 Cae Rhos HOLYHEAD Gwynedd LL65 2LF w 6277213

Joanne 29/07/2008 Warren House Veterinary Surgery Anchor Road Rochester Kent ME1 2PR **Tel:** (01634) 409988 w 6337790

Julie 23/02/2005 Elham Valley Referrals 24 Barham Business Park Elham Valley Road Barham Canterbury Kent CT4 6DQ **Tel:** (01303) 840499 w 6327406

Katherine Mary Ann 07/06/2005 The Old Golfhouse Veterinary Group The Old Golf House Brandon Road Thetford Norfolk IP24 3ND **Tel:** (01842) 764 244 w 6326933

Katherine Rachel 24/02/2004 St Austell Ongar Road Stondon Massey Brentwood Essex CM15 0EQ **Tel:** (01277) 821447 w 6293691

Kenneth Martin 05/02/2009 27 New Street Bierley BRADFORD West Yorkshire BD4 6AN **Tel:** 01274652872 m 6347107

Leonie Rose 28/09/2005 6 Cumberland Close Angmering LITTLEHAMPTON West Sussex BN16 4BH w 6305131

Louise Catherine 27/03/2009 16 Laurel Drive Tilehurst Reading Berkshire RG31 5DY **Tel:** 01189422664 w 6395991

HALL Mariarosa (see MAISTRELLO, Ms)

Nicola Jane 18/10/2005 53-55 Maidstone Road Footscray SIDCUP Kent DA14 5HB **Tel:** (020) 8300 8111 w 6345611

Suzanne Elizabeth 30/11/2005 80 Berkeley Road Shirley SOLIHULL West Midlands B90 2HU **Tel:** (0121) 744 7840 w 6301611

Valerie (nee Alderson) 16/08/1982 Rock Head Cottage Glaisdale Whitby North Yorkshire YO21 2PZ **Tel:** (01947) 897206 w 6091219

Victoria Ann 16/01/1996 The Veterinary Surgery Higher Trenant Wadebridge Cornwall PL27 6HB **Tel:** (01208) 813258 w 6040999

Victoria Louise 19/08/2008 549 Queensferry Road Edinburgh Midlothian EH4 7QE **Tel:** (07730) 555 688 w 6410643

HALLAM Emma Shirley (nee Ball) 14/09/2001 45 Overdale Avenue Buxton Derbyshire SK17 7PY w 6228153

HALLAS Claire Louise (nee Turner) 21/01/1999 (02/12/2008) Croft House Veterinary Clinic 378 Soothill Lane Batley West Yorkshire WF17 6EU **Tel:** (01924) 474300 w 6128207

HALLETT Felicity Dawn 13/11/2006 Flat 29, Grove Court The Grove Dorchester Dorset DT1 1XL **Tel:** (01300) 341467 w 6330354

Joanne Sian 19/09/2006 (23/11/2009) Putlands Veterinary Surgery Maidstone Road Paddock Wood Tonbridge Kent TN12 6DZ **Tel:** (01892) 835456 w 6295374

HALLIGAN Karen 01/02/1999 (23/10/2000) 20 Cwrt Eirlys Pencoedtre Village Barry Vale of Glamorgan Vale of Glamorgan CF63 1HL **Tel:** (01446) 739416 w 6107559

HALLS Gemma Frances 03/09/2002 48 Albert Road St Philips Bristol BS2 0XA **Tel:** (0117) 972 4567 w 6270976

Victoria Florence 26/08/1997 Rectory Cottage The Street Ickham Canterbury Kent CT3 1QN w 6038163

HALLWORTH Kelly Ann 08/11/2006 203 High Street West GLOSSOP Derbyshire SK13 8EX **Tel:** (01457) 852835 w 6345468

HALSEY Michelle (see YARDLEY, Mrs)

HAMBRIDGE Amelia Claire 10/04/2007 22 Fleetwood Court Freshbrook Swindon Wiltshire SN5 8QE **Tel:** (01793) 634717 w 6342080

HAMER Caroline Lucy 05/08/2009 10 Cheriton Close St. Albans Hertfordshire AL4 9HU **Tel:** (01727) 766147 w 6352794

HAMILL Laura Jane 11/03/2005 52 Woodburn Road GLENROTHES Fife KY7 5BA **Tel:** (01592) 757290 w 6318463

HAMILTON Janis Christine DipAVN(Surgical) (nee Harwood) 09/08/1991 16 Drymen Road Bearsden Glasgow G61 2RB **Tel:** (0141) 942 0369 w 6052508

Kelly Lorraine (nee Parsons) 20/09/2005 33 Mercer Drive St.Georges Park Lincoln Lincolnshire LN1 1AG **Tel:** (01522) 529956 w 6339220

Lorna Mary Mackay 03/02/1997 2 Beech Drive Caldercruix Airdrie Lanarkshire ML6 7QF **Tel:** (01236) 843962 w 6108031

Sarah Jayne 17/03/2003 2 McLaren Park Blairgowrie Perthshire PH10 6US w 6276784

HAMMER Susan Mary (see CAMPBELL, Mrs)

HAMMETT Nicola Jane 13/05/2003 119 Noreen Avenue Minster on Sea Sheerness Kent ME12 2EJ **Tel:** (01795) 873 571 w 6281756

HAMMOND Donna Marie 10/08/1984 (19/03/2003) 3 Kinlett Close Highwoods Colchester Essex CO4 9UE **Tel:** (01206) 822918 w 6052166

HAMMOND Elizabeth Leander (see ROSTRON, Mrs)

Phillip Keith 15/04/2004 27 Clough Court Nottingham Nottinghamshire NG8 3FJ **Tel:** (0115) 8543075 m 6289137

HAMMONDS Holly Jayne 17/11/2004 24 King Street Bradley BILSTON West Midlands WV14 8PQ **Tel:** 07714469147 w 6318309

HAMPSHEIR Kimberley Jane 22/03/2004 1-5 Hugh Street London SW1V 1QQ **Tel:** (020) 7932 2370 w 6303690

HAMPSHIRE-BOSWELL Kirsty 18/11/2008 Animed Veterinary Centre 24 Oxford Street Whitstable Kent CT5 1DD **Tel:** (01227) 273005 w 6443775

HANCOCK Amy Louise 22/09/2008 Mill House Veterinary Surgery & Hospital 20 Tennyson Avenue King's Lynn Norfolk PE30 2QG **Tel:** (01553) 771457 w 6407662

Karen Tracey 14/03/2006 13 Ashcroft Road Sea Mills Bristol Avon BS9 2NE **Tel:** (0117) 907 1885 w 6344819

Lisa Michelle 05/08/2008 32 Deadmans Lane Derby Derbyshire DE24 8WE **Tel:** (01332) 757484 w 6416506

Rebecca (nee Garton) 02/10/2001 (18/09/2006) 36 Boston Road Kirton Boston Lincolnshire PE20 1DS **Tel:** (01205) 722696 w 6229253

HANDLEY Jodi Kate 14/01/2008 14 Ash Crescent BIRMINGHAM B37 6AD w 6407101

HANDLEY Lara Amy (see PENNICOTTE-HENRIE, Mrs)

HANDSCOMB Lisa Marie (nee Keel) 24/09/1987 45 Mount Pleasant Heolgerrig Merthyr Tydfil Mid Glamorgan CF48 1RY w 6054356

HANKINS-MEADOWS Rebecca Jane 10/04/2007 New Lodge Veterinary Centre Red Lodge Road Polebrook Oundle Northamptonshire PE8 5LL **Tel:** (01832) 270201 w 6368711

HANLEY Lauren Jane 27/11/2009 3 Starling Close Droylsden MANCHESTER M43 7TY **Tel:** (0161) 371 9087 w 6464224

HANLON Kirsty Ann 04/08/2008 96 Tollgate Bretton PETERBOROUGH PE3 9XB **Tel:** (07533) 740265 w 6401480

HANN Kathryn Rachel 03/09/1997 (14/03/2005) 3 Orchard Walk NESTON CH64 9TT w 6116042

HANNAH Gemma 08/09/2009 173b Greenrigg Road Cumbernauld Glasgow Lanarkshire G67 2QD **Tel:** (077) 25855916 w 6437593

Kirsty Janice 20/09/2005 McKenzie Bryson & Marshall 21 Hill Street Kilmarnock Ayrshire KA3 1HA **Tel:** (01563) 522701 w 6324029

HANNETT Tracey Jane 17/12/1996 Quarry House Veterinary Centre 148 Teignmouth Road Torquay TQ1 4RY **Tel:** (01803) 324341 w 6032933

HANSEN Lisa Jane 14/02/2008 6 Osborne Drive Chandler's Ford Eastleigh Hampshire SO53 2ND **Tel:** (02380) 368 261 w 6373837

HANSHAW Kathryn Sarah (see CULLUM-HANSHAW, Mrs)

HANSON Kelly Ann 25/06/2009 133 Mountdale Gardens Leigh-on-Sea Essex SS9 4AE **Tel:** 01702524502 w 6375520

HARBAGE Sarah Margaret (see WANT, Mrs)

HARBER Laura June 21/05/2009 55 Manor Court Road Handsacre RUGELEY Staffordshire WS15 4TF **Tel:** 07929043152 w 6437241

HARDCASTLE Hilary 16/10/2000 (26/11/2007) 2 Clayborn View CLECKHEATON West Yorkshire BD19 5NP **Tel:** (01274) 870135 w 6191182

Nicola 29/10/2004 16 St. James Street CLITHEROE Lancashire BB7 1HH **Tel:** (01200) 427447 w 6301622

HARDING Alison Sarah (see MILES, Mrs)

HARDING Angela Clare (nee Baxter) 27/08/2004 3 The Dale Waltham Abbey Essex EN9 1SU **Tel:** (01992) 769 670 w 6267621

Emma Laura 26/04/2002 Hollycroft 66 Roston Drive Hinckley Leicestershire LE10 0XP **Tel:** (01455) 616012 w 6269139

HARDING Fiona Nicola (see HAZELL, Mrs)

Jane Alexandra (nee Cowden) 31/10/2003 (19/05/2009) The Old Well Station Approach Station Road Pershore Worcestershire WR10 2DB **Tel:** (01386) 553631 w 6264211

Kerry Ann 04/12/2003 inside Pets at Home Chelmer Village Retail Park Chelmer Village Way Chelmsford Essex CM2 6XE **Tel:** (01245) 228914 w 6272406

Nicola Claire 31/03/2003 Mount Veterinary Hospital 21 High Street Wellington Somerset TA21 8QS **Tel:** (01823) 662286 w 6278115

HARDLEY Danielle Clare 10/02/2004 Willows Veterinary Group 70 High Street Winsford Cheshire CW7 2AP **Tel:** (01606) 592714 w 6297706

HARDMAN Claire 18/03/2008 2 Welfare Crescent Blackhall Colliery Hartlepool Cleveland TS27 4LU **Tel:** 07711748041 w 6372869

HARDSTAFF Emma Louise 19/01/2001 41 Little Barn Lane MANSFIELD Nottinghamshire NG18 3JD **Tel:** (01623) 405221 w 6152353

HARDY Claire Liza 10/02/2005 (26/01/2010) C/o Royal College of Veterinary Surgeons 62-64 Horseferry Road LONDON SW1P 2AF w 6320916

HARDY Faye (see HORNSBY, Mrs)

HARDY Gayle Suzanne (see BALL, Mrs)

Jamie Michelle 16/02/2009 2 Marsh Green Kerswell CULLOMPTON Devon EX15 2ER **Tel:** 07748270598 w 6434964

Lyndsay Amy 22/12/2004 35 Eastern Circle Burnage Manchester M19 1QD **Tel:** (0161) 442 3507 w 6283054

HARE Kirsty Anne (see FURNIVAL, Mrs)

HARFORD Sharon Anne 21/10/2008 7 Kelyway House Ewen Crescent LONDON SW2 2PD w 6404505

HARGEST Mary Charlotte 21/01/2008 Firfield Maesbury Marsh OSWESTRY Shropshire SY10 8JA **Tel:** 07944976591 w 6350517

HARGRAVE Laura Ann 24/05/2006 RSPCA Putney Animal Hospital 6 Clarendon Drive London SW15 1AA **Tel:** (0300) 123 0716 w 6344830

HARIS Michelle Louise (nee Lowe) 05/09/2000 120 Lincroft Crescent Coventry West Midlands CV5 8GX w 6202270

HARKER Gemma 16/09/2009 26 Conyers Avenue DARLINGTON County Durham DL3 9DE **Tel:** (01325) 281060 w 6376026

Katherine 03/06/2004 51 West Street Hucknall Nottingham Nottinghamshire NG15 7BY **Tel:** (0115) 952 7271 w 6290545

HARKESS Nicola Jayne 13/11/2009 Zetland Veterinary Hospital 32 Zetland Road Bristol BS6 7AB **Tel:** (0117) 944 5111 w 6461287

HARKINS Peter 29/12/2003 38 Greenacres Drive Garstang Preston Lancashire PR3 1RQ **Tel:** (01995) 602 503 m 6285012

HARLAND Gemma Elizabeth 10/05/2007 90 Lakeside Road Douglas ISLE OF MAN IM2 7DD **Tel:** (07624) 463330 w 6379128

HARLEY Lynn Michelle 04/08/1981 MacQueen Veterinary Surgery 1 Hopton Park London Road Devizes Wiltshire SN10 2EY **Tel:** (01380) 728505 w 608939X

Sharon Margaret (nee Pook) 19/01/1996 10 Broad Park Road Plymouth PL3 4PX **Tel:** (01752) 250741 w 6035173

HARLIN Clare-Marie 17/11/2009 13 Ridgeway Avenue GRAVESEND Kent DA12 5BD **Tel:** (01474) 534481 w 6465951

HARLOW Caroline Mary (see HOLLIS, Ms)

HARNEY Claire Louise 11/04/2005 Grove Veterinary Centre 231-239 Rawlinson Street Barrow-in-Furness Cumbria LA14 1DW **Tel:** (01229) 820402 w 6268270

HARPER Adena Lesley 23/12/2003 3 Sedge Drive BROMSGROVE Worcestershire B61 0UL **Tel:** (01527) 872059 w 6288290

Debbie Josephine 08/08/2005 15 Malmesbury Road COVENTRY CV6 2HX **Tel:** (02476) 722118 w 6301633

Jane (nee Thacker) 26/08/1994 Warwickshire College Moreton Morrell Warwick Warwickshire CV35 9BL w 6036825

Joanne (nee Brewer) 02/02/1994 (27/07/1999) Eastfield Veterinary Clinic Ltd Station Road North Thoresby GRIMSBY Lincolnshire DN36 5QU **Tel:** (01472) 840209 w 6067354

Rosalind Sophia 30/06/2003 3 Park Farm Thorney Peterborough Cambridgeshire PE6 0SY **Tel:** (01733) 271026 w 6283120

Sarah Jane (nee Meakin) 28/01/1999 80 Lindsworth Road Kings Norton Birmingham West Midlands B30 3RR **Tel:** (0121) 4596891 w 6132315

Suzanne Elaine 10/12/2007 4 Brickiln Street Brownhills Walsall WS8 6AU **Tel:** (01543) 375154 w 6358789

HARRIES Rachel Nia 10/09/2008 Chaseview Veterinary Clinic The Patch Hildersley ROSS-ON-WYE Herefordshire HR9 7NJ **Tel:** 07815155645 w 6435734

HARRINGTON Amy 02/06/2004 (11/11/2008) Anglia Ancton Lane BOGNOR REGIS West Sussex PO22 6NN **Tel:** (01243) 585592 w 6300038

Catharine Sybilla 14/10/2009 Flat B 455 Northolt Road HARROW Middlesex HA2 8JN w 6491845

Helen Louise (nee Lyth) 23/09/1997 Willows Veterinary Group 70 High Street Winsford Cheshire CW7 2AP **Tel:** (01606) 592714 w 6035628

Kelly-Marie 23/02/2005 52 Friars Oak Road Hassocks West Sussex BN6 8PY **Tel:** (01444) 233472 w 6293031

Victoria Jane 15/09/1995 83 Edinburgh Way Banbury Oxfordshire OX16 0PA **Tel:** (01295) 273437 w 6032525

HARRIS Abigail Marie (see MCKAY, Mrs)

HARRIS Alexandra Louise 10/01/2007 70 Brinkley Lane Highwoods COLCHESTER Essex CO4 9XE **Tel:** (01206) 842608 w 6354664

Amanda Joan (nee McGregor) 09/11/1989 2 Carters Cottages REDHILL Surrey RH1 6QQ **Tel:** (01737) 762365 w 6056353

Catherine Clare Margaret 03/02/2005 (15/01/2008) 6A Tattenham Crescent Epsom Downs Surrey KT18 5QS w 6293141

HARRIS Chloe Louise (see ATKIN, Mrs)

Donna 20/01/1997 (31/07/2000) The Barn Back Street Modbury Ivybridge Devon PL21 0RF w 6099411

Emma Beatrice 02/01/2008 Valley Vets Ltd Oakfield Street Ystrad Mynach Hengoed Mid Glamorgan CF82 7AF **Tel:** (01443) 813137 w 6366170

Helen Louise (nee Knuckey, formerly Dingle) 19/08/1991 Rowan House 2 Raleigh Farm Mitchell Newquay Cornwall TR8 5AT w 6054684

Janet Lois DipAVN(Surgical) (nee Dedman) 15/01/1987 (30/03/2000) 38 Banks Road Pound Hill Crawley West Sussex RH10 7BJ **Tel:** (01293) 452141 w 6049029

HARRIS Katherine Claire (see BADMAN, Mrs)

HARRIS Louise (see MARSHALL, Mrs)

Melissa Louise (nee Furniss) 17/09/2007 28 Woodwards Crawley West Sussex RH11 9PL **Tel:** (01293) 562435 w 6339110

Nicola Lynette 23/12/2003 Wood Street Veterinary Hospital 74 Wood Street Barnet Hertfordshire EN5 4BW **Tel:** (020) 8449 0074 w 6275904

Peta Alexis 14/12/2007 21 Forge Close Fleckney Leicester Leicestershire LE8 8DA w 6402206

Philip Alan 25/04/2005 St Anne's Veterinary Group 6 St Anne's Road Eastbourne East Sussex BN21 2DJ **Tel:** (01323) 640011 m 6294648

Rosalind Wendy (nee Horne) 16/08/1982 Woodmancote Veterinary Surgery Station Road Woodmancote CHELTENHAM Gloucestershire GL52 9HN **Tel:** (01242) 676113 w 6091048

Samantha Kelly 13/03/2002 (10/02/2005) Holmer Veterinary Surgery Roman Road Holmer Hereford HR1 1LE **Tel:** (01432) 272468 w 6204591

Sonya 13/11/2009 174 Winchester Road Grantham Lincolnshire NG31 8RX **Tel:** (01476) 566960 w 6466050

Vikki Leanne 15/05/2008 40 Knights end road MARCH Cambridgeshire PE15 9PA **Tel:** (07793) 115940 w 6390425

HARRISON Catherine May Janet 28/01/1998 Dunkirk Road Dunkirk Nottingham NG7 2PH **Tel:** (01159) 785787 w 6129812

HARRISON Charlotte Elizabeth (see WILLIAMS, Mrs)

HARRISON Clare Joanne (see WEEKES, Mrs)

Donna Elizabeth 24/02/2004 238 Hollinsend Road Sheffield South Yorkshire S12 2EJ **Tel:** (0114) 265 1674 w 6275343

Emma Elizabeth (nee Oxtoby) 21/03/2006 Rudston Grange Rudston Driffield North Humberside YO25 4DW **Tel:** (01262) 420079 w 6347305

Helen Susanne 29/01/2001 34 Cloves Hill Morley Ilkeston Derbyshire DE7 6DH **Tel:** (01332) 882784 w 6211466

Jennifer Patrice 17/07/2003 8 Withy Close Wootton Bassett Swindon Wiltshire SN4 7JF **Tel:** (01793) 850298 w 6274023

Joanne Laura 27/02/2002 4 Saffron Walk Bourne Lincolnshire PE10 9NR w 6263529

Jodie Annette 31/03/2008 1 Recreation Avenue Corringham STANFORD-LE-HOPE Essex SS17 9BZ **Tel:** (01375) 677026 w 6343092

HARRISON Katherine Elizabeth (see RIDING, Mrs)

Kirsty Jane McLeod (nee Alvsaker) 05/09/1985 (30/03/2005) Elvendale House Milltown Muddiford Barnstaple Devon EX31 4HG **Tel:** (01271) 850622 w 6052417

Marie Louise 04/06/2009 8 Cromwell Crescent Lambley Nottingham Nottinghamshire NG4 4PJ **Tel:** (0115) 931 3773 w 6443698

Nicola Jane 30/03/2006 31 Thornham Lane Royton Oldham Lancashire OL2 6UW **Tel:** (01616) 202126 w 6348438

HARRISON-CLAY Emma Michelle 20/01/1999 (29/01/2008) 7 Portland Way Cardinal Grange Kings Clipstone MANSFIELD Nottinghamshire NG21 9FE **Tel:** (01623) 631925 w 6030630

HARROD Jennifer Emily 01/04/2009 39 Bell Road Warnham Horsham West Sussex RH12 3QJ **Tel:** 01403260072 w 6443742

HARRON Rachel Christina Mary 16/02/2009 14 Shamrock Way Southgate LONDON N14 5RY **Tel:** (07976) 437670 w 6354103

HART Andrea Karen (see JEFFERY, Mrs)

HART Angela Dawn (nee Williams) 23/12/2003 (01/01/2006) 8 Watchwood Grove Calverton Nottingham Nottinghamshire NG14 6HX **Tel:** (0115) 9107454 w 6271768

HART Charlotte Rebecca (see SWANSON, Mrs)

HART Emma Louise (see ROBERTS, Mrs)

Joanna Clare 03/12/2008 64 Chartwell Place Sutton Surrey SM3 9TD **Tel:** 02086414025 w 6419696

Katie-Jane 05/07/2006 2 Wren Park Close Findern Derby Derbyshire DE65 6QQ w 6322467

Melissa Emily 04/09/1996 (13/09/2004) 15 Acorn Way Hurst Green Etchingham East Sussex TN19 7QG **Tel:** (01580) 860 706 w 6099433

Nicola Louise 18/11/2008 40 Rainham Road Rainham Essex RM13 7RL **Tel:** 01708501394 w 6443841

Vanessa Ruth 10/09/2009 2 Brashland Drive East Hunsbury NORTHAMPTON NN4 0SS **Tel:** (01604) 768149 w 6494452

HARTELL Claire Louise 12/05/2006 20 Fitzhamon Park Ashchurch TEWKESBURY Gloucestershire GL20 8JL w 6331168

Holly Louise 30/01/2009 Chapel House Biddisham AXBRIDGE Somerset BS26 2RE **Tel:** 01934751227 w 6419949

HARTLEY Claire Louise 06/02/1995 77-81 Browgate Baildon Shipley West Yorkshire BD17 6BY **Tel:** (01274) 580785 w 6029862

Claire Marie 25/01/1999 Holdgate Hall MUCH WENLOCK Shropshire TF13 6LW **Tel:** (07870) 990319 w 6123344

HARTLEY Nicola Dawn (see SUMMERFIELD, Mrs)

Rachael Yvonne 06/08/2008 10 Stanways Road St Columb Minor NEWQUAY Cornwall TR7 3HF w 6370988

HARTLEY Sharon (see NEWSOME, Mrs)

HARTLEY Victoria (see CHADWICK, Mrs)

HARTNOLL Katie Elizabeth (nee Bridle) 06/08/2008 6 Hayhurst Avenue MIDDLEWICH Cheshire CW10 0BA **Tel:** 01606737992 w 6351166

HARTWELL Karen Ann 04/03/2003 Harvest Veterinary Clinic Maidenbower Square Maidenbower Crawley West Sussex RH10 7QH **Tel:** (01293) 884422 w 6262627

Rebecca Louise 11/11/2008 Honeywick Cottage Honeywick Lane Chiddingly Lewes East Sussex BN8 6HF **Tel:** 01825873256 w 6428947

HARTWRIGHT Clare Elizabeth Dorothy 03/06/2008 17 Trenholme Court Beechwood Road CATERHAM Surrey CR3 6NQ w 6334303

HARVEY Carole Lynda (nee Strand) 25/02/2003 29 Lower Meadow HARLOW Essex CM18 7RD **Tel:** (01279) 415016 w 6265344

HARVEY Christine Louise (see MUMUNI, Mrs)

Claire Debra 18/10/2005 70 Mission Road Diss Norfolk IP22 4HX **Tel:** (01379) 651183 w 6243487

HARVEY Deborah Elaine (see THOMAS, Mrs)

Gemma Fern 17/02/2009 Unit 10 Egremont Road Bearsted Maidstone Kent ME15 8LH **Tel:** (01622) 736 677 w 6433083

Gemma Louise 21/07/2008 9 Potter Close Market Weighton YORK YO43 3RF w 6376037

Jacqueline Ann (formerly Lingard) 31/01/1992 (17/01/2002) Oakmount House Trafalgar Street Burnley Lancashire BB11 1TP **Tel:** (01282) 423640 w 6052483

Kirsty 05/04/2005 Rathgael Veterinary Clinic 24 Brook Lane Bangor County Down BT19 1ST **Tel:** (028) 9145 4129 w 6283747

HARVEY Rebecca Aimee (see SAUNDERS, Mrs)

Samantha Dawn 22/09/2009 19 St. Davids Close Brandon Suffolk IP27 0UR **Tel:** 01842810110 w 6439738

Sarah 10/02/2004 1-5 Hugh Street London SW1V 1QQ **Tel:** (020) 7932 2370 w 6265289

Scarlett Elizabeth 11/11/2008 Park Veterinary Centre 256 Cassiobury Drive WATFORD Hertfordshire WD17 3PA **Tel:** (01923) 223321 w 6434469

Victoria Elizabeth 13/07/2007 10 Merlin Drive DALTON-IN-FURNESS Cumbria LA15 8QE **Tel:** (078) 2526 0526 w 6349395

HARWOOD Jan (see STEVENSON, Miss)

HARWOOD Janis Christine (see HAMILTON, Mrs)

HASKELL Rebecca Elizabeth (nee Kyte) 11/01/2005 380 Shortdale Road Aldershot Hampshire GU11 3RS **Tel:** (01252) 329947 w 6283670

HASKEY Eleanor 16/06/2008 3 Sandy Bank BEWDLEY Worcestershire DY12 2AY **Tel:** (07762) 705231 w 6380767

HASSEN Diane Marie 22/01/1996 (22/04/2003) 145 Green Drift Royston Hertfordshire SG8 5BL **Tel:** (01763) 247856 w 6040296

HASSETT Rachel Mary 14/03/2006 17 Goose Lane Lower Quinton Stratford-upon-Avon Warwickshire CV37 8TA **Tel:** (01789) 261875 w 6320069

HASSON Lydia 27/10/2000 4 Greenfield Park Portishead Bristol BS20 6RQ **Tel:** (01275) 842260 w 6203623

HASTE Beverley 28/03/2008 Walden Windsoredge Lane Nailsworth Stroud Gloucestershire GL6 0NP **Tel:** (01453) 839344 w 6420818

HASTIE Karen 09/09/2004 18 Trenholme Court Beechwood Road CATERHAM Surrey CR3 6NQ **Tel:** (0795) 618 9545 w 6374959

HASTINGS Elizabeth Ann 27/01/1997 Oak House Veterinary Centre Ltd 277 Woodborough Road Nottingham Nottinghamshire NG3 4JT **Tel:** (0115) 969 1222 w 6034974

HASTWELL Pamela Anne 13/03/2008 32 Cotefield Drive Leighton Buzzard Bedfordshire LU7 3DS **Tel:** (01525) 370424 w 6366313

HATCH Andrea Dawn 13/08/1992 (30/04/2004) 17-19 Church Road Leyland Lancashire PR25 3EJ **Tel:** (01772) 432039 w 600785X

Nichola Louise (nee Dann) 10/02/1995 Oak Tree Farm Theale Wedmore Somerset BS28 4SN **Tel:** (01458) 860030 w 602449X

HATCHER Kerry Ann 17/05/2005 Mount Veterinary Hospital 21 High Street Wellington Somerset TA21 8QS **Tel:** (01823) 662286 w 6305307

HATCHETT Anna Rachel 07/02/2006 8 Mill Court The Carrs Ruswarp WHITBY North Yorkshire YO21 1YL w 6347646

HATFIELD Amanda Clare 22/03/2004 9 Strathmore Close Eccleshill Braford West Yorkshire BD2 3DQ **Tel:** (01943) 873147 w 6279721

HATFIELD Susan Margaret (see SYMONDS, Mrs)

HATTON Amanda Jane (see RENSHAW, Mrs)

HATTON Victoria Jane 30/08/2006 18 East Lockinge WANTAGE Oxfordshire OX12 8QG w 6436658

HAUGHIAN Zoe 22/01/1998 (01/02/2005) Milan Veterinary Clinic Somerset Road Douglas Isle of Man IM2 5AQ **Tel:** (01624) 674076 w 6098280

HAUTZ Lisa Marie 28/06/2005 69 Milldale Road Long Eaton Nottingham Nottinghamshire NG10 3JB **Tel:** 07763688057 w 6316824

HAVARD Carys Rhian 14/02/2000 556 Bath Road Brislington Bristol Somerset BS4 3JZ **Tel:** (01179) 775911 w 6191248

HAVELIN Katie Louise (see BLACKERY, Mrs)

HAVERCROFT Emma Louise (see DARLING, Mrs)

HAWES Nicola Dianne (nee Manfield) 26/08/1992 3 Herbert Street Old Town Hemel Hempstead Hertfordshire HP2 5HP **Tel:** (01442) 255117 w 6005692

HAWES Rachel (see MAYDOM, Mrs)

HAWKEN Claire Louise (nee Benney) 03/02/1994 (12/06/2000) 7 Thornton Close Roche ST. AUSTELL Cornwall PL26 8TR **Tel:** (01726) 891 478 w 606773X

HAWKER Alison Susanne 02/06/2004 482 Green Lane New Eltham London SE9 3TF w 6288125

HAWKER Stephanie June (see NASH, Mrs)

HAWKES Gail Ann (see GLENWRIGHT, Mrs)

HAWKES Jayne Margaret (see MANLEY, Mrs)

HAWKETT Joanne 27/05/2003 106 Hazebrouck Road Faversham Kent ME13 7RB w 6285298

HAWKINS Amie Louise 09/10/2009 42 Dunsford Gardens St Thomas EXETER Devon EX4 1LN **Tel:** 07511253198 w 6492362

Beverley Clare (nee Hollis) 02/11/2004 35 Coppice Road Rugeley Staffordshire WS15 1LT **Tel:** (01889) 578643 w 6283659

Emma Clare 25/03/2009 15 Pebble Island Way LEAMINGTON SPA Warwickshire CV31 1AR **Tel:** (01926) 772926 w 6351771

Emma Jane 29/01/2010 Berry House Veterinary Practice 41 Nightingale Road Hitchin Hertfordshire SG5 1RE **Tel:** (01462) 432824 w 6460814

Joanna Fleur 13/11/2009 Stow Veterinary Surgeons Maugersbury Road Stow on the Wold Cheltenham Gloucestershire GL54 1HH **Tel:** (01451) 830620 w 6464389

Karen Elizabeth 19/12/2008 The Laurels Barry Lane Hardington Mandeville Somerset **Tel:** 01935862093 w 6441927

Kerry-Anne 06/05/2008 Harvest Veterinary Clinic Maidenbower Square Maidenbower Crawley West Sussex RH10 7QH **Tel:** (01293) 884422 w 6363244

Kirsty Patricia 29/09/2009 4 Gratwicke Road Tilehurst READING RG30 4TT **Tel:** (0118) 9418556 w 6264464

Laura Jade 28/01/2010 113 Moffats Lane Brookmans Park HATFIELD Hertfordshire AL9 7RP **Tel:** 01707653394 w 6455149

Laura Jayne 01/09/2009 Fern Cottage Veterinary Surgery 233-235 Park Road Sittingbourne Kent ME10 1ER **Tel:** (01795) 476411 w 6455160

Lindsay Anne (nee Barnes) 07/02/2007 Zetland Veterinary Hospital 32 Zetland Road Bristol BS6 7AB **Tel:** (0117) 944 5111 w 6378391

Lisa 10/10/2008 385 Leek Road Endon Stoke-on-Trent Staffordshire ST9 9BA **Tel:** (01782) 503166 w 6437780

Lisa Julie 29/06/2007 Kernow Casho Quarff SHETLAND ZE2 9EY **Tel:** (01950) 477 529 w 6303712

Victoria Grace 15/02/2005 9 Whitmore Close New Southgate London N11 1PB w 6322478

HAWKSWORTH Shoned 24/05/2006 Coed Offa Penycae Road Ruabon WREXHAM Clwyd LL14 6EB **Tel:** (07920) 097870 w 6347019

HAWLEY Sarah Louise 27/02/2006 6 Bellfield Road Morecambe Lancashire LA4 5NQ **Tel:** (01524) 424966 w 6349549

HAWORTH Tara Claire 08/05/2008 55 Raymere Gardens London SE18 2LB **Tel:** (0208) 8540670 w 6357480

HAY Ainsley 18/04/2008 21 Westway Road Raynes Park LONDON SW20 9LX w 6507245

Gillian 10/04/2003 73 Ravensby Park Gardens Carnoustie Angus DD7 7NY **Tel:** (01241) 858600 w 6283197

HAY Kirstie Olivia (see ADAMS, Mrs)

HAY Rachel Mary (see FORBES, Mrs)

HAYCOCK Tracey (see ORGAN, Mrs)

HAYCOCKS Joanne Kay 10/01/2007 Flat 1, Fox & Goose Whicham Millom Cumbria LA18 5LX **Tel:** (01229) 772 045 w 6351870

HAYDON Katherine Elizabeth (see THOMPSON, Mrs)

HAYDON Vikki Michelle 26/03/2002 (26/11/2007) Flat 2 Whitlock Court 19 The Square HOLSWORTHY Devon EX22 6AN **Tel:** (01409) 254795 w 6272241

HAYES Laura DipAVN(Surgical), DipAVN(Medical) (nee Brooks, formerly McDonough) 29/07/1998 28 High Street Madingley CAMBRIDGE CB23 8AB **Tel:** (01954) 210935 w 6097822

Samantha Dee 05/03/2009 51 Bawtry Road Bessacarr Doncaster South Yorkshire DN4 7AA **Tel:** (01302) 534999 w 6425757

Suzanne Meryl (nee Tarran-Jones) 02/10/2001 The Ashley Church Road Mannings Heath Horsham West Sussex RH13 6JE w 6229286

HAYLER Naomi Elaine 20/10/2009 52 Pender Gardens Rumford FALKIRK FK2 0BJ **Tel:** 01236890665 w 6373463

HAYNE Lucy 15/01/1996 Thameswood Veterinary Clinics Ltd 62-64 Purton Road Swindon SN2 2LZ **Tel:** (01793) 526780 w 604241X

HAYNES Kate Alison (see CUMMINGS, Mrs)

HAYNES Katie (see SHARMAN, Mrs)

HAYNES Katie (nee Rogers) 11/11/2004 8 St George's Parade Wolverhampton West Midlands WV2 1BD **Tel:** (01902) 425262 w 6283637

Lisa Jayne 01/06/2007 The Dogs Trust Shoreham Brighton Road SHOREHAM-BY-SEA West Sussex BN43 5LT **Tel:** (01273) 452 576 w 6355379

HAYSOM Katie 03/12/2003 37 Devon Road Cheam Surrey SM2 7PE **Tel:** (020) 8642 3373 w 6286189

HAYTER Victoria Rebecca (nee Nichols) 04/02/2002 6 Burghwood Close Mileham King's Lynn Norfolk PE32 2PR **Tel:** (01328) 701 993 w 6255092

HAYWARD Hilary Anne 28/07/1975 (17/03/2008) Pfizer Walton Oaks Walton-on-the-Hill TADWORTH Surrey KT20 7NS **Tel:** (01737) 332299 w 6052643

Kimberley Louise 09/06/2008 7 Mintys Top Bromham CHIPPENHAM Wiltshire SN15 2HB **Tel:** 01380859850 w 6404494

Louisa Jane 02/10/1985 5 Stowe Court Stantonbury Milton Keynes Buckinghamshire MK14 6AQ **Tel:** (01908) 220562 w 6052654

Sarah Jayne 03/10/2007 107 Tilstock Crescent Shrewsbury Shropshire SY2 6HQ **Tel:** (01743) 235934 w 6375124

HAYWOOD Lucy Claire 10/09/2009 9 Avebury Road Westcliff-on-Sea Essex SS0 7AE **Tel:** 07704652774 w 6443687

HAZELL Fiona Nicola (nee Harding) 27/08/1996 (21/06/2005) 3 Hillcrest Road CASTLEFORD West Yorkshire WF10 3QX **Tel:** (01977) 516215 w 6043548

Jessica Louise (nee Masters) 21/10/1994 (04/05/2005) Cogges Veterinary Surgery Cogges Hill Road Witney Oxfordshire OX28 3XY **Tel:** (01993) 772627 w 6034001

Karly 30/05/2006 1 Ensign Way Littlehampton West Sussex BN17 6RQ w 6355368

HAZELTINE Andrea Jane (nee Key) 13/08/2003 21 Roach Vale Colchester Essex CO4 3YN **Tel:** (01206) 514107 w 6278478

HAZZARD Natalie Samantha 09/11/2009 60a Stafford Road Caterham Surrey CR3 6JB **Tel:** 07947809026 w 6427253

HEAD Lucinda Jane 31/10/2006 69 Freshwater Road Chatham Kent ME5 7SZ **Tel:** (01634) 319 524 w 6366137

HEAL Catherine Ruth (see SHARPLES, Mrs)

HEALD Shelley Ann (see LYONS, Mrs)

HEALEY Gemma Louise (see ALDRED, Mrs)

HEALEY Stefanie Jean 07/06/2005 8 Copthorne Luton Bedfordshire LU2 8RJ **Tel:** (01582) 727487 w 6292602

HEAP Emma Jane (see WRATHALL, Mrs)

HEAPS Joanna (see JACKSON, Mrs)

HEARD Sarah Jane (see LEECH, Mrs)

HEARD Sharon Anne 18/04/2008 11 Hunts Farm Close Tollesbury Maldon Essex CM9 8QX **Tel:** 01621868851 w 6366797

HEARNE Louise Frances Michelle (nee Sexton) 18/04/2005 (22/02/2007) 9 Merton Close MAIDENHEAD Berkshire SL6 3HH w 6292679

HEATH Davine Marie (nee Thompson) 22/03/2004 27 Deanscroft Way Meir Hay Stoke-On-Trent Staffordshire ST3 5XW **Tel:** (01785) 712235 w 6295605

Heidi Etain Louise 30/11/2005 22 Shaftesbury Road Bournemouth Dorset BH8 8SS w 6331520

HEATH Tania Jane (see BENSON, Mrs)

HEATHCOCK Katie 17/07/2008 17 Woodhead Row Water Street Port Sunlight WIRRAL Merseyside CH62 5HG w 6407200

HEATHFIELD Tania Carole 24/09/2009 2 Vancouver Drive Gillingham Kent ME8 0DD **Tel:** 01634235572 w 6383847

HEATON Claire 24/11/2008 9 Lakeland Gardens Chorley Lancashire PR7 2LL **Tel:** 07966145042 w 6432830

Emma Frances 06/12/2004 78 Mansfield Crescent Armthorpe Doncaster South Yorkshire DN3 2AA **Tel:** (01302) 833434 w 6326889

Kelly Jayne 31/10/2003 18 Coco Parade Skye Victoria 3977 Australia w 6277873

HEAYNS Bethaney Jane 11/11/2008 Harper Adams University College Edgmond NEWPORT Shropshire TF10 8NB w 6410786

HECTOR Nikki Claire 08/11/2006 67 Church Street Burton Latimer Kettering Northamptonshire NN15 5LU **Tel:** (01536) 420 966 w 6375135

HEDDINGTON Kati 17/07/2003 103 Aylesbury Crescent Bristol Avon BS3 5NN **Tel:** (0117) 9638 940 w 6282042

HEDGES Stephanie Leona (nee Barrett) 06/04/1992 (23/10/2003) 39 High Street Long Buckby NORTHAMPTON NN6 7RE **Tel:** (01327) 843251 w 6008820

Victoria Elisabeth (nee Fox) 26/01/1995 (31/12/2002) Royal College of Veterinary Surgeons 62-64 Horseferry Road LONDON SW1P 2AF **Tel:** (020) 7202 0782 w 6034690

HEDLAND Leonie Alexis 04/12/2003 40 Watson Street Hoyland Barnsley South Yorkshire S74 0NX **Tel:** (01226) 351 598 w 6298069

HEDLEY Amanda Louise 24/01/2005 New Priory Veterinary Practice The Deneway London Rd Brighton East Sussex BN1 8QR **Tel:** (01273) 540430 w 6320245

HEELEY Victoria Lee 24/11/2004 Crawshaw Hill Pudsey Leeds LS28 7BW **Tel:** (0113) 255 9992 w 6284990

HEFFER Evonne Marie 30/01/1996 (16/05/2003) The Village Animal Hospital CVS (UK) Ltd Guards Avenue Coulsdon Road Caterham Surrey CR3 5ZD **Tel:** (01883) 348483 w 6038243

HEFFERMAN Ruth Joy 17/07/2003 Ferlys House Overton Park Road Cheltenham Gloucestershire GL50 3BP **Tel:** (01242) 522 429 w 6271185

HEGARTY Caroline Patricia 20/11/2009 11 St. Marys Terrace Middletown Armagh County Armagh BT60 4HU **Tel:** (028) 37 568 986 w 6446899

Lindsey Jane 27/04/2005 (06/03/2007) 16 Primrose Road Hersham WALTON-ON-THAMES Surrey KT12 5JD w 6301105

HEGGIE Helen Ruth 22/03/2004 The Lawrie Veterinary Practice Kenilworth Court Kenilworth Road Cumbernauld Glasgow G67 1BP **Tel:** (01236) 727876 w 6289368

HEIGHT Sharron 21/07/2004 207 Daventry Road Coventry West Midlands CV3 5HH **Tel:** (02476) 503000 w 6292360

HEILLING Nicola Jane 09/01/2009 3 Curtiss Drive Leavesden Watford Hertfordshire WD25 7GN **Tel:** 02089524881 w 6437340

HEJTMANKOVA Jirina 03/07/2008 76-77 Maison Dieu Road Dover Kent CT16 1RE **Tel:** (01304) 201617 w 6519697

HELDREICH Ruth 03/09/1999 44 Onslow Road Mickleover Derby Derbyshire DE3 9JH **Tel:** (01332) 516792 w 6129302

HELLAWELL Claire Louise 18/11/2008 2 Elm Avenue Sowerby Bridge West Yorkshire HX6 2HU **Tel:** (01422) 831390 w 6293295

HELLINGS Lisa-Marie Jayne (nee Millgate) 17/12/2007 43 Beatrice Road Margate Kent CT9 5SN **Tel:** (01843) 295613 w 6328220

HELLSEN Michelle 28/01/2010 2 Woodland Avenue Worlingham BECCLES Suffolk NR34 7EF **Tel:** 01502710748 w 6461309

HELPS Karen Marie 10/02/1997 (10/04/2000) 48 Albert Road St Philips Bristol BS2 0XA **Tel:** (0117) 9774567 w 6043650

HEMINGWAY Elaine DipAVN(Surgical) 31/08/1999 Netherfield House Salisbury Road Low Moor Bradford West Yorkshire BD12 0AA **Tel:** (01274) 679192 w 6185088

HEMMING Justine Laura 04/03/2009 3 High Land Road Walsall Wood Walsall West Midlands WS9 9ER **Tel:** (01543) 453502 w 6403339

HEMPENSTALL Kelly Jane 29/01/2010 109 New Forest Drive BROCKENHURST Hampshire SO42 7QW **Tel:** 07912058189 w 6497752

HEMPSALL Roseanne Louise 19/07/2004 50 Beatrice Ave Lipson Plymouth Devon PL4 8QB **Tel:** 01752240478 w 6283329

HEN-BOISEN Katy (nee Bishop) 02/10/2001 Wakefield Vets4Pets Limited 106-116 Horbury Road Wakefield West Yorkshire WF2 8UB **Tel:** (01924) 290555 w 6229297

HENDERSON Amanda Jayne 14/03/2008 6 Warwick Close Canvey Island Essex SS8 9YB **Tel:** (07870) 260340 w 6390194

Angela Jane 19/01/1998 Woodside Veterinary Group Woodside Road Torphins BANCHORY Kincardineshire AB31 4TR **Tel:** (01339) 882556 w 6115504

Claire Louise 17/07/2008 19 Banchory Green Glenrothes Fife KY7 6UA **Tel:** 01592745782 w 6409444

Colette Michelle 15/01/1996 Copeland Veterinary Surgeons Myton Park Myton Road Ingleby Barwick Stockton on Tees Cleveland TS17 0WA w 6031714

Jennifer Claire 05/03/2009 43 South Street Greenock Renfrewshire PA16 8QG **Tel:** (01475) 722 867 w 6436911

Kathryn 26/01/1999 (22/03/2004) 4 Vine Cottages Church Street Hampton Lucy Warwick Warwickshire CV35 8BD **Tel:** (01789) 840426 w 6142786

Leanne 05/09/1996 97 Chester Road East Shotton Deeside Clwyd CH5 1QB **Tel:** (01244) 830065 w 6098305

Lisa Marie 08/04/2009 40 Lawrie Drive Penicuik Midlothian EH26 0HQ **Tel:** (01968) 678 127 w 6436900

HENDERSON Sarah Louise (see BARNES, Mrs)

Tracy 27/05/2003 26 Hamilton Drive Radcliffe-on-Trent NOTTINGHAM NG12 1AG w 6272428

HENDERSON Tracy Jane (see DINNELL, Ms)

HENDRY Alice Elizabeth (see ADAMS, Mrs)

HENDRY Dawn Carol 21/07/2008 12 Ethelfield Road COVENTRY CV2 4BW **Tel:** 07949220979 w 6376048

Sally Rachael (nee Williams) 15/09/1989 Hannam House Lamberts Lane Midhurst West Sussex GU29 9EA **Tel:** (01730) 816833 w 6052756

HENDY Maria Ann 09/07/2007 Upper Row Farm Laverton BATH BA2 7RB w 6352596

HENEBERY Rachel Louise 18/11/2008 92 Juddfield Street Haydock ST. HELENS Merseyside WA11 0BD **Tel:** (01744) 613549 w 6426219

HENNESSEY Michelle Louise (nee Hill) 20/07/1993 Staynes Hall Lane Hammerwich Burntwood Staffordshire WS7 0JU **Tel:** (01543) 252535 w 6015157

HENNESSY Lucy Elizabeth 08/10/2008 Kings Head Inn Chetwynd End NEWPORT Shropshire TF10 7JJ w 6410797

HENSBY Lucy Jane 07/06/2005 46 Mokyll Croft Taverham Norwich Norfolk NR8 6UG w 6320091

HENSHALL Leah Kate 09/10/2009 99 Windham Road BOURNEMOUTH BH1 4RN **Tel:** (01202) 303983 w 6436405

HENSON Amy Ciara 12/07/2006 4 Church Terrace London NW4 4JU **Tel:** (020) 8203 2090 w 6322269

Linda 11/09/2008 12 Kayswood Road Marple STOCKPORT Cheshire SK6 6EW **Tel:** 01614845806 w 6522931

HENSTEAD Julie (nee Devlin) 24/06/2009 16 Belfry Crescent Standish Wigan Lancashire WN6 0XY **Tel:** (01257) 426494 w 6356677

HENWOOD Julia Elizabeth (nee Crangle) 15/07/2005 (03/05/2007) 52 Guernsey Way Kennington ASHFORD Kent TN24 9LW **Tel:** (01233) 640819 w 6293636

HEPHER Gillian Margaret 14/09/1998 4 Burch Place New Road Eyam Hope Valley Derbyshire S32 5QE w 6131537

HERBERT Jemma-Anne Louise 04/11/2005 41 Tydies Coed Eva CWMBRAN Gwent NP44 4TN **Tel:** (07817) 455 450 w 6323347

Michelle Louise 16/08/2002 17 Green Leys Maidenhead Berkshire SL6 7EZ **Tel:** (01628) 673583 w 6263727

Sarah Jane 13/05/2003 PDSA Pet Aid Hospital 64 Heyford Road Braunstone Leicester Leicestershire LE3 1SR **Tel:** (0116) 255 8731 w 6286112

HERDMAN Melanie Jane 08/07/2008 Ramparts Veterinary Centre Windmill Way West BERWICK-UPON-TWEED TD15 1TB **Tel:** (01289) 330066 w 6373474

HERMIT Julie 31/03/2003 (12/02/2008) 15 Auchinleck Terrace CLYDEBANK Dunbartonshire G81 6QY **Tel:** (01389) 383190 w 6281657

HERON Corrine (see MILLINGTON, Mrs)

HERON Donna Michelle (nee Start) 23/01/1996 85 Temple Park Road South Shields Tyne and Wear NE34 0PR **Tel:** (0191) 4217515 w 6037851

HERRINGTON Jennifer Dianne Michelle 05/03/2008 Wakefield Vets4Pets Limited 106-116 Horbury Road Wakefield West Yorkshire WF2 8UB **Tel:** (01924) 290555 w 6404417

HERRON Amy Elizabeth 28/02/2007 10 Doublegates Court RIPON North Yorkshire HG4 2TT w 6365741

HERSEY Kate Alison (see CUMMINGS, Mrs)

HERST Lisa Maria (see DOWLEY, Mrs)

HERTZ Emelie Manning 26/02/2009 35 Salcott Road London SW11 6DQ **Tel:** 02079785527 w 6445172

HERWORTH Natalie Marie 09/11/2005 35 Roker Park Road Roker Sunderland SR6 9PL **Tel:** (0191) 516 0056 w 6339121

HESSION Tracy 10/07/2003 Ashleigh Veterinary Centre 221 Upper Chorlton Road Manchester Greater Manchester M16 0DE **Tel:** (0161) 881 6868 w 6283230

HETHERINGTON Lee-Ann 11/04/2005 Alver Veterinary Group 148 Forton Road Gosport Hampshire PO12 3HG **Tel:** (023) 9258 2991/2 w 6268886

Victoria Ann 09/02/2009 6 Brown Street WORKINGTON Cumbria CA14 2NL w 6445227

HEWES Gemma Leanne (see MOULE, Mrs)

HEWES Nicola (see WILLIAMS, Mrs)

HEWISON Kelly Anne 08/04/2005 Moorview Vets Moorview Station Road Backworth NEWCASTLE UPON TYNE NE27 0AA **Tel:** (0191) 256 6990 w 6299004

HEWITSON Claire Louise 29/05/2009 Cecil Avenue Veterinary Centre 1 Cecil Avenue Sale Cheshire M33 5BW **Tel:** (0161) 973 0375 w 6372880

HEWITT Jessica Ellen Sally 06/10/2006 Magpies Hound Road Netley Abbey Southampton Hampshire SO31 5FZ **Tel:** (023) 804 58354 w 6377126

Kerry (nee Higginson) 01/09/1995 18 Eden Drive Loxley SHEFFIELD S6 6TE **Tel:** (07904) 530383 w 6035865

HEWSON Rachel Helen (nee Wilson) 13/05/2003 High Meadows Parton Wigton Cumbria CA7 0HE **Tel:** (01946) 861636 w 6280117

HEX Alison Frances (see MOUNTY, Mrs)

Rebecca Joan 30/11/2006 11 Honeymans Close Trowbridge Wiltshire BA14 7DW **Tel:** (01225) 761258 w 6379810

HEYWOOD Katie Jane 26/10/2006 The Veterinary Surgery Higher Trenant Wadebridge Cornwall PL27 6HB **Tel:** (01208) 813258 w 6350033

HIBBERT Amanda Ellen (see GOANE, Mrs)

HIBELL Karen Mary (nee Wood) 22/02/1994 (25/04/2003) College of Animal Welfare at the Royal (Dick) Royal School of Veterinary Studies 1 Summerhall Square Edinburgh Midlothian EH9 1QH w 6068391

Tina Patricia 22/03/1979 Cornerstone Veterinary Centre Northwood Park Road Bushbury Wolverhampton WV10 8ET **Tel:** (01902) 397227 w 6052847

HICKENBOTTOM Wendy 29/08/2000 9 Dracaena Crescent Hayle Cornwall TR27 4EN **Tel:** (01736) 754621 w 6128921

HICKEY Kathryn Ann 03/09/2002 Masefield House Veterinary Surgery MASEFIELD HOUSE Wells Road Malvern WELLS Worcestershire WR14 4PA **Tel:** (01684) 576464 w 6270536

HICKMAN Jennifer Rose 29/01/2007 Baddaford Farm Ashburton NEWTON ABBOT Devon TQ13 7NF **Tel:** (01364) 642264 w 6331949

Julie Elizabeth 18/07/2009 39 Peterdale Drive WOLVERHAMPTON WV4 5NY **Tel:** 07940596759 w 6447614

HICKS Carol-Ann (nee Owen) 18/01/1996 54 Leamington Close Great Sankey Warrington WA5 3PY **Tel:** (01925) 711316 w 6037104

HICKS Janette (see HUMPHREYS, Mrs)

HICKS Janice Lesley (see HUNSLEY, Mrs)

HICKS Nicola Jayne 19/03/2007 6 Bincomb Avenue Birmingham West Midlands B26 3AD **Tel:** (0121) 742 0161 w 6374629

Toni Elizabeth 05/10/2001 7 Bridge Court Bath Road Taplow Buckinghamshire SL6 0AS w 6229550

HICKTON Nicola Jayne 09/11/2005 15 Deacon Road Kimpton ANDOVER Hampshire SP11 8PB **Tel:** (01264) 773084 w 6285419

HIDDEN Philippa Mary 14/08/1968 14 Coverts Road Claygate Esher Surrey KT10 0LN **Tel:** (01372) 467299 w 6052858

HIGERTY Janet Diane (nee Goaten) 08/08/2005 2 Fane Way Gillingham Kent ME8 9TD **Tel:** (01634) 321247 w 6300445

HIGGINS Jennifer Caroline 05/04/2005 (30/01/2007) 51 Coningsby Road Scunthorpe Lincolnshire DN17 2HL **Tel:** 07746701136 w 6322280

Joanne Clare (nee Rogers) 07/06/2005 15 Stansfield Road Benfleet Essex SS7 4NA **Tel:** (01268) 793 399 w 6267632

HIGGINS Kerry Anne (see SAMPLE, Mrs)

Kerry Joanne 21/05/2003 31 Central Road RAMSGATE Kent CT11 7SB w 6266532

Louise Frances 04/12/2007 60 Lanhydrock Road Plymouth Devon PL4 9HG **Tel:** (01752) 660313 w 6378446

Marie Elizabeth 30/01/2008 Stoke Place Farm Stoke Road Stoke Poges SLOUGH SL2 4NL **Tel:** (07763) 808533 w 6413250

HIGGINS Michelle Louise (see HOLLIDAY, Mrs)

Rachel 22/10/2004 Kits Nest Pelynt LOOE Cornwall PL13 2QH **Tel:** (01503) 272058 w 6290556

Vari Sheena 13/05/2003 67 Talbot East Kilbride GLASGOW G74 3NN **Tel:** (01355) 525264 w 6286882

HIGGINSON Kerry (see HEWITT, Mrs)

HIGGS Laura Natasha (nee Baldwin) 29/01/2008 40 Cotswold Close Minster Lovell WITNEY Oxfordshire OX29 0SX **Tel:** (01993) 706853 w 6404395

Lisa Victoria 13/11/2009 49 Old Ford End Road Queens Park BEDFORD MK40 4PG **Tel:** 07854776515 w 6464037

HIGHWOOD Alice Pamela 06/05/2009 Horns Lodge Claygate Road Marden Tonbridge Kent TN12 9PT **Tel:** (01892) 835456 w 6408872

HIGMAN Michelle Lorraine 18/03/2008 4 Culford Road Ingham Bury St. Edmunds Suffolk IP31 1NP **Tel:** (01284) 729607 w 6404516

HILEY Gemma Louise 10/08/2007 62 Wesley Way Tamworth Staffordshire B77 3JF **Tel:** (01827) 67338 w 6389336

HILL Catherine 16/02/2009 Clare Veterinary Group 75 Ballynure Road Ballyclare County Antrim BT39 9AG **Tel:** (028) 9332 2223 w 6345963

Cheryl Annette 31/03/2003 171 Manchester New Road Middleton Manchester M24 1DE **Tel:** (0161) 643 3097 w 6278093

Danielle Nicola 14/01/2008 16 Wyvern Way POULTON-LE-FYLDE Lancashire FY6 7LR **Tel:** (078715) 13019 w 6390392

Davina St Clair 29/08/2008 2 Whiteways Thornhill Wootton Bassett SWINDON SN4 7RX **Tel:** 01793731553 w 6400655

HILL Debbie (see CAMERON, Mrs)

Evelyn Laura Marian 08/11/2006 Thruxton Farm House Cholderton Salisbury Wiltshire SP4 0EF **Tel:** (01980) 629516 w 6357975

Gemma Louise 23/12/2008 The Wheel House Veterinary Centre Amersham Road Chesham Buckinghamshire HP5 1NQ **Tel:** (01494) 782001 w 6329694

Jemma Claire 04/01/2006 The Veterinary Surgery Inns Park Valley Truckle Camelford Cornwall PL32 9RX **Tel:** (01840) 212229 w 6332576

Joanna Robyn 16/08/2007 (04/02/2010) 5 School Lane Aston STEVENAGE Hertfordshire SG2 7HA **Tel:** (01438) 880506 w 6374640

Julie Ann 05/04/2005 29 Station Road Langbank PORT GLASGOW Renfrewshire PA14 6YA **Tel:** (01475) 540714 w 6318474

HILL Linda Patricia (see FARR, Mrs)

HILL Lisa Jane (see BOND, Mrs)

Louise Marie 23/02/2005 South Road Veterinary Centre Mountfields Road Taunton Somerset TA20 1AF **Tel:** (01823) 327272 w 6278346

HILL Michelle Louise (see HENNESSEY, Mrs)

Nichole Anita Teresa DipAVN(Surgical), DipAVN (Medical) 18/09/1998 38 Oak Tree Road Ampthill BEDFORD MK45 2UH **Tel:** (01525) 405744 w 6135677

Nicola Louise 21/05/2007 115 Church Road Gateshead Tyne and Wear NE9 5XE **Tel:** (0191) 482 6914 w 6377687

HILL Tracy Louise (see MCLAUGHLIN, Mrs)

Victoria Sarah 02/10/2009 3 Stevens Road Eccles AYLESFORD Kent ME20 7SH **Tel:** (01622) 716519 w 6465236

HILLABY Rachel (see GIBSON, Mrs)

HILLEN Kirsty Nicola 20/11/2009 26 Maple Drive EAST GRINSTEAD West Sussex RH19 3UR **Tel:** (01342) 325480 w 6491790

HILLMAN Rebecca Mary 06/03/2006 Flat 10, Lowes Court 135 Elm Grove Bromsgrove Worcestershire B61 0DX **Tel:** (01527) 558 755 w 6333390

HILLS Georgina Brenda (nee Dennis) 19/01/1998 The Shippon Thongsleigh Farm Pennymoor TIVERTON Devon EX16 8NA w 6117308

Lisa Jane 06/03/2008 82 Winchester Street Taunton Somerset TA1 1QE **Tel:** (01823) 274981 w 6272142

HILTON Catherine Mary 17/09/2007 162 Bradshaw Meadows BOLTON BL2 4ND w 6273143

Donna Joanna 28/09/2009 Flat 4 3 Raphael Rd Hove East Sussex BN3 5QP **Tel:** (01273) 540430 w 6441905

Nicola 03/12/2003 5 Eastwood Lane South WESTCLIFF-ON-SEA Essex SS0 9XH **Tel:** (07816) 188 961 w 6289379

Samantha Louise 31/10/2008 7 Kingswood Chase Leigh-on-Sea Essex SS9 3BB **Tel:** (01702) 711 092 w 6402756

HINCHLIFFE Faye (nee Goldsmith) 11/05/2009 2 Bernhard Gardens POLEGATE East Sussex BN26 5JN **Tel:** 01323482387 w 6250219

HIND Laura 09/02/2009 48 Fieldway Wavertree LIVERPOOL L15 7LU **Tel:** (0151) 280 2232 w 6348460

HINDMARSH Lucy 17/07/2009 Caldew Veterinary Hospital Carlisle House Townhead Road Dalston Carlisle Cumbria CA5 7JF **Tel:** (01228) 710208 w 6432929

HINDRY Lucy Charlotte Mickel 09/01/2004 Barrow Hill Veterinary 2 Fort Road HYTHE Kent CT21 6JS **Tel:** (01303) 269000 w 6293702

HINE Nicola Elizabeth (see FRITH, Mrs)

HINE Sanne Claire 29/12/2008 Belmont Church Lane Awbridge ROMSEY Hampshire SO51 0HN **Tel:** 01794341389 w 6403031

HINKS Emma Jane 14/01/2008 4 Leyburn Road Chelmsley Wood BIRMINGHAM B37 5JZ w 6390172

HINTON Hayley Marie 11/04/2005 51 Wickham Road WITHAM Essex CM8 1XE **Tel:** 01245321879 w 6288026

HIPKIN Julie (nee Ogle) 20/01/1999 PDSA PetAid Hospital Stoneygate Lane Felling Gateshead Tyne & Wear NE10 0LX **Tel:** (0191) 4382881 w 6116370

HIPPERSON Leanne (see DELOOZE, Mrs)

HIPPISLEY Helen Louisa 12/09/2008 33 Marsh Way North Cotes GRIMSBY South Humberside DN36 5XJ w 6414493

HIRD Amanda Jane 09/02/2009 32 Glenmarkie Terrace Dundee Angus DD3 8DT **Tel:** 01382523531 w 6424085

HIRD Elizabeth Ann (see KNOX, Mrs)

HIRST Emma Catherine (nee Guthrie) 07/09/1998 3 Northhill Park Laurencekirk Kincardineshire AB30 1EW **Tel:** (01561) 378355 w 6135644

HISCOCK Lisa Emily 11/03/2008 21 Springfield Road Wincanton Somerset BA9 9BL **Tel:** (01963) 32361 w 6401216

HISTED Katie Emma 17/09/2008 158 Winkworth Road Banstead Surrey SM7 2QT **Tel:** 1737371900 w 6367633

HITCHINSON Carol Anne 29/01/1996 (28/06/2006) 6 Newton Lane Darlington County Durham DL3 9EX **Tel:** (01325) 259796 w 6025234

HOAD Maxine Teresa 10/04/2003 (28/06/2006) 1 Northcote Lane Honiton Devon EX14 1NH **Tel:** (01404) 44111 w 6276377

Sarah Rhiannon 30/10/2003 Ashleigh Veterinary Centre 221 Upper Chorlton Road Manchester Greater Manchester M16 0DE **Tel:** (0161) 881 6868 w 6283208

HOAKSEY Joanna Frances (see WELSBY, Miss)

HOBAN Che (nee Beesley) 21/03/2001 The Brewhouse 4 Balterley Court Balterley CREWE CW2 5SB **Tel:** (01270) 821546 w 6214348

HOBBS Jennifer Elizabeth 14/01/2009 21 West Way Stopsley LUTON Bedfordshire LU2 8DZ w 6420059

Joanna Louise (nee Wright) 04/03/1999 (23/10/2000) Woodlands Veterinary Clinic Salisbury Avenue Warden Hill Cheltenham Gloucestershire GL51 3GA **Tel:** (01242) 255133 w 6030925

Rebecca Louise 30/10/2003 93 Babbington Lane Kimberley NOTTINGHAM NG16 2PT w 6289390

HOBDEN Kerry Michelle 10/09/2009 Fielding & Cumber Veterinary Surgeons 176-178 Chickerell Road Weymouth Dorset DT4 0QR **Tel:** (01305) 784197 w 6429266

Melissa 17/07/2008 New House Giffords Farm Battle Road Dallington Heathfield East Sussex TN21 9LH **Tel:** 01424838529 w 6386828

HOBSON Claire Louise (nee Clough) 15/10/2004 Torrington Orthopaedic Referrals IES House Mission Street Brighouse West Yorkshire HD6 1NQ **Tel:** (01484) 404770 w 6303217

HOBSON Katy Rebecca (see TAYLOR, Mrs)

HOCKEY Tracey 17/05/2005 1 De Curcis Close Nether Stowey BRIDGWATER Somerset TA5 1JX **Tel:** (01278) 734856 w 6307177

HOCKING Kathryn Anne (nee Leyshon) 01/01/1993 (18/10/2005) 20 Viking Way Winch Wen Industrial Estate Winch Wen Swansea SA1 7DA **Tel:** (01792) 310974 w 6066339

Melody Jane (nee Logsdon) 11/09/1996 Anwell Veterinary Centre 41 Brighton Road Coulsdon Surrey CR5 2BF **Tel:** (020) 8668 6151 w 6041664

HOCKLEY Emily Louise 19/04/2005 1 St. Hildas Way Flackwell Heath HIGH WYCOMBE Buckinghamshire HP10 9DE **Tel:** (01628) 520952 w 6319552

HODDER Lauren Kara 22/02/2007 The Wylie Veterinary Centre 196 Hall Lane Upminster Essex RM14 1TD **Tel:** (01708) 251200 w 6313348

HODGE Andrea Jane (see EDWARD, Mrs)

HODGES Amanda Jane (nee Bakewell) 26/02/2003 67 High Street Rocester Uttoxeter Staffordshire ST14 5JU **Tel:** (01889) 590449 w 6286211

Carly Louise 04/11/2005 Severn Veterinary Centre Berkeley House Berkeley Way Worcester Worcestershire WR4 9UP **Tel:** (01905) 756156 w 6288136

Claire 11/03/2008 2 Clare Cottages North Cheriton Templecombe Somerset BA8 0AA **Tel:** (01963) 31748 w 6410126

Deborah Jane 13/07/2007 69 Lansdowne Road Seven Kings ILFORD Essex IG3 8NF **Tel:** (077) 838 96494 w 6347481

Michelle Catherine (nee Bowerman) 04/10/2005 (26/02/2008) 12 Bradfield Avenue BUCKINGHAM Buckinghamshire MK18 1PR w 6319992

HODGINS Louise 11/03/2005 The Coach House Veterinary Clinic Wroslyn Road Freeland Witney Oxfordshire OX29 8AQ **Tel:** (01993) 880551 w 6327648

HODGKISS Kerry Ann Christina 15/12/2009 421 Holcombe Road Helmshore Rossendale Lancashire BB4 4NF **Tel:** 07894240524 w 6451541

HODGSON Allison (nee Robbins) 29/08/1992 (14/06/1999) 4 Coral Way REDCAR Cleveland TS10 2JP w 6005750

Carly Jane 11/03/2008 Calverley New Mill Road HOLMFIRTH HD9 7SG **Tel:** (01484) 680666 w 6342608

HODGSON Rebecca Louise (see GAMBLE, Miss)

Rebecca Marie 26/10/2009 1 Bence Lane Darton Barnsley Yorkshire S75 5NX **Tel:** (01226) 382108 w 6489722

Stephanie (nee Marshall) 05/01/2001 Court Colman Pen-y-fai BRIDGEND Mid Glamorgan CF31 4NG **Tel:** (01656) 725219 w 6204415

Verity DipAVN(Surgical) 13/04/2004 30 Brookvale Wilby Wellingborough Northamptonshire NN8 2UJ **Tel:** (01933) 227276 w 6291205

HODSON Rebecca Teresa 01/02/1994 (17/04/2003) 2 Great Eppleton Farm Cottages Hetton-le-Hole HOUGHTON LE SPRING Tyne and Wear DH5 9NL **Tel:** (0191) 5260378 w 6067864

HOEKSTRA Anna Jessica Aaltje 28/11/2008 8 Redesdale Place MORETON-IN-MARSH Gloucestershire GL56 0EF **Tel:** 07854449924 w 6421764

HOGAN Daniel James 10/01/2007 37 Cedar Court Rye Street BISHOP'S STORTFORD Hertfordshire CM23 2HB m 6375289

HOGBEN Caroline 22/12/2004 39 Cambria Avenue Rochester Kent ME1 3HZ **Tel:** (07909) 995209 w 6287091

Gemma Louise 15/11/2005 Westlands Carvans Park Herne Common Herne Bay Kent CT6 7LE **Tel:** (01227) 283859 w 6322489

HOGGETT Richard Andrew 04/06/2009 220 Kirkley Run Lowestoft Suffolk NR33 0NW **Tel:** 07891102297 m 6408861

HOLBROOK Carolyn Joanne (nee Moore) 12/09/2008 20 Huntsmoor Road TADLEY Hampshire RG26 4DQ w 6387224

HOLBY Jayne Claire (nee Jarman) 31/12/2003 9 Rivers Road Teynham Nr Sittingbourne Kent ME9 9TD **Tel:** (01795) 521024 w 6296265

HOLDEN Kirsty Louise 04/01/2006 Summerhill Veterinary Centre 14 Queens Road Fakenham Norfolk NR21 8DB **Tel:** (01328) 855814 w 6328957

Sarah Amy (nee Barber) 27/10/2008 39 Pinewood Park Farnborough Hampshire GU14 9LB **Tel:** (01252) 671823 w 6417221

Tracey Christine 07/12/2005 39 Oxlip Road WITHAM Essex CM8 2XY w 6287806

HOLDER Abigail Ruth DipAVN(Surgical) (nee Jones) 07/08/1992 Brunswick Place Veterinary Clinic Brunswick Place Cranbourne Lane Basingstoke Hampshire RG21 3NN **Tel:** (01256) 473371 w 6007882

Hazel Lisa 05/07/2006 (25/02/2009) 5 Ashurst Close Horsham West Sussex RH12 4JN **Tel:** (01403) 268 858 w 6345600

Karen 22/10/2004 1 Kings Lane Norton EVESHAM Worcestershire WR11 4TJ **Tel:** (01386) 870752 w 6304779

HOLDING Karen Margaret Lorraine 09/09/1998 12 Osmere Close Whitchurch Shropshire SY13 1PZ **Tel:** (01948) 663370 w 6133691

Zoe 14/07/2008 Tideswell Station Road East Winch KING'S LYNN Norfolk PE32 1NR **Tel:** (07801) 815 608 w 6401051

HOLDSWORTH Tina (nee Holdsworth, formerly Philpott) 16/09/2004 42 Cromwell Road Hayes Middlesex UB3 2PR **Tel:** (07525) 857484 w 6293306

HOLE Cheryl Dawn (nee Stanton) 31/10/2003 Teignview Veterinary Group Hospital Hill Dawlish Devon EX7 9NS **Tel:** (01626) 862020 w 6280139

Sarah Elizabeth 31/01/1994 Oban Veterinary Surgeons 14 Tweeddale Street Oban Argyll PA34 5DD **Tel:** (01631) 562876 w 6067547

HOLGATE Albert Charles Peter 27/02/2007 411 Eccles New Road Salford M5 5NN **Tel:** (0300) 123 0711 m 6350726

HOLIDAY Claire Jayne 07/02/2006 2 Plover Drive Milford on Sea Lymington Hampshire SO41 0XF **Tel:** (01590) 645885 w 6339275

HOLLAND Claire Louise 10/04/2008 15 Danywern Drive Winnersh Wokingham Berkshire RG41 5NS **Tel:** 01189894321 w 6355401

Deborah 20/11/1981 28 Westfield Grove YEOVIL Somerset BA21 3DL **Tel:** (01935) 474653 w 6053057

Deborah Jane 07/02/2000 (15/11/2004) Veterinary Hospital Fyfield Barrow Walnut Tree Local Centre Milton Keynes Buckinghamshire MK7 7AN **Tel:** (01908) 397777 w 6190291

Donna May 08/06/2006 46 Cranesbill Drive Worcester Worcestershire WR5 3HX **Tel:** (01905) 353 736 w 6323633

Lucy Elizabeth 01/10/2008 30 Pound Lane Bowers Gifford BASILDON Essex SS13 2HF **Tel:** 01268590652 w 6316857

Lucy Georgina 28/02/2005 Whinhayes Forest Lane Hightown Hill RINGWOOD Hampshire BH24 3HF **Tel:** (01425) 473270 w 6318958

Rebecca (nee McCormick) 14/11/2000 22 Downshire Park North BELFAST BT6 9JS w 6134618

Zowie Joe 11/11/2004 27 Windmill Walk Sutton ELY Cambridgeshire CB6 2NH **Tel:** (01353) 777543 w 6321510

HOLLEY Imogen Samantha 25/02/2003 Elms Farmhouse Grove Road Grove Wantage Oxfordshire OX12 7PD **Tel:** (01235) 773341 w 6280942

HOLLIDAY Faye Louise 30/11/2006 44 Summerhill Road Seven Sisters LONDON N15 4HD w 6376455

Michelle Louise (nee Higgins) 01/09/2000 School Bungalow Coulson Way Burnham SLOUGH SL1 7NP **Tel:** (01753) 520353 w 6202611

Samantha Joanne (nee Eglin) 28/04/2006 39 Valley Drive CARLISLE Cumbria CA1 3TB w 6343708

Sarah Ann 09/02/2009 8 Lawrence Road Hampton Middlesex TW12 2RJ **Tel:** 02087831034 w 6438561

HOLLINGSWORTH Helen (formerly Gillard) 12/11/1997 The Workshop Little Curtis Knowle Halwell Totnes Devon TQ9 7JY w 6117498

HOLLINGWORTH Emma Louise 08/01/2008 Llwyndewi Rhydowen Llandysul Dyfed SA44 4QF **Tel:** (01545) 590 424 w 6409411

HOLLIS Beverley Clare (see HAWKINS, Mrs)

HOLLIS Caroline Mary DipAVN(Surgical) (nee Hollis, formerly Harlow) 10/01/1990 The Laurels Veterinary Centre 1 Homefield Road Bromley Kent BR1 3AW **Tel:** (020) 8460 2033 w 6053104

HOLLOWAY Joanne (see RICE, Mrs)

HOLLOWAY Leanne Emma (see ROBESON, Mrs)

HOLLOWAY Neil Richard 28/01/2010 32 Beresford Road DORKING Surrey RH4 2DF **Tel:** 07729864770 m 6424041

Shan 08/01/2008 7 Fenton Farm Crundale HAVERFORDWEST Dyfed SA62 4PY **Tel:** (07816) 454495 w 6406815

HOLLY Jenna Kay 18/10/2006 615 Wells Road Whitchurch Bristol BS14 9BE **Tel:** (01275) 832410 w 6290765

HOLLYOAK Ursula DipAVN(Surgical) 09/08/1993 34 Barkers Butts Lane Coventry West Midlands CV6 1DT **Tel:** (024) 76590298 w 6030390

HOLMAN Lauren Danielle 10/06/2009 17 Leycroft Way Harpenden Hertfordshire AL5 1JW **Tel:** 01582622557 w 6407816

Sian (nee Godfrey) 05/07/2006 9 Larch Close BRIDGWATER Somerset TA6 4UY w 6285595

HOLMES Amanda Louise 26/06/2008 27 Mill Road BURGESS HILL West Sussex RH15 8DN **Tel:** (01444) 239271 w 6403878

Caroline Elizabeth (nee Tomlinson) 25/02/2003 Veterinary Health Centre Daisy Street Blackburn BB1 5EW **Tel:** (01254) 53622 w 6281624

HOLMES Emma (see CARTER-WALLER, Mrs)

HOLMES Justine Amy 06/05/2009 13 Gassons Road Snodland Kent ME6 5RW **Tel:** 01634242743 w 6435338

Karina Dawn 08/08/2005 Warren House Veterinary Surgery Anchor Road Rochester Kent ME1 2PR **Tel:** (01634) 409988 w 6316835

Michelle (nee Wootten) 10/01/1986 Aardvark Vets 43 Chester Road Whitby Ellesmere Port Merseyside CH65 9BE **Tel:** (0151) 3559880 w 6053137

Paula DipAVN(Surgical) 21/07/2004 48a Sunnymead Werrington PETERBOROUGH PE4 5BY **Tel:** (01733) 578797 w 6303283

HOLMES Rachel Louise (see RUSSELL, Mrs)

HOLMES Sarah Louise 19/01/1996 Alnorthumbria Veterinary Practice Ltd Wagonway Road Alnwick Northumberland NE66 1QQ **Tel:** (01665) 510999 w 6036541

HOLROYD Susan Mary 16/01/1997 Abbeydale Veterinary Centre 91 Preston New Road Blackburn BB2 6AY **Tel:** (01254) 681811 w 6098316

HOLT Karen Jane 21/01/2008 13 Albany Road Worcester Worcestershire WR3 8EY **Tel:** (01905) 20953 w 6388984

Marie Louise 01/09/2009 Arnwood Veterinary Clinics Ltd The Veterinary Clinic Winchester Street Sherwood Nottingham NG5 4AJ **Tel:** (0115) 962 1010 w 6490679

Sian 02/06/2004 337 Carterhatch Ln Enfield Middlesex EN1 4AW **Tel:** (020) 8366 8155 w 6277444

Susan Louise 24/08/1994 29 Hopgood Close Devizes Wiltshire SN10 2UG **Tel:** (01380) 720042 w 603169X

HOLTAWAY Rebecca Elizabeth 27/04/2009 9 Bockhill Road BURY ST. EDMUNDS Suffolk IP33 3XD **Tel:** 07780744473 w 6434854

HOMER Amy Charlotte 05/06/2008 Langford Veterinary Services Ltd Langford House Bristol North Somerset BS40 5DU **Tel:** (01934) 852422 w 6403174

Karen Michelle 07/08/1990 134 Shrivenham Road SWINDON SN1 2NT w 6053170

Kelly Anne 18/09/2007 The Liphook Equine Hospital Forest Mere Liphook Hampshire GU30 7JG **Tel:** (01428) 723594 w 6363255

HONEY Karen Ann (see DECRUZ, Mrs)

HONEYWILL Samantha (see SIVYER, Ms)

HONOUR Kate (see ANDREWS, Mrs)

HONOUR Michelle (see SCOLLICK, Mrs)

HOOLE Charlotte Jane 17/07/2008 19 The Homelands Ball Lane Coven Heath WOLVERHAMPTON WV10 7EZ **Tel:** 07792516998 w 6350528

HOOPER Kelly Marie 10/10/2005 5 Kinnersley Close REDDITCH Worcestershire B98 0LB w 6330310

Rebecca Janine 21/03/2007 Ardlair High Street Conon Bridge Dingwall Ross-Shire IV7 8AZ **Tel:** (01349) 861203 w 6317198

HOPCROFT Marion Clare 19/01/1998 (31/01/2002) Sparsholt College Sparsholt WINCHESTER Hampshire SO21 2NF **Tel:** (01270) 613294 w 6022040

HOPE Lesley Ann 27/05/2008 Clitheroe Farm Kilham Road DRIFFIELD North Humberside YO25 4BA **Tel:** (01377) 259383 w 6342619

HOPE Sarah Louise (see GRAVETT, Mrs)

HOPKIN Tammy Marie (see JARVIS, Mrs)

HOPKINS Amy Rhonwen (see MARTIN, Mrs)

HOPKINS Angela Kay 22/09/2004 87 Watford Road Cotteridge Birmingham B30 1NP **Tel:** (0121) 459 4333 w 6259954

HOPKINS Dawn Elizabeth (see LYDEN, Mrs)

Emma Elizabeth 07/12/2005 27 St. Johns Road CHRISTCHURCH Dorset BH23 1LX **Tel:** (01202) 471534 w 6318969

Joanne Shirley 06/04/2009 Hockley Cottage Main Road Broughton Banbury Oxfordshire OX15 5EB **Tel:** (01295) 276628 w 6383880

Laura Christine 21/04/2008 Saiyan Penrose Lowlands Road Vale GUERNSEY GY3 5SZ w 6357766

Laura Ellen 02/06/2008 3 Wash Cottages Easthorpe COLCHESTER Essex CO5 9HA **Tel:** (01206) 210267 w 6401876

Nicola (nee Davies, formerly Davies) 18/01/1999 (24/10/2000) Heol DDU Cottage Cefneithin LLANELLI Dyfed SA14 7ET **Tel:** (01639) 842170 w 6138383

Sian Elizabeth DipAVN(Surgical) (nee James) 16/08/1982 5 Clos Rhiannon Thornhill Cardiff CF14 9HQ **Tel:** (029) 20619581 w 6053818

Zoe Elizabeth 19/03/2007 27 Tomlinson Road Ashton-on-Ribble PRESTON Lancashire PR2 2JY w 6384848

HOPKINSON Jane Matilda Margaret (see LAMONT, Mrs)

HOPLEY Lorraine Margaret DipAVN(Surgical) 30/01/1997 Nettlegate Barn Colliers Lane Aston by Budworth Northwich Cheshire CW9 6NF w 6042103

Maxine 04/08/1981 (01/03/2006) Hawthorn Cottage Penstraze Chacewater Truro Cornwall TR4 8PH **Tel:** (01872) 561318 w 6053239

HOPPER Gail (nee Errington) 06/12/2004 25 Errington Drive Tanfield Lea STANLEY County Durham DH9 9PD w 6307375

HORDER Madelaine Rose 12/09/2008 Eastfield Veterinary Clinic Ltd Station Road North Thoresby

GRIMSBY Lincolnshire DN36 5QU **Tel:** (01472) 840209 w 6435371

HORE-RUTHVEN Angela Dron 31/10/2006 (03/06/2009) Charter Veterinary Hospital Charter Court Roundswell Business Park Barnstaple Devon EX31 3FG **Tel:** (01271) 371115 w 6367644

HORLER Caroline Louise 25/02/2004 35 Alexander Street London W2 5NU **Tel:** (07717) 434 014 w 6202479

HORNE Deborah Mary 28/07/1986 (08/05/2006) 14 Craig Brown Avenue SELKIRK TD7 4NB w 6053272

HORNE Rosalind Wendy (see HARRIS, Mrs)

HORNER Alexis (nee Bruce) 28/08/1998 Waltham Centre for Pet Nutrition Freeby Lane Waltham on the Wolds MELTON MOWBRAY Leicestershire LE14 4RT **Tel:** 07739971203 w 6133760

HORNSBY Faye (nee Hardy) 16/05/2006 Ridgeway Veterinary Centre 47 The Ridgeway Flitwick MK45 1DJ **Tel:** (01525) 714892 w 6288279

HORNSBY Haley Karen (see COLLINS, Mrs)

Natasha Jayne (nee Cilia) 21/11/2005 18 Carman Walk Crawley West Sussex RH11 9LD **Tel:** (01293) 560905 w 6351199

HORNSEY Amy Emily (nee Wells) 28/09/2005 27 Lowry Court Artists Way Andover Hampshire SP10 3SX **Tel:** (01264) 323395 w 6301204

HORSCRAFT Helen Michaela (see QUARTERMAINE, Mrs)

HORSLEY Charlotte Joanne (nee Dibb) 14/01/1999 9 Mostyn Avenue Craig-y-don Llandudno Conwy LL30 1YS **Tel:** (01492) 877049 w 6042839

HORSPOOL Teresa Elizabeth (nee Thomas) 19/01/1983 Sundean Veterinary Clinic 11 High Street LYDNEY Gloucestershire GL15 5DP **Tel:** (01594) 840404 w 6075977

HORSWELL Victoria Mary (see VANNER, Mrs)

HORTON Karina Michelle (nee Land) 03/09/2002 Broad Lane Vets Ltd 255 Broad Lane Coventry West Midlands CV5 7AQ **Tel:** (024) 7646 4789 w 6264849

Lesley Joanne 03/09/1999 Rase View Church Street Market Rasen Lincolnshire LN8 3ET w 6185748

Lisa Marie 03/09/1998 48 Glanville Gardens Bristol Avon BS15 9WU **Tel:** (01179) 618437 w 6128353

HORWILL Claire Louise 06/11/2008 Clifton Veterinary Surgery Anstey Lane Alton Hampshire GU34 2RH **Tel:** (01420) 82163 w 6425702

HOSIE Clare Margaret (see SUTTON, Mrs)

HOSKING Lynn (see KERRIGAN, Miss)

HOSKINS Claire Elizabeth 01/10/1982 (03/11/2008) 15 Lysander Court Warkworth MORPETH Northumberland NE65 0UY **Tel:** (01665) 714253 w 605332X

Lisa Joan 23/02/2005 118 Clun Road Wick LITTLEHAMPTON West Sussex BN17 7ER w 6317242

HOTHERSALL Donna Jayne 30/07/2004 15 Russell Street SKIPTON North Yorkshire BD23 2DX w 6289786

HOTHI-ASHBERRY Angela Susan (nee Moody) 03/03/1997 (22/10/2003) 42 Paterson Place Shepshed Loughborough Leicestershire LE12 9RX **Tel:** (01509) 503558 w 6098520

HOTSTON MOORE Paula Jane 27/07/1988 32 Beech Road Shipham Winscombe Somerset BS25 1SB **Tel:** (01934) 844371 w 6053330

HOUGHTON Janine Fay (nee Skingle) 06/04/1995 St Anne's Veterinary Group 6 St Anne's Road Eastbourne East Sussex BN21 2DJ **Tel:** (01323) 640011 w 6095712

HOUGHTON-KENNEDY Nicola Joanne (see BREW, Mrs)

HOULDSWORTH Diane Susan 14/03/2006 37 Coppice Avenue Norwich Norfolk NR6 5RD **Tel:** (01603) 460 520 w 6342091

HOULIHAN Katy 13/05/2003 MacQueen Veterinary Surgery 1 Hopton Park London Road Devizes Wiltshire SN10 2EY **Tel:** (01380) 728505 w 6272439

HOUSEMAN Bethan Lorraine 30/08/2006 17 Ffordd Rhiannon LLANFAIRPWLLGWYNGYLL Gwynedd LL61 5QB w 6261241

HOUSTON Joanne Victoria 04/06/2003 (11/05/2005) 11 Russell Place Oare FAVERSHAM Kent ME13 0QF w 6205658

HOWARD Christopher 30/11/2006 273 Bakers Ground Stoke Gifford Bristol Avon BS34 8GE **Tel:** (07891) 621615 m 6328440

Helen Louise 03/12/2003 Alfreton Park Veterinary Hospital 216 King Street Alfreton Derbyshire DE55 7DF **Tel:** (01773) 832218 w 6293174

Jessica (nee Perry) 29/06/2007 157 Torquay Crescent STEVENAGE Hertfordshire SG1 2RL w 6371692

Katharyn Sarah 07/01/2010 213 Croydon Road Beckenham Kent BR3 3QH w 6489766

Katherine Sarah 26/08/2003 (27/04/2005) 1-5 Hugh Street London SW1V 1QQ **Tel:** (020) 7932 2370 w 6204228

HOWARD Kirsty Louise (see COWARD, Mrs)

Shauna 07/10/2009 31 Society Road South Queensferry Edinburgh EH30 9XP **Tel:** (0131) 331 1230 w 6574136

HOWARD Zoe Louise (see SUMMERS, Mrs)

HOWARTH Kathryn Susan 19/01/2001 6 Camm Street BRIGHOUSE West Yorkshire HD6 1UE w 6210784

Susan Dianne DipAVN(Surgical), DipAVN(Medical) (nee Edwards) 03/09/1997 The Old Joinery Workshop 22 Hollinwood Road Disley STOCKPORT Cheshire SK12 2EB **Tel:** 01663764000 w 6115898

Victoria Helen 22/06/2009 55 Barley Mill Crescent Consett County Durham DH8 8JX **Tel:** (01207) 507402 w 6351287

HOWBRIDGE Joanne 07/02/2007 26 Southfield Park Market Weighton YORK YO43 3QL w 6373727

HOWE Amy 21/05/2009 53 Heron Way Wallington Surrey SM6 9DX w 6452355

Deborah Mary 15/07/2005 115 Brook Gardens EMSWORTH Hampshire PO10 7LB **Tel:** (01243) 371974 w 6326922

Lisa Jayne (nee Fitz-Gerald) 15/04/2004 Ashworth Veterinary Group 60 Bridge Road Cove

Farnborough Hampshire GU14 0HP **Tel:** (01252) 542121 w 6286354

HOWE Sally-Ann (see ROBERTS, Mrs)

HOWELL Christina Jane 08/02/2008 39 Kerrfield Estate Northampton Northamptonshire NN5 6JY **Tel:** 07725589673 w 6383891

HOWELL Helen Mary (see CROFTS, Mrs)

Joy Sarah Helen DipAVN(Surgical) 01/08/1985 35 Ash Court Victoria Gardens NEWBURY Berkshire RG14 1EY **Tel:** (01635) 580292 w 6053385

Shelley Claire (nee Archer) 27/08/2008 2 Old Well Walk SALE Cheshire M33 4NY **Tel:** (0161) 9764495 w 6395969

HOWES Susan Emma 06/10/2006 4 Hiller Close BROADSTAIRS Kent CT10 1JG **Tel:** (01843) 869265 w 6334237

HOWLAND Caroline Ray 27/01/2009 59 Swepstone Close Lower Earley READING RG6 3EY **Tel:** 01189667488 w 6383198

HOWLETT Katherine Barbara Mary 08/01/2008 The Mewes Veterinary Clinic 4 Haywards Road Haywards Heath West Sussex RH16 4HT **Tel:** (01444) 456886 w 6391932

HOWSE Amy Louise Mary 23/01/2008 1 Winston Avenue Ipswich Suffolk IP4 3LS **Tel:** 01473712815 w 6400710

HOWSON Karen Louisa (see BELCHER, Mrs)

HOWTON Sarah Christine 08/02/2008 Havana House 33 Churchill Court Wilton Salisbury Wilts SP2 0HL **Tel:** (07917) 897649 w 6409576

HOY Andrea 12/01/1987 (02/11/2001) 70 Brinkley Lane Highwoods COLCHESTER Essex CO4 9XE **Tel:** (01206) 842608 w 605340X

Caroline Elizabeth 26/02/1988 (19/07/1999) 158 St. Albans Road Sandridge ST. ALBANS Hertfordshire AL4 9LP w 6053410

HOY Shona (see PURDY, Mrs)

HOYLE Megan Pearl 27/11/2008 98 Ashcroft Road IPSWICH Suffolk IP1 6AD **Tel:** (07538) 676727 w 6400974

HUBBARD Imogen Naomi 05/10/2000 27 Milborough Crescent London SE12 0RR **Tel:** (0208) 851 4773 w 6142800

HUBBLE Laura Jane (see HUBBLE EDWARDS, Mrs)

HUBBLE EDWARDS Laura Jane (nee Hubble) 30/09/1998 (21/01/2009) 52 Allbrook Hill EASTLEIGH Hampshire SO50 4LY **Tel:** (023) 806 15080 w 6137222

HUBBLEDAY Sarah Jane (see ELLIOT, Mrs)

HUBBOCKS Fiona Amy 23/03/2007 86 St. Johns Grove HARROGATE North Yorkshire HG1 3AH **Tel:** (01423) 526169 w 6301666

HUCKER Clair Anita 30/06/2003 Heathfield Hursley Hill BRISTOL BS14 0QZ **Tel:** (01275) 832594 w 6263716

HUDD Alison Mary (nee Mascall) 26/08/1970 Sloe Gin Cottage Fishwater Bourton Devizes Wiltshire SN10 2LJ w 6053443

HUDDLESTON Hayley Marie 12/07/2004 Coco Markus House Nelson street Grimsby North East Lincolnshire DN32 7SH **Tel:** (01472) 343278 w 6284374

Hazel Ann 07/12/2006 (09/02/2009) 69 Woodrow Gardens Saintfield BALLYNAHINCH County Down BT24 7WG w 6326394

HUDDLESTON Sarah Catherine (see BALDOCK, Mrs)

HUDSON Beverley May (see LEE, Mrs)

HUDSON Emma Louise 15/04/2008 7 Harvey Street Carlisle Cumbria CA2 7NX **Tel:** ((01228)) 528 288 w 6412348

Joanne Louise 01/04/2008 47 Westfield Road DUNSTABLE Bedfordshire LU6 1DN **Tel:** (077730) 25545 w 6402184

Katie 22/09/2006 50 Chapel Street Bolton-upon-Dearne ROTHERHAM South Yorkshire S63 8HY **Tel:** (01709) 898 580 w 6376477

Lucy Aileen 25/06/2004 86 Rivington Crescent Kingstanding Birmingham West Midlands B44 0PL w 6284517

Nancy Ruth 30/08/2006 Eastgate Veterinary Centre 133 Eastgate Pickering North Yorkshire YO18 7DW **Tel:** (01751) 472204 w 6347118

Natalie Diane 19/04/2005 7 The Hedges Wanborough Swindon Wiltshire SN4 0BJ **Tel:** (01793) 790836 w 6299026

Shelly Marie 30/07/2004 Church Walk Veterinary Centre Ltd St Mary's Place Church Walk Ulverston Cumbria LA12 7EN **Tel:** (01229) 583675 w 6296243

Suzanne Elizabeth 06/02/2002 (31/07/2006) 16 James Avenue BLACKPOOL Lancashire FY4 4LB w 6243718

HUDSPETH Vikkie Lesley 03/02/2005 22 Burghley Avenue BOREHAMWOOD Hertfordshire WD6 2JF **Tel:** (07970) 699240 w 6318001

HUFFINLEY Emma Jane 27/08/2004 (29/09/2008) 22 Wood Grove LEEDS LS12 5NN **Tel:** (0113) 252 5818 w 6279127

HUGGONSON Gemma 31/03/2009 4 Livingstone Road Teignmouth Devon TQ14 8NL **Tel:** (01626) 774718 w 6363266

HUGHES Annaliese Helen (see MAGEE, Mrs)

HUGHES Corinna Jessica 01/05/2008 17 Pound Street Carshalton Surrey SM5 3PG **Tel:** (0208) 7734918 w 6354037

Emma Jane 21/11/2007 Oakhurst Rectory Park Boxford SUDBURY Suffolk CO10 5JS **Tel:** (01787) 210 706 w 6332290

Gemma Candice 08/01/2008 17 Nash Lane Belbroughton STOURBRIDGE West Midlands DY9 9SW w 6392130

Hannah Jane 19/03/2007 (01/07/2009) Elizabeth Street Veterinary Clinic 55 Elizabeth Street London SW1W 9PP **Tel:** (020) 7730 9102 w 6373848

Helen DipAVN(Surgical) 14/12/2000 12 Tintern Crescent NORTH SHIELDS NE29 8PG **Tel:** (0191) 2894556 w 6205548

HUGHES Helen Pritchard (see PRENTICE, Mrs)

HUGHES Helen Rachael (see JESSHOPE, Mrs)

Jennifer Ruth 26/03/2002 74 Manor Road Cudworth Barnsley South Yorkshire S72 8DF **Tel:** (01226) 716164 w 6267918

Jenny Lynn 02/11/2004 51 Birmingham Road Whitacre Heath Coleshill BIRMINGHAM B46 2ET w 6287894

HUGHES Joanne (see LEWIS, Mrs)

Louise Jane 25/06/2004 (28/04/2009) 11 Purbeck Terrace Road SWANAGE Dorset BH19 2DE **Tel:** (01929) 426239 w 6284528

Rachael Louise 27/04/2006 68 Mallard Crescent Iwade Sittingbourne Kent ME9 8TJ **Tel:** (01795) 427910 w 6343235

Rachel 03/05/2005 28 Green Lane Mossley Hill Liverpool L18 6HB **Tel:** (0151) 724 2664 w 6328176

Rosemary Ann (nee Davies) 12/05/2004 6 Rhodfa Wen Llysfaen Colwyn Bay Conwy LL29 8LE **Tel:** (01492) 516998 w 6278654

HULLOCK Linda Anne 18/01/2002 (01/03/2007) Flat 22 Arbour House Arbour Square LONDON E1 0PP w 6266620

HULME Caroline Sarah 29/09/2004 14 Firethorn Drive Godley HYDE Cheshire SK14 3SN **Tel:** (07753) 761714 w 6305153

HULME Karen Louise (see FISH, Mrs)

HULSE Janet 03/09/1996 2 Thanet Walk Rowhedge Colchester Essex CO5 7EW **Tel:** (01206) 729372 w 6099535

HULSON Gemma (see ADDISON, Mrs)

HUMBLE Joanne Elizabeth 14/09/2005 56 Cornwall Crescent Rothwell Leeds West Yorkshire LS26 0RA **Tel:** (07739) 318246 w 6347129

HUME Susanna Nicola 31/10/2006 Queen Mother Hospital for Small Animals Hawkshead Lane North Mymms Hatfield Hertfordshire AL9 7TA **Tel:** (01707) 666366 w 6367655

HUMPHERSTON Laura Michelle 11/07/2007 27 Boraston Drive Burford Tenbury Wells Worcestershire WR15 8AG **Tel:** (01584) 811 655 w 6350638

HUMPHREYS Elizah Charlotte 04/06/2009 55 Linskill Terrace NORTH SHIELDS Tyne and Wear NE30 2EW **Tel:** (0191) 2586092 w 6415318

Janette (nee Hicks, nee Humphries) 28/06/1993 (26/11/2009) 9 Haydon Hill Close Charminster DORCHESTER Dorset DT2 9WP **Tel:** (01305) 263227 w 6066645

Louise Catherine (nee Spencer) 29/08/1996 River Cottage Old Hillcliff Lane Hillcliff Lane Turnditch BELPER Derbyshire DE56 2EA w 6098735

Nicola Jane 22/09/2004 Bridgefield Veterinary Surgery Central Carpark Wem Shropshire SY4 5AA **Tel:** (01939) 232291 w 6264046

HUMPHRIES Janette (see HUMPHREYS, Mrs)

HUMPHRIES Zoe Anna 15/12/2004 Castle Veterinary Surgeons Montalbo Road Barnard Castle County Durham DL12 8ED **Tel:** (01833) 695695 w 6267434

HUMPHRYS Gemma 07/12/2005 The Dell Pen y Fron Road Pantymwyn Mold Clwyd CH7 5EF **Tel:** 07984084315 w 6344203

HUNSLEY Janice Lesley (nee Hicks) 12/09/1972 The Blue Cross Animal Hospital Nelson Street Grimsby South Humberside DN32 7SH **Tel:** (01472) 343278 w 6053534

HUNT Carrianne Elizabeth 10/02/2004 59 Falcon Road Anstey Leicester Leicestershire LE7 7FY **Tel:** (0116) 235 1006 w 6283494

Clare Elizabeth 16/08/2007 St. David Veterinary Centre Pentwyn Shopping Precinct Pentwyn Drive Cardiff South Glamorgan CF23 7EY **Tel:** (029) 2073 3111 w 6349153

HUNT Emma Elizabeth (see MASLEY, Mrs)

Georgina Anne 25/08/1998 21 St. George Drive Hednesford CANNOCK Staffordshire WS12 0FB **Tel:** (01543) 682499 w 6037002

Georgina Elizabeth (nee Baker) 24/08/1999 29 Trysull Gardens WOLVERHAMPTON WV3 7LD **Tel:** (07702) 068325 w 6149001

Ingrid Sarah 29/08/2008 25A Park Road Mount Pleasant Exeter Devon EX1 2HS **Tel:** (01392) 216136 w 6439166

Janette Rosemary 21/01/1999 7/8 Sketty Avenue Sketty Swansea SA2 0TE **Tel:** (01792) 205515 w 6138689

Jodine 17/11/2000 New Era Veterinary Hospital Flat 3, Victoria Road St Saviour JERSEY JE2 7QG **Tel:** (01777) 710576 w 6204371

Kerry Lynn 12/12/2005 Shire Carr Farm Kirkby Lane Pinxton NOTTINGHAM NG16 6JA **Tel:** (07887) 546721 w 6348493

Kirsty 15/06/2009 19 Priestly Close STOWMARKET Suffolk IP14 1UJ w 6452146

Lisa Marie 13/05/2008 51 Broadoak Road Benchill Wythenshaw Manchester Lancashire M22 9NE **Tel:** (0161) 998 7382 w 6407167

Lucy Marie 05/04/2005 Copse View Springfield Gardens NEW MILTON Hampshire BH25 5RG **Tel:** (01425) 620793 w 6331179

Rachel Elizabeth 28/08/1996 85 Ansley common Nuneaton Warwickshire CV10 0PP w 603783X

Sarah Jane 07/04/2006 5 Woodland View CALDICOT Gwent NP26 4EE w 6320102

HUNT Susan June (see GREGSON, Mrs)

Suzanne Claire 13/04/2004 13 Chapel Ln Letty Green Hertfordshire SG14 2PA **Tel:** (01707) 261236 w 6279281

HUNT LACEY Christina Irene (see NICHOLS, Mrs)

HUNTER Amanda Jane 15/04/2008 8 Coniston Road COULSDON Surrey CR5 3BS **Tel:** (0208) 6607335 w 6409015

Jill 13/07/2004 Meadow Lane Veterinary Centre 9 Meadow Lane Loughborough Leicestershire LE11 1JU **Tel:** (01509) 212437 w 6283340

Karen Jane (formerly Coleman) 12/01/1987 Bowbridge Surgery Bowbridge Stroud Gloucestershire GL5 2LA **Tel:** (01453) 762350 w 6047906

Katie Louise 18/11/2009 53-55 Maidstone Road Footscray SIDCUP Kent DA14 5HB **Tel:** (020) 8300 8111 w 6465995

Kaye Louise 04/12/2003 Westside Veterinary Surgery West Side Bixter SHETLAND ZE2 9NA **Tel:** (01595) 810456 w 6275453

HUNTER Nicola Louise (see EDWARDS, Mrs)

HUNTING Katie Emma 07/06/2005 8 Somerset Gardens Bognor Regis West Sussex PO21 2AA **Tel:** 01243822796 w 6286365

HUNTLEY Angela Louise (see SHEPPARD, Mrs)

HURLEY Emma Charlotte 15/04/2004 12a The Precinct Westmeads Aldwick BOGNOR REGIS West Sussex PO21 5SB w 6293548

Julia Anne 05/04/2005 (05/03/2009) 25 Thornton Close ALRESFORD Hampshire SO24 9FE **Tel:** (01962) 732289 w 6328968

HURLOCK Georgia Beth 28/09/1999 (22/12/2003) Queen Mother Hospital for Small Animals Hawkshead Lane North Mymms Hatfield Hertfordshire AL9 7TA **Tel:** (01707) 666366 w 6185341

HURREN Kelly Ann 12/10/1999 (21/06/2005) 113 Station Road North Chingford London E4 7BU **Tel:** (020) 8529 4004 w 6185770

HURST Erica Jane 14/11/2008 Hillcrest Upton Cross LISKEARD Cornwall PL14 5BE **Tel:** (01579) 362201 w 6429915

Julie 12/12/1996 (20/09/2002) 2 Church Hill View Castlewellan Co Down BT31 9HZ **Tel:** (028) 437 26209 w 6098338

HUSSEY Rebecca Jane 31/12/2003 81 Arundel Road Wordsley West Midlands DY8 5EJ **Tel:** (01384) 838309 w 6271273

HUTCHENS Jessica Jon 29/01/2009 69 Copperfields Lydd ROMNEY MARSH Kent TN29 9UU **Tel:** (077567) 26599 w 6429233

HUTCHINGS Jennifer Ellen 05/03/2002 (15/11/2007) Davies Veterinary Specialists Manor Farm Business Park Higham Gobion Hertfordshire SG5 3HR **Tel:** (01582) 883950 w 6204525

Jessica (nee Vant) 14/01/2008 32 Willow Farm Way Broomfield HERNE BAY Kent CT6 7QH **Tel:** 07834983687 w 6402679

Yvette Helen (nee Todd) 10/02/2004 The Scott Veterinary Clinic 405 Goldington Road Bedford Bedfordshire MK41 0DS **Tel:** (01234) 261 622 w 6287938

HUTCHINS Louise 31/05/2001 (16/11/2004) 12 Shore Drive WIRRAL Merseyside CH62 4RW w 6219782

Sarah Louise 08/01/2008 384 Wood Lane SHEFFIELD S6 5LR **Tel:** (0114) 2344503 w 6366324

HUTCHINSON Cara Marie 18/11/2009 Braid Veterinary Hospital 171 Mayfield Road Newington Edinburgh EH9 3AZ **Tel:** (0131) 667 2478 w 6407596

Claire 28/04/2008 46 Barlborough Road Ilkeston Derbyshire DE7 8WJ **Tel:** (07984) 153855 w 6389787

Rachel Marie 15/06/2009 41 Harrop White Road Mansfield Nottinghamshire NG19 6SL **Tel:** 01623468590 w 6408839

Rosie Elizabeth 04/04/2008 Lower Mitchell Cottage Eastnor LEDBURY Herefordshire HR8 1EJ **Tel:** (01531) 630132 w 6378248

Samantha 16/07/2007 (03/02/2010) 74 Torrington Avenue Tile Hill COVENTRY CV4 9AR **Tel:** (02476) 473175 w 6349230

Sarah Louise 16/05/2008 Blastfurnace Cottage Underhill Glaisdale WHITBY North Yorkshire YO21 2PF **Tel:** (01947) 897002 w 6359746

HUTT Jacqueline Claire 30/03/2001 26 Stephen Street Redfield BRISTOL BS5 9DX **Tel:** (0117) 955 3088 w 6214601

Jolene Amy 02/10/2009 21 Edith Cavell Close THETFORD Norfolk IP24 1TJ **Tel:** (01842) 764244 w 6492131

HUTTON Gemma Louise 02/09/2008 4 Franklin Close Stapenhill BURTON-ON-TRENT Staffordshire DE15 9AN w 6414625

HUTTON Samantha Leigh (see ROBINSON, Mrs)

HVEDING Silje Christin 28/09/2005 Tanglewood 14 Merrow Chase Guildford Surrey GU1 2RY **Tel:** (01483) 858195 w 6354686

HYDE Jennifer Elizabeth 22/02/2007 11 Wolverton Gardens Horley Surrey RH6 7LZ **Tel:** (01293) 785 214 w 6343741

Lisa Marie 18/10/2005 9 The Drive MELTON MOWBRAY Leicestershire LE13 0BT **Tel:** (01664) 854032 w 6333973

HYGATE Hayley Denise (nee Sycamore) 27/02/2006 24 Kingswood Road GILLINGHAM Kent ME7 1DZ **Tel:** (01634) 329069 w 6327032

HYLAND Lynn Margaret (see TUDOR, Mrs)

HYLANDS Wendy Jane (see NEVINS, Mrs)

HYND Dawn (nee Adamson) 24/08/1999 57 Brandy Riggs Cairneyhill DUNFERMLINE Fife KY12 8UY w 6136794

HYNDMAN Lorna Elizabeth Doyle 03/12/2003 3 Spring Drive Farcet PETERBOROUGH PE7 3AJ w 6292613

HYNES Emma Jayne 19/12/2006 116 Hayes Lane Bromley Kent BR2 9EP **Tel:** (07944) 563728 w 6294263

I

IBBETSON Helen Mary 06/02/2002 Tower Wood Veterinary Group 27 Tinshill Road Leeds Yorkshire LS16 7DR **Tel:** (0113) 267 8419 w 6255235

IDDON Lisa 22/04/2008 17-19 Church Road Leyland Lancashire PR25 3EJ **Tel:** (01772) 432039 w 6403867

IGLESIAS Jayne Louise (nee Richens) 30/06/2003 (22/08/2006) 438 Hook Road Chessington Surrey KT9 1NA **Tel:** (020) 8397 1776 w 6260317

ILES Zoe Lynsey 20/01/1995 40 Victoria Park Kingswood Bristol Avon BS15 1SA w 6033256

ILETT Andrea Nicole 11/01/2005 83 Malards Way Bicester Oxfordshire OX26 6WT **Tel:** (01869) 242787 w 6283296

IMPEY Jacqueline 23/01/1990 (27/08/2009) St. Mary's Lodge 11 Hill Road Southend-on-Sea Essex SS2 6JT **Tel:** (01702) 313024 w 6053625

INCE Lucy Elizabeth (see DUNCAN-BROWN, Mrs)

INCLEDON-WEBBER Rosalind Amber 10/06/2003 Queen Mother Hospital for Small Animals Hawkshead Lane North Mymms Hatfield Hertfordshire AL9 7TA **Tel:** (01707) 666366 w 6286992

INGHAM Caroline (see WHATLING, Mrs)

INGHAM Sarah Rachel 25/09/2009 2 Rectory Cottage Grainsby Lane Grainsby GRIMSBY South Humberside DN36 5PT **Tel:** 01472841316 w 6460858

Zoe 07/10/2009 34 Flying Fields Road SOUTHAM Warwickshire CV47 1GA w 6439584

INGRAM Eleri Bethan 04/06/2009 4 Barley Croft BRISTOL BS9 3TF w 6415252

Kelly Marie 04/01/2006 38 Forrit Brae Bucksburn Aberdeen Aberdeenshire AB21 9SL **Tel:** (01224) 714719 w 6342630

Laura Jayne Parry (nee Bryant) 04/12/2003 Wingrave Veterinary Surgery 84 Mulgrave Road Sutton Surrey SM2 6LZ **Tel:** (020) 8642 9100 w 6284649

Sharon Anne 27/04/2001 (31/03/2006) Marches Veterinary Group Ryelands Road Leominster Herefordshire HR6 8PN **Tel:** (01568) 612266 w 6129335

Vicki Marie 14/10/2008 80 Ventonlace Grampound Road Truro Cornwall TR2 4EQ **Tel:** (01726) 882760 w 6378105

INGRAM-LUCK Joanne Maria 25/11/2008 The Bungalow Welsh Road Little Sutton Ellesmere Port Merseyside CH66 4QR **Tel:** (01503) 398 082 w 6418475

INMAN Emma Jayne 24/10/2008 28 Marshfoot Lane HAILSHAM East Sussex BN27 2JW **Tel:** (07917) 123294 w 6363277

INNES Cassie Joanne 21/06/2005 Ivybank Veterinary Clinic 2 Low Green Road Irvine Ayrshire KA12 8RA **Tel:** (01294) 273161 w 6291337

INNS Rachel Julie 03/07/2009 29 Summer Hill Avenue Kidderminster Worcestershire DY11 6BY **Tel:** 01299822423 w 6400688

ION Victoria (see DODD, Mrs)

IREDALE Jennine Marie (nee Stanley) 13/12/2001 15 Close Head Drive Thornton Bradford West Yorkshire BD13 3QQ **Tel:** (01274) 830513 w 6274771

IRELAND Lucinda Charlotte (nee Pearsall) 03/03/2005 West Midlands Safari & Leisure Park Spring Grove Bewdley Worcestershire DY12 1LF **Tel:** (01299) 402114 w 6321554

IRESON Jo (formerly Stewart, formerly Richmond) 06/12/2004 (25/03/2009) 93 High Street Wrestlingworth SANDY Bedfordshire SG19 2EJ w 6308057

IRONS Julie Faye Elizabeth 20/09/1999 19 Green Leys Badsey Evesham Worcestershire WR11 7XE **Tel:** (01386) 47860 w 6184736

IRONSIDE Jennifer Elizabeth 29/12/2009 The Nurses House 5 Inshes Holdings Inshes INVERNESS IV2 5FF **Tel:** 07900861846 w 6437142

Rebecca Jane 05/07/2006 132 Elmers End Road Beckenham Kent BR3 4TA **Tel:** (07904) 315865 w 6321521

IRVINE Catriona Claire 08/08/2008 22 Thurston Place LIVINGSTON West Lothian EH54 6RU **Tel:** (01506) 494474 w 6318485

Chantel Tanya 04/12/2003 2 Dene Close WORCESTER PARK Surrey KT4 7HQ **Tel:** (020) 82245071 w 6266169

IRVINE Jenny Caryl Mary (see COOKE, Mrs)

Julia 20/11/2000 76 Spa Road BALLYNAHINCH County Down BT24 8PP w 6038152

IRVING Laura Ann 22/09/2006 944 Aikenhead Road Kings Park Glasgow Lanarkshire G44 4QG **Tel:** (0141) 563 4448 w 6350737

Lynn 30/10/2003 27 Laceys Lane Exning NEWMARKET Suffolk CB8 7HL **Tel:** 07795073635 w 6277400

IRWIN-PORTER Gemma (nee Dix) 25/02/2003 5 Taynton Close Bitton BRISTOL BS30 6JZ **Tel:** (07834) 761191 w 6274562

ISAAC Linda Maria (see KING, Mrs)

ISAACS Michelle (see CRESSWELL, Miss)

ISAACS Michelle Claire 10/02/2004 82 Bruce Street SWINDON SN2 2EN w 6286387

IVENS Tracy Joanne (nee Barrow) 06/12/2004 31 Norfolk Road Turvey Bedford Bedfordshire MK43 8DU **Tel:** (01234) 881381 w 6301248

IVES Cheryl Diana 30/05/2006 17 St. Andrews Close Sutton ELY Cambridgeshire CB6 2QU **Tel:** (01954) 781 256 w 6353828

IVES Deborah (see WATTS, Mrs)

IVEY Amanda Louise 27/09/2006 Clifton Veterinary Surgery Anstey Lane Alton Hampshire GU34 2RH **Tel:** (01420) 82163 w 6377698

IZARD Julie (nee Reid) 12/01/1989 (30/05/2008) 31 Norbury Drive LANCING West Sussex BN15 0QQ **Tel:** (01903) 530884 w 6059547

IZZARD Hannah Clare (see PERRY, Mrs)

J

JACK Rachel Elizabeth 14/09/2009 Alver Veterinary Group 148 Forton Road Gosport Hampshire PO12 3HG **Tel:** (023) 9258 2991/2 w 6492087

JACKMAN Morna Lucy 03/04/2009 3 Spruce Cove Tramore Co. Waterford Ireland **Tel:** (00353) 51 390060 w 6414471

JACKSON Ann 31/07/1987 (25/04/2007) Ashley Vets Pet Hospital 6 Hersham Road Walton-on-Thames Surrey KT12 1JZ **Tel:** (01932) 248941 w 6053705

JACKSON Becky Kuiama (see WASHINGTON, Mrs)

Emma Louise 07/02/2007 Hillcrest Animal Health Ltd Water Street Chorley Lancashire PR7 1EX **Tel:** (01257) 262448 w 6343752

Gemma 22/03/2004 16 Steeplands Bradley HUDDERSFIELD West Yorkshire HD2 1QQ **Tel:** (0148) 4530985 w 6286002

Helen Jane 29/07/2009 14 Dewfalls Drive Bradley Stoke BRISTOL BS32 9BT **Tel:** (07736) 420 747 w 6319299

Jane Caroline Kay Sheila Pat 28/01/2009 19 Clifton Street Greenbank PLYMOUTH PL4 8JA **Tel:** 07903018044 w 6445128

Joanna (nee Heaps) 22/03/2004 (10/04/2007) Scarsdale Veterinary Hospital 45-47 Kedleston Road Derby DE22 1FN **Tel:** (01332) 345191 w 6279116

Katie Anne 10/12/2007 24 Reeves Road Birmingham West Midlands B14 6SQ **Tel:** (0121) 443 2612 w 6324249

Kerry Ann (nee Crewe) 20/11/2002 (06/09/2007) 176 Jeremy's Green Edmonton London N18 2NE **Tel:** (020) 8807 4668 w 6281426

Laura Marie 04/10/2005 61 The Links Kempston Bedford Bedfordshire MK42 7LT **Tel:** (01234) 855046 w 6352079

Leah 12/12/2007 Sileby Hall Cossington Road Sileby Loughborough Leicestershire LE12 7RS **Tel:** (01509) 812445/6 w 6410390

Lisa Marie 11/05/2004 4 Goyt Road Vernon Park Stockport Cheshire SK1 2EZ **Tel:** (0161) 429 6553 w 6278588

Louise Josephine 19/01/1998 Petwell House 319 Station Road South Hayes Middlesex UB3 4JF **Tel:** (020) 8848 1818 w 6108643

JACKSON Louise N G (see GLYSEN, Mrs)

Mandy 06/02/2008 36 Chapelfield Crescent Thorpe Hesley Rotherham South Yorkshire S61 2TP **Tel:** 01142457687 w 6406155

JACKSON Maxine Louise (see KETLEY, Mrs)

Nadine Emily DipAVN(Surgical) 04/12/2003 11 Tudor Road Welwyn Hertfordshire AL6 9JU **Tel:** (01438) 717043 w 6288400

Naomi 04/06/2009 151 Taylor Road Hindley Green Wigan Lancashire WN2 4TJ **Tel:** 07812806558 w 6436537

JACKSON Nicola Louise (see EDWARDS, Mrs)

Nicola Rose 25/09/2000 12 Ascot Avenue Runcorn Cheshire WA7 4YW **Tel:** (01928) 569291 w 6115785

JACKSON Penelope Sarah (see JACKSON-SMITH, Mrs)

Sara Louise 12/03/2009 215 Soundwell Road BRISTOL BS15 1PT **Tel:** (0117) 9571110 w 6434931

Sarah Caroline 06/12/2004 12A Milespit Hill Mill Hill London NW7 2PL **Tel:** (0208) 906 8394 w 6293713

Sarah Lesley 10/02/2009 11 Rock Farm Close Little Neston Neston Merseyside CH64 4DX **Tel:** 01513361888 w 6412007

Susan Lynda 04/10/2005 (29/06/2007) 81 Hulton Close Southampton SO19 9TY w 6324051

Timothy Daniel Frank 14/01/2008 142 Imeary Street SOUTH SHIELDS Tyne and Wear NE33 4EL **Tel:** (07882) 185 356 m 6376488

Victoria Louise 21/02/2002 4 Kingswell Avenue WAKEFIELD West Yorkshire WF1 3DY w 6205768

Zoe Eve 03/05/2005 Forevergreen Lindrick Lane Tickhill Doncaster South Yorkshire DN11 9RA **Tel:** (07974) 215829 w 6300071

JACKSON-SMITH Penelope Sarah (nee Jackson) 01/09/1987 Mill House Veterinary Surgery & Hospital 20 Tennyson Avenue King's Lynn Norfolk PE30 2QG **Tel:** (01553) 771457 w 605375X

JACOB Suzanne Elizabeth 11/03/2005 Green Farm Folly Lane Bramley Tadley Hampshire RG26 5BB **Tel:** (01256) 881 304 w 6285100

JAFFRAY Hazel Marie (formerly Bain) 22/06/2001 Ardene House Veterinary Hospital Kingswells Aberdeen AB15 8PJ **Tel:** (01224) 740700 w 6223544

JAGAIT Nikki Ravinder 09/09/2009 12 Rosemullion Close Exhall COVENTRY CV7 9NQ **Tel:** 02476317174 w 6381152

JAMEISON Christine Elizabeth 30/10/2003 80 Main Street Albert Village Swadlincote Derbyshire DE11 8EN **Tel:** (07811) 946793 w 6288884

JAMES Amanda Susan 11/11/2004 Summerhill Veterinary Centre 43 Summerhill Avenue Newport Gwent NP19 8FQ **Tel:** (01633) 255394 w 6325987

JAMES Debra Amanda (see KENNEDY, Mrs)

Gillian 07/05/2009 20 Anstey Road ALTON Hampshire GU34 2RB **Tel:** 07939323351 w 6421269

Jane Anouska (nee Taylor) 24/08/1998 (07/09/2005) 2-3 Trentham District Centre Stanley Matthews Way Trentham Lakes STOKE-ON-TRENT Staffordshire ST4 8AD **Tel:** (075983) 15605 w 6122362

Joanna Elizabeth Emilia (nee Barnard) 11/03/2005 (09/09/2009) Highfield Veterinary Surgery Highfield Stables White Stubbs Lane Broxbourne Hertfordshire EN10 7PZ **Tel:** (01992) 440738 w 6294098

Katie Sue 06/12/2004 (25/11/2009) 9 Malcolm Drive Bucknall Stoke on Trent Staffordshire ST2 8LQ **Tel:** (01782) 535496 w 6272989

Kay Amanda (nee Phillips) 14/01/1999 6 Attlee Close NORTHAMPTON NN3 6FF **Tel:** (01604) 671850 w 6118516

Louise 17/05/2005 (21/01/2009) Moorside Skelsceugh Rd Winder Frinzington Cumbria CA26 3UE **Tel:** (01946) 861778 w 6286310

Louise 18/10/2005 21 Pheasant Way Yaxley Peterborough Cambridgeshire PE7 3HN **Tel:** (07960) 058887 w 6350044

Philippa Jane 16/06/2008 Coedcae Farm LLANDOVERY Dyfed SA20 0HQ **Tel:** (01550) 720 849 w 6380778

JAMES Sian Elizabeth (see HOPKINS, Mrs)

Stephanie Emma 11/09/1998 25 Hallam Drive Shrewsbury Shropshire SY1 4YE w 6137787

JAMESON Emma Louise (nee Garland) 20/01/2009 Rossdales Equine Hospital Cotton End Road Exning Newmarket Suffolk CB8 7NN **Tel:** (01638) 577 754 w 6403999

JAMESON Karen (see WAKEFIELD, Mrs)

Katherine Jane DipAVN(Medical) (nee Waldie) 15/11/2001 63 Nedd Road Ballykelly Limavady Co Londonderry BT49 9HZ w 6261406

JAMIESON Lauren 09/06/2009 Warlands Green Holmside Edmondsley Durham County Durham DH7 6EX **Tel:** 01913719632 w 6443478

Leeann (nee Reilly) 13/01/2004 5 Skye Quadrant WISHAW Lanarkshire ML2 8XJ **Tel:** (01698) 386663 w 6257897

Nicola Anne 15/09/2009 Ardene House Veterinary Hospital Kingswells Aberdeen AB15 8PJ **Tel:** (01224) 740700 w 6439716

JANES Laura Yvonne 17/01/2006 Ark Veterinary Practice 41 Connaught Road Fleet Hampshire GU51 3LR **Tel:** (01252) 616 185 w 6330200

JANSMA Kerry Deborah Joanne 17/01/2008 20 Hertford Road Clare Sudbury Suffolk CO10 8QH **Tel:** 07990824584 w 6377709

JAPPY Karen Ann 04/09/2009 Top Floor Flat 122 Auchmill Road Bucksburn ABERDEEN AB21 9LS **Tel:** 07709110166 w 6349241

JAQUES Barbara Mary (nee Jaques, formerly Boughey) 04/08/1989 Clinical Investigations Centre Royal Veterinary College Hawkshead Lane North Mymms HATFIELD Hertfordshire AL9 7TA **Tel:** (01707) 666605 w 6046006

Sally Rebecca 13/11/2009 3 Pykes Farm Cottages Forest Road WOKINGHAM Berkshire RG40 5QS w 6489414

JARDIM Katrina Maria 11/07/2005 311 Main Street PO Box 140 Gibraltar Gibraltar w 6299708

JARMAN Charlotte Anne 09/09/2008 Hollybank Manston Court Road Margate Kent CT9 4LE **Tel:** 01843823544 w 6406188

JARMAN Jayne Claire (see HOLBY, Mrs)

Marisa Lucinda 13/07/2007 16 Cathcart Crescent PAISLEY Renfrewshire PA2 7EB **Tel:** (0141) 562 6599 w 6350055

JARVIS Athena Dawn 23/03/2007 3 Raleigh Grove LUTON Bedfordshire LU4 8RE **Tel:** (01582) 758525 w 6304053

Hannah Lydia 26/04/2007 88 Royston Avenue Southend-on-Sea Essex SS2 5LA **Tel:** 01702614291 w 6373738

Lisa Kay 05/01/1989 Lantra Lantra House Stoneleigh Park KENILWORTH Warwickshire CV8 2LG **Tel:** (01935) 826418 w 6094300

Tammy Marie (nee Hopkin) 23/10/2001 R S P C A Block Fen Animal Centre Block Fen Drove Wimblington March Cambridgeshire PE15 0FB **Tel:** (0870) 906 1426 w 6263859

JARVIS Victoria Jane (see JARVIS-HORN, Mrs)

JARVIS-HORN Victoria Jane (nee Jarvis) 04/02/2002 54a Stakes Hill Road Waterlooville Hampshire PO7 7LB **Tel:** (023) 9226 2346 w 6269194

JASPER Carolyn Sarah (see POWLES, Mrs)

JAUNCEY Nicola Clare 26/04/2002 Lamb House 17 Newport Street Hay-on-Wye Hereford HR3 5BG **Tel:** (01497) 820863 w 6275486

JAYE Isabel Charlotte 20/09/2005 North End Cottage North End Ravenstone OLNEY Buckinghamshire MK46 5AN **Tel:** (01908) 551467 w 6332301

JAYNE Jacqueline Kim (nee Allaway) 06/08/1991 13 Porthycarne Street Usk Monmouthshire NP15 1RZ **Tel:** (01291) 672637 w 6044541

Rachel Victoria (nee Morris) 14/05/2007 41 Laurel Drive Penperlleni Pontypool Gwent NP4 0BQ **Tel:** (01873) 882 909 w 6351375

JEFCOATE Emma Catherine (see OPPERMAN, Mrs)

JEFFERD Jane Louise (see LEWIS, Mrs)

JEFFERIES Emma Vivienne 22/03/2004 37 South Rd Grassendale Park Liverpool L19 0LS **Tel:** (0151) 427 6737 w 6269007

Lyndsey Ann 26/02/2008 111 Godwin Road Stratton Swindon Wiltshire SN3 4XF **Tel:** (01793) 330960 w 6348504

Phillipa Caroline 12/05/2008 3 Front Street Sunnybrow Crook County Durham DL15 0NF **Tel:** (01388) 748416 w 6411556

Shelly Ann 06/09/2000 (12/11/2007) Tom Cobley Tavern Spreyton CREDITON Devon EX17 5AL w 6203150

JEFFERIS Carina Natalie Ellen 16/06/2008 43 Charlton Road Keynsham BRISTOL BS31 2JG **Tel:** (07792) 648 735 w 6380789

JEFFERSON Elizabeth Ann 13/08/2003 109A Pedmore Road Lye Stourbridge West Midlands DY8 8DG **Tel:** (01384) 897632 w 6262022

JEFFERSON Rachel Ann (see ANDERSON, Mrs)

JEFFERY Andrea Karen DipAVN(Surgical) (nee Hart) 23/08/1990 (19/05/1999) University of Bristol School of Veterinary Nursing Veterinary Nursing Unit Langford House Langford Somerset BS40 5DU **Tel:** (0117) 9289517 w 6052428

Hayley Lorraine 16/07/2001 Bridge House Veterinary Surgery Pilton Bridge Barnstaple Devon EX31 1PG **Tel:** (01271) 342119 w 6144557

Vicky Louise 20/08/1999 2 Prince Charles Close Exmouth Devon EX8 4RG **Tel:** (07887) 588175 w 6133250

JEFFERYES-WHITE Sally 30/03/2006 (13/03/2009) Penygraig Farm Rhydyfelin ABERYSTWYTH Dyfed SY23 4QA w 6324777

JEFFREY Amy Caroline 15/11/2005 (11/01/2010) 24 Bogarde Drive Wainscott ROCHESTER Kent ME3 8GR **Tel:** (01634) 726078 w 6339132

JEFFREYS Jessica 13/07/2007 31 Fitzalan Road Littlehampton West Sussex BN17 5ET **Tel:** (01903) 713806 w 6349560

JEMMETT Ann 28/08/1996 (25/09/2006) 14 Cambridge Grdens Tunbridge Wells Kent TN2 4SE **Tel:** (01892) 549285 w 6041449

JENKIN Donna Mary 25/02/2004 8 Trecarrell Close LAUNCESTON Cornwall PL15 9DG w 6290138

JENKINS Claire Amanda 19/02/2001 6 Greenhill Close Dosthill Tamworth Staffordshire B77 1NA **Tel:** (01827) 260538 w 6116530

Elizabeth Mary 25/02/2003 12 Cedar Road Hatfield Hertfordshire AL10 8NY **Tel:** (01707) 890610 w 6279006

Emma 09/01/2004 The Flat Fernlea Vets Blackhorse Road Kingswood Bristol BS15 8DZ w 6293724

JENKINS Emma Louise (see CLARE, Miss)

Helen Elaine (nee Kirby) 12/01/2004 Hillside Hicksmill Polyphant NR Launceston Cornwall PL15 7PT **Tel:** (01566) 86719 w 6290149

Helen Louise (nee Ranger) 29/08/1997 21 Maple Avenue Glenover Fields Haverfordwest Pembrokeshire SA61 1EF **Tel:** (01437) 760772 w 6100112

Kirsty 10/02/2004 11 Buckfast Close Lower Ham Plymouth Devon PL2 2HD **Tel:** (01752) 567567 w 6276245

JENKINS Nina (see MAXWELL, Mrs)

Victoria 10/04/2007 27 Mill Street OTTERY ST. MARY Devon EX11 1AB w 6382406

JENKINSON Aimee Louise 19/03/2007 (11/02/2009) 8 Bramshaws Acre Cheadle STOKE-ON-TRENT ST10 1BE **Tel:** (01538) 752383 w 6298784

Alison Jane (nee Baxter) 11/05/2004 (17/03/2006) Mill House Ormiston Road Pathhead Lothian EH37 5XD w 6267874

Sharon (formerly Curry) 22/07/1993 (06/05/2003) 36 Olivet Road Woodseats Sheffield South Yorkshire S8 8QS **Tel:** (0114) 250 7733 w 6066532

JENNER Sarah Joanne 30/07/1992 (19/11/1998) 14 Burlington Road New Malden Surrey KT3 4NY **Tel:** (020) 8942 2202 w 6053909

JENNINGS Amy Elizabeth 18/11/2008 13 Bratten Court 34 Westbury Road CROYDON CR0 2ES w 6410676

Cathryn Lesley (formerly Cooper) 22/01/1985 Holme Veterinary Centre Unit 6, Imex Business Park Crossley Mill, New Mill Road Honley Holmfirth West Yorkshire HD9 6QB **Tel:** (01484) 660900 w 6092041

Kelly Ann (nee Martin) 31/10/2003 32 Campbell Road Caterham Surrey CR3 5JL **Tel:** (01883) 372664 w 6280337

Lauren 31/10/2006 47 Fennels Way Flackwell Heath HIGH WYCOMBE Buckinghamshire HP10 9BX w 6370999

Rosalind Anne Elizabeth 17/09/2007 2 Croft Bank Millbrook Stalybridge Cheshire SK15 3HR w 6353839

Shelley Marie 14/03/2006 Manchester Street Veterinary Surgery Manchester Street Oldham OL8 1UF **Tel:** (0161) 624 4596 w 6347151

JERMEY Victoria Jayne DipAVN(Medical) (nee Snelgrove) 05/02/1999 Bramble Field Cottage Coombe Road Compton NEWBURY Berkshire RG20 6RQ **Tel:** (01635) 578991 w 6138521

JERVIS Claire Jane (nee Field) 16/08/2006 Pool House Veterinary Group Fosseway Lane Lichfield Staffordshire WS13 8JY **Tel:** (01543) 262464/262433 w 6345446

JESSHOPE Helen Rachael (nee Hughes) 15/07/2005 31 Lavender Road East Malling West Malling Kent ME19 6EE **Tel:** (07709) 432889 w 6296749

JIGGINS Joanna Elizabeth (see GREENHOUGH, Mrs)

JOHANSSON Anna Karin Elisabeth 01/06/2007 Third House Craymere Road Briston MELTON CONSTABLE Norfolk NR24 2LS **Tel:** (0781) 8833790 w 6380646

JOHNSON Donna Marie (nee Charlton) 27/08/2003 12 Boundary Close New Edlington Warmsworth Doncaster South Yorkshire DN12 1SF **Tel:** (01709) 858234 w 6282988

Elizabeth Ann 27/02/2006 31 Birkburn Road Kelloholm Sanquhar Dumfriesshire DG4 6SE w 6324062

Elizabeth Susan 06/03/2006 32 Bachelor Gardens Harrogate North Yorkshire HG1 3EL **Tel:** 07776652203 w 6343587

Emma Jeanne DipAVN(Medical) (nee Simpkins) 14/09/2001 23 Wentworth Close Ash Vale ALDERSHOT Hampshire GU12 5NB w 6228285

Frances Louise 13/05/2003 36 Boston Road Kirton Boston Lincolnshire PE20 1DS **Tel:** (01205) 722696 w 6270965

Gemma Louise 29/09/2004 3 Elm Tree Walk Farnborough Hampshire GU14 9FG w 6326416

Graeme Henry 28/06/2002 Falkland Veterinary Clinic 214 Newtown Road Newbury Berkshire RG14 7ED **Tel:** (01635) 46565 m 6272076

JOHNSON Hayley Rebecca (see WOOD, Mrs)

Helen Jane 14/05/2007 Prince Bishop Veterinary Hospital 1 Plantation Street Leadgate Consett County Durham DH8 7PP **Tel:** (01207) 590340 w 6376510

Jemma (nee Simpson) 23/12/2003 Limekiln Cottage Ixworth Road Stowlangtoft Bury St. Edmunds Suffolk IP31 3JU w 6290886

Jodie Leanne 13/04/2004 75 High Street Moxley Wednesbury WS10 8RT **Tel:** (01902) 409502 w 6292624

Julie Ann DipAVN(Surgical) 05/03/2002 53 Wansbeck Close STEVENAGE Hertfordshire SG1 6AA w 6262264

Katrina Joanne (nee Smith) 16/09/1991 Scarsdale Veterinary Hospital 45-47 Kedleston Road Derby DE22 1FN **Tel:** (01332) 345191 w 6054028

JOHNSON Katy Elizabeth (see COLEMAN, Mrs)

Kelly Leanne 14/09/1998 Beechwood Veterinary Group Ltd 132 Austhorpe Road Leeds LS15 8EJ **Tel:** (01132) 645422 w 6132767

Kimberley Sarah Dawn 22/10/2004 Cromwell Veterinary Hospital 36-36a St. Johns Street HUNTINGDON Cambridgeshire PE29 3DG **Tel:** (01480) 52601/52222 w 6318023

Lindsay Barbara 08/11/2006 Dovecote Veterinary Hospital 5 Delven Lane Castle Donington Derby DE74 2LJ **Tel:** (01332) 810395 w 6367666

Lisa Marie 05/08/2008 3 Merton Walk BICESTER Oxfordshire OX26 4UF w 6416396

Marc Vicente 14/09/1998 5 Grey Friars Wybers Wood Grimsby South Humberside DN37 9QT **Tel:** (01472) 509221 m 6132428

Nichola (formerly Brett) 23/08/1999 107 Leeson Drive FERNDOWN Dorset BH22 9RD w 6185308

Nicola Anne (nee Day) 06/09/1999 52 Derwent Drive Mitton TEWKESBURY Gloucestershire GL20 8BB **Tel:** (01684) 273 831 w 6128400

Nicola-Jayne (nee Biggs) 25/01/1993 Warwickshire College Moreton Morrell Warwick CV35 9BL **Tel:** (01926) 318372 w 6065517

Paula Margaret 26/08/1994 414-416 Leach Lane Sutton Leach St. Helens Merseyside WA9 4NA **Tel:** (01744) 820505 w 6032230

Samantha 29/07/2008 9 Butterworth Way Egham Surrey TW20 8JT **Tel:** 01784438264 w 6367094

Stacey Helen 21/04/2008 27 Portland Road EAST GRINSTEAD West Sussex RH19 4EB **Tel:** (01342) 327799 w 6357392

Tanya Rachel 06/10/2006 The Shirley Chart Hill Road Staplehurst TONBRIDGE Kent TN12 0RL **Tel:** (01580) 892051 w 6326955

Wendy Dorothy 12/05/2006 36 Boston Road Kirton Boston Lincolnshire PE20 1DS **Tel:** (01205) 722696 w 6311753

Zana Eluise (nee McGuinness) 06/10/2006 11 Mendip Crescent Bristol Avon BS16 6UF **Tel:** (0117) 904 4679 w 6326438

JOHNSTON Claire Louise 05/07/2006 17 Charlock Road Locking Castle Weston-super-Mare Avon BS22 8NQ **Tel:** (07890) 322356 w 6321532

Jolene Anne 16/07/2007 69 Ladysmith Road EDINBURGH EH9 3EY **Tel:** (07825) 048557 w 6317693

Tamara Lorraine 19/01/1998 (06/02/2002) Midsummer Veterinary Group Soskin Drive Stantonbury Fields MILTON KEYNES Buckinghamshire MK14 6DT **Tel:** (01908) 321115 w 6117895

JOHNSTONE Catherine (see EDGAR, Miss)

JOHNSTONE Hayley Leslie 06/08/2008 89/1 Polwarth Terrace EDINBURGH EH11 1NW w 6324535

Lucy Alice 19/01/2000 Robson Veterinary Hospital Laurencekirk Business Park Aberdeen Road Laurencekirk Kincardineshire AB30 1EY **Tel:** (01561) 377314 w 6190434

JOINER Catherine Louise 07/02/2006 The Veterinary Surgery Janet Street Thurso Caithness KW14 7EG **Tel:** (01847) 892387 w 6349582

JOLLIFFE Marion 01/09/1997 Blue Cross Animals Hospital Argyle Place London W6 0RQ **Tel:** (020) 8748 5150 w 611791X

JONAS Angela Dawn (nee Crossley) 09/11/2005 The Veterinary Surgery Higher Trenant Wadebridge Cornwall PL27 6HB **Tel:** (01208) 813258 w 6351221

Michelle Emma 05/10/2009 8 Westwood Gardens WYMONDHAM Norfolk NR18 0DP **Tel:** (01953) 605538 w 6492120

JONES Abigail Ruth (see HOLDER, Mrs)

JONES Alice Cecilia (nee Wolf) 02/09/1997 3 Mill Lane Ampleforth North Yorkshire YO62 4DJ **Tel:** (01439) 788181 w 6119065

Allison Jayne (nee Bryan) 09/05/2005 Clent Hills Veterinary Group 34 Stourbridge Road BROMSGROVE Worcestershire B61 0AE **Tel:** (01527) 872488 w 6259943

Amy 05/12/2008 5 Britannia Way Westward Ho BIDEFORD Devon EX39 1UP w 6412887

Angela Louise 24/11/2005 Alan Croft Thimble Lane St. Martins Oswestry Shropshire SY11 3BW **Tel:** (07866) 624806 w 6320113

Anna Louise 24/04/2009 13 Garden Close Ashford Middlesex TW15 1LH **Tel:** 01784247955 w 6440519

Anna May 04/04/2008 The Horseshoe Cottage 39 The Homend Ledbury Herefordshire HR8 1BP **Tel:** (01531) 636591 w 6398268

JONES Annette Louisa (see BRISBOURNE, Mrs)

Barbara Anne (nee Copeland) 12/09/1995 (15/05/2008) 123 Woodvale Kingsway Quedgeley GLOUCESTER GL2 2BU w 6038254

Camilla Anne 20/09/2006 27 Evans Close TIPTON West Midlands DY4 8BG **Tel:** (01564) 774122 w 6272186

Caroline Mary 07/02/2000 North Radworthy Farm Heasley Mill South Molton Devon EX36 3LF **Tel:** (01598) 740 200 w 6190577

Catherine Gail 05/11/2007 Abington Park Veterinary Surgery 427 Wellingborough Road Northampton NN1 4EZ **Tel:** (01604) 628 685 w 6366808

Claire Anne (nee Pirnie) 07/06/2005 The Frederick Jennings Centre Hepton Court York Road Leeds LS9 6PW **Tel:** (01132) 408818 w 6285551

Clare Amanda 24/12/2002 Derlwyn Cwmgwili Llanelli Dyfed SA14 6PS **Tel:** (01269) 832592 w 6270547

Corinna (nee Nickisson) 30/08/2006 Bron Heulog Cwm Road Trelawnyd Rhyl Clwyd LL18 6EF **Tel:** (01745) 571 737 w 6355764

Deborah Louise 31/08/1999 13 Bourne Court 60 Pampisford Road PURLEY Surrey CR8 2NE w 6129073

Eleanor Louise 25/02/2003 Creamery House Chapel Lane Brvera Chester Cheshire CH3 6EW **Tel:** (01244) 620287 w 6273880

Elena Sian 21/07/2008 Rousden House Crown Hill Llantwit Fardre PONTYPRIDD Mid Glamorgan CF38 2NA w 6377500

Elizabeth Anna (nee Jones, formerly Lakeman) 01/09/2008 Teignview Veterinary Group Hospital Hill DAWLISH Devon EX7 9NS **Tel:** (01626) 778507 w 6390128

Emma Michelle 04/12/2003 3 Hoghton Road Hale Village LIVERPOOL L24 4BW w 6277774

Esther Jayne (nee Stocks, formerly Smith) 10/04/2003 14 Frome Park Bartestree Hereford Herefordshire HR1 4BF **Tel:** (01432) 850351 w 6282152

Gillian Yvonne (formerly MacPherson) 19/01/1983 14 Brooklands Avenue MACCLESFIELD Cheshire SK11 8LB **Tel:** (01625) 263614 w 6090408

Gina 24/08/1998 9 First Avenue Astley Tyldesley Manchester M29 7JH **Tel:** (01942) 886141 w 6037942

Hannah Marie (nee Stanley) 30/07/2004 34 Manor Park Longlevens Gloucester Gloucestershire GL2 0HG **Tel:** (01452) 543045 w 6291964

Heledd Mai 17/01/2006 9 Meadow Park Treffgarne HAVERFORDWEST Dyfed SA62 5PQ **Tel:** (01437) 741415 w 6323369

Holly Victoria 06/08/2008 24 Tindall Close Harold Wood Romford Essex RM3 0PB **Tel:** (01708) 500165 w 6409180

Jane Mary 28/09/2005 Grove Cottage Hatherleigh OKEHAMPTON Devon EX20 3NA **Tel:** (01837) 810167 w 6342124

Jennifer Clare 04/11/2008 167 Hampton Road SOUTHPORT Merseyside PR8 5DJ **Tel:** 01704545750 w 6378116

Jenny Louise 17/11/2004 9 Granby Close REDDITCH Worcestershire B98 0PJ **Tel:** (01527) 529766 w 6288158

Joanne Alison 08/03/1989 (04/09/2000) Roscoes Farm Moss Lane Whittle Le Woods Chorley Lancashire PR6 8AA **Tel:** (01257) 276956 w 6054196

Josephine (nee Cullen) 09/03/1994 Cottage Pie Higher Metcombe Ottery St. Mary Devon EX11 1SR **Tel:** (01404) 812366 w 6029997

Julie 24/08/1999 7 Arnolds Close Barton on Sea New Milton Hampshire BH25 7JW w 6123730

Karen Elizabeth (nee Lowman) 05/02/1992 (31/10/2000) 238 Bute Street Cardiff CF10 5HT **Tel:** (029) 2048 0990 w 6055429

Karen Laura (nee Williams) 04/11/2008 14 Oak Road Acrefair WREXHAM Clwyd LL14 3HY **Tel:** 07595393456 w 6416451

Karen Stephanie 21/07/1993 24 Charlton Road Midsomer Norton RADSTOCK BA3 4AE w 6015259

Karen Susan 25/02/2003 142 Liverpool Road Aughton Ormskirk Lancashire L39 3LW **Tel:** (01695) 422862 w 6271438

Kathryn Helen (formerly Lee, nee Lee) 06/02/1997 Park House Veterinary Centre 5 & 6 Park Street Stafford Staffordshire ST17 4AL **Tel:** (01785) 252846 w 6098440

Kathryn Louise 18/10/2006 Chester Gates Referral Hospital Unit F Telford Court Chester Gates Chester Cheshire CH1 6LT **Tel:** (01244) 853 823 w 6366874

Katie Michelle 28/10/2008 Tremain Veterinary Practice Ltd 1 Farm Mill Lane WITNEY Oxfordshire OX28 4BJ **Tel:** (01993) 703146 w 6435492

Kelly Anne (nee Jones) 17/08/2005 3 Lake View Maidenhead Berkshire SL6 8TX w 6281558

JONES Kerry Nicola (see MADDOX, Mrs)

JONES Kirsty (see NIXON, Miss)

Kirsty Ann (nee Matthews) 27/08/1997 Abbeydale Vetlink Veterinary Training Ltd Wyastone Business Park Wyastone Leys Monmouth NP25 3SR w 6110743

JONES Krisia Elizabeth (see REID, Mrs)

JONES Laura Anne (see FARNWORTH, Mrs)

Laura Elizabeth 10/10/2008 6 Brouder Close Bardon Coalville Leicestershire LE67 4GF w 6444270

Leanne Elizabeth 06/03/2006 31 Wrexham Close Callands WARRINGTON WA5 9RL **Tel:** (01925) 470 619 w 6328187

Lucy Ann (nee Clark) 14/01/1991 Milford Veterinary Surgery 37 New Road Milford Godalming Surrey GU8 5BE **Tel:** (01483) 414747 w 6095304

JONES Lynn (see DARBY, Mrs)

Lynne 23/08/1999 (16/05/2003) Bridgnorth Veterinary Centre 52 Whitburn Street Bridgnorth Shropshire WV16 4QP **Tel:** (01746) 711561 w 6144251

Marie DipAVN(Medical) (nee Boxall) 03/09/1997 2 Wentworth Cottages Haultwick WARE Hertfordshire SG11 1JG w 6097505

Melanie 20/04/2005 8a Rutters Close WEST DRAYTON Middlesex UB7 9AL **Tel:** (01895) 449925 w 6321763

Michelle Louise 03/03/2003 Abbotsfield Road St Helens Lancashire WA9 4HU **Tel:** (01744) 853510 w 6269095

Monique 11/01/2005 Meadow View Ash Hey Lane Picton Gorse CHESTER CH2 4HD **Tel:** (01244) 300420 w 6283560

Nicola Louise 18/09/2007 Marches Veterinary Group Ryelands Road Leominster Herefordshire HR6 8PN **Tel:** (01568) 612266 w 6375157

Rachael Louise 28/02/2005 P D S A Woolfall Heath Avenue Liverpool Merseyside L36 3YD **Tel:** (0151) 480 2288 w 6322225

Rachael Victoria 29/01/2007 Cromwell Veterinary Hospital 36-36a St. Johns Street HUNTINGDON Cambridgeshire PE29 3DG **Tel:** (01480) 52601/52222 w 6357788

Rachel 10/02/2004 20 Brunswick Avenue Waterloo Street Hull HU2 9AY **Tel:** (01482) 224452 w 6288895

Rachel Margaret (nee Blaber) 12/02/1997 87 Sandpiper Road Whitstable Kent CT5 4TP **Tel:** (01227) 772660 w 6097469

Rebecca Lorainne Joanne (formerly Tandy) 02/02/2001 (26/02/2009) 54 Coriander Close Rubery Rednal Birmingham West Midlands B45 0PD **Tel:** (0121) 624 2008 w 6211950

Rhian Eirwen 07/02/2006 The Bungalow Lilleshall National Sports Centre Lilleshall Newport Shropshire TF10 9AT **Tel:** 07974071915 w 6332312

Ruth Diane 01/06/1980 Stone House Farm Peckforton Tarporley Cheshire CW6 9TJ **Tel:** (01829) 260354 w 6054265

Ruth Gwendoline 03/06/2003 112 Culfor Road Loughor SWANSEA SA4 6UA **Tel:** (01792) 897898 w 6277829

JONES Sally (see SIMPSON, Mrs)

Sarah Elisabeth 16/08/2006 Church Lane Llanbadarn Fawr Aberystwyth Dyfed SY23 3QU **Tel:** (01970) 612526 w 6297288

Sarah Elizabeth 04/11/2005 Mount Veterinary Hospital 21 High Street Wellington Somerset TA21 8QS **Tel:** (01823) 662286 w 6343763

Sarah Louise (nee Gerrard) 03/02/1999 The Veterinary Surgery Hallfield Lane WETHERBY West Yorkshire LS22 6JU **Tel:** (01937) 582025 w 6098189

Sarah Louise Rowena 27/10/2008 28 King Street Avonmouth BRISTOL BS11 9AW w 6431829

Sharon Louise 02/09/2008 Parkland Bungalow Colenso Terrace Rhymney TREDEGAR Gwent NP22 5NQ **Tel:** (01685) 843142 w 6343774

Shelly Anne 30/10/2003 Orchard Veterinary Centre 21 Church Street Oldbury West Midlands B69 3AF **Tel:** (0121) 544 8951 w 6280348

Shelly Elizabeth 18/11/2009 21 Cios Crvcywell Parcgwernfadog Morriston SWANSEA SA6 6RD w 6465984

Susan Elizabeth (nee Jones, nee Dickinson) 08/08/2002 Carmarthen Veterinary Centre Llysonnen Road Llanllwch Carmarthen Carmarthenshire SA31 3SA **Tel:** (01267) 220 404 w 6255741

Tina Elizabeth 17/01/2007 Seers Croft Veterinary Surgery Tower Road Faygate Horsham West Sussex RH12 4SD **Tel:** (01293) 851122 w 6375542

Tracy Margaret (nee Ballingall) 01/09/1998 8 Elm Avenue Lenzie Glasgow G66 4HJ **Tel:** (0141) 578 5966 w 6028381

Victoria 13/08/2004 South View Steeles Row Burneside Kendal Cumbria LA9 6PY **Tel:** (01539) 725 656 w 6295429

Yolanda Jane Louise (nee Tucker) 04/10/2005 7 Burrough Road Northam BIDEFORD Devon EX39 1BU **Tel:** (01237) 420725 w 6344423

Yvonne Marie 10/09/2009 125 Wroslyn Road Freeland Witney Oxon OX29 8HP **Tel:** 01993881426 w 6466798

JONES-HUGHES Dollores 20/09/2000 Maes Uchaf Llanbedrgoch Gwynedd LL76 8TZ **Tel:** (01248) 450085 w 6077453

JORDAN Emma Mary 13/03/2002 (20/01/2005) NKR Veterinary Specialists Warren Road Bluebell Hill Chatham Kent ME5 9RD **Tel:** (01634) 666655 w 6255796

Hannah Fay 05/07/2006 Mill House Veterinary Surgery & Hospital 20 Tennyson Avenue King's Lynn Norfolk PE30 2QG **Tel:** (01553) 771457 w 6329705

Hannah Rachael 11/12/2009 50 Croft Avenue Bromborough Wirral CH62 2BR **Tel:** 01513348910 w 6451816

Hellen Paula (formerly Davis) 03/09/1996 (14/05/2004) 36 Wentworth Road Blacker Hill BARNSLEY South Yorkshire S74 0RU **Tel:** (01226) 360 145 w 6041325

JORDAN Sharna Louise (see CLARKE, Miss)

JORGENSEN Heidi Susannah 25/02/2003 Clinica Veterinaria Sana Sana Avda. Ramon Ortega 9A 03700 Alicante Spain w 6276839

JOUBERT Gillian Mary 29/09/2004 12 Birchend Place Germiston Glasgow Lanarkshire G21 2BJ **Tel:** (0141) 763 0800 w 6295451

JOUGHIN Valerie Frances 05/10/2001 14 Cranbourne Avenue Birkenhead Merseyside CH41 0BU **Tel:** 0151-652-4944 w 6229649

JOVANOVIC Anna Louise 25/02/2003 22 Mason Close Headless Cross Redditch Worcestershire B97 5DF **Tel:** (01527) 450266 w 6279864

Nadia Kaylee 24/11/2009 20 Sker Walk Nottage Porthcawl Mid Glamorgan CF36 3RA **Tel:** (0783) 448 3802 w 6440794

JOY Caroline Sarah 14/09/1999 87 Kenilworth Road St Leonards on Sea East Sussex TN38 0JD **Tel:** (01424) 437328 w 6134425

JOYCE Belinda Lorraine 23/02/2005 8 Doris Street Newmarket Suffolk CB8 0LD w 6323380

Emma Jane 04/12/2003 34 Barkers Butts Lane Coventry West Midlands CV6 1DT **Tel:** (02476) 590298 w 6286409

Rebecca Ann (nee Logan) 29/12/2003 13 Clifton Close Caterham Surrey CR3 5NX w 6274826

Tracey Louise 13/07/2007 Swanspool Veterinary Clinic 1 London Road Wellingborough Northamptonshire NN8 2BT **Tel:** (01933) 222145 w 6349406

JUDD Hayley 24/09/2009 47a Winchester Road Chandlers Ford Eastleigh Hampshire SO53 2GF **Tel:** (023) 8025 2543 w 6489799

JUDGE Alison Marie 02/02/2001 Pet Care Veterinary Surgery 355 Bexley Road Erith Kent DA8 3EZ **Tel:** (01322) 346173 w 6101670

JUKES Lisa (see WILLSHER, Mrs)

JUKES Louise Mary (see MOON, Mrs)

JULIAN Aimee Lauren 06/08/2008 193 Canterbury Road Bapchild Sittingbourne Kent ME10 4UL **Tel:** (07766) 495 659 w 6402723

K

KANE Helen Joanne 05/07/2006 22 Willetts Way Dawley Telford Shropshire TF4 2RR w 6288169

Sarah Emma 27/02/2006 The Veterinary Surgery Maple Street Huddersfield HD5 9AX **Tel:** (01484) 421512 w 6342663

KASATKIN Emma 19/02/2001 1 West Block Witton Gilbert Durham County Durham DH7 6TD w 6131581

KATTENHORN Hayley Louise 07/02/2006 4 Prospect Row St. Neots Cambridgeshire PE19 1JS **Tel:** (01480) 407891 w 6347668

KAVANAGH Janine Rachel 07/10/2009 2 Applegarth South Milford LEEDS LS25 5BL **Tel:** (01977) 681769 w 6440772

KAY Pamela 22/06/2009 8 Kings Inn Terrace Carnwath Lanark Lanarkshire ML11 8EL w 6412469

KEABLE Gemma 14/11/2008 20 Brunswick Avenue Waterloo Street Hull HU2 9AY **Tel:** (01482) 224452 w 6377720

KEARSEY Emma Joanne 07/02/2006 64 Ashfield Road CARTERTON Oxfordshire OX18 3QZ **Tel:** (01993) 867711 w 6344896

KEARVELL Rosemary Anne (see MILLARD, Mrs)

KEAY Nicola Claire (see ROBERTS, Mrs)

KEEFE Susan Jane 03/01/2008 37 The Paddocks WITHAM Essex CM8 2DR **Tel:** (01376) 519905 w 6332587

KEEL Lisa Marie (see HANDSCOMB, Mrs)

KEELING Claire Helen (nee Keeling, formerly Pedley) 01/09/2000 67 High Street Rocester Uttoxeter Staffordshire ST14 5JU **Tel:** (01889) 590449 w 6143950

Penelope Jane 14/09/2004 (01/02/2007) Calweton Veterinary Centre 79 Tavistock Road Callington Cornwall PL17 7RD **Tel:** (01579) 383231 w 6282482

KEEN Jennifer Ann (nee King) 18/01/2002 23 Gentian Close CHATHAM Kent ME5 0RP **Tel:** (01634) 319956 w 6259734

KEENAN Siobhan Marie 31/01/2000 (26/09/2007) Flat 2 Aireworth Veterinary Centre Aireworth Road Keighley West Yorkshire BD21 4DJ **Tel:** (01236) 733 543 w 6190335

KEENE Katherine Elizabeth (nee Venning) 02/02/1999 (26/06/2004) Cats Protection National Cat Centre, Veterinary Clinic Chelwood Gate Haywards Heath RH17 7TT **Tel:** (0870) 770 8255 w 6121992

Zoe Louise 29/06/2007 18 Niven Close WICKFORD Essex SS12 9QJ **Tel:** (01268) 730907 w 6380327

KEENES Selina Irene 23/07/2007 15 Highfield Field Dalling HOLT Norfolk NR25 7LF **Tel:** 07736769245 w 6368645

KEEP Natasha Claire 01/05/2009 16 Farleys Way Peasmarsh RYE East Sussex TN31 6PZ **Tel:** 01797230369 w 6435965

KEHOE Claire Marie 19/01/2005 (20/11/2009) Twickenham Veterinary Surgery 58 Hampton Road Twickenham Middlesex TW2 5QB **Tel:** (020) 8898 0528 w 6318947

KEITH Michelle Lesley 09/05/2005 69 Main Street Methven PERTH PH1 3QJ **Tel:** (01738) 840423 w 6318496

KELLETT Claire (nee O'Brien) 04/11/2005 Bramley Vets4Pets Limited Old School House Lower Town Street Bramley Leeds Yorkshire LS13 4BN **Tel:** (0113) 255 4466 w 6324667

KELLY Adelaide Faith 23/12/2008 Top Floor Flat 593 Wandsworth Road LONDON SW8 3JD **Tel:** 07905292711 w 6436702

Anne Theresa 23/07/2009 18 Glenville Drive Clonsilla Dublin 15 Ireland **Tel:** 0035318214277 w 6408707

Audrey DipAVN(Surgical) 02/03/1992 17 Foxdale Place Bonnybridge Stirlingshire FK4 2FB **Tel:** (01324) 819366 w 6054389

Claire Elaine 29/09/2009 Swanspool Veterinary Clinic 1 London Road Wellingborough Northamptonshire NN8 2BT **Tel:** (01933) 222145 w 6463938

KELLY Emma Angela (see REED, Mrs)

Emma Louise 04/02/2009 40 Woodcote Road Leigh-on-Sea Essex SS9 3NP **Tel:** 07931914681 w 6403647

Hayley Nicole (nee West) 28/06/2005 34 Queens Crescent Horndean WATERLOOVILLE Hampshire PO8 9ND **Tel:** (07834) 405759 w 6270734

Helen Louise 26/10/2005 Fairwater Veterinary Surgery Fairwater Square Cwmbran Gwent NP44 4TA **Tel:** (01633) 869300 w 6316417

Lynsay Anne 18/10/2006 (03/02/2010) 48 Collingwood Avenue CORBY Northamptonshire NN17 2SB w 6367677

Sarah Margaret 10/02/2004 55 Barlanark Place Glasgow Lanarkshire G33 4PS **Tel:** (0141) 573 5578 w 6300489

Sharon Louise 16/08/2007 405-407 Hollinwood Avenue New Moston Manchester M40 0JQ **Tel:** (0161) 684 9449 w 6268105

KELSALL Alison May 05/11/1996 (23/02/2000) 58 Ballater Crescent Vicars Cross CHESTER CH3 5JE **Tel:** (01244) 403928 w 6098382

Julie Margaret (nee Slack) 10/02/2004 2 Repton Drive Haslington Crewe Cheshire CW1 5SA **Tel:** (01270) 252486 w 6291887

KELSEY Leah Harriet 15/12/2008 106 Belvoir Way Peterborough Cambridgeshire PE1 4TQ **Tel:** (01733) 709594 w 6434359

Lisa Ann 30/11/2005 16 Chatsworth Gardens Billingham Cleveland TS22 5JW **Tel:** (01642) 659842 w 6324557

KELSO Amanda Cameron (nee Forsyth) 25/02/1992 Crooklands Bungalow Haywood By Forth Lanarkshire ML11 8ES **Tel:** (01555) 811541 w 6050635

KEMBLE Lorna Marie 27/01/2009 749 Chester Road Erdington Birmingham B24 0BY **Tel:** (0121) 373 4415 w 6351793

KEMP Amy (see RILEY, Mrs)

KEMP Andrea 24/05/2005 20 Hepworth Croft College Town SANDHURST Berkshire GU47 0GH w 6329716

KEMP Emma Louise (see BRICE, Mrs)

Lucy Catherine 17/11/2004 Miramar Veterinary Centre 15 Holt Road Sheringham Norfolk NR26 8NA **Tel:** (01263) 822293 w 6326427

Megan Burton 11/09/2008 10 Vale Mills Boyer Street Derby Derbyshire DE22 3TE w 6420840

Rebecca Jill 20/05/2009 Flat 5 Dove Court London Road UCKFIELD East Sussex TN22 1HU **Tel:** 07784171671 w 6380580

KEMPSHALL Samantha Joy 18/01/2002 (23/02/2009) Flat 3 46 North Road East PLYMOUTH Devon PL4 6AY w 6269524

KEMPSON Claire Madeleine 06/02/1995 10 Harrington Place Brighton East Sussex BN2 3LR **Tel:** (01273) 883609 w 6036428

KENDALL Catherine Mary Christine 15/07/2005 12 Haycroft Road Stevenage Hertfordshire SG1 3JJ **Tel:** (01438) 356116 w 6295484

Emma Patricia 05/10/2004 Inside Pets at Home Middlebrook Retail Park Middlebrook Bolton Lancashire BL6 6JA **Tel:** (01204) 469478 w 6273286

Kimberley Anne 09/09/2008 73 Devonshire Park Bideford Devon EX39 5HZ **Tel:** (01271) 375356 w 6434656

KENDHAMMER Sarah Louise 04/03/2008 137 The Moors Kidlington Oxfordshire OX5 2AQ **Tel:** (01865) 377461 w 6405055

KENDRAY Anna Louise 13/07/2007 503 Norwich Road IPSWICH IP1 6JT **Tel:** (07732) 087952 w 6347503

KENEHAN Lauren Patricia 14/12/2007 (18/02/2009) 18 Hollingbourne Tower Westwell Close ORPINGTON Kent BR5 4QU **Tel:** (01689) 837229 w 6412953

KENNEDY Claire 24/11/2004 18 Grundisburgh Road Woodbridge Suffolk IP12 4HG **Tel:** (01394) 380083 w 6320883

Debra Amanda (nee James) 19/01/1983 Easter Bush Veterinary Centre University of Edinburgh Easter Bush Roslin Midlothian EH25 9RG **Tel:** (0131) 650 7650 w 6090372

KENNEDY Jacqueline (see LAMB, Mrs)

Laureen Ruth 05/03/2002 Clare Veterinary Group 75 Ballynure Road Ballyclare County Antrim BT39 9AG **Tel:** (028) 9332 2223 w 6270866

Lorna Ann 26/01/2010 9 Parr Street Douglas ISLE OF MAN IM1 1BJ **Tel:** (01624) 613406 w 6465478

KENNEDY Shirley (see NOTMAN, Mrs)

Tammy Ann 13/01/2004 Paws Veterinary Health Centre Edward Street Nuneaton Warwickshire CV11 5RP **Tel:** (024) 7638 4064 w 6268930

KENNETT Samantha 13/11/2009 Lower Flat 55 New Road LITTLEHAMPTON West Sussex BN17 5AU **Tel:** (07768) 529612 w 6493330

KENNY Gayle Michelle 12/01/2009 24 Elderwood Road Tranmere BIRKENHEAD Merseyside CH42 5PL **Tel:** 01516419536 w 6434755

KENNY Kate Louise (see MAIL, Ms)

Samantha Victoria 19/08/1992 The Flat 195 Bowerham Road LANCASTER LA1 4HT w 6007929

Sarah Joan 06/03/2006 5 Thames Road St. Helens Merseyside WA9 4HB **Tel:** (01744) 609 697 w 6253299

KENT Claire Elizabeth (formerly Richards) 10/08/1992 (31/05/2000) Penmellyn Veterinary Group Station Road St. Columb Major Cornwall TR9 6BX **Tel:** (01637) 880307 w 6015882

KENT Emma Louise (see RANCE, Mrs)

KENT Jane (see ROEBUCK, Mrs)

Suzanne Mary 02/11/1990 (09/01/2007) Guide Dogs For ther Blind Association Edmondscote Manor Warwick New Road Leamington Spa Warwickshire CV32 6AH **Tel:** (01926) 337244 w 6054480

KENWRIGHT Sarah-Jane (nee Price) 08/03/1998 94 Milton Street MAIDSTONE Kent ME16 8LL **Tel:** (01622) 729446 w 6129492

KENYON Claire Lewis (see ALLISON, Mrs)

KENYON Elizabeth Victoria (see WILCOX-WOOD, Mrs)

KENYON Samantha Jane Lisa (nee Watson) 03/09/1996 (23/10/1998) PDSA Petaid Hospital Acklam Road Middlesbrough Cleveland TS5 4EB **Tel:** (01642) 825793 w 6098859

Sarah Louise (nee Shinn) 29/10/2004 43-47 Holme Lane Hillsborough Sheffield South Yorkshire S6 4JP **Tel:** (0114) 234 3013 w 6262715

KEOGHANE Carrie Ann (see DAVIES, Mrs)

KERKHOFF Nicola Anne 10/07/2009 Flat 12 Kingsdown 115a Ridgway LONDON SW19 4RL **Tel:** 07792686426 w 6560463

KERLEY Michelle 03/09/2002 Queen Mother Hospital for Small Animals Hawkshead Lane North Mymms Hatfield Hertfordshire AL9 7TA **Tel:** (01707) 666366 w 6274595

KERR Clare Frances Elizabeth 01/08/2002 (28/03/2008) 70 Main Street Doune Perthshire FK16 6BW **Tel:** (01786) 841304 w 6271603

Jemma Claire 26/04/2007 126 Main Street Blantyre Glasgow Lanarkshire G72 0EW **Tel:** (01698) 309803 w 6348669

Joan Linda 25/01/2000 19 Chyngton Road Seaford East Sussex BN25 4HL **Tel:** (01323) 899 755 w 6191303

Joanne Lesley (nee Spry) 23/01/1998 Robson Veterinary Hospital Laurencekirk Business Park Aberdeen Road Laurencekirk Kincardineshire AB30 1EY **Tel:** (01561) 377314 w 611556X

Julie-Anne 17/01/2008 14 Binley Road Chelmer Village CHELMSFORD CM2 6XJ **Tel:** (01245) 284 991 w 6386531

KERRIAGE Sasha Joanne 06/12/2004 259 Bilton Road Rugby Warwickshire CV22 7EQ **Tel:** (01788) 812650 w 6258546

KERRIDGE Sally Elizabeth (nee Rose) 10/04/2003 Copperbeech Cottage Carron Aberlour Banffshire AB38 7QP **Tel:** (01340) 810610 w 6277642

KERRIGAN Lynn (formerly Hosking) 08/09/1997 (22/04/2005) 43 Channels Farm Road Swaythling Southampton SO16 2PF **Tel:** (023) 80559872 w 6099502

KERROD Gillian Samantha (nee Arnold) 01/09/1992 Abbey House Veterinary Hospital Commercial Street Morley Leeds West Yorkshire LS27 8AG **Tel:** (0113) 252 5818 w 6005717

KERRY Emma Louise 14/10/2008 24 Offmore Road KIDDERMINSTER Worcestershire DY10 1SA w 6443852

Jenna Rowe 18/11/2009 25 Fairmuir Road Muir of Ord Ross-Shire IV6 7TB **Tel:** (01463) 871 078 w 6403889

KERVELL Jennifer Anne Louise 01/02/2008 C/o Royal College of Veterinary Surgeons 62-64 Horseferry Road LONDON SW1P 2AF w 6382868

KETLEY Maxine Louise (nee Jackson) 22/01/1997 9 Eagle Gardens Bedford Bedfordshire MK41 7FE **Tel:** (01234) 269 076 w 6041347

KEUTENIUS Lucy Madeline 18/04/2005 Flat 1/3 1393 Dumbarton Road Glasgow G14 9XT **Tel:** (0141) 581 6331 w 6317209

KEVAN Emma Elizabeth 11/09/2003 410 Eaton Road West Derby Liverpool L12 3HG **Tel:** (0151) 220 4668 w 6283967

KEY Andrea Jane (see HAZELTINE, Mrs)

KEY Tracey Michelle 11/09/2008 36 Balmoral Road Borrowash DERBY DE72 3FZ **Tel:** 01332672422 w 6429024

KEYTE Angelina Dawn 06/02/2009 350 Peterbrook Road Shirley Solihull West Midlands B90 1HY **Tel:** 01214308724 w 6445436

KEYTER Lea Jade 21/03/2007 489 Kingston Road Wimbledon LONDON SW20 8JP w 6452388

KEYTES Gemma Louise 06/05/2009 16 Queensway Mossley ASHTON-UNDER-LYNE Lancashire OL5 9PA **Tel:** 07590385730 w 6440090

KIBBLE Helen 31/03/2003 38 Deerhurst Chase Bicknacre CHELMSFORD Essex CM3 4XG w 6273539

KIDD Justine Mary 03/10/2004 Davies Veterinary Specialists Manor Farm Business Park Higham Gobion Hertfordshire SG5 3HR **Tel:** (01582) 883950 w 6328209

KILB Estelle Frances (see SMITH, Mrs)

KILBANE Hayley Jayne DipAVN(Surgical) 15/02/2002 University of Bristol School of Veterinary Nursing Veterinary Nursing Unit Langford House Langford Somerset BS40 5DU **Tel:** (0117) 9289517 w 6267665

KILBY Carly Marie 18/10/2006 4 Brae Rise WINSCOMBE Avon BS25 1LW **Tel:** 07793820915 w 6305868

Sarah Louise 03/09/2004 102 Malpas Road Newport Gwent NP20 5PL w 6288774

KILGOUR James Andrew 01/12/2008 Abbey Veterinary Centre 2 Augusta Street Grimsby Lincolnshire DN34 4TA **Tel:** (01472) 347054 m 6411083

KILL Deborah Anne 11/07/2005 CVS (UK) Ltd Animed Veterinary Hospital & Equine Unit Botley Road Shedfield Southampton Hampshire SO32 2JG **Tel:** (01329) 833112 w 6293449

KILLNER Josephine DipAVN(Surgical), DipAVN(Medical) (nee Medland) 03/02/1988 (30/10/2000) 54 Belmont Road Sutton Surrey SM2 6DW w 6093566

KILMURRAY James John 24/06/2009 166 Battersby Lane Warrington Cheshire WA2 7EU **Tel:** 07979298779 m 6379942

KIMBERLEY Sarah Jane 24/01/1993 86 Woodway Lane Coventry CV2 2EJ **Tel:** (024) 76411652 w 6065481

KIN WAI Tung 07/04/2009 Flat 3 2/F, Block N Tai Po Garden Tai Po N.T. Hong Kong **Tel:** (852) 96425999 w 6547967

KINCH Sarah-Jane 13/11/2006 Anchor Lane AYLESBURY Buckinghamshire HP20 1AJ **Tel:** (01296) 745377 w 6273363

KING Alison Jane Remony 12/09/1997 12 Burstellars St. Ives Huntingdon Cambridgeshire PE27 3XY **Tel:** (01604) 635835 w 6117975

Bridget Hazel 04/12/2003 Queen Mother Hospital for Small Animals Hawkshead Lane North Mymms Hatfield Hertfordshire AL9 7TA **Tel:** (01707) 666366 w 6270074

Claire Louise 16/01/2008 15 Fernmoor Drive Irthlingborough Wellingborough Northamptonshire NN9 5TL **Tel:** (01933) 650974 w 6406254

Emily Jane DipAVN(Surgical) 28/11/2000 (04/09/2003) New Priory Veterinary Practice The Deneway London Rd Brighton East Sussex BN1 8QR **Tel:** (01273) 540430 w 6203667

Helen Sarah Elizabeth 25/06/2004 299a St Albans Road Hemel Hempstead Hertfordshire HP2 4RP **Tel:** (01442) 213110 w 6283395

KING Jennifer Ann (see KEEN, Mrs)

Kate Samantha (nee Brown) 07/10/1991 (17/04/2003) South Mudges Farm Ilton Ilminster Somerset TA19 9HL **Tel:** (01460) 57505 w 6046527

Katherine 06/02/2009 33 Lapins Lane Kings Hill WEST MALLING Kent ME19 4LA **Tel:** 07730954632 w 6404868

Laura Louise 18/02/2008 9 Blake Street Wyesham MONMOUTH Gwent NP25 3TH **Tel:** (01600) 711995 w 6406991

Linda Maria (nee Isaac) 24/12/2002 26 Chalfield Close Warminster Wiltshire BA12 8PR **Tel:** (01985) 846759 w 6281030

Natalie Jayne 19/07/2006 115 Manor Hall Road Southwick BRIGHTON West Sussex BN42 4NL **Tel:** (01273) 884356 w 6318045

Pamela Dawn 27/12/2001 Bowbridge Surgery Bowbridge Stroud Gloucestershire GL5 2LA **Tel:** (01453) 762350 w 6263947

Victoria Louise 22/03/2004 106 Hendford Hill Yeovil Somerset BA20 2RF **Tel:** (01935) 474690 w 6275552

KINGDON Cerys (nee Phillips) 15/02/2005 5 Ralph Close Braunton Devon EX33 1DN **Tel:** (01271) 813515 w 6320157

Natalie Louise (nee Scribbins) 06/02/2009 3 Obridge Crescent TAUNTON Somerset TA2 7PZ w 6406023

KINGSCOTT Kayleigh 09/06/2009 24 Caldicot Close Willsbridge BRISTOL BS30 6UU **Tel:** 07825250971 w 6438660

KINGSTON Emma 15/09/2009 129 George Frederick Road Sutton Coldfield B73 6TE **Tel:** (0121) 6053350 w 6490426

Hayley Marie 11/03/2008 Rock Cottage Tresham WOTTON-UNDER-EDGE Gloucestershire GL12 7RW **Tel:** (07791) 224792 w 6405396

Sally Jeanette (nee Moore) 04/06/2009 3 Theo House Bastins Close Park Gate SOUTHAMPTON SO31 1DY **Tel:** (01489) 885167 w 6407783

KINKADE Hannah Louise Jayne 29/06/2007 Burghley Veterinary Centre Ltd St. Leonards Street

Stamford Lincolnshire PE9 2HU **Tel:** (01780) 762109 w 6372385

KINNEAR Ashley Victoria 12/12/2005 Alphavet Veterinary Centre 62 Muirs Kinross KY13 8AU **Tel:** (01577) 863328 w 6264530

Laura May 24/01/2005 29 Main Street Kirkliston West Lothian EH29 9AE **Tel:** (0131) 333 3203 w 6299565

KINSON Lindsay Dawn (see BARKER, Mrs)

KIRBY Ellen Thomasina 10/04/2007 Armac Veterinary Clinic 147 The Rock Bury Lancashire BL9 0ND **Tel:** (0161) 764 4618 w 6333412

Gemma 07/04/2006 4 Swallow Close DUDLEY West Midlands DY2 9TD **Tel:** (01384) 560421 w 6342135

KIRBY Helen Elaine (see JENKINS, Mrs)

Suzanne Maria (nee Clout) 20/11/2002 22 Lyngs Close Yalding Maidstone Kent ME18 6JS **Tel:** (01622) 872050 w 6282966

KIRK Alison Beverley 19/09/2006 3a Illingworth Place Oldbrook Milton Keynes Buckinghamshire MK6 2NP **Tel:** (01908) 234 146 w 6332389

Darren Richard 10/04/2003 2.15, 285 - 305 Centre Road Bentleigh Victoria 3204 Australia **Tel:** (00) 61 395 577 309 m 6285485

Jayne Michelle 12/12/2005 (17/02/2009) Rushcliffe Veterinary Centre Collington Way West Bridgford Nottinghamshire NG2 7LR **Tel:** (0115) 982 1717 w 6337834

Naomi Jane 20/09/2005 4 Orchard Cottages Berrycroft Soham ELY Cambridgeshire CB7 5BL w 6330211

Sarah Ann (nee Foster) 18/01/1993 (26/09/2007) 10 Sandown Road Toton Beeston Nottingham NG9 6GN **Tel:** (01159) 176005 w 606538X

KIRKALDY Andrea Lyn 29/10/2004 54 Dovercourt Road Rotherham South Yorkshire S61 1TG **Tel:** (01709) 324126 w 6317704

KIRKBY Jacqueline Louise 06/12/2004 1a Grimsby Road Waltham GRIMSBY South Humberside DN37 0PS w 6307892

KIRKHAM Hannah Louise 10/09/2009 Donnington Grove Veterinary Surgery Oxford Road NEWBURY Berkshire RG14 2JB **Tel:** (01635) 47170 w 6418607

Sian Ellen 10/02/2009 11 Churn Way Wirral Merseyside CH49 2RS **Tel:** 01516259916 w 6394319

KIRKNESS Karla Yvonne (see NEALE, Mrs)

KIRWAN Elizabeth Jane 12/05/2004 Summerfield Lodge Veterinary Surgery 24 Eridge Road Tunbridge Wells Kent TN4 8HJ **Tel:** (01892) 515885 w 6290160

KISSICK Katherine Elizabeth 09/08/1983 Animal Academy Myerscough College Bilsborrow Preston Lancashire PR3 0RY **Tel:** (01995) 642366 w 6054607

KITCHEN Claire Joanne (see MOULIN, Mrs)

KITCHING Sarah Louise 06/10/2009 Flat 2 9A Westgate Patrington Hull North Humberside HU12 0NA w 6420004

Victoria Louise 13/02/2009 53 Flyford Close Lodge Park Redditch Worcestershire B98 7LX **Tel:** 01527452052 w 6451530

KLEIN Rachel (see LEAVIS, Mrs)

Tanja 22/07/2008 6 Shears Drive Amesbury SALISBURY SP4 7YA w 6519829

KLIEM Hayley Louisa 22/02/2007 17 West Meadow Road Braunton Devon EX33 1EB **Tel:** 07909774115 w 6372891

KLIMAS Sharon (nee Klimas, formerly Scobbie) 27/05/2003 (08/01/2009) Thorny Cottage Gaultiquoy Milton Wick Caithness KW1 5SR **Tel:** (01955) 602 989 w 6285111

KLYN Sarah Michelle (see COLLINS, Mrs)

KNAPP Kerry Louise 23/12/2003 (03/02/2009) 30 Chennells Way HORSHAM West Sussex RH12 5TW **Tel:** (01403) 251581 w 6267709

KNEESHAW Michelle 20/03/2008 27 Churchfields BRADFORD West Yorkshire BD2 3JN **Tel:** 07940970017 w 6344214

KNESL Bronwyn Mary 23/11/2001 60 Woodbine Drive Mahopac New York 10541 USA w 6298938

KNIFTON Louise Margaret 26/10/2006 Sileby Hall Cossington Road Sileby Loughborough Leicestershire LE12 7RS **Tel:** (01509) 812445/6 w 6370581

KNIGHT Amy Elizabeth 08/01/2008 103 Melrose Road Thringstone Coalville Leicestershire LE67 8NH w 6401931

Emily Jayne 05/04/2005 (29/06/2009) The Willows Wolverton Road Norton Lindsey Warwick Warwickshire CV35 8JL **Tel:** (01926) 842013 w 6302095

Gemma Louise 24/05/2006 Flat 4 Chilterns 11 Chislehurst Road SIDCUP Kent DA14 6TS w 6288917

Katie 27/04/2006 22 Parc-An-Tansys Pengegon Camborne Cornwall TR11 4DD **Tel:** (01209) 717773 w 6348548

Katie Emma (nee Rimmington) 17/09/1998 (19/04/2002) Abington Park Veterinary Surgery 427 Wellingborough Road Northampton NN1 4EZ **Tel:** (01604) 628 685 w 6113380

KNIGHT Laura (see ANSELL, Mrs)

Leigh Patricia DipAVN(Surgical) 30/01/2001 PDSA Pet Aid Hospital Campus Way Gillingham Business Park Gillingham Kent ME8 0RR **Tel:** (01634) 376347 w 6211565

Lindsay Patricia (nee Penny) 15/02/2002 33 Withy Close ROMSEY Hampshire SO51 7SA w 6268908

Lisa Marie 18/02/2009 97b Main Road Pye Bridge ALFRETON Derbyshire DE55 4NW **Tel:** (01773) 604552 w 6346139

Rachael Susan 31/10/2003 13 Campbell Close RUGELEY Staffordshire WS15 2PP **Tel:** (01889) 585988 w 6286046

Zelda Louise 26/11/2009 Seers Croft Veterinary Surgery Tower Road Faygate Horsham West Sussex RH12 4SD **Tel:** (01293) 851122 w 6489359

KNIGHTLEY Samantha Jane 02/07/2004 (06/11/2008) 33 Clayway ELY Cambridgeshire CB7 4GD w 6290589

KNIGHTS Leila Vivienne 04/08/1992 Ambleside Veterinary Centre 19 Sidney Road Walton-on-Thames Surrey KT12 2NA **Tel:** (01932) 228915 w 6007940

KNOWLER Kimberley Jayne 15/04/2008 Lynwood Veterinary Group Station Road Wimborne Dorset BH21 1RQ **Tel:** (01202) 882101 w 6417177

KNOWLES Louise Anne 13/09/2000 185 Hawthorn Way Lindford BORDON Hampshire GU35 0RJ w 6140563

KNOWLES Melanie Ann (see PESTER, Mrs)

Natalya Rhianna 06/10/2006 17 White Horse Way WESTBURY Wiltshire BA13 3AH **Tel:** (01373) 823857 w 6333423

KNOWLSON Sarah Louise 22/10/2004 615 Wells Road Whitchurch Bristol BS14 9BE **Tel:** (01275) 832410 w 6272263

KNOX Elizabeth Ann (nee Hird) 01/09/1998 (05/01/2010) Old Wheelhouse Whittingham ALNWICK Northumberland NE66 4UP **Tel:** (01665) 574992 w 612188X

Helen Elizabeth 15/12/2004 Dawlea Farm Stogursey Nr Bridgwater Somerset TA5 1PR **Tel:** (01278) 732 910 w 6286420

Laura Jane Mary 27/11/2009 5 Pottery Villas New Road GILLINGHAM Dorset SP8 4JW **Tel:** (01747) 833683 w 6457690

KNUCKEY Helen Louise (see HARRIS, Mrs)

KOLTHAMMER Louise Ann 10/01/2007 90 Percy Road Romford Essex RM7 8RA **Tel:** (01708) 742 227 w 6359812

KORNELUK Jody 24/03/2009 124 High Street Loscoe Heanor Derbyshire DE75 7LG **Tel:** (01773) 761612 w 6371626

KORTAS Rebecca Louise 30/06/2008 4 Victoria Avenue Bredbury Stockport Cheshire SK6 1SD **Tel:** (0161) 6123482 w 6410379

KOSYLO Nichola Stacy 10/01/2007 166 Nottingham Road Eastwood Nottingham NG16 3GG **Tel:** (01773) 769298 w 6331971

KRAMER Lucy Clare 17/02/2009 109 The Knares Basildon Essex SS16 5SB **Tel:** (01268) 543616 w 6417518

KRUG Verena Dagmar 24/01/2008 9 Balmoral Drive Ramsey Forty Foot Ramsey HUNTINGDON Cambridgeshire PE26 2YR w 6404527

KUIPERS Anje Janna Willemina 05/09/2008 6a Clarendon Drive LONDON SW15 1AA **Tel:** (07934) 304663 w 6522348

KUNKEL Susanne 14/03/2005 104 Garthorne Road LONDON SE23 1EN w 6388577

KYLE Laura Jayne 30/03/2006 Capontree Veterinary Centre Greenhill Brampton Cumbria CA8 1SU **Tel:** (01697) 72318 w 6313634

KYTE Rebecca Elizabeth (see HASKELL, Mrs)

L

LA MONICA Christina Jane 25/06/2004 Marches Veterinary Group Ryelands Road Leominster Herefordshire HR6 8PN **Tel:** (01568) 612266 w 6269304

LACE Sara Alexandra 10/04/2003 11 Fletchers Drive Burscough Ormskirk Lancashire L40 5UY **Tel:** (01704) 821242 w 6262473

LACEY Amy Jayne 29/06/2007 Riverside Veterinary Practice Cradge Bank Spalding Lincolnshire PE11 3AB **Tel:** (01775) 723066 w 6382769

Katheryne Helen 18/10/2005 36 Olivet Road Woodseats Sheffield South Yorkshire S8 8QS **Tel:** (0114) 250 7733 w 6323391

Laura Caroline 22/03/2004 85 Lavender Hill Battersea London SW11 5QL **Tel:** (020) 7228 0648 w 6302128

Sarah Joanne 02/11/2004 32 Cumberland Road Chafford Hundred Grays Essex RM16 6DS **Tel:** (01375) 480544 w 6311379

LACK Teresa Jane (nee Lack, formerly Purssord) 23/01/1996 32 Brook Street Colne Engaine Colchester ESSEX CO6 2JD **Tel:** (01787) 224450 w 6033620

LACKEY Janine Ann (see BRADY, Mrs)

LADKIN Catherine Gillian 15/07/2005 42 Rancliffe Crescent LEICESTER LE3 1NQ w 6294296

LAGNA Charlotte Elizabeth 17/07/2003 53 Farm Hill EXETER EX4 2LW w 6274298

LAING Michelle Margaret 28/02/2007 48 Pine Court Cumbernauld GLASGOW G67 3AY **Tel:** (0141) 777 6947 w 6345677

Samantha 09/07/2007 50 Windsor Drive Wingerworth CHESTERFIELD Derbyshire S42 6TJ w 6352607

LAIRD Heather Morag (see PACKHAM, Mrs)

LAKEHAL Samantha Lesley 19/02/2001 Fremantle Post Shop PO Box 293 Fremantle Western Australia 6959 Australia **Tel:** (00) 61 8 042 427 1903 w 6212368

LAKEMAN Elizabeth Anna (see JONES, Miss)

LAKEMAN Nicola Anne (see ACKERMAN, Mrs)

LAKIN Faye 28/04/2009 54 Larch Road Liverpool Merseyside L36 9TZ **Tel:** (0151) 489 7674 w 6437021

LALL Sheila Margaret 31/10/2003 12 Lincoln Drive Waddington LINCOLN LN5 9NH **Tel:** (01522) 722209 w 6277752

LAMB Catherine Margaret 24/08/1998 29 York Place Knaresborough North Yorkshire HG5 0AD **Tel:** (01423) 862 121 w 6128433

Jacqueline (nee Kennedy) 10/12/2002 6 Cairnsgarroch Way Bourtreehill South IRVINE Ayrshire KA11 1EW **Tel:** (01294) 216 452 w 6282394

Kathryn Alexandra 29/01/2009 3 Fordwich Street Butler Perth Western Australia 6036 Australia w 6417067

Sophie Charlotte 01/06/2007 59 Barfields Bletchingley REDHILL RH1 4RD w 6374684

LAMBERT Nicola Jane 23/02/2005 43 Chambers Road ST. LEONARDS-ON-SEA East Sussex TN38 9HY **Tel:** (07717) 884269 w 6320124

Ruth Ann (nee Bennett) 30/01/1996 3 Poundbury Business Centre Poundbury Dorchester Dorset DT1 3WA **Tel:** (01305) 267083 w 6037239

LAMBIE Alison Jane (see LAMBIE-DAMER, Mrs)

LAMBIE-DAMER Alison Jane (nee Lambie) 31/10/2003 9 Montrose Street Brierfield NELSON Lancashire BB9 5BZ w 6277686

LAMBTON Donna 02/03/1988 (24/04/2006) 28 Woodlands Road Ansdell Lytham St Annes Lancashire FY8 4EP w 6052676

LAMONT Jane Matilda Margaret (nee Hopkinson, formerly Craven) 18/10/1990 Beechwood Veterinary Group 430 Dewsbury Road Leeds LS11 7LJ **Tel:** (01132) 700325 w 6048444

Joanna Rosamund 15/09/2009 Ardene House Veterinary Hospital Kingswells Aberdeen AB15 8PJ **Tel:** (01224) 740700 w 6436262

LAMOURY Joanne (see MCCARTNEY, Mrs)

LAMPARD Angela Jane (see CHAPMAN, Miss)

LAMSLEY Deborah Ann 18/07/2002 12 Guildford Road West FARNBOROUGH Hampshire GU14 6PU **Tel:** (0870) 040 0014 w 6316626

LANCASTER Elizabeth Grace (see STACKHOUSE, Mrs)

LAND Ceri (nee Williams) 03/09/1999 79-81 Poplar Road Redditch Worcestershire B97 6NY **Tel:** (01527) 67402 w 6135371

LAND Karina Michelle (see HORTON, Mrs)

Natalie 14/05/2007 24 Heathway Seaham County Durham SR7 7UX **Tel:** (01915) 815 662 w 6374695

LANDAIS Annick Martine Louise 16/01/1996 (17/09/1999) Sir Harold Harmsworth Memorial Hospital 22 Sonderburg Road London N7 7QD **Tel:** (0870) 753 8081 w 6034646

LANDER Jocelyn Christie 29/12/2003 5a Elcombe Swindon Wiltshire SN4 9QL **Tel:** (01793) 814960 w 6353564

Kate Elisabeth 08/11/2006 (06/08/2009) Veterinary Health Centre 52 Clarendon Street Leamington Spa Warwickshire CV32 4PE **Tel:** (01926) 330179 w 6375553

Laura Anne (nee Cornwell) 22/09/2004 The Vale Veterinary Centre Station Road Tiverton Devon EX16 4LF **Tel:** (01884) 253355 w 6319530

LANDSBERG Claire Louise (nee Parker) 22/03/2004 56 Tweseldown Road Church Crookham FLEET Hampshire GU52 8DF **Tel:** (01252) 616513 w 6303767

LANE Gillian Linda (nee Edgar) 29/06/2007 (19/01/2010) 40 Echline Terrace SOUTH QUEENSFERRY West Lothian EH30 9XH **Tel:** (0131) 331 2206 w 6347008

Leanne 03/06/2004 281 Hempstead Road Gillingham Kent ME7 3QJ **Tel:** 07747712405 w 6292173

Nicola (nee Windeatt) 17/09/2003 49 Sutton Close TORQUAY Devon TQ2 8LL w 6272824

Sarah Rebecca (nee Quinn) 24/01/2005 121 Lower Street Pulborough West Sussex RH20 2BP **Tel:** (01798) 872089 w 6291029

Stephanie Victoria 29/06/2007 2 Buttercrambe Road Stamford Bridge York YO41 1AN **Tel:** (01759) 371066 w 6345996

Victoria 15/02/2008 10 Laird Drive SHEFFIELD S6 4BW **Tel:** 07739139949 w 6410357

LANG Aileen Elizabeth 28/10/2003 60 Willson Croft BIRMINGHAM B28 0SS **Tel:** (0131) 449 3967 w 6282350

Tracy Angela 03/03/2005 78 David Street Grimsby South Humberside DN32 9NN **Tel:** (01472) 319406 w 6319167

LANGHAM-HOBART Karen Jean 26/08/2003 (01/09/2009) 23 Milton Abbas BLANDFORD FORUM Dorset DT11 0BL **Tel:** (020) 8561 2123 w 6282647

LANGLEY Rebecca Louise 07/04/2009 51d Fleet Road Rochester Kent ME1 2QA **Tel:** 01634405939 w 6448461

LANGNER Karen Eleanor 24/02/2009 Argoed Brymbo Road Bwlchgwyn Wrexham Clwyd LL11 5UB **Tel:** 01978757859 w 6447185

LANGRIDGE Alison Jayne 23/08/2004 Clinical Skills Centre Royal Veterinary College Hawkshead Lane North Mymms Hatfield Hertfordshire AL9 7TA w 6297299

LANGRISH Natasha Jayne (see GOODERHAM, Mrs)

LANGSTON Dulcie 29/08/2008 26 Gannel View Close Lane NEWQUAY Cornwall TR8 4NH **Tel:** 01637852088 w 6410973

LANGVAD Trine 01/04/2008 6 Oxford Street Exning NEWMARKET Suffolk CB8 7EW **Tel:** (01638) 578127 w 6510281

LANHAM Karin Rebecca 21/11/2005 4 Proctor Close Maidenbower CRAWLEY West Sussex RH10 7JW **Tel:** (01293) 413592 w 6342146

LANSLEY Sarah Jane Louise (nee Cooke) 28/01/2009 4 Coombe Lane Whiteley Village Hersham WALTON-ON-THAMES Surrey KT12 4EL **Tel:** (01932) 854278 w 6339033

LARKIN Jane Elizabeth 10/02/2005 The Barn Veterinary Surgery Wenham Road Copdock Ipswich IP8 3EY **Tel:** (01473) 730213 w 6295506

LARKINS Emma Louise (see MIDGLEY, Mrs)

LARMOUR Emma Jane 07/02/2006 Cedarmount Veterinary Clinic 67 Bryansburn Road Bangor County Down BT20 3SD **Tel:** (02891) 271364 w 6326064

Lisa Claire (nee Martin) 28/08/1997 28 Frensham Close Banbury Oxfordshire OX16 1FQ **Tel:** (0795) 81 3496 w 6034555

LARNDER Lorna Mary (nee Blackburn) 27/08/2003 52 The Green Freethorpe Norwich Norfolk NR13 3AH **Tel:** (01603) 713269 w 6272417

LASHLEY Helen Marjorie (nee Dunn) 07/02/2006 14 Petterson Dale Coxhoe Durham DH6 4HA **Tel:** (0191) 384 7609 w 6253750

LASHMAR Tineka Cherree 14/09/2001 11 Marlborough Road MARGATE Kent CT9 5SU w 6139660

LAST Emma Jane 10/11/2008 49 Peppard Road Caversham READING RG4 8NH **Tel:** (0118) 972 3562 w 6427165

LATHAM Lesley Jayne (nee Corbett, formerly Swaine) 17/01/1991 Mercia Veterinary Surgery 28 Marmion Street Tamworth Staffordshire B79 7JG **Tel:** (01827) 54343 w 6048207

LATTER Zoe Clare (nee Brown) 28/08/1991 53 Westway Gardens Redhill Surrey RH1 2JB **Tel:** (01737) 761563 w 6046593

LATTO Rona Carmel 23/01/1995 (13/03/2002) Meadows Veterinary Centre Station Road Oldmeldrum Inverurie Aberdeenshire AB51 0EZ **Tel:** (01651) 872481 w 6029126

LAUGHLIN Denise Margaret 13/04/2004 30 Bellrock Avenue PRESTWICK Ayrshire KA9 1SQ w 6291348

LAUNDON Cally Ann 09/03/2005 41 Friar Walk WORTHING West Sussex BN13 1BL w 6290809

LAVERY Amanda Claire 14/05/2007 3 Danaway Cottages Maidstone Road Borden Sittingbourne Kent ME9 7PT **Tel:** (07815) 092044 w 6342652

LAVIGNE Julie 20/10/2008 44 Lower Dagnall Street ST. ALBANS Hertfordshire AL3 4PY w 6537143

LAVIN Samantha Jane (see ATKINS, Mrs)

LAW Claire Louise 06/02/2002 28 Peregrine Drive Tile Kiln Farm Estate CHELMSFORD Essex CM2 8XY w 6273000

Emma Margaret 10/03/2009 11 Carlton Road EASTBOURNE East Sussex BN22 7EN **Tel:** 07747094978 w 6449396

LAW Karen Louise (see MCQUOID, Mrs)

Stacey Ann 06/08/2008 10 Methuen Avenue Hoghton Preston Lancashire PR5 0JN **Tel:** (01254) 853767 w 6413283

LAWES Carly Phillipa 08/12/2008 22 Sovereign Court RUSHDEN Northamptonshire NN10 6EZ **Tel:** (07956) 222782 w 6438253

Nicola Anne (nee Causer) 10/05/2007 32 Winter Drive Hawkinge Folkestone Kent CT18 7QX **Tel:** (01303) 893 442 w 6383671

LAWLESS Louise Claire 22/09/2006 25 Gainsborough Road Warrington Cheshire WA4 6DA **Tel:** (01925) 636 474 w 6332356

LAWLEY Shelly Marie (see THORNE, Mrs)

LAWRENCE Briony Dawn 11/02/2008 94 Apollo Walk HULL HU8 0TT **Tel:** (01482) 374 0139 w 6416495

Doreen Molly (nee Greaves) 06/02/1979 (23/01/2007) 6 Hollycombe Close Liphook Hampshire GU30 7HR **Tel:** (01428) 723415 w 6003345

LAWRENCE Joanna (see LEWIS, Mrs)

Lindsey Jane 20/11/2008 20 Montpelier WESTON-SUPER-MARE Avon BS23 2RH w 6394297

Michelle 08/11/2006 2 Wyndcliffe Court Cottages St Arvans Chepstow Gwent NP16 6EY w 6301930

Rowena Clare 18/04/2008 The Veterinary Hospital 4 Bath Road Hungerford Berkshire RG17 0HE **Tel:** (01488) 682193/683999 w 6351628

LAWRENCE Tracy Anne (see GREENSMITH, Mrs)

LAWS Elizabeth Rosina 02/11/2000 West Court Farm Cliffe Rochester Kent ME3 7ST **Tel:** (01634) 220238 w 6202710

LAWSON Amy Claire 20/11/2008 3 Washpit Cottage Choppards Lane Holmfirth West Yorkshire HD9 2RE w 6411611

Eleanor Judith 24/01/1989 Culverden Veterinary Group 11 Culverden Park Road Tunbridge Wells Kent TN4 9RD **Tel:** (01892) 520296 w 6094366

Gail Carolyn 04/05/1966 Wild Rose Cottage 19 Watergates Lane Broadmayne Dorchester Dorset DT2 8HA **Tel:** (01305) 854205 w 6001097

LAWSON Heather Elizabeth (see MCINTYRE, Mrs)

Victoria Christine 04/02/2009 Hinton Farm Hinton Chippenham Wiltshire SN14 8HG **Tel:** 01179373649 w 6410368

LAWTON Claire Marie 06/07/2004 (21/07/2008) Kiln Cottage Stokes Marsh Lane Coulston Wetybury Wiltshire BA13 4NZ **Tel:** (013870) 830603 w 6288422

LAYE Lisa Karen (nee Fell) 04/12/2003 72 Woodlands Avenue Rustington Littlehampton West Sussex BN16 3EY **Tel:** (01903) 785762 w 6287872

LAYEN Dawn Catherine (see BODE, Mrs)

LAZENBY Kate Dawn 21/05/2007 18 Fairways Whitley Bay Tyne and Wear NE25 9YG **Tel:** (0191) 2513177 w 6373309

LE BER Demelza Jayne 29/04/2009 Mandeville Braye Road Vale Guernsey Channel Islands GY3 5PA **Tel:** 01481244291 w 6409367

LE CORNU Rebecca Clare 10/02/2009 Meadowvale La Rue Es Philippes Grouville Jersey Channel Islands JE3 9UZ **Tel:** 07700339138 w 6421654

LE COUILLIARD Samantha Laura 20/11/2009 Highview House La Rue Militaire St. John Jersey Channel Islands JE3 4DP **Tel:** 07797778588 w 6420851

LE GALLOUDEC Nicola Marie 26/08/1999 Isabelle Vets Route Isabelle St. Peter Port Guernsey GY1 1QR **Tel:** (01481) 723863 w 6185880

LE PAGE Alison Elaine (see LE PAGE-BRIDGE, Mrs)

LE PAGE-BRIDGE Alison Elaine (nee Le Page) 20/03/1991 (07/10/2003) 25 St James Close Lostock Hall Preston Lancashire PR5 5RJ **Tel:** (01772) 311046 w 6054913

LE QUELENEC Tracey (nee Leetham) 25/08/1999 (28/08/2003) End Cottage Veterinary Clinic Boothferry Road Howden Goole DN14 7TA **Tel:** (01430) 434861 w 6145404

LEA Karen Margaret 28/03/2008 22 Glen Park Drive Hesketh Bank Nr Preston Lancashire PR4 6TA w 6263364

Samantha 29/01/2007 Fern Cottage Veterinary Surgery 233-235 Park Road Sittingbourne Kent ME10 1ER **Tel:** (01795) 476411 w 6371637

LEACH Diane (see WYNN, Mrs)

LEACH Victoria Lorraine 09/09/2004 109 Ash Hill Road Ash ALDERSHOT Hampshire GU12 5DN w 6274496

LEADBEATER Bethany Clare (nee Leonard-Williams) 08/01/2008 Ashfield Veterinary Group 118 Queens Road Halifax West Yorkshire HX1 3XY **Tel:** (01422) 365306 w 6358811

Wendy 30/01/2001 16 Ely Crescent WEST BROMWICH West Midlands B71 2SD **Tel:** (07786) 860228 w 6152717

LEAHY Eibhlin 26/04/2007 64 Fallow Rise HERTFORD SG13 7NL w 6454500

LEAKE Alison Clare 10/10/2005 Archenfield Veterinary Surgery Archenfield Road Ross-on-Wye Herefordshire HR9 5AZ **Tel:** (01989) 562115 w 6332400

Tina Rebecca 26/09/1999 (28/04/2004) 6 Folkestone Road Walthamstow LONDON E17 9SD **Tel:** 07717643084 w 6185517

LEAR Tracey Elizabeth DipAVN(Surgical) 28/07/1992 Top Floor Flat Nempnett Farm Nempnett Thrubwell Blagdon BRISTOL BS40 7UZ **Tel:** (01761) 462081 w 6054957

LEATHAM Claire Louise 22/02/2008 110 Lindsey Avenue York North Yorkshire YO26 4RL **Tel:** (01904) 341 694 w 6404428

LEATHERLAND Amy Louise 13/08/2007 15 Nuttall Street ALFRETON Derbyshire DE55 7AY w 6331245

LEAVENS Sarah Louise (see ADAMSON, Mrs)

LEAVER Caroline (see THORNBORROW, Mrs)

LEAVIS Rachel (nee Klein) 22/03/2004 27 Chiltern Drive Edith Weston OAKHAM Rutland LE15 8HN w 6250725

LEDBURY Heather Frances (nee Willey) 01/06/2007 Flat 5 Waterside House The Wharf Pangbourne READING RG8 7DS **Tel:** (0188) 984 1818 w 6355346

LEDWARD Amanda Claire 18/10/2006 5 Lyncroft Close Crewe Cheshire CW1 6HP **Tel:** (01270) 584862 w 6374706

LEE Adweena Tsoi Ling 21/07/2008 The Veterinary Surgery Kenyon Street Accrington Lancashire BB5 1BE **Tel:** (01254) 231703 w 6381867

Angharad Elizabeth 05/07/2006 20 Charles Street Griffithstown Pontypool Gwent NP4 5HQ **Tel:** (01495) 752327 w 6301688

Beverley May (formerly Hudson) 31/03/2003 Cromwell Veterinary Hospital 36-36a St. Johns Street HUNTINGDON Cambridgeshire PE29 3DG **Tel:** (01480) 52601/52222 w 6275860

Helen Barbara 28/02/2008 23 Plumpton Walk Bradford West Yorkshire BD2 1PB **Tel:** (01274) 780 250 w 6388731

Joanne Tracey (formerly Lee) 13/08/2004 (05/02/2009) The Granary Bunstead Barns Poles Lane Hursley Winchester Hampshire SO21 2LL **Tel:** (01962) 767920 w 6291700

LEE Kathryn Helen (see JONES, Mrs)

Laura Elizabeth 31/10/2005 Silva House Veterinary Clinic Silver Street Midsomer Norton Radstock Somerset BA3 2ET **Tel:** (01761) 412223 w 6346568

Maggie Mei Ki 01/04/2009 G/F No. 5 Wang Che Village Sai Kung Hong Kong **Tel:** (852) 63380465 w 6547307

Michelle 21/08/1998 (21/01/2009) 28 Broad Lane Brinsley Nottingham NG16 5BD **Tel:** (01773) 780622 w 611337X

Michelle Lorraine 21/12/2005 Stirling Lodge Clinic 2 Stirling Road CHICHESTER West Sussex PO19 7DJ **Tel:** (01243) 786101 w 6308233

Nicole Leeann (nee Chambers) 04/12/2003 28 Dupre Close Chafford Hundred Grays Essex RM16 6RA **Tel:** (01375) 481 917 w 6273627

Susan Evelyn 17/07/2003 25 Baker Street POTTERS BAR Hertfordshire EN6 2DZ **Tel:** (01707) 658 508 w 6284957

Victoria Louise 18/05/2009 9 Watery Lane Northolt Middlesex UB5 6QL **Tel:** 07768737677 w 6434447

LEE FALCONER Rebecca 01/07/2008 Cogges Veterinary Surgery Cogges Hill Road Witney Oxfordshire OX28 3XY **Tel:** (01993) 772 627 w 6367116

LEECH Rachel Ann (nee Pellow, nee Pellow) 10/06/2003 (19/04/2005) 101 Barrington Road Loughton Essex IG10 2AX **Tel:** (0208) 508 9084 w 6268831

Sarah Jane (nee Heard) 13/05/1997 (12/05/2008) 6 Woodseaves Close Irlam MANCHESTER M44 6RQ w 6108585

LEEDHAM-HAWKES Chantelle 16/09/2004 19 Mountside Street Hednesford Staffordshire WS12 4DD **Tel:** (01543) 879 768 w 6294351

LEEKS Samantha Jane 18/02/2008 78 Rigbourne Hill Beccles Suffolk NR34 9JH **Tel:** (01502) 712 134 w 6401854

LEESON Jill Tracey 21/03/2007 213 Melton Road Edwalton Nottingham Nottinghamshire NG12 4AF **Tel:** (01159) 145002 w 6351298

LEETHAM Tracey (see LE QUELENEC, Mrs)

LEGG Jane Louise Alice 24/01/2006 33 Pear Tree Close Alderholt FORDINGBRIDGE Hampshire SP6 3ER w 6348449

Ruth Elizabeth (nee Selleck) 13/11/2006 5 Ruffets Wood Gravesend Kent DA12 5JQ **Tel:** (077) 911 90873 w 6368766

LEGGO Diane Mary (nee Tripp) 24/01/1997 (05/03/2002) Mead Barn Butcombe BRISTOL BS40 7XF **Tel:** (01761) 462771 w 6109137

LEHRER Ceri Marie 25/09/2008 18 White Road Methwold THETFORD Norfolk IP26 4PA **Tel:** 01366727097 w 6388742

LEIGH Charlene Zoe 24/09/2009 43 Gladstone Street Loughborough Leicestershire LE11 1NR w 6489458

LEIGH Debra Kay (see SMITH, Mrs)

Emma 22/05/2001 (20/12/2004) Alnorthumbria Veterinary Practice Ltd Belvedere Terrace Alnwick Northumberland NE66 2NX **Tel:** (01665) 602516 w 6218253

LEIGHTON Liza Jane (nee Weller) 24/02/2004 73 Halcyon Road Newton Abbot Devon TQ12 2LY **Tel:** (01626) 365425 w 6273418

Zoe Michelle 22/10/2009 Booth Cottage Cinder Lane St. Michaels TENBURY WELLS Worcestershire WR15 8PN **Tel:** (01584) 810227 w 6466930

LEIVERS Samantha Jane 11/11/2008 3 Coronation Road Hucknall Nottingham Nottinghamshire NG15 7EJ **Tel:** 01159529360 w 6410720

LEMKE Tracy Leigh Dawn (see GRIFFITHS, Mrs)

LENNIE Suzanne Donna 16/08/2007 8 Lochinvar Place Bonnybridge Stirlingshire FK4 2BL **Tel:** (01324) 880 545 w 6373496

LENNOX Gemma Louise 31/10/2006 1 Manley Gardens Longlevens Gloucestershire GL2 0HY **Tel:** (01452) 506223 w 6276696

LENTON Wendy Ann (see PARKINSON, Mrs)

LEONARD Deborah Anne 22/04/2008 2 Wessex Way Highworth Swindon Wiltshire SN6 7NT **Tel:** (07730) 532818 w 6405308

Debra Fiona 04/02/2002 3 Amy Close Longford Coventry West Midlands CV6 6NZ **Tel:** (02476) 360470 w 6272461

LEONARD-WILLIAMS Bethany Clare (see LEADBEATER, Mrs)

LESZCZYNSKI Zoe Angela (nee Gravenor) 06/04/2001 97 Brendon Grove Bingham NOTTINGHAM NG13 8TN w 6215151

LETCH Fiona Elizabeth Joyce 15/05/2009 27 Winchester Drive Midway Swadlincote Derbyshire DE11 7LR **Tel:** (01283) 223101 w 6405924

LEVENSCOTE Michelle Anne (see LEVESCONTE, Miss)

LEVER Sarah 29/08/2008 106 Ellington Drive BASINGSTOKE Hampshire RG22 4EX w 6412854

LEVER-BECK Hannah Lisa 30/01/1996 (08/01/2009) Newnham Court Veterinary Group Bearsted Road Weavering Maidstone Kent ME14 5EL **Tel:** (01622) 734555 w 6020280

LEVESCONTE Michelle Anne (formerly Levenscote) 19/03/2007 (18/11/2009) 18 Oaktree Garth WELWYN GARDEN CITY Hertfordshire AL7 3UZ w 6320949

LEVETT Sharon Joanne (see SIMS, Mrs)

LEVIN Jo Ann 26/02/2000 (19/05/2004) 2 Broadway Bebington Wirral Merseyside CH63 5NH **Tel:** (0151) 608 7822 w 6041267

LEVITT Amie Jane (see ATKINS, Mrs)

LEVITT Jenifer Davina 15/04/2004 (26/05/2009) Inside Pets at Home Wessex Gate Retail Park Broadstone Way Poole Dorset BH15 3TE **Tel:** (01202) 677675 w 6264299

LEVITT Louise Marie (see DRISCOLL, Mrs)

LEWCHENKO Tracy 17/12/2007 The Veterinary Hospital 23 Wellington Street Thame Oxfordshire OX9 3BW **Tel:** (01844) 212000 w 6371054

LEWENDON Karen Louise (nee Taylor) 17/08/1990 (18/11/1999) 29 Sand Hill Shrivenham Swindon Wiltshire SN6 8BQ **Tel:** (01793) 784 724 w 6061760

LEWINGTON Lisa Victoria 11/02/2008 28 Sloe Close WESTON-SUPER-MARE Avon BS22 7DG w 6366335

LEWINS Alexandra Gentle (see SPENCELEY, Mrs)

LEWIS Ana Alicia 28/02/2007 238 Chelmsford Avenue Grimsby South Humberside DN34 5DF **Tel:** (079) 514 28191 w 6349736

Bernadette Anne Marie (nee Martin) 06/08/1991 (18/07/2001) The Old Post Office Yeolmbridge Launceston PL15 8TH **Tel:** (01566) 777087 w 6055917

Donna Leigh 28/02/2001 Pet Care Veterinary Surgery 355 Bexley Road Erith Kent DA8 3EZ **Tel:** (01322) 346173 w 6213325

Elisabeth Anne 14/01/1991 (18/06/2001) The Veterinary Surgery Redmans Hill Blackford Wedmore Somerset BS28 4NG **Tel:** (01934) 712229 w 6001100

Gemma Louise 11/09/2009 18 Birch Grove Birchmoor Tamworth Staffordshire B78 1AP **Tel:** (01827) 892246 w 6434634

Gemma Suzanne 23/02/2005 11 Fairhaven Avenue Croydon Surrey CR0 7RX **Tel:** (020) 8656 5600 w 6320135

Jane Louise (nee Jefferd) 23/07/2009 40 Clarendon Road Aylesham Kent CT3 3AG w 6389281

Joanna (nee Lawrence) 13/10/1998 (18/12/2009) The Croft Lower Vexford Lydeard St. Lawrence Taunton Somerset TA4 3QJ **Tel:** (01984) 667454 w 6133851

Joanna Isabel 29/01/2001 53 Queens Road Tewkesbury Gloucestershire GL20 5EL **Tel:** (01684) 273412 w 6211356

Joanne (nee Hughes) 31/12/2003 9 Pen-y-Gam Terrace Haested Nr Bridgend Mid Glamorgan Wales CF34 9AU **Tel:** (01656) 735458 w 6289159

Karlene Diane 07/12/2009 29 De Havilland Close Upper Cambourne CAMBRIDGE CB23 6BP **Tel:** 01954715785 w 6431928

Kathryn Amanda 10/01/2007 Salisbury Bungalow Newton in Bowland Clitheroe Lancashire BB7 3DZ **Tel:** (01200) 446 366 w 6353861

Kelly Ann 28/06/2005 10 Pearmain Close Willand Cullompton Devon EX15 2TD **Tel:** (01884) 820 986 w 6399984

Laura 31/10/2003 4 Manby Street LINCOLN LN5 8NW w 6257237

Lucinda Jo 28/02/2007 The Lodge Aintree Hospital Gate Longmoor Lane Liverpool Merseyside L9 7LQ **Tel:** (0151) 525 0847 w 6352805

Mandy Nicola (nee Crutchley) 06/07/2004 Broad Lane Vets Ltd 255 Broad Lane Coventry West Midlands CV5 7AQ **Tel:** (024) 7646 4789 w 6290820

LEWIS Michelle Rose (see THOMAS, Mrs)

Rebecca Louise (nee Tannahill) 15/02/2005 The Oak Veterinary Group, Prendergast Farm Well Lane Haverfordwest Dyfed SA61 2PL **Tel:** (01437) 760111 w 6301864

LEWIS Sarah Peggy (see WYATT, Mrs)

Tracey Ann 17/04/2008 53 Waterside Mews NEWPORT Shropshire TF10 7PA w 6400028

LEWITT Christie Suzanne (see LEWITT-SMITH, Mrs)

LEWITT-SMITH Christie Suzanne (nee Lewitt) 12/05/2004 5 The Cygnets FELTHAM Middlesex TW13 6NA **Tel:** (020) 8898 9684 w 6266488

LEWORTHY Joanna 08/11/1999 (01/03/2006) 17 Oakford Villas North Molton South Molton Devon EX36 3HN **Tel:** (01598) 740079 w 6186364

Katie May DipAVN(Surgical) 04/12/2003 Shallowford Farm Lynton North Devon EX35 6PH **Tel:** (01271) 866770 w 6270294

Richard Gordan 10/02/2004 122 Pennine Road Bromsgrove Worcestershire B61 0TN **Tel:** (01562) 883621 m 6275101

LEY Rebecca Sandra (see MILLS, Mrs)

LEYSHON Kathryn Anne (see HOCKING, Mrs)

LIDDLE Marion Tait (see WEDDERBURN, Ms)

LIDDON Sarah Georga 24/01/2005 29 Redwood Way BARNET Hertfordshire EN5 2RU w 6291227

LIDSTER Sarah Helen (see SILVER, Mrs)

LIFFEN Tara Lynn 27/04/2006 2 Euston Court FELIXSTOWE Suffolk IP11 2YD **Tel:** (07917) 411276 w 6329023

LIGGINS Clare Louise 14/09/2009 177 Long Furrow East Goscote LEICESTER LE7 3ST w 6453180

LIGHT Charlotte Ivy 02/10/2009 Forest Veterinary Centre Hemnall Street Epping Essex CM16 4LQ **Tel:** (01992) 575790 w 6452729

Emma Jane (nee Cooke) 10/04/2003 6 Scotter Square Bishopstoke EASTLEIGH Hampshire SO50 6DP w 6284946

Stephanie 04/06/2009 4 Highfield Close Angmering LITTLEHAMPTON West Sussex BN16 4BQ w 6407805

LIGHTFOOT Deborah 16/04/2007 University of Glasgow Veterinary School Garscube Estate Glasgow G61 1QH **Tel:** (0141) 330 5848 w 6453477

Sarah June 03/03/2005 19 Sandhill Road Farndon Newark Nottinghamshire NG24 4TE **Tel:** (01636) 686514 w 6319178

LIGHTOWLER Tina (see NASH, Mrs)

LILLEY Emma Louise 21/01/2009 The Lane Veterinary Clinic 374 Moston Lane Old Moston MANCHESTER M40 9JS **Tel:** (0161) 682 2122 w 6374717

LIMBRICK Tracy Jane (see GROOMBRIDGE, Mrs)

LIMEBEAR Katherine Ann (nee Syckelmoore) 21/08/1995 2 Hartley Cottage Hartley Wespall Hook Hampshire RG27 0BB **Tel:** (01256) 883151 w 6036461

LIMENTANI Alison 04/08/2009 Wood Green Animal Shelter Kingbush Farm London Road Godmanchester Huntingdon Cambridgeshire PE29 2NH **Tel:** (0844) 2488181 w 6436207

LIN Bik Kei 17/08/2005 SPCA (HK) No 5 Wan Shing St Wai Chai Hong Kong **Tel:** (+852) 28020501 w 6339154

LINDLEY Karen Yvette (nee Swain) 04/08/1981 51 Priory Drive Plymouth Devon PL7 1PX **Tel:** (01752) 330703 w 6003265

LINDO Mary Dominique 30/08/2000 Watkins & Tasker Veterinary Group 2a Chescombe Road Yatton BRISTOL BS49 4EJ **Tel:** (01934) 833 685 w 6204074

LINDON Rebecca Louise 11/08/2009 39 Weston Road Aston Clinton Aylesbury Buckinghamshire HP22 5EJ **Tel:** 01296632714 w 6437076

LINDOP Holly Louise 14/01/2008 38 Downlands Road Devizes Wiltshire SN10 5EB **Tel:** (01380) 724307 w 6366346

LINDSAY Denise 14/03/2006 Unit 1, Asda Shopping Centre Jesmond Drive Bridge of Don Aberdeen AB22 8UR **Tel:** (01224) 826121 w 6257611

LINDSAY Rachel Marianne (see SHARMA, Mrs)

LINES Lisa Vicky 25/02/2003 2 Sunbury Court Manor Road BARNET Hertfordshire EN5 2JH **Tel:** (07980) 029 882 w 6280304

Rebecca Jane 23/05/2008 85b Gammons Lane WATFORD WD24 5HU **Tel:** (01923) 774 955 w 6403020

LINEY Lynda Anne (formerly Alexander) 29/08/1996 2 Hornage Cottage Bicester Road Brill Aylesbury Buckinghamshire HP18 9SE **Tel:** (01844) 238768 w 6042544

LINGARD Jacqueline Ann (see HARVEY, Miss)

LINLEY Sarah Louise 16/01/2008 Springfield Veterinary Group 1 Stubbin Lane Sheffield South Yorkshire S5 6QG **Tel:** (0114) 2422 815 w 6366357

LIPSCOMBE Andrew James 04/10/2005 24 Abbeydale Road South Sheffield South Yorkshire S7 2QN **Tel:** (0114) 2363391 m 6281063

LIPTROTT Sophie Ruth 30/07/2002 11 Sidford Close Darcy Lever BOLTON BL3 1RW **Tel:** (01204) 380881 w 6268127

LISHER Jonathan Michael 07/05/2009 97 Downland Court Stonery Road Portslade Brighton East Sussex BN41 2PS **Tel:** (01273) 426 100 m 6443885

LISTER Julie Alexia Dawn 26/01/1999 44 Lakeside Close Old Whittington CHESTERFIELD Derbyshire S41 9TD **Tel:** (07866) 450047 w 6170645

Samantha 08/02/2008 1 Eastwood Terrace Ossett West Yorkshire WF5 9LQ **Tel:** (01924) 260057 w 6403713

LITCHFIELD Claire Elizabeth 20/11/2002 4 Hall Lane Cottage Main Street Little Brington NORTHAMPTON NN7 4HS **Tel:** (07775) 597 644 w 6273451

Sarah Louise 21/12/2005 7 Phillips Field Road Great Cornard SUDBURY Suffolk CO10 0JH w 6317440

LITHGO Rachel (nee Neale, formerly Atkins) 27/08/1996 1 Saffron Walk Hartlepool Cleveland TS25 1AE **Tel:** (01429) 294 840 w 6036745

LITTEN Janet Mary 22/02/1999 The Annexe Parsonage Farm Oakford TIVERTON Devon EX16 9JD **Tel:** (01398) 351232 w 6144513

LITTLE Georgina Ann 28/09/2005 9 Heronslade WARMINSTER Wiltshire BA12 9HR **Tel:** (01985) 215540 w 6343136

Kim Michelle 30/01/2009 Stonepit Glanfield Terrace Limington Yeovil Somerset BA22 8EP **Tel:** 01935840438 w 6419960

LITTLE Lisa Marie (see WINTER, Mrs)

LITTLEHALES Allison Valerie (nee Furness) 06/09/1996 (21/01/2008) Abbey Veterinary Centre 16 Holywell Street Shrewsbury SY2 5DB **Tel:** (01743) 232713 w 6038888

LIVERMORE Emma Marie 28/01/1997 27 Suffolk Road Maldon Essex CM9 6AX **Tel:** (01621) 841113 w 6041642

LIVERSEDGE Laura Emma Victoria 22/12/2000 88-92 Merton High Street Merton London SW19 1BD **Tel:** (020) 8254 1400 w 6204481

LIVINGSTONE Amanda Louise 08/01/2008 9 Polmont Road Laurieston Falkirk FK2 9QQ **Tel:** (01324) 623359 w 6370592

Zara Pauline 16/09/2008 1 Shannon Road Fareham Hampshire PO14 3RL **Tel:** 01329513459 w 6382428

LLOYD Holly Anne-Marie 28/09/2005 13 Railway Cottage Stamford Road Essendine STAMFORD Lincolnshire PE9 4LG w 6345490

LLOYD Stacy Marie (see BROOK, Mrs)

Susan 03/08/2006 Fishergill Aikton Wigton Cumbria CA7 0JP **Tel:** (01697) 342683 w 6351309

LLOYD-TAYLOR Nicole Sara 17/01/2006 48 Old School Close Codicote HITCHIN Hertfordshire SG4 8YJ w 6327439

LOBB Sarah Elizabeth 08/01/2008 Fair View The Mounts East Allington Totnes Devon TQ9 7QJ w 6403350

LOCK Amanda Jane (see DAY, Mrs)

LOCK Joanne Louise 26/01/1999 106 Hendford Hill Yeovil Somerset BA20 2RF **Tel:** (01935) 474690 w 6137754

Katie Robyn 04/02/2008 Wilbury Veterinary Surgery 20 Wilbury Avenue Hove East Sussex BN3 6HR **Tel:** (01273) 737924 w 6402800

Michelle Gillian 23/08/2000 Westway Veterinary Centre 426-428 West Road Newcastle upon Tyne NE5 2ER **Tel:** (0191) 274 7910 w 6202732

Rebecca Elizabeth (nee Lock, formerly Sewell) 26/08/1999 The Old Piggery Chapel Hill Porthtowan TRURO Cornwall TR4 8AS w 6142662

LOCKE Jenny Deborah (nee Reader) 11/09/1998 24 Millmead Way Hertford Hertfordshire SG14 3YH w 6139580

LOCKETT Emma Clair 05/08/2008 50 Frithwood Drive DRONFIELD Derbyshire S18 2DA w 6411072

LOCKEY Natalie Joy (nee Baker) 03/02/1997 Ridgeway Veterinary Centre 47 The Ridgeway Flitwick MK45 1DJ **Tel:** (01525) 714892 w 6040911

LOCKITT Sarah Jane 28/01/1997 43 The Knole Faversham Kent ME13 7QH w 6108698

LOCKWOOD Elizabeth Kate (nee Andrews) 25/09/1996 (17/03/2006) 3 Pavilion Gardens Market Lavington DEVIZES Wiltshire SN10 4EB w 6097378

Kay Leslie 06/05/2009 77 Kingston Road Ipswich Suffolk IP1 4BG **Tel:** 07933439045 w 6449099

LOFT Amy Eloiza 19/01/1998 (01/03/2001) 13 Falkland Road DORKING Surrey RH4 3AB **Tel:** (01306) 640299 w 6099728

LOFTHOUSE Samantha Jayne 02/09/2009 71 Fecitt Brow Blackburn Lancashire BB1 2AT **Tel:** (01254) 725 876 w 6437626

LOFTUS Elizabeth Clare 30/05/2008 5 Wistaria Close Pilgrims Hatch Brentwood Essex CM15 9PR **Tel:** (01277) 232934 w 6376092

Emma Jane 14/12/2006 Veterinary Centre Princess Avenue Clitheroe Lancashire BB7 2AL **Tel:** (01200) 423256 w 6371846

LOGAN Beverley (nee McAlpine) 24/01/1994 Grahams Road Veterinary Clinic 53 Grahams Road Falkirk Central FK2 7DJ **Tel:** (01324) 623163 w 6066168

Helen Elizabeth 04/06/2009 Grove House Halton Holegate SPILSBY Lincolnshire PE23 5PA **Tel:** 07952786867 w 6407794

LOGAN Rebecca Ann (see JOYCE, Mrs)

LOGSDON Melody Jane (see HOCKING, Mrs)

LOIS Regina Silvia 10/01/2007 Beech House Veterinary Clinic 35 Harrington Road Brighton BN1 6RF **Tel:** (01273) 505071 w 6376675

LOMAS Jennifer Clare (see CARTWRIGHT, Miss)

LONDON Thomas Paul 09/07/2007 14 Doulton Way Ashingdon ROCHFORD Essex SS4 3BX **Tel:** (01702) 540 841 w 6352618

LONG Michelle (see COCKLIN, Mrs)

LONG Sherene Laura Marie (formerly Thompson) 06/01/2009 14 The Pines LEEDS LS17 8GB **Tel:** 01132695954 w 6418530

LONGBOTTOM Helen Louise 14/05/2008 94 Blakemere Crescent PORTSMOUTH PO6 3SH **Tel:** 078702985568 w 6371109

LONGMORE Sonia Louise 27/05/2009 52 Sherwood Road Birmingham West Midlands B28 0HB **Tel:** (07515) 896276 w 6413514

LONGRIDGE Karen Marie 27/08/1996 (08/10/1999) Acorn House Veterinary Surgery Linnet Way BEDFORD MK41 7HN w 6042351

LONGSHAW Claire Louise (see SLATTER, Mrs)

LONSDALE Elaine Marie (see POLLOCK, Mrs)

LONSDALE Samantha Allison (nee Lonsdale) 11/01/2005 Station House Trimdon Station County Durham TS29 6BN w 6287575

Samantha Allison (nee Lonsdale) 11/01/2005 Station House Trimdon Station County Durham TS29 6BN w 6287575

Yvonne Marie 03/05/2005 35 Collett Way Priorslee TELFORD Shropshire TF2 9SL **Tel:** (01902) 292781 w 6301699

LOPEZ Joanna 23/06/2009 33 Langley Burrell Chippenham Wiltshire SN15 4LQ **Tel:** 01249445672 w 6419421

LORD Fiona Jane 22/03/2004 Upton Manor Farmhouse Uploders Bridport Dorset DT6 4PQ **Tel:** (01308) 485220 w 6277510

Karen 31/08/1999 32 Winston Avenue NEWTON-LE-WILLOWS Merseyside WA12 9RW w 6184945

Kirsty Jane 17/01/2008 60 Rowell Way CHIPPING NORTON Oxfordshire OX7 5BD **Tel:** (01608) 643511 w 6403680

LOTT Jill 06/10/2006 68 Main Road HOCKLEY Essex SS5 4RF **Tel:** 07968669323 w 6329738

LOTTER Nicola Sian 11/10/2004 38 Courtlands Avenue Lee LONDON SE12 8HZ w 6284825

LOUGHHEAD Gillian 05/04/2005 15 Derwent Road HEXHAM Northumberland NE46 1DL **Tel:** (01434) 609956 w 6327571

LOUGHLIN Karen 09/02/2009 14 Waverley Terrace Bonnyrigg Midlothian EH19 3BE **Tel:** (0131) 663 2604 w 6437131

LOVATT Lucinda Anna 05/10/2009 Rushcliffe Veterinary Centre Collington Way West Bridgford Nottinghamshire NG2 7LR **Tel:** (0115) 982 1717 w 6457745

Rebecca Elizabeth 10/09/2009 106 Barrows Lane Yardley Birmingham BS6 1SD **Tel:** (0121) 7852865 w 6466842

LOVE Jody Janet 10/09/2009 The Farm House New Rides Farm Eastchurch Sheppey Kent ME12 4DD **Tel:** (01795) 880134 w 6488875

LOVEDAY Samantha Louise (nee Gill) 06/03/1991 27 Monk Ings Avenue Birstall Batley West Yorkshire WF17 9HY w 6051264

LOVELL Marie 06/10/1994 3 Longfield Road Meopham GRAVESEND Kent DA13 0EW **Tel:** (07952) 816331 w 6031656

LOWDEN Emma Louise 01/09/2000 Thrifts Farm Farnham Green Bishops Stortford Hertfordshire CM23 1HL **Tel:** (01279) 771313 w 6202853

LOWE Carol Elaine (see MACK, Mrs)

LOWE Hannah Lucy 02/06/2008 18 Beaconsfield Road Altrincham Cheshire WA14 5LQ **Tel:** (0161) 23304 w 6387851

Jennie Louise 23/01/2003 6 Hinton Close London SE9 4SE w 6253475

Jennifer Alice 24/08/2009 54 Haslemere Avenue East Barnet Hertfordshire EN4 8EU w 6417672

Joanne Elisabeth 24/11/2004 57 Callowbrook Lane Rubery Birmingham B45 9HW **Tel:** (0121) 460 1762 w 6293482

Lianne Amy 10/02/2004 Abbeydale Veterinary Centre 91 Preston New Road Blackburn BB2 6AY **Tel:** (01254) 681811 w 6288455

LOWE Michelle Joanne (see AINSWORTH, Mrs)

LOWE Michelle Louise (see HARIS, Mrs)

Sharron Amanda 05/11/2008 5 Hawthorne Avenue New Arley COVENTRY CV7 8HF w 6443984

LOWERISON Claire Frances (nee Bryant) 14/11/2008 Lanwades Park Kentford Newmarket Suffolk CB8 7UU **Tel:** (01638) 552700 w 6433149

LOWES Harriet Anna 24/02/2004 3 Chapel Cottages Crowell Road Kingston Blount Chinnor Oxfordshire OX39 4RT **Tel:** (01844) 353893 w 6294593

LOWICK Kelly Elizabeth 29/07/2005 Green Lane Veterinary Centre Leachfield Estate Green Lane West, Cabus Garstang Preston Lancashire PR3 1PR **Tel:** (01995) 603349 w 6320960

LOWMAN Karen Elizabeth (see JONES, Mrs)

LOWRY Rachel Louise 18/10/2006 75 Valley Road STOCKPORT Cheshire SK4 2DB **Tel:** (01614) 313521 w 6345501

LOWTHER Christine Irene 17/05/2005 6 Western Way GOSPORT Hampshire PO12 2NG **Tel:** (07909) 851970 w 6314679

Clare 06/07/2004 5 Ladies Walk Caton Road Lancaster Lancashire LA1 3NX **Tel:** (01524) 67777 w 6295517

Kelly Marie 13/11/2009 14 Easington Street Peterlee County Durham SR8 3LD **Tel:** (07786) 366702 w 6429101

LOWTON Claire Louise (see POCKLINGTON, Mrs)

LOXLEY Claire Danielle 04/11/2008 26 Greens Road Coventry West Midlands CV6 2FH **Tel:** 02476334297 w 6437901

LOYND Holly Victoria (nee Phillips) 17/07/2008 1 Shoemaker Close Astcote TOWCESTER Northamptonshire NN12 8AT **Tel:** 07768915794 w 6413415

LUCAS Hannah Louise 18/06/2009 Brelades Veterinary Surgeons 20 Knoll Road Dorking Surrey RH4 3EP **Tel:** (01306) 883086 w 6415219

Lauren 20/04/2009 5 Dukes Avenue DORCHESTER Dorset DT1 1EN **Tel:** 01305262913 w 6457954

LUCKETT Yvette (nee Moore) 04/02/2002 71 Kimberley Road Solihull West Midlands B92 8PX **Tel:** (0121) 743 8660 w 6272329

LUDLOW Paul James 13/04/2004 Flat 7 Lauderdale House 155 Gresham Road STAINES Middlesex TW18 2AQ **Tel:** (07515) 941 524 m 6261153

LUFF Lucy Rose 05/01/2005 32 Gorse Lane Upton Poole Dorset BH16 5RS **Tel:** (01202) 620488 w 6296947

LUFFINGHAM April Jodie 08/01/2008 The Veterinary Clinic School Way Okehampton Devon EX20 1EU **Tel:** (01837) 52148 w 6392460

LUKE Dominique Audrie Helen 04/01/2006 57 Russell Way LEIGHTON BUZZARD Bedfordshire LU7 3NF w 6416143

LUM Sharon Tracey 20/09/2006 24 Bader Drive Upper Heyford BICESTER Oxfordshire OX25 5TN **Tel:** (01869) 233 643 w 6344445

LUMB Judith Mary (nee Scott) 09/03/1983 (23/05/2006) Yew Tree Cottage Dean Head Barkisland Halifax West Yorkshire HX4 0EA **Tel:** (01422) 822 406 w 606036X

LUMBIS Rachel Helen 20/11/2002 Department of Veterinary Clinical Sciences The Royal Veterinary College Hawkshead Lane North Mymms Hertfordshire AL9 7TA **Tel:** (01707) 666881 w 6270789

LUMLEY Josie Paula 09/09/2008 Milford Main Road Cutthorpe CHESTERFIELD Derbyshire S42 7AG **Tel:** 07725340852 w 6419674

LUMSDEN Fiona Jean (see WATSON, Mrs)

LUND Tracey Louise 23/02/2005 150 Moorview Way SKIPTON North Yorkshire BD23 2LN w 6324095

LUNDIE Elizabeth Leanne 23/02/2005 51 Townfield Lane Frodsham Cheshire WA6 7RF **Tel:** (01928) 730051 w 6318320

LUNDSTROM Sarah Marjorie (nee Bradford) 31/07/1992 Lear House 16 Waterloo Street Stoke Plymouth Devon PL1 5RP **Tel:** (01752) 510075 w 6008376

LUNGLEY Lisa Michelle (nee Mitson) 24/01/2008 8 The Street Boxted Bury St. Edmunds Suffolk IP29 4JP **Tel:** (01284) 830075 w 6374882

LUNN Kathryn Mary 25/02/2003 123 New Street ANDOVER Hampshire SP10 1DR w 6262033

Stacey Elizabeth 10/04/2003 34 Crescent Road Kidderminster Worcestershire DY11 6RW **Tel:** (01562) 742178 w 6277994

LUNNISS Sarah Louise 14/04/2008 16 Rayford Close Dartford Kent DA1 3AJ **Tel:** (01322) 277163 w 6403064

LUNNON Rebekah Charlotte 23/01/2009 123 Old Birmingham Road Lickey End Bromsgrove Worcestershire B60 1DF **Tel:** (01527) 873256 w 6349076

LUPETTI Janine (see BOYCE, Mrs)

LUSTY Joanne Louise 01/04/2003 43 The Mall Ealing London W5 3TJ **Tel:** (020) 8567 2724/ 0711 w 6270228

LUTLEY Carina Nicole 09/03/2009 9 Heron Way Coley Park Reading Berkshire RG1 6DY w 6418618

LUTWYCHE Tracy Anne DipAVN(Surgical) 19/02/1999 2 Prince of Wales Close London NW4 4QN **Tel:** (0208) 3606603 w 6140417

LYDEN Dawn Elizabeth (nee Hopkins) 04/09/1996 (27/01/2009) Pencoed College Pencoed Bridgend Mid Glamorgan CF35 5LG **Tel:** (01656) 863015 w 6099499

LYE Justine Hazel 05/12/2007 179 Main Street Witchford ELY Cambridgeshire CB6 2HP **Tel:** (0775) 1232479 w 6403812

LYNCH Claire Elizabeth 15/11/2005 The Old Moat House 42 Earlswood Common Earlswood SOLIHULL West Midlands B94 5SL **Tel:** (01564) 703890 w 6317220

Debra Anne 04/08/1981 (30/03/2000) 13 Eastcote Lane Hampton-in-Arden Solihull West Midlands B92 0AS **Tel:** (01675) 442826 w 605551X

James Alan 24/05/2006 24 St. Johns Street Farncombe Godalming Surrey GU7 3EJ **Tel:** (01483) 421833 m 6268721

Mandy 29/12/2008 5 Roman Vale Old Harlow HARLOW Essex CM17 0JB **Tel:** 07534909112 w 6420026

Tara (nee Foggo) 26/07/1993 1 Pen-Y-Glyn Bryn-y-Maen Colwyn Bay LL28 5EW **Tel:** (01492) 532 991 w 6066565

LYNN Debra Louise 30/11/2006 143 Lucas Avenue Chelmsford Essex CM2 9JR **Tel:** 01245283030 w 6353872

LYON Jacqueline 16/06/2006 11 Cherry Orchard ASHTEAD Surrey KT21 1HS w 6354697

LYONS Carly Jane 16/02/2000 20 Derwent Close WATERLOOVILLE Hampshire PO8 0DH **Tel:** (02392) 571971 w 6135509

Lesley-Ann Elizabeth (nee Boyd) 01/02/1994 (06/08/1999) 48 Hillside The Spa Ballynahinch Co Down BT24 8PS **Tel:** (028) 97563259 w 6067343

Michelle Alison 06/08/2008 23 Old Garden Close Locks Heath Southampton Hampshire SO31 6RN **Tel:** (01489) 580 200 w 6403900

Shelley Ann (nee Heald) 17/11/1992 Millstones Peel Cottage Road TODMORDEN Lancashire OL14 7QJ **Tel:** (0161) 745 7214 w 6064488

LYONS Victoria Samantha (see CLARK, Ms)

LYTH Helen Louise (see HARRINGTON, Mrs)

LYTTLE Deborah Catherine (see ARMSTRONG, Mrs)

M

MACALISTER Gemma Irene DipAVN(Medical) (nee Cunliffe) 03/12/2003 26 The Chase Boroughbridge YORK North Yorkshire YO51 9JT w 6287454

MACAUSLAND Lindsay (nee Gardner) 23/08/2004 1 Avon View STRATHAVEN Lanarkshire ML10 6GG w 6276960

MACCOY Susan Elizabeth Gay 22/03/2004 41 South Ave South Shields Tyne & Wear NE34 6RA **Tel:** (0191) 4557558 w 6276509

MACCUISH Lynne 25/06/1975 (29/06/2007) The Avenue Veterinary Group 241 Bingley Road Shipley West Yorkshire BD18 4DN **Tel:** (01274) 583397 w 6055531

MACDONALD Andrea 05/04/2005 23 Carseggie Crescent GLENROTHES Fife KY7 5DJ **Tel:** (01592) 752722 w 6318529

Debbie Ann (nee Burns) 13/01/2004 80 Bellshill Road Uddingston GLASGOW Lanarkshire G71 6NR **Tel:** (01698) 817999 w 6244774

Donna 04/02/2009 Moorpark House 5 Orton Place Glasgow G51 2HF **Tel:** (0141) 445 6869 w 6425724

MACDONALD Donna Elaine (see GAYLOR, Mrs)

Faye Alexandra 22/09/2009 Checkley Hall Farmhouse Checkley Lane Checkley NANTWICH Cheshire CW5 7QA **Tel:** 01270520468 w 6461078

Gemma Catherine 06/05/2008 Dykeside Harray Orkney Orkney KW17 2LQ **Tel:** (01856) 771385 w 6377522

Isla Glenda 25/02/2003 Queen Mother Hospital for Small Animals Hawkshead Lane North Mymms Hatfield Hertfordshire AL9 7TA **Tel:** (01707) 666366 w 6274947

Jill Mary Fiona DipAVN(Surgical) 03/09/1999 2 Tarvin Mews Church Street Tarvin CHESTER CH3 8EB **Tel:** (01772) 493502 w 6186331

MACDONALD Kerrie-Ann (see GALLAGHER, Mrs)

Lauren Louisa 05/03/2009 71 Wester Broom Drive Edinburgh Midlothian EH12 7RF **Tel:** 01315390182 w 6439672

Lianne Heather 21/07/2008 133 Valley Drive HARROGATE North Yorkshire HG2 0JS w 6403086

Louise Rebecca 04/02/2009 5 Beauchamps Close Chelmsford Essex CM1 6ZP **Tel:** 01245469861 w 6403603

Lucy Jane 05/01/2005 19 Sun Hill Royston Hertfordshire SG8 9AU w 6261362

Rebecca Nyland 26/11/2009 2 Meadow Way Caversham READING RG4 5LY w 6389292

Sharon 22/10/2004 (21/01/2008) Flat Ground Right 8 Blackwood Street Barrhead GLASGOW G78 1JX w 6291359

Victoria Naomi 02/09/2008 24 Weaverham Road Sandiway NORTHWICH Cheshire CW8 2NJ **Tel:** (01606) 301872 w 6431719

MACE Donna Claire 19/07/1999 (18/04/2007) 17 Court Lane Seaton Devon EX12 2AR **Tel:** (01297) 24087 w 6134957

Donna Marie 05/09/1996 (27/02/2003) 851 Home Farm TIDWORTH Hampshire SP9 7AQ w 6103893

Melanie Ann (nee Borrmann) 07/08/2002 Mill House Veterinary Surgery & Hospital 20 Tennyson Avenue King's Lynn Norfolk PE30 2QG **Tel:** (01553) 771457 w 6267478

MACE Suzanne Marie (see WILDMAN, Mrs)

MACEACHERN Erin Yvonne (formerly McEachern) 09/05/2005 16 Keills Cottages Keills ISLE OF ISLAY PA46 7RF **Tel:** (01496) 840678 w 6318518

MACEDO Emmeline Louisa 01/12/2000 67 Alma Road Carshalton Surrey SM5 2PQ **Tel:** (0208) 6423928 w 6204943

MACFADYEN Kelly Jane 22/03/2004 17a Coniston Road BEXLEYHEATH Kent DA7 6PX w 6298696

MACFARLANE Clara Kim (nee Pemberton) 10/01/2008 3 Lamport Close WIDNES Cheshire WA8 3RQ **Tel:** (0151) 5100781 w 6296364

Karen Jill 03/08/2006 Oakfield Veterinary Group 2 Margaret Road Atherstone Warwickshire CV9 1EE **Tel:** (01827) 713 149 w 6355214

MACHIN Amie 25/06/2004 385 Leek Road Endon Stoke-on-Trent Staffordshire ST9 9BA **Tel:** (01782) 503166 w 6270756

Joanne 19/03/2007 Wilson Veterinary Group 5-11 Tenters Street BISHOP AUCKLAND County Durham DL14 7AD **Tel:** (01388) 602707 w 6349098

MACINTYRE Gillian Ruth (formerly Andrew) 06/12/2004 41 Woodbridge Hill GUILDFORD Surrey GU2 9AD w 6286563

MACK Carol Elaine (nee Lowe) 17/08/1995 10 Westcots Drive Winkleigh Devon EX19 8JP **Tel:** (01344) 483191 w 6026952

MACKAY Karen Helen Wilma 03/09/2002 21 Briargrove Gardens Inshes INVERNESS IV2 5AH **Tel:** (01463) 235986 w 6261340

Laura Sadie Katie 04/12/2003 Barnfield House Veterinary Centre 405 Pinner Road Harrow Middlesex HA1 4HN **Tel:** (020) 8427 7360 w 6279083

Yvonne 12/01/2009 Reay House Doll Brora Sutherland KW9 6NJ **Tel:** 01408621672 w 6439804

MACKENZIE Gareth John 25/02/2003 56 Manchester Road Shaw Oldham Lancashire OL2 7DE **Tel:** (01706) 840936 m 6277312

Irene Evelyn (nee McCormick) 23/11/2001 (24/04/2006) Newsome House No. 20 Holding Woodside Farm Woodside Coupar Angus Perthshire PH13 9LP **Tel:** (01828) 670595 w 6241980

Joanna 22/05/2009 c/o Balmoral Veterinary Centre 140 Stockmans Lane BELFAST BT9 7JE **Tel:** 02890666881 w 6440321

Joanna Louise 15/01/2009 17 Bluebell Walks Paddock Wood Tonbridge Kent TN12 6BL **Tel:** (01892) 837687 w 6414438

Joanne Alison 22/03/2004 23 Cranbrook Road East Barnet Hertfordshire EN4 8UP **Tel:** (0208) 4403385 w 6289808

MACKEY Gwen Peggy 06/08/2008 East Cottage Weybridge Farm Woolley Road Alconbury HUNTINGDON Cambridgeshire PE28 4HN **Tel:** (01480) 890 365 w 6378688

MACKIE Dawn Kelly 01/04/2003 St Clair Veterinary Group 2 Pottery Street Kirkcaldy Fife KY1 3ET **Tel:** (01592) 599500 w 6282262

Elizabeth Marion 15/06/2009 Goodockhill Farm Newhouse Motherwell Lanarkshire ML1 5NE **Tel:** (01698) 870231 w 6408751

Layla Frances (nee Wate, nee Wate) 10/12/2002 Avonvale Veterinary Centres Ltd 88 Coventry Street Southam Warwickshire CV47 0EA **Tel:** (01926) 812826 w 6279622

MACKIN Karen Nicola 16/10/2007 Holly Cottage Common Side Brailsford Ashbourne Derbyshire DE6 3AX **Tel:** (01335) 360735 w 6403372

MACKINNON Catherine 06/02/1992 9 Hillhead Avenue Burnside Rutherglen Glasgow G73 4NJ **Tel:** (0141) 583 5317 w 6055600

MACKINNON Kirsty Jacqueline (see MCNICHOLL, Mrs)

MACKINNON Nicola Jane (see WATSON, Mrs)

MACLAREN Gillian 03/02/2009 3 Dunnottar Street Bishopbriggs GLASGOW G64 1PR w 6439595

MACLEAN Diane Irene (see SMILLIE, Mrs)

Kelly Dawn (formerly Mears, nee Mears) 19/04/2005 Mill House Veterinary Surgery & Hospital 20 Tennyson Avenue King's Lynn Norfolk PE30 2QG **Tel:** (01553) 771457 w 6291128

Laura 15/02/2002 Royal(Dick)School of Veterinary Studies Easter Bush Roslin Midlothian EH25 9RG **Tel:** (0131) 650 6253 w 6271636

Rachel Helen 22/03/2004 52 Boscundle Avenue Goldenbank Falmouth Cornwall TR11 5BX **Tel:** (01326) 317662 w 6299037

MACLENNAN Johan Alice 26/04/2007 37 Balnakyle Road Inverness Inverness-Shire IV2 4BT **Tel:** (01463) 224763 w 6383231

MACLEOD Gillian (see MORTON, Mrs)

MACLEOD Janice 15/06/2009 49 Prestwick Road AYR KA8 8LF **Tel:** (01292) 265955 w 6408762

MACNAUGHTON Kirsty Sarah (see GRANT, Mrs)

MACNEILL Miranda 06/08/2007 Coach House Achany LAIRG Sutherland IV27 4EE **Tel:** (01549) 402 118 w 6334721

MACPHEE Lucy Anne 08/11/2006 (24/08/2009) 34 Leaves Green Crown Wood Bracknell Berkshire RG12 0TF w 6342157

MACPHERSON Gillian Yvonne (see JONES, Mrs)

MACPHERSON Janet Louise 12/05/2004 Chattan House Glaick Ardross Ross-Shire IV17 0XW **Tel:** (01349) 882129 w 6299048

Josie Lauren 08/04/2005 35 Bournemead Avenue Northolt Middlesex UB5 6PU **Tel:** (07876) 502603 w 6291711

MADDEN Lisa Jayne (nee Maguire) 04/08/1987 Broad Lane Vets Ltd 255 Broad Lane Coventry West Midlands CV5 7AQ **Tel:** (024) 7646 4789 w 6055644

MADDOCKS Emma Louise (see WHITLOCK, Mrs)

MADDOCKS Tracey Yliana 26/02/2009 244b Gordon Avenue CAMBERLEY Surrey GU15 2NU **Tel:** 01276512126 w 6436757

MADDOX Kerry Nicola (nee Jones) 27/05/2003 87 Woolpitch Wood CHEPSTOW Gwent NP16 6DR w 6269711

Laurie Kaye 20/02/2009 39 Highburn Cramlington Northumberland NE23 6AZ **Tel:** 01670738254 w 6449572

MADELEY Lisa Marie 28/11/2008 56 Rookery Road Wombourne Wolverhampton WV5 0JQ **Tel:** (01902) 324551 w 6356270

MADELEY Samantha (see BELDING, Mrs)

MADEN Christina Marie (nee Paull) 16/07/2002 144 Russells Ride Cheshunt WALTHAM CROSS Hertfordshire EN8 8UH **Tel:** (01992) 306745 w 6266246

MAGARINOS Jesus Angel Miguez 08/09/1995 (13/09/1999) 30 Tileston Road Winthrop MA 02152 USA m 6032310

MAGEE Annaliese Helen DipAVN(Surgical) (formerly Hughes, nee Morgan) 27/01/1997 (04/03/2005) Fuchsia Pet Boutique and Spa 15 Bradford Road BRIGHOUSE West Yorkshire HD6 1RW **Tel:** (01484) 530516 w 610975X

MAGUIRE Elaine Rosaleen 17/09/2007 Derrynacloy Rosslea Enniskillen County Fermanagh Northern Ireland BT92 7AZ **Tel:** (028) 677 51593 w 6386542

MAGUIRE Lisa Jayne (see MADDEN, Mrs)

Melissa 09/03/2009 147 Midhurst Road LONDON W13 9TJ **Tel:** 07703104215 w 6540696

Ruth Ailsa 07/04/2006 39 Shore Mount LITTLEBOROUGH Lancashire OL15 8EN **Tel:** (01706) 379 938 w 6305318

MAHER Laura Anne 04/12/2003 Pool House Veterinary Group Fosseway Lane Lichfield Staffordshire WS13 8JY **Tel:** (01543) 262464/262433 w 6262726

MAHON Abigail Jessica Louise 04/11/2008 Freshwater Cranbrook Road Benenden Cranbrook Kent TN17 4ET **Tel:** 01580240784 w 6378699

MAIDMENT Emma Jane 03/08/1989 3 Dodford Court Fockbury Road Dodford Bromsgrove Worcestershire B61 9AP **Tel:** (01527) 832651 w 6055677

MAIDWELL Hannah Judith 12/12/2005 (29/02/2008) 5 Rosliston Road Walton-on-Trent SWADLINCOTE Derbyshire DE12 8NQ **Tel:** (01827) 281284 w 6325151

MAIL Kate Louise (nee Mail, formerly Kenny) 11/09/2003 238 Bute Street Cardiff CF10 5HT **Tel:** (0292) 048 0990 w 6286915

MAIN Fiona Margaret 19/01/1998 Clyde Veterinary Group By The New Lanark Market Hyndford Road Lanark ML11 9AX **Tel:** (01555) 660000 w 6115537

MAINWARING Louise Marie 13/08/2008 16 Massey Avenue LYMM Cheshire WA13 0PJ **Tel:** 07747744928 w 6418090

Sarah Jane (nee Bowen) 06/08/1992 (17/01/2003) 6 Lodge Road Bourne Lincoln Lincolnshire PE10 9BP **Tel:** (01778) 424516 w 6008707

MAISTRELLO Mariarosa (formerly Hall) 21/02/1992 (27/03/2002) 167 Wakefield Road Garforth LEEDS LS25 1NE **Tel:** (0113) 2875617 w 6052086

MAKEPEACE Ellen Elizabeth (nee Rutherford) 19/03/2007 Coomara Veterinary Practice Coomara Carleton Carlisle Cumbria CA4 0BU **Tel:** (01228) 524740 w 6272549

MALACHOWSKI Elizabeth 06/03/2006 20 Yew Tree Avenue Ockbrook DERBY DE72 3TB **Tel:** (079) 1539 0089 w 6340397

MALE Raymond Sean 13/04/2004 24 Mill Meadow IVYBRIDGE Devon PL21 0AW m 6273198

MALEED Emma Ruth 16/01/1996 53 Searchlight Heights The Willows Chattendon Rochester Kent ME3 8NF **Tel:** (01634) 252854 w 6033482

MALIK Aneesa 11/09/2008 105 Bilton Road Rugby Warwickshire CV22 7AS **Tel:** (01788) 560 067 w 6441113

MALLABAR Beverley (nee Blackett) 22/08/2000 (16/11/2004) 10 Calderwood Crescent Low Fell GATESHEAD Tyne and Wear NE9 6PH **Tel:** (0191) 422 3081 w 6137481

MALLARD Rebecca Anne (nee Prangley) 19/03/2007 Hale House 19 Langley Road Chippenham Wiltshire SN15 1BS **Tel:** (01249) 653561 w 6332048

MALLORD Lauren Marie 19/03/2007 94 Woodview Gadebridge Hemel Hempstead Hertfordshire HP1 3HS **Tel:** (01442) 211 865 w 6373749

MALONE Karen Deborah (nee Wells) 03/05/2005 (05/02/2008) 101 Victoria Avenue WESTGATE-ON-SEA Kent CT8 8BQ w 6304152

MALPUS Kezia Margaret 24/12/2002 80 Shelley Street LEIGH Lancashire WN7 5EX w 6277356

MALTBY Sally Emily Charlotte 29/01/2009 15 Haglane Copse Pennington Lymington Hampshire SO41 8DT **Tel:** 07871055280 w 6340408

MALTON Deborah Fiona (see FOGARTY, Mrs)

MALYON Terri Ann 15/11/2005 11 Oriole Way Larkfield AYLESFORD Kent ME20 6LN w 6350308

MANFIELD Lisa (nee May) 01/08/1989 71a Plymouth Road BUCKFASTLEIGH Devon TQ11 0DH **Tel:** (01364) 643368 w 6055735

MANFIELD Nicola Dianne (see HAWES, Mrs)

MANLEY Jayne Margaret (nee Stevenson, formerly Hawkes) 08/07/1993 (10/03/2004) 20 Leiros

Parc Drive Bryncoch NEATH West Glamorgan SA10 7EW **Tel:** (01639) 632262 w 6015124

MANN Abigail Louise 26/03/2002 21 Falcon Drive Crewe Cheshire CW1 3RX **Tel:** (01270) 505993 w 6266774

MANN Alison (see COLLINS, Mrs)

Fiona Jane (nee Bowers) 07/10/2008 46 Dulverton Drive Furzton MILTON KEYNES MK4 1DF w 6438462

James Gavin 01/04/2009 142 Hatch Road Brentwood Essex CM15 9QB **Tel:** 07881574282 m 6405660

Nicola Jane (nee Sealey) 11/08/1987 (21/01/2009) 218 Lower Farnham Road Aldershot Hampshire GU46 6QQ **Tel:** (01252) 343088 w 6093646

Nicole Louise 19/12/2007 232 Allerton Road Allerton Bradford West Yorkshire BD15 7AA **Tel:** (01274) 480031 w 6330343

Susan Mary 27/07/1979 Hexworthy Barton Lawhitton Launceston Cornwall PL15 9NL **Tel:** (01566) 772755 w 6055746

MANNING Karen Michelle (nee Olley) 29/12/2003 179 The Broadway North Shields Tyne and Wear NE30 3DQ **Tel:** (01603) 431091 w 6128932

MANSFIELD Lisa (see CROWE, Mrs)

MANSFIELD Lisa Ann (nee Cox) 30/05/2003 Stocton Veterinary Centre Stocton Close Woodbridge Road Guildford Surrey GU1 1HR **Tel:** (01483) 575155 w 6262682

MANSFORD Katie Narelle 06/08/2003 59 Cranleigh Close Sanderstead SOUTH CROYDON Surrey CR2 9LH w 6283923

MANSO Cristina Ana (see FARRELL, Mrs)

MANSON Jessica Helen (nee Poulter) 19/02/1996 C/o Royal College of Veterinary Surgeons 62-64 Horseferry Road LONDON SW1P 2AF w 6040977

Lorraine Denoon 18/02/2009 Park Head Canisbay WICK Caithness KW1 4YH w 6411523

Nicola (nee Welsh) 18/09/2000 Moray Coast Veterinary Group West Road Greshop Estate Forres Morayshire IV36 2GW **Tel:** (01309) 672243 w 6203502

MANSTON Nichola Anne 03/02/2009 6 Midgham Farm Cottages Midgham Fordingbridge Hampshire SP6 3DA **Tel:** 01425652083 w 6443896

MANT Joy Leah 03/12/2003 3 Kirby Close Middle Barton CHIPPING NORTON Oxfordshire OX7 7HJ w 6282185

MANTON Louise 04/12/2009 1 Vale View Road DOVER Kent CT17 9NP **Tel:** (01304) 219606 w 6494870

MANUEL Emma Jane 14/09/2009 125 Lingfield Road East Grinstead Sussex RH19 2EL **Tel:** (1342) 323 072 w 6466864

MAPE Kerry 04/02/2009 The Avenue Veterinary Clinic 33 St. Peters Avenue Kettering Northamptonshire NN16 0HB **Tel:** (01536) 512200 w 6446085

MAPLE Caroline Louise 04/09/2008 3 Roding Drive Kelvedon Hatch Brentwood Essex CM15 0XA **Tel:** (01277) 374651 w 6353883

Jodie Maria 04/02/2009 Briar House Veterinary Surgery 13-15 St Peters Road Broadstairs Kent CT10 2AG **Tel:** (01843) 863395 w 6440717

MAPLESDEN Claire Louise 17/02/2009 1 Bury Road Tottington Bury Lancashire BL8 3HD **Tel:** (01204) 886655 w 6449154

MAPP Nicola Jayne 19/03/2007 14 Ashmore Drive Trench TELFORD Shropshire TF2 7EN w 6366819

MARCHANT Laura Mary 22/03/2004 44 Staithes Lane Morpeth Northumberland NE61 1TD **Tel:** (01670) 512275 w 6265597

MARGAN Victoria Louise 17/01/2008 49 Chatteris Way Lower Earley Reading Berkshire RG6 4JA **Tel:** 01189671385 w 6385684

MARKHAM Janet Ann (see MILLER, Mrs)

MARKLAND Andrea Phillippa 29/01/2007 35 Vicarage Lane Elworth Sandbach Cheshire CW11 3BW **Tel:** 01260290282 w 6374090

MARKLEW Shelley Jean 30/11/2009 22 Bashkir Road WESTBURY Wiltshire BA13 3GY **Tel:** (01373) 825126 w 6496278

MARKS Elizabeth Caroline (nee Emby) 13/05/2003 Unit 10 Egremont Road Bearsted Maidstone Kent ME15 8LH **Tel:** (01622) 736 677 w 6270921

Jessica Beth 22/05/2009 Foldhill Farm Foldhill Lane Martock Somerset TA12 6PQ **Tel:** 07790302480 w 6444281

Natalie Claire 19/09/2006 288 Robin Hood Lane BIRMINGHAM B28 0EQ **Tel:** (0121) 2442219 w 6301710

MARLIN Laura Theresa 28/07/2008 12 Swanwick Lane Broughton MILTON KEYNES MK10 9LB **Tel:** 01234391119 w 6377753

MARLOW Claire (see GREEN, Mrs)

MARLOW Sara Elisabeth 27/04/2006 Oakfield Veterinary Group 2 Margaret Road Atherstone Warwickshire CV9 1EE **Tel:** (01827) 713 149 w 6334248

MARNER Katherine Mary 02/06/2004 48a Heath Row Bishop's Stortford Hertfordshire CM23 5DE w 6264618

MARR Cheryl Anne (nee England) 26/08/1998 34 Goulden Street CREWE CW1 3LA **Tel:** (01270) 250930 w 6041926

MARRINGTON Hayley Elizabeth 20/03/2009 18 Lincoln Place Haslingden Rossendale Lancashire BB4 5DS **Tel:** 01706229899 w 6297596

MARRIOTT Elizabeth Julie Mary 19/03/2007 21 Olive Grove STOURPORT-ON-SEVERN Worcestershire DY13 8XY w 6334314

MARSDEN Anna Elizabeth 07/11/2008 Edgemoor Veterinary Practice Station Road Helmsley North Yorkshire YO62 5BZ **Tel:** (01439) 771166 w 6434502

Katy Anne 14/10/2002 6 Blackfirs Lane Somerford Congleton Cheshire CW12 4QQ **Tel:** (01260) 278914 w 6277246

Kerry Anne 30/11/2005 Bray House Veterinary Practice 36 Asfordby Road Melton Mowbray Leicestershire LE13 0HR **Tel:** (01664) 562054 w 6270932

Victoria Ellen 02/06/2004 180 Renacres Lane Halsall Ormskirk Lancashire L39 8SQ **Tel:** (01704) 821204 w 6299587

MARSH Catherine Claire 07/02/2006 31 Selway Drive BURY ST. EDMUNDS Suffolk IP32 7PL **Tel:** (01284) 760052 w 6344874

Hayley Ann 17/05/2005 73 Bancombe Road Somerton Somerset TA11 6JE **Tel:** (01458) 850438 w 6323193

Kristina Louise 10/02/2004 10 Tinshill Drive Cookridge LEEDS LS16 7DH **Tel:** (0113) 281 7567 w 6289456

MARSH Michelle Louise (see OPENSHAW, Mrs)

MARSH Sonia Catherine (see TAYLOR, Ms)

MARSHALL Catherine Mary DipAVN(Surgical) (nee Billington) 27/08/1997 19 White Stone Close The Ings Redcar Cleveland TS10 2PS **Tel:** (01642) 511330 w 6101717

Charlotte Catherine Jane 15/01/2008 21 Buckley Place Crawley Down CRAWLEY West Sussex RH10 4JG **Tel:** (01342) 718624 w 6363288

Claire Christine Alice 28/07/2008 42 Icknield Way TRING Hertfordshire HP23 4HZ w 6395980

Hannah Jayne 08/11/2006 51 Brecks Road Ordsall RETFORD Nottinghamshire DN22 7UA w 6350649

Helen Joy (nee Marshall) 20/01/1997 (27/07/1999) Corner House Veterinary Practice Ltd 84 Withycombe Village Road Exmouth Devon EX8 3AG **Tel:** (01395) 277775 w 6039167

Kelly Lea 28/04/2003 79 Cherry Tree Walk BECKENHAM Kent BR3 3PE **Tel:** (0208) 6587977 w 6270283

Kelly Trixie 19/04/2005 (07/07/2009) 9 Thurlestone Parade High Street SHEPPERTON Middlesex TW17 9AR w 6275321

MARSHALL Lara Jane (see MITCHELL, Mrs)

Laurie 01/12/2008 5 Lynemouth Road Ellington Morpeth Northumberland NE61 5HN **Tel:** 01670861703 w 6419685

Lisa (nee Sharples) 23/08/2000 Pennington House Veterinary Centre Newlands Road LEIGH Lancashire WN7 4HA **Tel:** (01942) 673777 w 6136783

Louise (nee Harris) 01/12/2000 232 Allerton Road Allerton Bradford West Yorkshire BD15 7AA **Tel:** (01274) 480031 w 6205647

Nicola Jane (nee Tierney) 27/08/1996 34 Boundary Road Walsall Wood Walsall West Midlands WS9 9QZ w 6039360

Racheal Mary 22/03/2004 5 Portland Street Rawcliffe Bridge GOOLE DN14 8NN w 6289467

Rebecca Anne 23/10/2008 Sandhole Veterinary Centre Malling Road Snodland Kent ME6 5LG **Tel:** (01634) 242502 w 6436416

Sally Louise 16/03/2007 19 School Road Tilehurst Reading Berkshire RG31 5AR **Tel:** (0118) 942 8240 w 6383242

MARSHALL Stephanie (see HODGSON, Mrs)

MARSHALL Tracy Deborah (see CAMPBELL, Mrs)

MARSON Hannah Jane 31/03/2003 53 Daffodil Way CHELMSFORD CM1 6XE w 6260955

MARTIN Amy Rhonwen (nee Hopkins) 08/11/2006 (18/03/2009) 4 Rotherham Close Cawston RUGBY Warwickshire CV22 7TG w 6367083

Arlene Elizabeth 13/01/2004 (02/11/2009) Royal School of Veterinary Studies College of Animal Welfare 1 Summerhall Square EDINBURGH EH9 1QH **Tel:** (0131) 650 7947 w 6290985

MARTIN Bernadette Anne Marie (see LEWIS, Mrs)

Carole DipAVN(Surgical) (formerly Bowden) 14/09/1987 19 Polglase Walk Trispen St Erme Truro Cornwall TR4 9BP **Tel:** (01872) 242173 w 6046017

Claire 14/09/2009 5 Meadowcroft Close Glenfield Leicester LE3 8QX **Tel:** (0116) 2311635 w 6453323

Danielle Tracey 10/01/2007 4 Southerden Close HAILSHAM East Sussex BN27 2AF w 6276971

Emily May 22/12/2009 Dove House Bishopstone AYLESBURY Buckinghamshire HP17 8SH w 6459450

Emma Jane 24/09/2009 17 Newholme Close Croxheath Park LIVERPOOL L12 0JG **Tel:** (0151) 5474519 w 6284748

Emma Jane 02/09/2008 2 Hall Cottages The Hall London Road Six Mile Bottom NEWMARKET Suffolk CB8 0UF w 6435305

Faye Denise 17/09/2009 28 Lorraine Road Aylestone Leicestershire LE2 8ER w 6493374

Jean Sheila (nee Rapley) 22/08/1994 (19/01/1999) Crofts Veterinary Surgery Collards Lane Haslemere Surrey GU27 2HU **Tel:** (01428) 653056 w 602895X

Jenna Shaula 09/02/2009 1/3 358 Perth Road Dundee Angus DD2 1EN **Tel:** (01382) 660398 w 6436812

Joanna Kathleen 13/05/2003 79 Cherry Gardens HERNE BAY Kent CT6 5QY **Tel:** (01227) 742 344 w 6266543

MARTIN Karen Susan (see SADDLETON, Mrs)

Kate Louise 19/09/2006 534 Sutton Road SOUTHEND-ON-SEA Essex SS2 5PW w 6347184

MARTIN Kelly Ann (see JENNINGS, Mrs)

Laura Jane Ellen 29/06/2007 The Harbour Veterinary Group 34 Manor Close Havant Hampshire PO9 1BD **Tel:** (023) 9248 4788 w 6325965

Lisa 08/11/2006 Flat 3 Shernwood House 2 Hermitage Walk LONDON E18 2DE w 6442840

MARTIN Lisa Claire (see LARMOUR, Mrs)

Lyndsay Jane (nee Pinsard) 20/04/2009 Heritage House La Grande Rue St. Martin Guernsey Channel Islands GY4 6LH **Tel:** (01481) 239101 w 6302590

Rachael Elizabeth 13/07/2007 239 Upper Grosvenor Road Tunbridge Wells Kent TN1 2EJ **Tel:** (07743) 672496 w 6349626

MARTIN Rachael Sarah (see WILLIAMS, Mrs)

Rhea Felicity 07/02/2007 (03/07/2009) Eton Veterinary Clinic 31 London Road Tonbridge Kent TN10 3AB **Tel:** (01732) 352004 w 6367270

Sarah Isabel 10/06/2009 17 St. Modwena Way Penkridge Stafford Staffordshire ST19 5ST **Tel:** (01785) 714 623 w 6440145

Tracey 08/09/2005 Winton Lodge Veterinary Clinic 36 Ashley Road Epsom Surrey KT18 5BH **Tel:** (01372) 722313 w 6263826

MARTINS Claire Louise 05/07/2006 26 Nottingham Close Leavesden Watford Hertfordshire WD25 7QT **Tel:** (01923) 465056 w 6345050

MARTLAND Helen Elizabeth 18/11/2009 Grove Farm High Lane Ormskirk Lancashire L40 7SW w 6439562

MASCALL Alison Mary (see HUDD, Mrs)

MASKELL Lisa Anne (see BROOKS, Mrs)

MASKELL Michelle Jean 11/07/2005 45 Buckhurst Crescent Swindon Wiltshire SN3 3DA **Tel:** (01793) 542753 w 6282746

MASLEY Emma Elizabeth (nee Hunt) 31/03/2003 3 Puffin Close Weston-super-Mare Avon BS22 8TU **Tel:** (01934) 515 539 w 6263925

MASON Audrey (nee McNair) 30/07/1992 19 Winton Gardens Uddingston Glasgow G71 6AQ **Tel:** (01698) 305075 w 6004779

Colette 18/10/2005 30 Eva Street Leigh Lancashire WN7 5EZ **Tel:** (01942) 261720 w 6313656

Helen Elizabeth 15/10/2008 83 Holly Lane Walsall Wood WALSALL WS9 9JQ w 6287003

Helena Lucy 11/03/2005 16 Legion Close Norton Canes Cannock Staffordshire WS11 9TG **Tel:** (01543) 277049 w 6292646

Joanne Elizabeth (formerly Daniell, nee Richardson) 17/08/1981 Corner House Veterinary Practice Ltd 84 Withycombe Village Road Exmouth Devon EX8 3AG **Tel:** (01395) 277775 w 6061352

Julia Mary 04/09/1989 (08/11/2001) 107 East Barnet Road New Barnet Barnet Hertfordshire EN4 8RF **Tel:** (020) 8440 5742 w 6055983

Molly Ansley 17/01/2008 14 Garforth Road Keighley West Yorkshire BD21 4DR **Tel:** (01535) 675 809 w 6381295

Vicki Michelle 29/06/2007 1A Monks Pond Street Northampton NN1 2LF **Tel:** (020) 8527 1556 w 6371648

MASSA Kerry Ann 12/09/2008 1 Roseburn Place Flat 2f2 EDINBURGH EH12 5NP **Tel:** 07963471204 w 6405110

MASSEY Abigail Beth (nee Driver, formerly Dutton) 09/09/1998 Moreton Hall Veterinary Centre Easlea Road Moreton Hall Bury St. Edmunds Suffolk IP32 7BS **Tel:** (01284) 747000 w 6135236

Samantha Leigh (nee Poulton) 21/07/2008 34 Chesterfield Road Eckington SHEFFIELD S21 4BD w 6376147

MASSIE Louise 07/10/2008 Lyn-Lea Cottage Nether Kinmundy Peterhead Aberdeenshire AB42 4YP **Tel:** 01779821189 w 6381284

MASSYN Katherine Olga 27/06/2003 (26/10/2006) 1 Augustus Mews 76 Augustus Road LONDON SW19 6LZ w 6340276

MASTERS Carly Lynn 13/03/2008 1 Stenbury Way Netley Abbey Southampton Hampshire SO31 5PU **Tel:** (023) 804 54052 w 6401436

MASTERS Jessica Louise (see HAZELL, Mrs)

Joanne Mary (formerly Sandry) 09/08/1991 (30/06/2000) Manor Farm Hambridge Langport Somerset TA10 0AY **Tel:** (01460) 281207 w 6060213

Stacy Louise 18/09/2009 7 Creswell Place Warwickshire CV22 7G2 **Tel:** 07515472301 w 6377764

MASTERSON Kristy Louise 08/09/2005 15 St. Marys Walk Steeple Bumpstead HAVERHILL Suffolk CB9 7EX **Tel:** (01440) 730857 w 6326042

MATAN Claire Leanne (nee Rymell) 14/12/2007 Riverside Veterinary Centre Unit 3, Goods Wharf Goods Road Belper Derbyshire DE56 1UU **Tel:** (01773) 829 544 w 6391910

Stefan William 27/05/2003 (22/02/2005) 10 Hollyhouse Drive South Normanton Alfreton Derbyshire DE55 2LB **Tel:** (01773) 605270 m 6278764

MATANLE Eleanor (Ellie) 25/02/2003 8 The Coppice Sturry CANTERBURY Kent CT2 0JU w 6269645

MATHER Rebecca Claire 22/03/2004 53-55 Maidstone Road Footscray SIDCUP Kent DA14 5HB **Tel:** (020) 8300 8111 w 6291898

MATHESON Stanley John 13/11/2006 Hykeham Green Lincoln Road North Hykeham Lincoln Lincolnshire LN6 8NH **Tel:** (01522) 683300 m 6381900

MATSON Melanie Jane (see O'BRIEN, Mrs)

MATTHEWS Anna Jane 05/10/2009 Fairfax House Warwick Road Stratford-upon-Avon Warwickshire CV37 0NZ **Tel:** (01789) 292354 w 6387213

Barbara Ann 12/07/2006 Hope Vets Shantock Hall Lane Bovingdon Hertfordshire HP3 0NQ **Tel:** (01442) 833198 w 6351342

Helen Jane 14/03/2006 Hook Veterinary Centre Bell Meadow Road Hook Hampshire RG27 9HG **Tel:** (01256) 764771 w 6353113

Joanna DipAVN(Surgical) 26/01/1994 (02/03/2007) 176 Moseley Wood Gardens Cookridge LEEDS LS16 7JE **Tel:** (0113) 2160306 w 6067911

Kelly Anne 21/04/2009 80 Northorpe Thurlby Bourne Lincolnshire PE10 0HJ **Tel:** (01778) 394633 w 6445414

MATTHEWS Kirsty Ann (see JONES, Mrs)

Leanne Marie 27/02/2006 79 Seymour Way Sunbury-on-Thames Middlesex TW16 7NL **Tel:** (01932) 765953 w 6332620

Melissa 24/11/2009 6 Petit Road BOURNEMOUTH BH9 3JE **Tel:** (01202) 522235 w 6496190

MAUBANE Molefe Patrick 20/05/2003 Inside Pets at Home Unit 1 Bourges Boulevard Peterborough

Cambridgeshire PE1 1NG **Tel:** (01733) 865924 m 6334600

MAUD Katie 24/11/2008 Tower Wood Veterinary Group 27 Tinshill Road Leeds Yorkshire LS16 7DR **Tel:** (0113) 267 8419 w 6438297

MAUDE Charlotte 21/12/2005 20 Parker Avenue Calow CHESTERFIELD Derbyshire S44 5AY **Tel:** (01246) 200987 w 6337526

MAUNDER Alison Jane 24/02/2004 95 Maple Crescent Penketh Warrington WA5 2LQ **Tel:** (01925) 726378 w 6292382

MAUNDERS Hannah Eve 16/04/2007 7 Selborne Way Whitehill BORDON Hampshire GU35 9BQ **Tel:** (01420) 488 158 w 6290182

MAURICE Jane Ann 17/05/2005 23 Burnett Square Hertford Hertfordshire SG14 2HB **Tel:** (01992) 303176 w 6272802

MAWER Gayle 03/10/2007 Clyde Veterinary Group New Lanark Market Hyndford Road Lanark Lanarkshire ML11 9SZ **Tel:** (01555) 660000 w 6349263

MAWER Tracey Louise (see DAVIES, Mrs)

MAXWELL Jennifer Louise 30/07/1992 Heritage House La Grande Rue St. Martin Guernsey Channel Islands GY4 6LH **Tel:** (01481) 239101 w 6007441

Nina DipAVN(Surgical) (nee Jenkins) 30/08/1979 Lady Margaret House St. Anns Road Prestwich Manchester M25 9LF **Tel:** (0161) 773 1198 w 6056069

Ria Virginia 27/01/2005 171 Little Brays Harlow Essex CM18 6EY **Tel:** (01279) 422 066 w 6267313

MAY Claire Louise 08/11/2006 13 Harcourt Road Bracknell Berkshire RG12 7JH **Tel:** (01344) 305646 w 6358833

Ellen 24/02/2009 21 Wren Court Ash ALDERSHOT Hampshire GU12 6AX **Tel:** 01252320071 w 6433545

Jane Elizabeth 15/10/2008 22 Wynsome Street Southwick TROWBRIDGE Wiltshire BA14 9RE **Tel:** 01225755714 w 6441938

Jessica Louise 07/10/2008 8 North Street Wickwar Wotton-under-Edge Gloucestershire GL12 8NQ **Tel:** (07843) 445 906 w 6437384

MAY Laura Louise (see BROWNLOW, Mrs)

MAY Lisa (see MANFIELD, Mrs)

MAY Louise (see DALLY, Mrs)

Rebecca Jayne 02/09/2009 1 Stowe Road Barholm STAMFORD Lincolnshire PE9 4RD **Tel:** 01778560586 w 6249713

Suzanne Kirsty 06/11/1998 2 Barton Lane Wall Heath KINGSWINFORD West Midlands DY6 9EZ **Tel:** (01384) 298298 w 6140574

MAYALL Natasha Margaret 26/10/2006 31 Burton Avenue NORTH WALSHAM Norfolk NR28 0EP w 6345732

MAYDOM Rachel (nee Hawes) 24/05/2005 81 Elmdale Drive Carlton Colville Lowestoft Suffolk NR33 8DQ w 6320927

MAYELL Cheree 16/12/2009 37 Woodland Walk LIMAVADY County Londonderry BT49 9EP **Tel:** 07779540086 w 6441773

MAYES Christine Mary Margaret 03/08/1972 13 Charter Road Kingston upon Thames Surrey KT1 3PY **Tel:** (0208) 3909446 w 6056091

MAYNARD Donna-Marie (nee Cook) 10/04/2008 Newnham Court Veterinary Group Bearsted Road Weavering Maidstone Kent ME14 5EL **Tel:** (01622) 734555 w 6410236

MAYNE Tracy Anne (nee Roberts) 14/02/1994 (13/01/2005) 10 Ettingley Close Wirehill Redditch Worcestershire B98 7UF **Tel:** (01527) 853 389 w 6068198

MAYOR Victoria 20/08/2009 8/4 Hailesland Grove Edinburgh Midlothian EH14 2QQ **Tel:** (0131) 478 7361 w 6437659

MCADAM Wendy Ann 29/01/2009 84 Miller Road Bedford Bedfordshire MK42 9NZ **Tel:** 01234304678 w 6438286

MCALEER Hayley Jayne 21/10/2009 24 Reigate Road Urmston Manchester Lancashire M41 6PT **Tel:** 01617477235 w 6438649

MCALINDEN Kelly 29/10/2004 110 Elder Street Govan Glasgow G51 3NG **Tel:** (0141) 445 2735 w 6291370

MCALLISTER Laura Linda (nee Stanfield) 22/09/2000 (25/06/2008) 28 Brentwood Park BELFAST BT5 7LR **Tel:** (02890) 659725 w 6203062

MCALPINE Beverley (see LOGAN, Mrs)

MCAUSLAND Seona Margaret 01/04/2003 Forest Lodge Veterinary Practice 14 Barton Court Road New Milton Hampshire BH25 6NP **Tel:** (01425) 614482 w 6266950

MCCABE Marese 13/01/2004 'Hillview' Clontoe Ballinode Co Monaghan Ireland **Tel:** (02830) 252000 w 6279611

MCCALL Bridget Rachel 01/09/1992 36 High Street Cranford Kettering Northamptonshire NN14 4AA **Tel:** (01536) 330453 w 6005739

MCCALL Samantha Leigh (see ROBINSON, Mrs)

MCCALLUM Fiona 05/08/2008 13 Loch Torridon East Kilbride Glasgow Lanarkshire G74 2EU **Tel:** (01355) 221 560 w 6405143

Lynsey (nee McKee) 23/08/2005 (24/11/2008) 51 Thrashbush Crescent WISHAW Lanarkshire ML2 8LW **Tel:** (01698) 387027 w 6273550

MCCALMAN Aileen Catherine (see MCCALMAN-HART, Mrs)

MCCALMAN-HART Aileen Catherine (nee McCalman) 16/01/2002 1 Kyle Court High Street Earlston Berwickshire TD4 6BS w 6271614

MCCARRON Andrea Victoria 23/02/2005 20 Avon Road REDCAR Cleveland TS10 1NW **Tel:** (01642) 288353 w 6267027

MCCARTHY Alyson Mary Ellen 19/08/1988 Lucan Veterinary Hospital Chapel Hill Lucan Co Dublin Ireland **Tel:** (00) 353 1 6282840 w 6056149

Megan Jane 03/06/2004 20 Vanguard Street Deptford LONDON SE8 4DP **Tel:** (020) 8694 0693 w 6306154

MCCARTHY Megan Lucy (see BESTBIER, Mrs)

MCCARTNEY Joanne (nee Lamoury) 24/02/2004 (19/11/2007) 38 Chequers Avenue Lancashire LA1 4HZ **Tel:** (01524) 64649 w 6288301

MCCLEAN Sarah 11/11/2004 27 Newstead Way HARLOW Essex CM20 1BW **Tel:** (07769) 972741 w 6318056

MCCLEMENTS Laura Jayne 06/10/2009 9 Grove Side High Street Yoxford Saxmundham Suffolk IP17 3HT **Tel:** (01728) 668921 w 6434172

MCCLENAGHAN Alison Roberta (nee Peak) 30/01/1990 2 Killyleagh Road Killinchy Newtownards Co Down BT23 6TA **Tel:** (02897) 542111 w 6058485

MCCLUSKEY Emma Marion 18/02/2008 1 Craigower Crescent PITLOCHRY Perthshire PH16 5HS **Tel:** 07816123911 w 6318507

Michelle 29/06/2007 12 Fern Grove Bedworth Warwickshire CV12 0GA **Tel:** 07793436032 w 6368722

MCCOLL Karin 04/10/2005 11 Steeple Street Kilbarchan Johnstone Renfrewshire PA10 2JF **Tel:** (01505) 704248 w 6279204

Lisa Marie 16/04/2007 33 Drum Brae South EDINBURGH EH12 8DT **Tel:** (0131) 317 7113 w 6327450

MCCOMISKIE Tanya Fay 14/05/2007 81 Tudor Way HERTFORD SG14 2DY **Tel:** (07904) 315366 w 6342685

MCCONNELL Paula Joan 14/09/2001 480 Manchester Road Bury Greater Manchester BL9 9NY **Tel:** (0161) 763 6333 w 6228263

MCCONVILLE Vicky Anne 17/01/2006 66 Studland Road MANCHESTER M22 5AN w 6333907

MCCOOEY Rachael Dawn (nee Edwards) 03/09/2008 Langrick House Didbrook CHELTENHAM Gloucestershire GL54 5PF w 6437868

MCCOOKE Donna Marie 02/10/2001 2 Foundry Cottage Foundry Lane Summerbridge HARROGATE North Yorkshire HG3 4JN w 6229275

MCCORMACK Rachel Bridget 03/09/2008 71 Riverway LONDON N13 5JU **Tel:** 02088869340 w 6434898

MCCORMICK Irene Evelyn (see MACKENZIE, Mrs)

MCCORMICK Rebecca (see HOLLAND, Mrs)

MCCORRY Roberta 27/02/2006 151 Ballyboley Road LARNE County Antrim BT40 2SY **Tel:** (02828) 260153 w 6333709

MCCOURT Angela Mary (see MCNELLAN, Mrs)

MCCOWLIFF Iain Joseph 06/08/2008 33 Gerald Street South Shields Tyne and Wear NE34 8RG **Tel:** (0191) 519 2725 m 6387884

MCCOY Jennifer Louise 18/11/2008 Willows 3 Upper Pitching Chilcompton RADSTOCK BA3 4HS **Tel:** 01761232272 w 6437274

MCCRAE Julie 17/01/2006 c/o The Veterinary Hospital 169-170 High Street Lowestoft Suffolk NR32 1HU **Tel:** (01502) 513376 w 6337801

MCCREIGHT Karen Wilson 03/09/2008 74 Marches Drive Armadale BATHGATE West Lothian EH48 2PH **Tel:** 01501733120 w 6373518

MCCRICKARD Alison Mariecia (nee Burchill, nee Burchill) 17/03/2003 "Carseview" Leetown Perth Perthshire PH2 7NN **Tel:** (01738) 861160 w 6288653

MCCRONE Jacqueline (see GALLACHER, Mrs)

MCCULLOCH Paul Robert 13/01/2004 36 Girtford Crescent Sandy Bedfordshire SG19 1HR **Tel:** (01767) 222127 m 6266895

MCCUTCHEON Amanda Louise 04/01/2006 26 Springfields WIGTON Cumbria CA7 9JT w 6300577

MCDAID Ciara Brigid 02/06/2008 1 Eaves Avenue Chapel-en-le-Frith HIGH PEAK Derbyshire SK23 0LS **Tel:** 07731526604 w 6387323

MCDERMOTT Laura Jayne 16/04/2008 74 Whitburn Street Glasgow Lanarkshire G32 6RE **Tel:** (0141) 778 2090 w 6373529

MCDONALD Claire Louise 18/10/2006 2 Bishops Way Newport Isle of Wight PO30 5WT **Tel:** (01983) 522804 w 6339176

Margaret 30/09/1983 Jammaj President Kennedy Drive Plean Stirling FK7 8AY **Tel:** (01786) 811609 w 6056240

Susan Vanessa (nee Green) 03/09/2002 17 Langmuir Way TAPPING WA 6065 Australia w 6276443

Teresa 22/12/2004 Chapel Garth Trumfleet Lane Moss Doncaster DN6 0EB **Tel:** (01302) 701 268 w 6278412

MCDONALD-BELL Samantha Dawn 25/01/2000 17 Warwick Avenue EGHAM Surrey TW20 8LW w 6190764

MCDONOUGH Laura (see HAYES, Mrs)

MCDOUGALL Claire 21/11/2005 127 Devonshire Street KEIGHLEY West Yorkshire BD21 2LU **Tel:** (01535) 602731 w 6343807

Kirsty Anne 30/11/2009 21 Sneddon Street Burnbank HAMILTON Lanarkshire ML3 0QX **Tel:** (01698) 828574 w 6405000

MCDOWALL Nicola Mary 11/05/2004 21 Lutton Place Edinburgh Midlothian EH8 9PD **Tel:** (0131) 668 1026 w 6291381

MCDOWELL Nichola Ann 24/11/2004 4 Woodlands Avenue WHITEHAVEN Cumbria CA28 6TF **Tel:** (01946) 695112 w 6325107

MCEACHERN Erin Yvonne (see MACEACHERN, Miss)

MCELHILL Catriona 15/11/2005 4 Union Street ALEXANDRIA G83 9AH **Tel:** (01360) 441078 w 6291392

MCENTEE Helen Frances 15/11/2001 7 Warwick Road South Old Trafford Manchester M16 0JW **Tel:** (0161) 881 0222 w 6264365

MCEWEN Joanna Lucie 22/03/2000 Chester Gates Referral Hospital Unit F Telford Court Chester Gates Chester Cheshire CH1 6LT **Tel:** (01244) 853 823 w 6134491

MCFADZEAN Zena Maxine (nee Flanagan) 15/01/1996 Hale House 19 Langley Road Chippenham Wiltshire SN15 1BS **Tel:** (01249) 653561 w 6036494

MCFARLANE Jennifer Elizabeth 16/09/2009 11-17 The Precinct West Meads Bognor Regis West Sussex PO21 5SB **Tel:** (01243) 842832 w 6379513

MCGARRAGH Stephanie 19/03/2007 52 Park Lane Abram Wigan Lancashire WN2 5XJ **Tel:** (01942) 514506 w 6363376

MCGARTY Gemma Elizabeth 25/09/2009 20 Rainton Close Gateshead Tyne and Wear NE10 8RW **Tel:** 01914691221 w 6437736

MCGEAGH Danielle Louise 05/09/2008 7 Cambridge Street Carlton NOTTINGHAM NG4 3JS **Tel:** 01159538411 w 6417012

MCGEE Louise Kathleen 21/11/2005 (25/02/2009) 6 Senior Drive Salisbury Wiltshire SP2 8QD **Tel:** (01722) 332030 w 6297310

MCGILL Elizabeth Agnes 18/06/2009 48 Kingsacre Road Glasgow Lanarkshire G44 4LP **Tel:** (0141) 649 0221 w 6345688

Laura Jane 30/05/2006 25 Calais View Dunfermline Fife KY11 4NR **Tel:** (01383) 842 357 w 6296782

MCGIMPSEY Kim Alexandra (see FERGUS, Mrs)

Michelle 14/09/2009 53 Beechcroft Park NEWTOWNARDS County Down BT23 8QL **Tel:** 07929371706 w 6492747

MCGIVERN Anne-Marie 22/03/2004 215 Lancaster Road Salford Lancashire M6 8WA **Tel:** (07952) 564865 w 6295528

MCGLOGAN Karen 17/04/2008 54a Colliers Road Fallin STIRLING FK7 7HU **Tel:** (07926) 538580 w 6264684

MCGRATH Kelly Ann 09/02/2009 6 Marlowe Place Leeholme HOUGHTON LE SPRING Tyne and Wear DH5 8HS **Tel:** 01915841548 w 6435503

Kelly Anne 14/01/2008 45 Lionheart Way Bursledon SOUTHAMPTON SO31 8HF **Tel:** 07860362269 w 6340386

Laura Alison 21/06/2005 Flat 3 32 Atherley Road SOUTHAMPTON SO15 5DQ w 6303745

MCGREGOR Amanda Joan (see HARRIS, Mrs)

MCGREGOR Fiona Elizabeth (see SIRRELL, Mrs)

Phillipa Jane 08/09/2009 Briar Cottage Main Street Farnsfield NEWARK Nottinghamshire NG22 8EF **Tel:** 01623882855 w 6460880

MCGUIGAN Carol Jean 01/10/1970 (21/07/1999) 114 Starling Place Boundary Way Watford WD25 7SP **Tel:** (01923) 671188 w 6056364

MCGUINNESS Doreen Margaret 10/02/1994 2A Deramore Drive BELFAST BT9 5JQ w 6067922

MCGUINNESS Zana Eluise (see JOHNSON, Mrs)

MCHUGH Dawn Patricia DipAVN(Surgical) 01/08/1977 65 High Street Stetchworth Newmarket Suffolk CB8 9TH **Tel:** (01638) 507768 w 6056386

Helen (nee Stephenson) 07/04/2003 Ash Field House Ash Tree Garth Barkston Ash TADCASTER North Yorkshire LS24 9ET w 6266400

MCILVEEN Clare Margaret 17/02/2009 2 Manor Lane Killinchy NEWTOWNARDS County Down BT23 6NS **Tel:** 07711224352 w 6429035

MCINARLIN Michele Linda 29/08/2000 92 Pendeen Road Barlanark Glasgow G33 4UF **Tel:** (0141) 771 8628 w 614570X

MCINDOE Caroline Dean 16/06/2006 47 Old Rome Drive KILMARNOCK Ayrshire KA1 2RU w 6349021

MCINTOSH Aimee Patricia 12/05/2009 3 Ward Road Rosehearty FRASERBURGH Aberdeenshire AB43 7NN **Tel:** 01346571204 w 6319794

MCINTOSH Jillian (see ANDERSON, Mrs)

MCINTYRE Fiona Louise (see WHYTE, Mrs)

MCINTYRE Heather Elizabeth (nee Lawson) 22/02/1993 Lower Nuide Farm Cottage Nuide KINGUSSIE Inverness-Shire PH21 1NR w 6014426

MCINTYRE Jane Barbara (see RUSSELL, Mrs)

Kayleigh Ann 26/11/2009 Higher Clough Farm Keasdon Road Dalehead Slaidburn Lancashire BB7 4TS w 6452718

MCIVER Ellie 06/10/2006 Fivehills Fairmoor Morpeth Northumberland NE61 3JL **Tel:** (01670) 512 038 w 6372396

MCKAY Abigail Marie (nee Harris) 28/06/2005 Donnington Grove Veterinary Surgery Oxford Road NEWBURY Berkshire RG14 2JB **Tel:** (01635) 47170 w 6323336

Johann Elizabeth 15/01/1990 (07/06/2007) 15 Walkers Close Burnham Market Kings Lynn Norfolk PE31 8EP **Tel:** (01328) 738 703 w 6056433

Lynsey Janet 30/07/2004 South Kilduff Farm Fossoway Kinross Kinross-shire KY13 0PN **Tel:** (01577) 840022 w 6301138

Rosalind Katherine (nee McKeown) 10/09/1998 15 Earl Drive Dundonald Kilmarnock KA2 9DE **Tel:** (01563) 851 053 w 6108086

MCKEANEY Sarah Louise 13/07/2007 34 Old Manor Road Mansfield Woodhouse Mansfield Nottinghamshire NG19 9LX **Tel:** (01623) 424771 w 6347514

MCKEATING Sandra Dawn (nee Wilson) 18/03/2003 Millcroft Veterinary Group Wakefield Road Cockermouth Cumbria CA13 0HR **Tel:** (01900) 826666 w 6280150

MCKEE Kirsty Ann 06/10/2006 Eye Vet 59 Main Street Frodsham Warrington Cheshire WA6 7DF **Tel:** (01928) 734 040 w 6288818

MCKEE Lynsey (see MCCALLUM, Mrs)

MCKELLAR Korina Lee 04/08/1981 College Road CULLOMPTON Devon EX15 1TG **Tel:** (01884) 32228 w 6089301

MCKENZIE Cheryl 13/04/2004 10 Backdean Road Danderhall Edinburgh EH22 1RE **Tel:** (0131) 663 3583 w 6291590

Rachael (nee Pickard) 17/01/1991 (14/03/2005) Daventry Veterinary Clinic Stephenson Close Drayton Fields Daventry Northamptonshire NN11 8RF **Tel:** (01327) 877767 w 6058758

MCKEON Jacqueline-Anne Bridget 16/07/2007 (03/06/2009) 26 Albert College Drive Glasnevin Dublin 9 Ireland **Tel:** (003531) 837 8272 w 6266345

MCKEOWN Gemma Ann 16/09/1996 27 Beechwood Avenue MIRFIELD West Yorkshire WF14 9LG **Tel:** (01924) 490515 w 6043424

Linsey Marie 10/04/2003 Mintlaw Veterinary Surgery Ivy Court Station Road Mintlaw Peterhead Aberdeenshire AB42 5EB **Tel:** (01771) 624001 w 6286255

MCKEOWN Rosalind Katherine (see MCKAY, Mrs)

MCKEOWN Victoria Louise (see PERRIS, Mrs)

MCKINLAY Fiona Margaret (see ROBB, Mrs)

MCKINLEY Olive Frances (see SEMPLE, Mrs)

MCKINNON Janice Lynette 28/07/2008 18a Rocky Bank Road Birkenhead Merseyside CH42 7LB **Tel:** 01516524425 w 6412513

MCLAIN Emma Louise 24/02/2004 The Veterinary Surgery Maple Street Huddersfield HD5 9AX **Tel:** (01484) 421512 w 6276795

MCLAREN Fiona Elaine 13/08/2008 47 Cortachy Crescent Northmuir Kirriemuir Angus DD8 4TP **Tel:** (01575) 574687 w 6404747

Laura Joy 16/06/2006 39 Station Road Whittlesford Cambridge CB2 4NL **Tel:** (01223) 833651 w 6261329

MCLAUGHLIN Tracy Louise (nee Hill) 15/12/2004 21 Aeron Place Gilfach BARGOED Mid Glamorgan CF81 8JA w 6277169

MCLEAN Emma Louise (nee Coleman) 27/08/2004 Dundas Veterinary Group 99 Dundas Street Edinburgh EH3 6SD **Tel:** (0131) 557 1819 w 6290314

MCLEAN Natasha Ann (see FIELDSON, Mrs)

Sarah Isobel 12/05/2004 Vets Now (Liverpool) Woolfall Heath Avenue Huyton Liverpool Merseyside L36 3YD **Tel:** (0151) 480 2040 w 6299576

MCLEARY Sandra (nee Paterson) 23/01/1995 (15/06/2007) 11 Graham Terrace Airth Falkirk FK2 8LF **Tel:** (01324) 831428 w 6022696

MCLENNAN Natalie Jill (nee Thornhill) 24/05/2005 82 Bailies Drive Elgin Morayshire IV30 6JJ **Tel:** (01343) 556135 w 6304130

MCLEOD Hayley Louise 21/11/2000 Shutts Farm Shutts Lane BAKEWELL Derbyshire DE45 1JA w 6204580

MCMAHON Jacqueline Ann 14/10/2002 John Hankinson Veterinary Surgery 9 Shardeloes Road London SE14 6NZ **Tel:** (020) 8692 3030 w 6253365

Leigh Norma 21/04/2005 Jocks Lodge Watling Street Radlett Hertfordshire WD7 7HL **Tel:** 07709433443 w 6288939

MCMANUS Ashley Mary 28/03/1983 (26/11/2007) Portman Veterinary Clinic 86 York Street London W1H 1QS **Tel:** (020) 7723 2068 w 6056466

Kelly Joanne 19/07/2006 Priory Veterinary Group 17 Market Place Bridlington East Yorkshire YO16 4QJ **Tel:** (01262) 674085 w 6326977

MCMATH Linsay 22/06/2001 (26/09/2003) Dalblair Veterinary Surgery 52-54 Dalblair Road Ayr KA7 1UQ **Tel:** (01292) 263744 w 6146102

MCMEECHAN Elaine Lisa 31/10/2007 2/2 10 Leyden Court Maryhill GLASGOW G20 9LY **Tel:** 07740986451 w 6373540

MCMILLAN Samantha Jane DipAVN(Medical) (nee Burke) 05/11/2003 16 Ullswater Close Stevenage Hertfordshire SG1 6AF **Tel:** (01438) 312 384 w 6291161

MCMINN Charleen 29/06/2007 Parkside Veterinary Group 5 Kings Cross Road Dundee Angus DD2 3PT **Tel:** (01382) 810777 w 6339286

MCMURRAN Rebecca Rose 11/04/2008 15 De Courcy Park Greyabbey NEWTOWNARDS County Down BT22 2SA **Tel:** (028) 427 88531 w 6324139

MCNAIR Audrey (see MASON, Mrs)

MCNALLY Roisin Mary 29/09/1999 (17/04/2003) 12 Moor Park Gardens Blacks Road Dunmurry Belfast BT10 0QG **Tel:** (028) 908 76258 w 6042180

MCNAMARA Lisa Joanne 08/03/1996 26 Lingwood Road Great Sankey Warrington Cheshire WA5 3EN **Tel:** (01925) 723120 w 6033529

MCNAMEE Katherine Anne 01/09/2008 Tinkers Lodge Slaidburn Clitheroe Lancashire BB7 4TD **Tel:** (07968) 055334 w 6287586

MCNELLAN Angela Mary DipAVN(Surgical) (nee McCourt) 21/01/1998 49-51 Stockiemuir Avenue Bearsden Glasgow G61 3JJ **Tel:** (0141) 942 7070 w 6108064

MCNICHOL Joanne Susan (nee Whitaker) 08/09/2005 (20/11/2009) 1 Wood Street Haworth KEIGHLEY West Yorkshire BD22 8BJ **Tel:** (01535) 644466 w 6312083

MCNICHOLL Kirsty Jacqueline (nee Mackinnon) 04/10/2005 175 Glencoats Drive Paisley Renfrewshire PA3 1RR **Tel:** (01415) 637508 w 6313359

MCNICOL Alanna Thornton 01/07/2008 Equipet Veterinary Hospital 24 Nicol Street Kirkcaldy Fife KY1 1NY **Tel:** (01592) 641333 w 6381889

MCNULTY Linda Ann 20/09/1999 (24/03/2004) 9 Pangbourne Avenue Urmston Manchester Lancashire M41 0GF **Tel:** (0161) 7482767 w 6185495

MCPHAIL Gillian Frances (nee Graham) 20/11/2002 24 St. Margaret Street Dunfermline Fife KY12 7PE **Tel:** (01383) 732897 w 6273341

MCPHEE Alyson Margret 27/03/2008 Ashgate Station Road Portbury Bristol Avon BS20 7TN w 6348790

MCQUEEN Stuart 21/01/2008 Coombefield Veterinary Hospital Coombe Lane Axminster Devon EX13 5AX **Tel:** (01297) 630500 m 6382439

MCQUOID Karen Louise (nee Law) 02/02/1998 35 Landseer Drive DOWNHAM MARKET Norfolk PE38 9NG **Tel:** (01366) 384552 w 610836X

MCSKIMMING Joanne Elizabeth 03/12/2003 (19/09/2006) 15 Chesterfield Road Basingstoke Hampshire RG21 3BQ **Tel:** (01256) 460755 w 6283846

MCVEIGH Catherine Nora 09/12/2002 11 Cairn Park Gortin Omagh Co Tyrone BT79 8NB w 6277125

MEAD Katy Alice 19/03/2007 33 Hammonds Lane Totton Southampton Hampshire SO40 3LF **Tel:** (023) 8066 1887 w 6381482

Ruth Elizabeth 01/04/1982 51 Kings Meadow Wigmore Leominster Herefordshire HR6 9UY **Tel:** (01568) 770 382 w 6056590

MEADE Kerry Anne 12/05/2004 Wingrave Veterinary Surgery 84 Mulgrave Road Sutton Surrey SM2 6LZ **Tel:** (020) 8642 9100 w 6287696

MEADOWS Lucy Ann (see TURNER, Mrs)

MEADOWS Mary Jane 24/08/1998 Paddystone Sandhurst Lane Sandhurst Gloucester GL2 9PB **Tel:** (01452) 730478 w 6137299

MEAKIN Sarah Jane (see HARPER, Mrs)

MEAKINGS Jane (see RUSSELL, Mrs)

MEALOR Lisa Clare 27/04/2006 31 Gilbert Grove EDGWARE Middlesex HA8 0HJ **Tel:** (02089) 062678 w 6311709

MEARS Justine (see THORNE, Mrs)

MEARS Kelly Dawn (see MACLEAN, Mrs)

MEDCALF Lynda Janice 30/01/1990 7 Hurst Road Croydon CR0 1JT **Tel:** (020) 8686 3972 w 6056637

MEDLAND Josephine (see KILLNER, Mrs)

MEDLAND Tracey Louise (see EAST, Mrs)

MEE Laura Elizabeth 31/10/2003 5 Club Street London Road Stoke-on-Trent ST4 5RQ **Tel:** (01782) 413415 w 6291722

MEECH Samantha Lucy 16/06/2008 272 Down Road Portishead BRISTOL BS20 8HZ **Tel:** (07790) 158 989 w 6380811

MEECHAM Alison Joanne 07/08/1997 (07/01/2004) Sparsholt College Sparsholt Winchester Hampshire SO21 2NT **Tel:** (01962) 797 388 w 6108767

MEGAW Michelle Mary (nee Stevenson) 31/08/1999 38 Carnacally Road NEWRY Co Down BT34 1LS **Tel:** (028) 4065 1609 w 6115446

MEHTA Antonia Jean 21/08/1998 The Barn Animal Hospital Great Binfields Road Old Basing BASINGSTOKE Hampshire RG24 8AD **Tel:** (01256) 329522 w 6036359

MEIN Bonnie Marie (see CARTWRIGHT, Mrs)

Charlotte Anne 13/05/2003 Rosebank 43 Brooklynn Close Waltham Chase Southampton Hampshire SO32 2RZ **Tel:** ((01489)) 896176 w 6278148

MELLING Joanna Ruth (see ELLIS, Mrs)

MELLOR Jemma Natalie 08/06/2009 131 Station Road Hatton Derby Derbyshire DE65 5EJ **Tel:** (01283) 520323 w 6434579

Joanne 08/07/2003 (19/01/2010) Unit T Viking House Daneholes Roundabout Stanford Road Grays Essex RM16 2XE **Tel:** (01375) 385129 w 6275948

Kayleigh Marie 15/11/2007 14 Springfield Drive Stafford Staffordshire ST17 9LG **Tel:** 07866668832 w 6382450

Louise 14/10/2008 9 Lee Close Stoney Stanton Leicester Leicestershire LE9 4ED **Tel:** (01455) 272 556 w 6434513

MELTON Della 02/03/2001 36 Boston Road Kirton Boston Lincolnshire PE20 1DS **Tel:** (01205) 722696 w 6213512

MELVILLE Kerry Lorraine 20/09/1999 (06/11/2003) 12 Kippielaw Medway Easthouses Dalkeith Midlothian EH22 4HX **Tel:** (0131) 663 0250 w 6135757

MERCER Aimee Rebecca 24/04/2009 Solton Manor East Langdon Dover Kent CT15 5JB **Tel:** 01304852248 w 6412975

Helen Louise 16/06/2004 35 Buckstone Oval Leeds West Yorkshire LS17 5HF **Tel:** (0113) 2930781 w 6298102

MERRETT Michelle Ann (nee Wilson) 17/09/1999 (20/01/2010) 29 Manley Avenue Golborne Warrington WA3 3XA **Tel:** (01942) 713417 w 6186386

MERRIFIELD Karen Valerie 10/02/2009 2 St. Austell Road St. Blazey Gate Par Cornwall PL24 2EE **Tel:** 01726816856 w 6426318

MERRIS Sharada Louise 08/03/1999 (24/10/2000) Fennis Fields Farm King's Newnham Rugby Warwickshire CV23 0JJ **Tel:** (01788) 833185 w 6039600

MERRITT Helen Louise (see BOYD, Mrs)

MERRYWEATHER Jayne Isabel 04/01/2006 2 Bishops Way Newport Isle of Wight PO30 5WT **Tel:** (01983) 522804 w 6346150

MESSAGE Sara Jasmine 06/08/2009 29 Rotunda Road Eastbourne East Sussex BN23 6LE **Tel:** (01323) 648895 w 6403130

MESSENGER Lucy Rebecca 18/01/2002 2 Pennine Way Stalmine POULTON-LE-FYLDE Lancashire FY6 0QU **Tel:** (01253) 702462 w 6191435

METCALF Michelle Louise 01/08/2008 16 Stubbins Lane Chinley HIGH PEAK Derbyshire SK23 6AE **Tel:** 01162108443 w 6359735

METCALFE Claire 13/04/2004 6 Skelgillside Nenthead Road Alston Cumbria CA9 3TR **Tel:** (01434) 381792 w 6268017

Heather Eve 31/10/2005 Nantwich Veterinary Hospital Crewe Road End Nantwich Cheshire CW5 5SF **Tel:** (01270) 610349 w 6351364

Rebekah Helen 20/04/2005 Bishopton Veterinary Group Mill Farm Studley Road Ripon North Yorkshire HG4 2QR **Tel:** (01765) 602396 w 6304812

Sarah Louise 03/09/2008 Grange Vets Victoria Road Darlington County Durham DL1 5SJ **Tel:** (01325) 465371 w 6415494

METHERELL Victoria 27/09/2004 Flat 3 Bridport House 200 Heritage Way GOSPORT Hampshire PO12 4WF **Tel:** (023) 9258 2991 w 6285034

MICHAEL Angiy 28/11/2003 (09/02/2009) 10 Alder Drive Wardley Swinton MANCHESTER M27 9QG **Tel:** (0161) 793 7042 w 6296309

Kelly Victoria 30/05/2008 12 Duncan Court New Farm Loch Kilmarnock Ayrshire KA3 7TF **Tel:** (07786) 042535 w 6412359

MIDDLETON Karen Elsie 21/06/2005 Old Mill Cottage 268 Dunkirk Lane Leyland Lancashire PR26 7SN **Tel:** (01772) 510340 w 6320993

Natasha Elaine 30/11/2007 5 Clover Avenue Bishop's Stortford Hertfordshire CM23 4BW **Tel:** (01279) 504193 w 6383253

Toni Melanie (nee Snart) 11/01/1988 65 Marsh Lane Misterton Doncaster South Yorkshire DN10 4DL **Tel:** (01427) 890415 w 6056750

MIDGLEY Emma Louise (nee Larkins) 17/07/2003 (01/09/2006) 35 High Street Yelling St. Neots Cambridgeshire PE19 6SB **Tel:** (01480) 880593 w 6275090

MIDGLEY Victoria Claire (see PEDDER, Mrs)

MIDSON Lianne Frances (nee Twyman) 29/07/1992 4 Burnan Road WHITSTABLE Kent CT5 2QD **Tel:** (01227) 266762 w 6008263

MILDON Shelley Rachel 25/03/2002 83 Stafford Road Seaford East Sussex BN25 1UA w 6275112

MILEES Lindsey Jane (see MILES, Miss)

MILES Alison Sarah (nee Harding) 19/01/1995 Cornerstone Veterinary Centre Northwood Park Road Bushbury Wolverhampton WV10 8ET **Tel:** (01902) 397227 w 6034861

Carly Chelsea 29/04/2009 2 Ridgeway Close Hemel Hempstead Hertfordshire HP3 9TB **Tel:** 01442248348 w 6426439

Joanna Jacquie 27/11/2009 Windmill Farm Burwardsley Road Tattenhall Nr Chester Cheshire CH3 9NS **Tel:** (01829) 770228 w 6496168

Laura Diane 26/08/2008 14 Avenue Road LONDON N12 8PY **Tel:** (079045) 29523 w 6204437

Lindsey Jane (formerly Milees) 24/11/2004 285 Quemerford Calne Wiltshire SN11 8LB **Tel:** (01249) 815556 w 6286057

Lisa Ann Mary 10/04/2007 18 Heath Close Hessett Bury St. Edmunds Suffolk IP30 9BL **Tel:** (01359) 270905 w 6376521

MILES Megan Claire (see ALLISON, Mrs)

Ruth Ellen 03/05/2007 The Barn Animal Hospital Great Binfields Road Old Basing BASINGSTOKE Hampshire RG24 8AD **Tel:** (01256) 329522 w 6353124

Tammy Louise 15/07/2005 (21/01/2010) 266 Harrogate Road Eccleshill Bradford Yorkshire BD2 3RH **Tel:** (01274) 400500 w 6326999

MILLAR Ava (formerly Mortensen, nee Mortensen) 10/05/1999 11 Gardenston Street Laurencekirk Kincardineshire AB30 1UG **Tel:** (01561) 378246 w 6134593

Bonny 15/01/1996 (14/07/1999) Rossdales Equine Hospital Cotton End Road Exning Newmarket Suffolk CB8 7NN **Tel:** (01638) 577 754 w 6097119

MILLARD Jemma Helen Deborah 28/02/2001 (17/04/2003) The Philippa & George Adams Centre 6 Amersham Vale New Cross London SE14 6LD **Tel:** (020) 8691 0577 w 6213336

MILLARD Leanne Jane (see MURPHY, Mrs)

Rosemary Anne (nee Kearvell) 17/07/2003 Pykelle The Greenway West Hendred Wantage Oxfordshire OX12 8RG **Tel:** (01235) 833621 w 6263881

MILLER Amanda Jane 10/02/1997 95 Kings Road Hayling Island Hants PO11 0PE **Tel:** (023) 92463228 w 6041380

Caroline Ann 09/10/2008 Alton Carron Aberlour Banffshire AB38 7QT w 6377533

Catherine Victoria 30/09/2008 Woodpeckers 8 Highridge ALTON Hampshire GU34 1QN w 6412799

Colleen Louise 20/02/2009 6 Eleanora Gardens Douglas Isle of Man IM2 3NR **Tel:** 07624200611 w 6439573

Debbie Fraser 29/06/2007 86 Viewfield Terrace Lumphinnans Cowdenbeath Fife KY4 8AB w 6372913

Janet Ann (nee Markham) 14/02/1977 12 Langley Park Road Iver Buckinghamshire SL0 9QN **Tel:** (01753) 672593 w 6086253

Karen Julie (nee Pateman) 12/05/2004 Berry House Veterinary Practice 41 Nightingale Road Hitchin Hertfordshire SG5 1RE **Tel:** (01462) 432824 w 6293768

Kerry-Ann 26/10/2006 Toachim House Veterinary Surgery Toachim House South Road Faversham Kent ME13 7LR **Tel:** (01795) 531313 w 6347206

Patricia 01/02/2010 2 Harrow House Harrow Road WICK Caithness KW1 5TW **Tel:** (01955) 606455 w 6465588

Polly Anna (nee Elmer) 13/05/2003 (14/05/2007) 1 Boytens View Old Barn Road Brumstead NORWICH NR12 9HA **Tel:** (01692) 580171 w 6280106

MILLER Wendy Jane (see MILLER-SMITH, Mrs)

MILLER-SMITH Wendy Jane (nee Miller) 22/03/1988 The Closes Kirkcowan Newton Stewart Wigtownshire DG8 0EL **Tel:** (01671) 830865 w 6056819

MILLETT Lucy Charlotte 19/02/2009 Scesaplana Gorse Avenue Kingston Gorse East Preston Littlehampton West Sussex BN16 1SF **Tel:** (01903) 784353 w 6389006

MILLETT Naomi Jane (see SADLER, Mrs)

MILLGATE Lisa-Marie Jayne (see HELLINGS, Mrs)

MILLINER Jenny Anne 14/04/2008 17 Larchfield YORK YO31 1JS **Tel:** (01904) 412448 w 6388753

MILLINGTON Corrine (nee Heron) 13/08/2003 109 West Road Westcliff on Sea Essex SS0 9AZ **Tel:** (01702) 305 736 w 6278038

MILLINGTON Jacqueline (see GOULDING, Mrs)

MILLS Alison Clare (see ROBINSON, Mrs)

MILLS Aron-Louise 21/03/2007 (21/04/2009) 22 Woodland Way Devizes Wiltshire SN10 5LA **Tel:** (01380) 721453 w 6382802

Clare Elizabeth 16/06/2009 8 St George's Parade Wolverhampton West Midlands WV2 1BD **Tel:** (01902) 425262 w 6378798

Gail Louise 25/08/2009 Percheron Lodge Gull Farm Deeping High Bank Deeping St. Nicholas Spalding Lincolnshire PE11 3DY **Tel:** 01733554953 w 6437758

Hannah Louise 22/03/2004 Morar Gussage St Michael Wimborne Dorset BH21 5JE w 6301160

Kate 21/01/2008 39 Stonechat Gardens Bristol Avon BS16 1UQ **Tel:** (0117) 965 2447 w 6401392

Kelly Eva 12/08/2003 5 Club Street London Road Stoke-on-Trent ST4 5RQ **Tel:** (01782) 413415 w 6285925

Kerri Tace 27/10/2008 70 Elmdon Lane Marston Green BIRMINGHAM B37 7EQ w 6410764

Rebecca Louise (nee Gunsman) 23/07/2007 34 Southgate Street Bury St. Edmunds Suffolk IP33 2AZ **Tel:** (01284) 701444 w 6352783

Rebecca Sandra (nee Ley) 15/09/1994 (07/06/1999) East Greadon Farm Bradworthy HOLSWORTHY Devon EX22 7RB **Tel:** (01409) 241347 w 6031907

Tamzin Joelle 13/05/2003 Brambledene Chivers Road Stondon Massey Nr Brentwood Essex CM15 0LJ **Tel:** (01277) 823206 w 6286453

Tanya Louise 15/01/1987 25 Long Furlong Over CAMBRIDGE CB24 5PG **Tel:** (01954) 203016 w 6056841

MILNE Emma Louise (nee Christie) 13/05/2003 Wardhill Cottage East Pitforthie BRECHIN Angus DD9 7PE w 6278698

Louise DipAVN(Surgical) 13/10/1993 40 Guernsey Road Norwich Norfolk NR3 1JJ **Tel:** 07765430141 w 6065743

Sarah Elizabeth 01/08/2002 Sparsholt College Sparsholt WINCHESTER Hampshire SO21 2NF **Tel:** (01962) 797545 w 6260779

Sarah Michelle 28/06/2002 57 Fenton Road Warboys Huntingdon Cambridgeshire PE28 2SL **Tel:** (01487) 822886 w 6259965

Victoria (nee Cutler) 20/09/1999 (13/12/2001) 48 Parkfield Rank Pucklechurch Bristol Avon BS16 9NP **Tel:** (0117) 9326369 w 6129186

MILNER Caroline Louise 15/09/2009 39 Sandgate Drive Kippax Leeds West Yorkshire LS25 7EX **Tel:** (0113) 2862510 w 6439683

Tanya Louise Jane (nee Swift) 15/02/2002 17 Green Lane SELBY North Yorkshire YO8 9AN **Tel:** (01757) 241358 w 6264134

MINCHER Kathryn Mandy (formerly Bracey) 22/01/1985 2 Hibbert Street New Mills High Peak Derbyshire SK22 3JJ **Tel:** (01663) 745294 w 6046083

MINETT Emily Jane 25/06/2008 26 Woodside Close Knaphill Woking Surrey GU21 2DD **Tel:** (07912) 762708 w 6381306

Rachel (nee Molsher, nee Minnett) 25/02/2003 7 Stagshaw Drive Peterborough Cambridgeshire PE2 8NG **Tel:** (01733) 340417 w 6281503

MINNETT Rachel (see MINETT, Mrs)

MINNEY Carol Elizabeth (see TECKMAN, Mrs)

MINTER Fiona Ruth 15/07/2008 65 The Glade Coulsdon Surrey CR5 1SS **Tel:** (01737) 552 135 w 6416429

MINTERN Kerry Denise 02/11/2004 309 The Ridge Hastings East Sussex TN34 2RA **Tel:** (01424) 751595 w 6321015

MISKELLY Louise Dorothy (nee Diack) 11/07/2005 Woodside Veterinary Group Woodside Road Torphins BANCHORY Kincardineshire AB31 4TR **Tel:** (01339) 882556 w 6289852

MISS HODSON Emma Louise (see COOPER, Mrs)

MISSEY Rebecca Louise (nee Missey, formerly Glicksman) 01/02/1999 (26/10/2000) 154 High Street Ramsgate Kent CT11 9TT **Tel:** (01843) 591899 w 6118152

MITCHELL Amy Galina Eva 12/05/2008 23 Hawkcliffe View Silsden Keighley West Yorkshire BD20 0BS **Tel:** (01535) 654 603 w 6403097

Carolanne 27/03/2008 22 Atholl Way LIVINGSTON West Lothian EH54 8TH **Tel:** (07806) 415157 w 6405154

Deborah Ruth 15/01/2008 15 Langton Lea High Shincliffe Durham County Durham DH1 2QF **Tel:** (0191) 386 3747 w 6384859

MITCHELL Fiona (see VAN WEZEL, Mrs)

Joanne Lesley (nee Suter) 13/08/1990 (17/03/2006) 2 The Witheys Wanborough Swindon Wiltshire SN4 0BQ **Tel:** (01793) 790 141 w 6061534

Judith Susan 27/08/2004 3 Ancrum Gardens Dundee DD2 2HU **Tel:** (01382) 669 023 w 6276025

Lara Jane (nee Marshall) 24/02/2004 (13/01/2010) Dairy Cottage Ovington Alresford Hampshire SO24 0RB **Tel:** (01420) 82163 w 6303811

MITCHELL Lisa Caroline (see MULCOCK, Mrs)

Nicola Julie Rebecca 24/10/2008 The Black Mountain Caravan & Camping Park Llanddeusant LLANGADOG Dyfed SA19 9YG **Tel:** 01550740217 w 6391899

Nicole Mary Susan Liz 11/08/2008 125 Preston Crescent Prestonpans East Lothian EH32 9RB **Tel:** (07842) 792843 w 6386938

Sarah Louise 17/04/2009 10 Corner Brake Plymouth Devon PL6 7QP **Tel:** 07970966989 w 6441795

MITCHELMORE Jean 22/09/1978 142 Chatteris Avenue Harold Hill Romford RM3 8EU **Tel:** (01708) 341659 w 6056921

MITSON Lisa Michelle (see LUNGLEY, Mrs)

MOATE Hannah Jane 10/01/2007 12 Belvedere Gardens Chineham Basingstoke Hampshire RG24 8GB **Tel:** (01256) 351244 w 6353135

Helen Laura 16/06/2008 11 Highfield Close FARNBOROUGH Hampshire GU14 0HW **Tel:** (07884) 458 358 w 6380822

MOCK Katherine Ann 27/04/2006 Providence House Black Dog Crediton Devon EX17 4QS **Tel:** (01884) 860569 w 6353894

MODESTOU Jennifer 29/06/2007 30 Browning Road ENFIELD Middlesex EN2 0EL **Tel:** (020) 8367 2544 w 6344885

MOFFATT Nicola Ann 06/02/2009 25 Walton Drive Choppington Northumberland NE62 5EG **Tel:** 01670829825 w 6445568

MOGFORD Sarah Elizabeth (see BOLTON, Mrs)

MOGRIDGE Dayna Louise 09/03/2009 93 Hillside Road Northwood Middlesex HA6 1PZ **Tel:** 01923822889 w 6435844

Gemma Catherine DipAVN(Medical) 02/03/2001 (19/04/2006) 59 The Elms Haslingfield CAMBRIDGE CB23 1ND w 6213523

MOHAN Kim Kathleen 10/08/2001 (18/11/2008) Queen Mother Hospital for Small Animals Hawkshead Lane North Mymms Hatfield Hertfordshire AL9 7TA **Tel:** (01707) 666366 w 6227086

MOIR Elaine (nee Slater) 23/01/1997 (08/08/2001) 22 Kershope Drive Oakwood Derby Derbyshire DE21 2TQ **Tel:** (01332) 677433 w 6031248

MOIR Kirsty Alexandra (see CROUCH, Mrs)

MOIR Louise Edwina (see MOORE, Miss)

MOLD Katie Jean (see GAZEY, Mrs)

MOLE Joanne Rose 29/07/2008 11 Orchard Avenue Mitcham Surrey CR4 4JD w 6416374

MOLLOY Kerry Georgina 12/09/2008 3 Rossall Street Ashton-on-Ribble PRESTON PR2 2RS **Tel:** 07939205251 w 6435415

MOLSHER Rachel (see MINETT, Mrs)

MOLYNEUX Helen Louise (nee Butcher) 22/03/2004 Hollybank Veterinary Centre Chester Road Sandiway NORTHWICH Cheshire CW8 2DX w 6299455

MOMMERSTEEG Chelsey 13/11/2009 Raddenstiles Veterinary Surgeons Liverton Business Park Salterton Road Exmouth Devon EX8 2NR **Tel:** (01395) 264747 w 6574125

MONAGHAN Amanda Rachel 01/04/2009 20 Mason Close Redditch Worcestershire B97 5DF **Tel:** (01527) 450271 w 6379205

Genna Elizabeth (formerly Monoghan) 27/02/2007 27 Gleanings Avenue Norton Tower HALIFAX West Yorkshire HX2 0NU w 6366830

MONAGHAN Victoria Louise (see BOSWELL, Mrs)

MONAN Lisa 15/11/2001 7 Essex Road SOUTHPORT Merseyside PR8 4NA **Tel:** (01704) 567326 w 6265388

MONCRIEFF Wendy Jacqueline (see RATTRAY, Mrs)

MONEY Lisa Ann (see TOWART, Mrs)

MONGER Hannah Louise 08/05/2001 (11/06/2009) 4 Flexditch Cottages Little London Road Silchester Reading Hampshire RG7 2PT **Tel:** (01189) 700700 w 6116982

MONK Heather Elizabeth 07/02/2006 6 Ashley Drive Bramhall Stockport Cheshire SK7 1EW **Tel:** (0161) 440 9801 w 6292206

Michelle Nadene 19/09/2006 2 Duncryne Place Bishopbriggs Glasgow G64 2DP **Tel:** (0141) 772 1019 w 6438715

Polly Louise 17/07/2003 4 Tillbrooks Hill Cowlinge NEWMARKET Suffolk CB8 9QF w 6280722

MONKMAN Nicola Louise 23/03/2006 7 North End Cottages Hilston Road Roos HULL HU12 0JA **Tel:** (01964) 670904 w 6340430

MONOGHAN Genna Elizabeth (see MONAGHAN, Miss)

MONRO Susan Ann 11/10/2000 Northleigh Farm Main Road Birdham Chichester West Sussex PO20 7BY **Tel:** (01243) 513514 w 6203513

MONTAGUE Gillian Hazel (nee Morrow) 22/04/2002 All Creatures Veterinary Health Centre Greystone Road Limvady BT49 0PB **Tel:** (028) 777 69777 w 6204613

Lucy Margaret 21/07/2008 Fitzpatrick Referrals Ltd Halfway Lane Eashing Godalming Surrey GU7 2QQ **Tel:** (01483) 423761 w 6376136

Maura (nee Doherty) 24/11/1999 199 Whitebridge Road Carrickmore OMAGH County Tyrone BT79 9EH w 6186210

MONTGOMERY Denise Cora 02/06/2004 Jubilee Veterinary Centre 3 Jubilee Road Newtownards County Down BT23 4YH **Tel:** (02891) 812226 w 6270668

Judith Mary (nee Taylor) 09/08/1983 30b Lancaster Road LONDON SE25 4AF **Tel:** (020) 8653 2407 w 6061738

Sharon Alexandra 09/11/2009 27 Carmoney Road Eglinton LONDONDERRY BT47 3JJ **Tel:** (028) 71 810390 w 6325294

MOODY Angela Susan (see HOTHI-ASHBERRY, Mrs)

MOODY Anne Marie (see WILLSON, Mrs)

MOODY Claire Elizabeth 06/08/2008 Orchard House Gribthorpe GOOLE North Humberside DN14 7NT **Tel:** (01757) 289623 w 6344236

Jennifer 05/02/2009 99 Westmorland Avenue Blackpool Lancashire FY1 5PF **Tel:** 01253838862 w 6447790

Lucy Rachel 02/10/2009 54 Oakway Woking Surrey GU21 8TR w 6425669

MOON Janine Louise 28/01/1994 51 Roedale Road Brighton East Sussex BN1 7GB **Tel:** (01273) 566284 w 6067944

Louise Mary DipAVN(Surgical) (nee Jukes) 06/01/1989 (07/11/2003) The Stable Barn Woodford Blackawton Totnes Devon TQ9 7AA **Tel:** (01803) 712768 w 6054301

MOONEY Kelly Bridgette (see ROBERTS, Miss)

MOORE Alison Liane 21/12/2009 3 Dene Royd Close Stainland HALIFAX West Yorkshire HX4 9QP w 6464356

Barbara Jill 18/02/1998 (27/02/2009) 1 Crossways Venelle de Simon Alderney Guernsey Channel Islands GY9 3TN **Tel:** (01481) 822616 w 6118185

MOORE Carolyn Joanne (see HOLBROOK, Mrs)

Clare Louise 13/12/2007 11 Blendworth Lane SOUTHAMPTON SO18 5GY **Tel:** (02380) 447797 w 6357997

Clare Louise (nee Boughton) 04/12/2003 30A Sandon Road Meir Stoke-on-Trent ST3 7DL **Tel:** (01782) 599280 w 6268809

Danielle Louise 19/03/2007 18 Tregarrian Road Tolvaddon Camborne Cornwall TR14 0HD **Tel:** (01209) 610 228 w 6385618

Donna-Marie 27/11/2009 26 Woodhead Road Carmountside Stoke-on-Trent Staffordshire ST2 8DJ **Tel:** (07505) 397 811 w 6434920

Heather Louise 03/05/2005 Begoade Farm Begoade road Onchan Isle of man IM4 6AU **Tel:** (01624) 624531 w 6282130

Jacqueline Ruth 07/09/1998 (24/07/2001) 672 City Road Sharrow Sheffield South Yorkshire S2 1GH w 6101681

MOORE Joanne Sharron (see RUSSELL, Mrs)

Katherine Lucy 10/12/2007 3 Coot Hide Sampford Peverell TIVERTON Devon EX16 7SN **Tel:** (07737) 948488 w 6334523

Kim Elizabeth 04/04/2006 Galemire Veterinary Hospital Galemire CLEATOR MOOR Cumbria CA25 5QX **Tel:** (01946) 810295 w 6327659

Leonie Ruth 25/11/1999 Zetland Veterinary Hospital 32 Zetland Road Bristol BS6 7AB **Tel:** (0117) 944 5111 w 6185066

Lisa Mary 24/08/1990 (06/09/2007) RSPCA Putney Animal Hospital 6 Clarendon Drive London SW15 1AA **Tel:** (020) 8789 8252 w 6057073

Louisa Maria 25/03/2002 (21/01/2009) Dogs Trust Rescue Centre Honiley KENILWORTH Warwickshire CV8 1NP **Tel:** (01926) 484398 w 6268589

Louise Edwina (formerly Moir) 19/09/2000 84 Sibson Road Birstall Leicester Leicestershire LE4 4NA **Tel:** (0116) 267 3518 w 6202633

Margaret Elizabeth 30/03/1992 (22/08/2005) 74 Cleobury Meadows Cleobury Mortimer KIDDERMINSTER Worcestershire DY14 8EY **Tel:** (01299) 271894 w 6057095

Marianne Louise 21/06/2005 4 Richmond Green CARLISLE CA2 6SY **Tel:** (01228) 380 458 w 6332631

MOORE Sally Jeanette (see KINGSTON, Mrs)

MOORE Sarah Karen (see WHITE, Mrs)

MOORE Sharon Suzanne (see PARYLO, Mrs)

MOORE Shenade Lucinda (see DUGGAN, Mrs)

MOORE Susan Anne (see BARBER, Ms)

MOORE Yvette (see LUCKETT, Mrs)

MOORES Sarah Jane 25/03/2009 48 Stockholm Road STOCKPORT Cheshire SK3 9QS **Tel:** 01612821747 w 6431851

MOORHOUSE Erica Ghislaine 16/06/2008 Highmoor Clearbrook YELVERTON Devon PL20 6JB **Tel:** (01822) 854 277 w 6380833

MOOTIEN Hayley (nee Dunn) 24/06/2004 PDSA Kings Road Southwick Sunderland SR5 2LH **Tel:** (0191) 516 0636 w 6296694

MORAN Lillian Christina 14/05/2003 Ballybrown Clarina Co Limerick Ireland **Tel:** 00353-61-353337 w 6255554

Michelle 26/04/2007 18 Eton Drive Liverpool Merseyside L10 2JZ **Tel:** (0151) 531 1480 w 6378149

MORAWSKI Angela Alexandra 18/12/2007 148 Whittingham Lane Goosnargh PRESTON PR3 2JL **Tel:** (01772) 861660 w 6404351

MORDEY Stefanie Victoria 11/02/2008 13 Hillfoot Drive Pudsey West Yorkshire LS28 7QL **Tel:** (07866) 712788 w 6401458

MORE Jane Helen 22/11/1976 (03/11/2008) 3 Pittornie Farm Cottage Dairsie Cupar Fife KY15 4SW w 6057142

MOREAU Carol Anne 19/01/2005 37 Churchill Avenue Wyton on the Hill St Ives Cambridgeshire PE28 2EG w 6319563

MORETON Katherine Ann 07/02/2006 62 Matley Moor SWINDON SN3 6NL **Tel:** (07810) 348254 w 6342168

MORGAN Annaliese Helen (see MAGEE, Mrs)

MORGAN Chrissie 11/11/2009 3 Drovers Way Burton CARNFORTH Lancashire LA6 1HU **Tel:** 07824332882 w 6436504

MORGAN Clare Agnes (see SMITH, Mrs)

Donna 25/02/2003 Cartref Southend Road Stanford-le-Hope Essex SS17 8HW **Tel:** (01375) 674104 w 6261989

MORGAN Fritha Jane (see QUIRK, Mrs)

Helen Joy 12/05/2004 10 Water Lane Ospringe Faversham Kent ME13 8TS w 6272483

Karen Marie 11/07/2005 2a Cecil Street Flat 3 LIVERPOOL L15 1HR w 6275651

Leanne 10/07/2008 126 Salisbury Avenue Barking Essex IG11 9XU **Tel:** 02085945801 w 6379216

Louise Paula 18/10/2005 Isabelle Vets Route Isabelle St. Peter Port Guernsey GY1 1QR **Tel:** (01481) 723863 w 6283703

Lydia Claire (nee Williams) 10/12/2002 The Croeso Veterinary Hospital Ltd 111 Whitchurch Road Cardiff CF14 3JQ **Tel:** (029) 2061 9899 w 6257578

Mark 14/05/2007 NKR Veterinary Specialists 4 Park Road EAST MOLESEY Surrey KT8 9LE **Tel:** (01634) 666655 m 6365752

Michelle Louise 19/01/2009 8 Rufford Road Bootle Merseyside L20 5EP **Tel:** 07917665895 w 6376532

Nicola 01/08/2002 23 Rodwell Gardens Old Farm Park MILTON KEYNES Buckinghamshire MK7 8QP w 6272032

Rachael Elizabeth 17/07/2003 24 Bakers Piece WITNEY Oxfordshire OX28 1PQ w 6274650

Rachel Ann 06/02/2002 51 Bawtry Road Bessacarr Doncaster South Yorkshire DN4 7AA **Tel:** (01302) 534999 w 6271746

Samantha Francis DipAVN(Medical), DipAVN(Surgical) 31/08/1999 The Cottage Coldbrook Farm Argae Lane BARRY Vale of Glamorgan CF63 1BL **Tel:** (07711) 333023 w 6185935

Sara Dawn 19/09/2006 Westway Veterinary Centre 426-428 West Road Newcastle upon Tyne NE5 2ER **Tel:** (0191) 274 7910 w 6323413

Susan Ann 15/11/2005 Abbots Leigh Chapel Road Keeston Haverfordwest Dyfed SA62 6HL **Tel:** (01437) 710556 w 6347624

MORLEY Faye Elizabeth 12/09/2008 509 Lordship Lane London SE22 8JY **Tel:** (020) 8693 4677 w 6411468

Gemma Katerina 14/03/2008 3 Oaklands Caravan Site Hatherleigh Road OKEHAMPTON Devon EX20 1LG **Tel:** 07718761082 w 6276982

Jeannie Maureen 14/01/1982 (22/04/2002) 10 Back Street Lakenheath Brandon Suffolk IP27 9HB **Tel:** (01842) 861199 w 6057164

Katie Louise (nee Tart) 23/02/2005 4 Chapel Row Praze An Beeble Camborne Cornwall TR14 0LA w 6272351

Louise 29/06/2007 6 Southend Road STANFORD-LE-HOPE Essex SS17 0PG w 6357425

Victoria Kate 17/11/2004 20 Albert Road Colne Lancashire BB8 0AA **Tel:** (01282) 863892 w 6300115

MORRALL Suzanne Elizabeth 27/04/2006 28 Eastwood Drive Donnington TELFORD Shropshire TF2 7LY w 6345523

MORRELL Karen 12/05/2004 Karrick House 12A Jubilee Close Kirton Boston Lincolnshire PE20 1XB w 6291909

Katrina Anne 11/03/2008 16 Carroll Drive Crewe Cheshire CW2 8DH **Tel:** (01270) 662389 w 6391954

MORRIES Sally-Anne 16/08/2007 29 Lent Green Lane Burnham SLOUGH SL1 7AS **Tel:** (07759) 239 707 w 6285386

MORRIS Amanda Lorraine 12/03/2008 10 Peach Street Heanor Derbyshire DE75 7GU **Tel:** (01773) 719957 w 6411545

Carrie 06/05/2009 80 Victoria Street Kirkwall Orkney KW15 1DQ **Tel:** (01856) 870112 w 6405176

Charlotte Amy 24/06/2004 7 Woodfield Avenue GRAVESEND Kent DA11 7QQ w 6288466

Georgina Anne 25/06/2004 34 Southgate Street Bury St. Edmunds Suffolk IP33 2AZ **Tel:** (01284) 701444 w 6285562

Jenna Clare 10/04/2007 Woodlands Warwick Road Wolston Coventry West Midlands CV8 3HB **Tel:** (024) 76542568 w 6350660

Julie Elizabeth (nee Summerhill) 11/09/1995 23 Netherton Place Whitburn West Lothian EH47 8JG **Tel:** (07811) 994204 w 6038753

Julie Marie 05/02/1999 (27/10/2000) Pype Hayes Veterinary Centre 1066 Chester Road Pype Hayes Erdington Birmingham B24 0SA **Tel:** (0121) 350 2303 w 6123286

MORRIS Kirstie Louise (see STANISLAS, Mrs)

Leanne Rachel 01/04/2003 (10/04/2008) 27 Lancaster Street Six Bells ABERTILLERY Gwent NP13 2NW w 6262847

Louise (nee Pritchard) 21/03/2007 9 Newark Road Sutton-in-Ashfield Nottinghamshire NG17 5JP **Tel:** (01623) 455 852 w 6372935

Nicola Jane 11/11/2008 Denbies View Veterinary Centre Westcott Road Dorking Surrey RH4 3DP **Tel:** (01306) 882996 w 6444325

MORRIS Rachel Victoria (see JAYNE, Mrs)

Rebecca 06/08/2008 Home Bush Brox Lane Ottershaw CHERTSEY Surrey KT16 0LN **Tel:** (01932) 873050 w 6342179

Ruth Elizabeth 30/05/2006 180 Merthyr Road Whitchurch CARDIFF CF14 1DL **Tel:** (02920) 529446 w 6327670

Susan Elizabeth 10/01/2003 (19/04/2005) Lynwood Veterinary Group 1 Dunbar Road Bournemouth Dorset BH3 7AY **Tel:** (01202) 555553 w 6191479

Victoria Louise (nee Slater) 19/04/2006 39 Wayfarers Drive Tyldesley Manchester Lancashire M29 8RP **Tel:** (01942) 895 513 w 6297662

MORRISON Kerrie Elizabeth Ann 06/10/2009 14 Manor Lodge MAGHERAFELT County Londonderry BT45 6QL w 6415824

Leanne (nee Petrie) 31/10/2003 Meadows Veterinary Centre Station Road Oldmeldrum Inverurie Aberdeenshire AB51 0EZ **Tel:** (01651) 872481 w 6278841

Lynne 22/03/2004 67 Webster Avenue Carronshore FALKIRK FK2 8BA **Tel:** (01324) 873517 w 6291414

MORROW Gillian Hazel (see MONTAGUE, Mrs)

Kelly Ann 18/09/2007 Ardene House Veterinary Hospital Kingswells Aberdeen AB15 8PJ **Tel:** (01224) 740700 w 6372924

MORSE Helen Claire (see WAYLEN, Mrs)

MORTELL Sarah 16/09/2008 Sileby Hall Cossington Road Sileby Loughborough Leicestershire LE12 7RS **Tel:** (01509) 812445/6 w 6434535

MORTENSEN Ava (see MILLAR, Mrs)

MORTIMER Gemma Ann 10/12/2009 59 Telham Avenue RAMSGATE Kent CT12 6EB **Tel:** 07782306558 w 6464290

MORTON Amy Amanda 27/11/2008 29 Duddon Grove Longhill Estate HULL HU8 9NX w 6434612

Gillian (nee MacLeod) 08/08/2002 Ardmohr Stirling Road Milnathort Kinross KY13 9XR **Tel:** (01577) 863494 w 6261307

Karen Jane 30/03/2006 2 Brooke Street Dudley West Midlands DY2 8RB **Tel:** (01384) 252817 w 6354708

Nicole Halina 11/01/2005 4 Glebe Meadow Callington Cornwall PL17 7JB **Tel:** (01579) 382973 w 6271339

Sally Louise 27/07/1988 (04/10/2002) Aston Fruit Farm Stoney Lane Kilcot Newent Gloucestershire GL18 1PB **Tel:** (01989) 720208 w 6013783

MORWOOD Joanna Ellen (see REYNOLDS, Mrs)

MOSELEY Linda Louise 15/04/2004 1 Old Eign Hill Hampton Park Hereford Herefordshire HR1 1TU **Tel:** (01432) 357222 w 6296320

MOSLEY Jane Harriett 18/04/2005 10 Tattershall Drive HEMEL HEMPSTEAD Hertfordshire HP2 7QE w 6333720

MOSS Emma Jane 10/04/2003 128 Wickhay Lee Chapel North Basildon Essex SS15 5AQ **Tel:** (01268) 442404 w 6282218

Emma Jane 06/08/2008 29 Coombe Road HAMPTON Middlesex TW12 3PB w 6388247

Jennifer 09/09/2008 94 Appledore Avenue BEXLEYHEATH Kent DA7 6QH **Tel:** (01322) 335234 w 6318353

Laura Diane 25/02/2009 78 Garry Way Romford Essex RM1 4AW **Tel:** (01708) 742440 w 6396255

Laura Elizabeth 02/09/2008 5 Rowton Drive Skirlaugh HULL HU11 5DZ **Tel:** 07730618157 w 6435745

MOSSOP Lesley 06/07/2004 Owler Hall Cottage Birds Lane Tattenhall Chester Cheshire CH3 9NL **Tel:** (01244) 330 151 w 6287498

MOTHERSDALE Susan DipAVN(Surgical) 22/01/1987 19 Philip Drive Flackwell Heath Buckinghamshire HP10 9JD **Tel:** (01628) 523071 w 6058204

MOTT Natalie Samantha 26/03/2008 46 High Street Whitwell HITCHIN Hertfordshire SG4 8AG **Tel:** 07789394945 w 6349417

MOULE Gemma Leanne (nee Hewes) 22/03/2004 1 Thrift Farm Cottages Baldock Road ROYSTON Hertfordshire SG8 9NN w 6295407

MOULES Leanne Sarah 13/07/2007 34 Hyde Valley WELWYN GARDEN CITY Hertfordshire AL7 4NA **Tel:** (01707) 327090 w 6349428

MOULIN Claire Joanne (nee Kitchen) 05/09/1996 Barnsley Vets4Pets Limited 161 Wilthorpe Road Barnsley South Yorkshire S75 1JQ **Tel:** (01226) 289000 w 6041030

MOULTON Sallyann (see REED, Mrs)

MOUNT Lorna Fairroligh 11/11/2008 113 Chambersbury Lane Hemel Hempstead Hertfordshire HP3 8BE **Tel:** (01442) 213271 w 6409158

MOUNTIER Rebecca Samantha (see WOOD, Mrs)

MOUNTY Alison Frances (nee Hex) 23/12/2003 4 Church Fields TROWBRIDGE Wiltshire BA14 0EJ **Tel:** (01225) 761393 w 6292822

MOUZER Helen Frances (see FROST, Mrs)

MOWAT Amanda (nee Phillips) 18/04/2008 Kirk Cottage St. Margarets Hope ORKNEY KW17 2TJ **Tel:** (01856) 831433 w 6388764

MOWBRAY Kathryn Elizabeth 04/02/2009 10 Parkfield Road North Manchester Lancashire M40 3TA **Tel:** 01616823561 w 6413338

MOYLAN Kelly Rearne 24/08/2009 C/O 99 Conway Drive Fulwood PRESTON PR2 3ER **Tel:** 07747410078 w 6563499

MOYNIHAN Keira Alanna 02/07/2008 31 The Green Bathgate West Lothian EH48 4DA w 6355225

MUDDLE Jennifer Claire 09/10/2009 2 Windmill Place Rectory Lane Ashington PULBOROUGH West Sussex RH20 3LF **Tel:** (01903) 892083 w 6428958

MUIR Susan (see WINWOOD, Mrs)

MULCAHY-HAWES Katie Louise 30/11/2005 The Oxford Cat Clinic 78A Westway Botley Oxford Oxfordshire OX2 9JU **Tel:** (01865) 243000 w 6344401

MULCASTER Jade Louise 26/04/2007 12 Burrow Walls Northside WORKINGTON Cumbria CA14 1BB w 6379238

MULCOCK Lisa Caroline (nee Mitchell) 12/02/1997 Unit 4, Burraton Yard Burraton Square Poundbury DORCHESTER Dorset DT1 3GR w 6017154

MULDER Tanya Ingrid 13/12/2002 65 Oakley Road Caversham Reading Berkshire RG4 7RN **Tel:** (0118) 947 9298 w 6327164

MULDOON Paula Mary (see QUINN, Mrs)

MULHALL Lisa Joanne (nee Rutland) 03/10/1994 52 Morpeth Avenue Borehamwood Hertfordshire WD6 4BN **Tel:** (0208) 9537311 w 6028858

MULLALLY Corinne Morven 27/01/1999 (26/10/2000) Wildbore Veterinary Group 5 Newcastle Street Worksop Nottinghamshire S80 2AS **Tel:** (01909) 472059 w 6138350

MULLEN Catherine Elizabeth 25/01/1999 2 Rockwood Cottages Severn Crescent CHEPSTOW Gwent NP16 5DZ w 6129470

MULLINEUX Yvonne Veronica 29/07/2005 (14/07/2009) 116 Edgemoor Drive Crosby LIVERPOOL L23 9UQ w 6304823

MULLINGS Carly Morgan 16/08/2006 Lynwood Veterinary Group 1 Dunbar Road Bournemouth Dorset BH3 7AY **Tel:** (01202) 555553 w 6354719

Kelly Jayne 12/05/2006 71 Eanleywood Lane Norton Runcorn Cheshire WA7 6SP **Tel:** (01928) 719086 w 6350748

MULLINS Jennifer Elisabeth 30/05/2003 Stowe Veterinary Group 54 Bury Road Stowmarket Suffolk IP14 1JF **Tel:** (01449) 613130 w 6262363

Tracey Louise 14/01/2008 8 Stableford Close Shepshed LOUGHBOROUGH Leicestershire LE12 9BT **Tel:** 01509504265 w 6383792

MUMUNI Christine Louise (nee Harvey) 01/04/2003 7 Hurst Road Croydon CR0 1JT **Tel:** (020) 8686 3972 w 6280502

MUNDY Claire Lorraine (see STANLEY, Mrs)

MUNN Lisa Mary (see BARKER, Mrs)

MUNNERY Lisa Maria (see DOWLEY, Mrs)

MUNRO Caroline Ann 21/03/2006 85 Somerville Drive Carnwath Lanark Lanarkshire ML11 8JW **Tel:** (01501) 785432 w 6318551

Jennifer 20/11/2009 67 Station Road Hatfield DONCASTER South Yorkshire DN7 6QN w 6456370

Karen Lesley 17/01/2006 Levalsa Meor Farm Levalsa Meor London Apprentice ST AUSTELL Cornwall PL26 6DN w 6291425

MUNRO Laura Anne (see BLACK, Mrs)

MURBY Helen Elizabeth (nee Murby) 31/08/1999 (01/11/2002) Glenthorne Veterinary Centre 71 Derby Road Uttoxeter Staffordshire ST14 8EB **Tel:** (01889) 562164 w 6152841

Helen Elizabeth (nee Murby) 31/08/1999 (01/11/2002) Glenthorne Veterinary Centre 71 Derby Road Uttoxeter Staffordshire ST14 8EB **Tel:** (01889) 562164 w 6152841

MURDOCH Catriona Allison Louise 12/10/2009 Fisherie Green Cottage Fisherie Turrriff Aberdeenshire AB53 5GU **Tel:** 07976577426 w 6489469

MURLEY Rebecca 28/04/2008 70 Moormead BUDLEIGH SALTERTON Devon EX9 6PY **Tel:** (07813) 097219 w 6305340

MURPHY Cheryl Ann 30/04/2001 Priory Veterinary Surgeons Limited 10 Evesham Road Reigate Surrey RH2 9DF **Tel:** (01737) 242190 w 6031929

Christine Mary 02/12/1992 Feldon Veterinary Centre 1 Guy Street Leamington Spa Warwickshire CV32 4RX **Tel:** (01926) 423161 w 6057379

Claire Louise 04/08/2008 39 Oval Road South Dagenham Essex RM10 9DP w 6381317

Claire Marie 07/06/2005 13 Moncrieffe Street Walsall West Midlands WS1 2LA **Tel:** (01922) 724454 w 6319574

Gemma-Ann 21/03/2006 112 Katherine Street Ashington Northumberland NT63 9DW **Tel:** (079) 226 74030 w 6342190

Katie Marie 11/07/2005 CVS (UK) Ltd Animed Veterinary Hospital & Equine Unit Botley Road Shedfield Southampton Hampshire SO32 2JG **Tel:** (01329) 833112 w 6327087

Leanne Jane (nee Millard) 13/01/2004 4 Inwood Court Rodney Road WALTON-ON-THAMES Surrey KT12 3NF w 6288950

Michelle Susan 31/08/2005 10 Belmont Road Aberdeen Aberdeenshire AB25 3SR **Tel:** (01224) 492048 w 6313678

Steven Peter 22/01/2001 (03/12/2008) 11 Northampton Road Lavendon OLNEY Buckinghamshire MK46 4EY **Tel:** (01234) 241573 m 6203051

Suzanne Louise 21/03/2000 95 Weoley Castle Road Birmingham West Midlands B29 5QD **Tel:** (0121) 4446847 w 6149351

Victoria Elizabeth 12/05/2004 (24/03/2006) 43 Ridgeway Drive Bromley Kent BR1 5DG **Tel:** (0208) 857 9343 w 6289522

MURRAY Cheryl Linda DipAVN(Surgical) (nee Skeoch) 14/10/2002 107 Linton Woods Lane Linton on Ouse YORK YO30 2TF **Tel:** (01347) 848850 w 6278720

Eilidh Morven 23/09/2009 Bard Vets Ltd 15 Catherine Street Dumfries DG1 1JF **Tel:** (01387) 255295 w 6286277

Elaine (nee Crombie) 02/09/1998 Esk Valley Veterinary Surgery 21 Eskbank Road Dalkeith Midlothian EH22 1HG **Tel:** (0131) 654 1232 w 6041303

Helen 24/03/2009 54 Winford Grove WINGATE County Durham TS28 5DU **Tel:** 01429835530 w 6426351

Helen (nee Myers) 25/01/1995 132 Netherfield Widnes Cheshire WA8 8BU **Tel:** (0151) 4220845 w 6029476

Judy Violet 19/01/2001 (23/02/2009) RSPCA Putney Animal Hospital 6 Clarendon Drive London SW15 1AA **Tel:** (0300) 123 0716 w 6130646

MURS Fay 11/05/2004 65 Carrallays Witham Essex CM8 1XW w 6287762

MURSELL Jolene Marie 09/09/2008 18 Tredegar Road BRISTOL BS16 4BS w 6435525

MURTAGH Terri Ann 20/11/2009 28 East Holme ERITH Kent DA8 3NR **Tel:** 01322401966 w 6498577

MUSK Victoria Louise (nee Noble) 06/11/2000 21 Elm Road Farncombe Godalming Surrey GU7 3SW **Tel:** (01483) 417994 w 6144284

MUSTAFA Lynsey Anne 03/09/2008 182 Birdsfoot Lane LUTON LU3 2DL w 6379337

MYBURGH Hannah Victoria (nee Allen) 11/09/2008 Summerhill Veterinary Centre 14 Queens Road Fakenham Norfolk NR21 8DB **Tel:** (01328) 855814 w 6264431

MYERS Helen (see MURRAY, Mrs)

MYLES Catherine Johan 20/01/1995 (06/07/2006) 55 Portland Road South Norwood London SE25 4UN **Tel:** (020) 8656 8367 w 6025278

N

NADEN Kay Lesley 05/09/2000 37 Nottingham Road Belper Derbyshire DE56 1JG **Tel:** (01773) 599014 w 6204063

NAIRN Carly Anne 28/09/2005 Seymour Cottage Veterinary Surgery Weston Road Totnes Devon TQ9 5BT **Tel:** (01803) 866283 w 6339198

Julie 21/01/2008 1/236 Willcock Drive Mahomets Geraldton 6530 Western Australia Australia **Tel:** (00) 61 8 996 46961 w 6386861

NARRAWAY Susan Victoria 07/02/2006 Palo Alto Sulhamstead READING RG7 4BE w 6344863

NARTEY Gertrude Dede-Ofoley DipAVN(Surgical) 26/01/1998 82 Danebury New Addington Croydon Surrey CR0 9EW **Tel:** (01689) 842248 w 614319X

NASH Cheryl 05/06/2006 (04/12/2008) 21 Cornelia Terrace SEAHAM County Durham SR7 7RZ **Tel:** (0191) 581 7520 w 6329771

Claire Louise (nee Clifford) 01/04/2003 (19/11/2007) 32 Marlborough Road Gloucester Gloucestershire GL4 6GE **Tel:** (01452) 300432 w 6272395

NASH Jessica Amy (see BARRON, Mrs)

Lindsay Grace 04/11/2005 12 Grayshot Drive Blackwater CAMBERLEY Surrey GU17 0EW w 6329056

NASH Samantha Louise (see BORLAND, Mrs)

Sharon 05/04/2005 84 Trowbridge Road Romford Essex RM3 8YW w 6261274

Stephanie June (nee Hawker) 11/09/2003 (01/06/2009) 20 Breamore Close New Milton Hampshire BH25 5QZ **Tel:** (01425) 611143 w 6259767

Tina (nee Lightowler) 05/04/2005 14 Macaulay Road Shakespeare Gardens RUGBY Warwickshire CV22 6HE **Tel:** (01788) 816 869 w 6304075

NASTALY Kelly Dawn (formerly Brown) 26/01/2000 6 Seaview Cottages Breach Lane Lower Halstow NR. Sittingbourne Kent ME9 7DG **Tel:** (01795) 841469 w 6149012

NATHAN Samantha Rachal 19/03/2008 Wellpets Animal Hospital 211 High Street Sheerness Kent ME12 1UR **Tel:** (01795) 662243 w 6401953

NAVOTNI Michael 26/10/2005 Torrington Orthopaedic Referrals IES House Mission Street Brighouse

West Yorkshire HD6 1NQ **Tel:** (01484) 404770 m 6326075

NEAL Emma Ruth 18/12/1986 (07/03/2001) The Shepton Veterinary Group Allyn Saxon Drive Shepton Mallet Somerset BA4 5QH **Tel:** (01749) 343955 w 6057539

Hannah Louise 11/03/2005 (08/01/2009) Flat 64 Central Walk Station Approach EPSOM Surrey KT19 8BY **Tel:** (01372) 722351 w 6327010

Louise Elizabeth 29/09/2008 30 Homefield Road Warlingham Surrey CR6 9HQ **Tel:** (01883) 627819 w 6389028

NEALE Karla Yvonne (nee Kirkness) 30/01/1996 (29/10/2001) 52 Vermont Close Great Sankey Warrington Cheshire WA5 8WX **Tel:** (01925) 714297 w 6041289

NEALE Rachel (see LITHGO, Mrs)

NEAME Leasa Marie 23/12/2003 Walnut Lodge Canterbury Road Selsted Dover Kent CT15 7HL **Tel:** (01303) 844574 w 6289687

NEBEL Catherine Mary 20/11/2008 Yew Cottage Brook Street Kingston Blount CHINNOR Oxfordshire OX39 4RZ w 6421676

NEEDHAM Vicky 24/12/2003 19 Brockley Avenue Shuttlewood CHESTERFIELD Derbyshire S44 6RB w 6289951

NEILD Victoria Kathleen 13/01/1993 (28/08/2003) 283 Alcester Road South Kings Heath BIRMINGHAM B14 6EB **Tel:** (01214) 444388 w 6065492

NEILES Gemma Louise (see WHITE, Mrs)

NEILL Catherine Anne (nee Bazley) 04/04/2006 39 Station Road Whittlesford Cambridge CB2 4NL **Tel:** (01223) 833651 w 6272285

NELMES Joanna Louise 17/08/2009 17 Wharrad Close Bidford-on-Avon ALCESTER Warwickshire B50 4FR **Tel:** 01789772838 w 6277092

NELSON Anne Margaret (see FELSTEAD, Mrs)

NELSON Anthea Margaret 18/04/2008 88-92 Merton High Street Merton London SW19 1BD **Tel:** (020) 8254 1400 w 6507256

Caroline 26/10/2006 6 Moor Lane Thornton LIVERPOOL L23 4TW **Tel:** (0151) 924 4771 w 6279072

Clair Marie (nee Poulter) 10/02/2004 (13/11/2007) 24 Houfton Crescent Bolsover CHESTERFIELD Derbyshire S44 6BP **Tel:** (01246) 828437 w 6295561

Debbie Kay 06/08/2007 44 Church Road Stockingford Nuneaton Warwickshire CV10 8LD **Tel:** (02476) 386855 w 6378468

Kirsty Maria 24/04/2008 19 Cox Green Road Egerton BOLTON BL7 9HF **Tel:** (01204) 597912 w 6330772

NELSON Sarah Amanda (see SCHOLES, Mrs)

NELSON Susan Jane (see SCOTT, Mrs)

NESBITT Julie Kay (nee Benney) 28/08/1997 19 Monaton Close Helston Helston Cornwall TR13 8GB **Tel:** (01326) 221646 w 6112649

NESS Sheila Brechin 02/01/1990 (18/05/2007) 11 Sidlaw Avenue North Shields Tyne and Wear NE29 9EA **Tel:** (0191) 2911987 w 6057561

NESTOR Christine Eileen (see WILLIAMSON, Mrs)

NETHERTON Tracey Elizabeth (formerly Van-De-Vyver) 21/08/1985 (28/03/2008) 8 West Villas Burstwick Hull HU12 9EE **Tel:** (01964) 623261 w 6092267

NETTLESHIP Michelle Claire 22/03/2004 8 Waldorf Avenue Alvaston DERBY DE24 8UE w 6291546

NETTLETON Kathryn Margaret 22/02/2007 93 Parker Road Horbury Wakefield West Yorkshire WF4 5JR **Tel:** (01924) 785 379 w 6363794

NEVILL Tina Louise 04/03/2008 4 Linden Close Benfleet Essex SS7 4BD **Tel:** (01268) 753642 w 6379315

NEVINS Wendy Jane (nee Hylands) 15/03/1994 (24/07/2000) 49 Balfour Road SOUTHPORT Merseyside PR8 6LE w 6029578

NEW Bethan 29/06/2007 35 Newcombe Road Bournemouth Dorset BH6 5LX **Tel:** (07816) 075999 w 6348515

NEWALL Sarah Jane (see COMBOY, Mrs)

NEWBERY Emma Joanne 18/01/2010 Seadown Veterinary Hospital Frost Lane Hythe Southampton Hampshire SO45 3NG **Tel:** (023) 8084 2237 w 6440728

Gillian Patricia 01/11/1984 (09/09/2003) 1 Stone Court West Lane Emberton OLNEY Buckinghamshire MK46 5ND **Tel:** (0208) 2054405 w 6057572

NEWBOLD Charlotte Lisa 05/09/2008 66 Bucklebury Hanworth BRACKNELL Berkshire RG12 7YJ w 6389798

NEWBURY Tracy Emma 15/07/2005 322 Margate Road Ramsgate Kent CT12 6SQ **Tel:** (01843) 582050 w 6296331

NEWBY Rachel Hannah 26/10/2005 23 Ash Grove Skegby SUTTON-IN-ASHFIELD Nottinghamshire NG17 3FH w 6355819

NEWELL Laura Michelle 30/11/2007 The Veterinary Hospital 118 Victoria Drive Bognor Regis West Sussex PO21 2EJ **Tel:** (01243) 841111 w 6396244

Lindsay Maria 09/04/2008 15 Lincoln Road Burton-on-Trent Staffordshire DE15 9HP **Tel:** (01283) 534191 w 6376554

NEWELL Sharon Vanessa (see ADAMS, Mrs)

NEWHAM Susan Lilian (formerly Cozens) 05/08/1976 Laurel Farm Thorpland Road FAKENHAM Norfolk NR21 8NH **Tel:** (07954) 563903 w 6000311

NEWINGTON Sarah Louise (nee Whittingham) 16/01/1996 Abbey Veterinary Centre 16 Holywell Street Shrewsbury SY2 5DB **Tel:** (01743) 232713 w 6039032

NEWMAN Eve Therese 10/01/2007 5 Darent Place DIDCOT Oxfordshire OX11 7UQ w 6317759

Felicity Megan (nee Stewart) 14/10/2008 18 Aspen Walk HAYWARDS HEATH West Sussex RH16 3RB w 6405418

Lisa Anne 21/11/2008 25 Ellesmere Road Berkhamsted Hertfordshire HP4 2EX **Tel:** 07754690513 w 6438275

Louise Clare 29/07/2005 1-5 Hugh Street London SW1V 1QQ **Tel:** (020) 7932 2370 w 6290600

Rachel 20/11/2002 54 Wear Road Bicester Oxford HP18 2FF **Tel:** (01869) 245680 w 6276223

NEWSOME Sharon (nee Hartley) 27/02/2006 14 Nacton Close Sutton WOODBRIDGE Suffolk IP12 3TF **Tel:** (07940) 480064 w 6333379

Teresa Mary 20/10/2009 4 Douglas Street DEWSBURY West Yorkshire WF12 9DX **Tel:** 01132779174 w 6418486

NEWTON Karen Claire 09/05/2006 Flat 3, 20 High Street MALMESBURY Wiltshire SN16 9AU **Tel:** (01666) 822 847 w 6261120

Rosalyn Elizabeth 10/04/2001 10 Jubilee Villas Hassall SANDBACH Cheshire CW11 4XR w 6205834

NICCOLLS Tania Michelle 25/03/2002 Forest Veterinary Clinic 7 Park Road Fordingbridge Hampshire SP6 1EQ **Tel:** (01425) 652221 w 6275123

NICE Gemma Hayley 05/04/2005 78 Ashurst Road Brighton East Sussex BN2 4PH **Tel:** (01273) 695531 w 6290853

NICHOL Eilis Maire 05/11/1982 20 The Downs Highlands Rathmullen Road Drogheda Co Meath Ireland **Tel:** (00353) 87 6998211 w 6057652

NICHOLAS Megan Louise (see RYDER, Mrs)

NICHOLAS Sarah Louise 09/11/2009 The Veterinary Centre Wellington New Road Taunton Somerset TA1 5LU **Tel:** (01823) 333722 w 6446987

NICHOLAS Sian Julie (see BROWN, Mrs)

NICHOLLS Bronwyn Anne 12/08/1971 (23/01/2006) Hillbrow Church Road Otley IPSWICH IP6 9NP **Tel:** (01473) 890899 w 6057674

Caroline Ann 19/01/2009 Manor Farm Buckland Aylesbury Buckinghamshire HP22 5HU **Tel:** 07876575678 w 6397718

Cathryn Jaime 10/02/2009 15 Nicholsfield Loxwood Billingshurst West Sussex RH14 0SP **Tel:** 07944042277 w 6436966

Claire Elaine 03/10/2007 93 Southbourne Grove WESTCLIFF-ON-SEA Essex SS0 9UN **Tel:** (01702) 301153 w 6379832

Claire Ellen 19/12/2006 14 Albion Street Rugeley Staffordshire WS15 2BY **Tel:** (01889) 582459 w 6365763

Helen Marie 13/05/2003 Westwood House 106 High Street Boston Spa Wetherby West Yorkshire LS23 6DR **Tel:** (01937) 842210 w 6281327

Lara Jane 03/12/2008 Flat 2 83 Lorna Road HOVE East Sussex BN3 3EL **Tel:** (07782) 206 272 w 6441124

NICHOLS Christina Irene (nee Hunt Lacey) 10/04/2003 (16/01/2007) Greenways Lawfords Hill Road Worplesdon GUILDFORD Surrey GU3 3QB **Tel:** (01483) 237 334 w 6277455

Katie 17/11/2004 Tysul Veterinary Group Pencader Road Pontwelly Llandysul Dyfed SA44 4AE **Tel:** (01559) 363318 w 6326009

Katy Ann DipAVN(Surgical) 27/02/1996 (07/03/2002) 2 New Cottages Hawkshead Lane North Mymms HATFIELD Hertfordshire AL9 7TF **Tel:** (01707) 643071 w 6042271

NICHOLS Nicola (see NICHOLS-EVANS, Mrs)

NICHOLS Victoria Rebecca (see HAYTER, Mrs)

NICHOLS-EVANS Nicola (nee Nichols) 17/11/2004 Gwernant Farm Rhydlewis Llandysul Ceredigion SA44 5QJ w 6318067

NICHOLSON Kerry Margaret (nee Wallace) 10/09/1997 (03/08/2001) 17 Litton Way Whinmoor Leeds LS14 2DL **Tel:** (0113) 295 9981 w 6098815

NICKISSON Corinna (see JONES, Mrs)

NICKOLLS Nicola Gayle 31/10/2003 Briar House Veterinary Surgery 13-15 St Peters Road Broadstairs Kent CT10 2AG **Tel:** (01843) 863395 w 6268545

NICOLSON Jenna 14/08/2008 The Stables Ardbeg Croft Heights of Brae STRATHPEFFER Ross-Shire IV14 9AF w 6400787

NIELSEN Joanne Jacqueline 04/10/2005 21 Tweedale Crescent Madeley Shropshire TF7 4DZ w 6306374

NIGHTINGALE Joanne Carole (see WATTS, Mrs)

NIMMO Danielle Samantha Diane 24/11/2009 North Park Veterinary Group 64 Fore Street North Tawton Devon EX20 2DT **Tel:** (01837) 82327 w 6497708

Gemma Louise 02/11/2004 Coombe Cottage Rake LISS Hampshire GU33 7JD w 6286464

Lynne Christina (nee Fotheringham) 12/09/2000 Clyde Veterinary Group 331 Lanark Road Auchenheath Lanarkshire ML11 9UU **Tel:** (01555) 860880 w 6130500

NINNES Elaine Michelle 10/01/2007 219 Lee Street Hull North Humberside HU8 8NR **Tel:** (01482) 223688 w 6280403

NIVEN Jolie Ann 03/09/1998 5 Darwell Avenue Eccles Manchester Lancashire M30 7AB **Tel:** (0161) 281 2364 w 6122045

NIX Lisa Joanne 05/07/2006 55 Meadow Drive Thorpe Willoughby Selby North Yorkshire YO8 9PN **Tel:** (01757) 708509 w 6342707

NIXON Georgina 05/04/2005 Copperfield Green Lane Prestwood GREAT MISSENDEN Buckinghamshire HP16 0QA **Tel:** (01494) 866056 w 6323435

Kirsty (nee Nixon, formerly Jones) 30/01/1996 91 Halesworth Drive Havelock Park SUNDERLAND SR4 8DJ w 6031339

NOBLE Olivia Fern Parry 09/12/2009 15 Agbrigg Road Wakefield West Yorkshire WF2 6AA **Tel:** 07779214638 w 6398147

Shirley Elaine 21/01/1980 New Priory Veterinary Practice The Deneway London Rd Brighton East Sussex BN1 8QR **Tel:** (01273) 540430 w 6057743

NOBLE Victoria Louise (see MUSK, Mrs)

NOCK Rachel Claire (nee Pirie) 15/09/1997 6 Brooklands Wordsley Stourbridge West Midlands DY8 5UN **Tel:** (01384) 75548 w 6132031

NOLAN Katie Jayne (see GOODES, Mrs)

NOONE Christopher 11/09/1992 (02/11/2000) Inside Pets at Home Centre Retail Park Broadway Royton Oldham Lancashire OL2 5HX **Tel:** (0161) 624 7539 m 6006721

NORMAN Lana Ruth (see GOULDING, Mrs)

NORMAN Louise 04/09/1997 2 Regents Court Finkle Street COTTINGHAM North Humberside HU16 4AB **Tel:** (01482) 645897 w 6112558

NORRIS Beverley Caren 03/02/1999 (26/01/2010) 16 Darnley Road ASHINGTON Northumberland NE63 8BB w 6132596

Deborah 11/11/2009 24 Church Lane East Carlton MARKET HARBOROUGH Leicestershire LE16 8YA w 6460902

Emma Jayne 08/11/2006 3 Factory Lane Penwortham Preston Lancashire PR1 9TD **Tel:** (01772) 748302 w 6371021

NORTH Angela 30/09/1991 (22/04/2003) Warwickshire College Moreton Morrell Warwick Warwickshire CV35 9BL **Tel:** (01926) 318000 w 6022685

Danielle Stacey 23/02/2005 Chase Veterinary Group 89-91 Seaside Eastbourne East Sussex BN22 7NL **Tel:** (01323) 639331 w 6313744

Helen Jane (nee Benney) 08/11/2006 Station Farm London Road Six Mile Bottom Newmarket Suffolk CB8 0UH **Tel:** (01638) 572012 w 6382274

NORTHROP Lynn 27/09/2004 Abbey Veterinary Group 89 Dodworth Road Barnsley South Yorkshire S70 6ED **Tel:** (01226) 242217 w 6324326

NORTON Kelly Dee 07/12/2005 7 Wagbullock Rise Easthampstead BRACKNELL Berkshire RG12 7QD **Tel:** (01344) 453675 w 6325129

Laura Louise 09/03/2009 No 1 Bramston Way Southfields Laindon Essex SS15 6TP **Tel:** (01268) 564664 w 6404879

Maryanne 11/03/2008 19 Clayfields Penn High Wycombe Buckinghamshire HP10 8AT **Tel:** (01494) 814988 w 6412535

NORWELL Wendy Anne 07/06/2005 181 Strathtay Road Perth PH1 2JU **Tel:** (01738) 626933 w 6296804

NOTMAN Shirley (nee Kennedy) 22/08/1990 (02/02/2000) Shannonhill Galston Ayrshire KA4 8PH **Tel:** (01560) 700212 w 6054447

NOTON Sarah Helen 20/11/2009 23 The Shires Paddock Wood Tonbridge Kent TN12 6YD **Tel:** 07926160793 w 6436977

NOYES Leanne 11/01/2005 Severn Veterinary Centre Berkeley House Berkeley Way Worcester Worcestershire WR4 9UP **Tel:** (01905) 756156 w 6327472

NUGENT Mary Josephine (see DALLOW, Mrs)

NUNN Abigail Victoria 01/02/2008 75 Melford Road STOWMARKET Suffolk IP14 2PR **Tel:** (01449) 673234 w 6406903

Laura 08/01/2008 241 New Road Croxley Green Rickmansworth Hertfordshire WD3 3HE **Tel:** 01923774775 w 6401018

NURSE Eloise Layla (nee Payne) 28/02/2005 32 Wensum Walk Drayton Norwich Norfolk NR8 6AS **Tel:** (01603) 866233 w 6327681

Nicola Jane 20/10/2009 26 Downham Road Runcton Holme KING'S LYNN Norfolk PE33 0AD **Tel:** 01553811247 w 6415329

Rachel 05/10/2001 The Paddock 53 Cherrydown West Basildon Essex SS16 5AW **Tel:** (01268) 533636 w 6229671

Rachel Marie 02/03/2007 29 Oak Crescent Clehonger HEREFORD HR2 9RG **Tel:** (01684) 575 910 w 6371659

NUTLEY Laura Rachel 03/09/2008 Grove Lodge Veterinary Group Ltd 18 Upper Brighton Road Worthing West Sussex BN14 9DL **Tel:** (01903) 234866 w 6406529

NUTT Lucy 07/11/2008 45 Woods Road Street Somerset BA16 9PS **Tel:** 07779157711 w 6431873

NUTTALL Joanne Mary 12/08/1991 (15/05/2008) 90 Church Road Roberttown Liversedge Yorkshire WF15 8BE **Tel:** (01924) 507448 w 6057856

Linzi Angela DipAVN(Surgical) (nee Evans) 18/01/1996 7 The Sutherland Muxton Telford Shropshire TF2 8NH **Tel:** 07970153735 w 6042511

NUTTING Kate Susannah 30/05/2003 Rase Veterinary Centre Gallamore Lane Industrial Estate MARKET RASEN Lincolnshire LN8 3RX **Tel:** (01673) 842448 w 6279347

NYE Nicola Jayne (see GOUGH, Mrs)

O

O'CONNOR Clare Emily Beatrice (see O'CONNOR, Miss)

OAG Julie Fiona (see ROBERT, Mrs)

OAKES Emily Clare 21/07/2008 48 Swallow Walk Biddulph Stoke-on-Trent Staffordshire ST8 6TY **Tel:** (01782) 520461 w 6278016

Kelly Marie 15/11/2005 74 Homefield Rise Orpington Kent BR6 0RW **Tel:** (01689) 890655 w 6343169

OAKLEY Harriet Elizabeth 04/06/2009 35 The Manor Drive Worcester Park Surrey KT4 7LG **Tel:** 02083378081 w 6407651

OAKLEY Michelle 02/12/2009 Swanzdale Veterinary Care Centre 99 Scalby Road Scarborough North Yorkshire YO12 5QL **Tel:** (01723) 363006 w 6490954

OAKMAN Faye Joanne 18/11/2009 21 Greville Starkey Avenue NEWMARKET Suffolk CB8 0BX **Tel:** (01638) 668922 w 6491471

OATES Victoria Elizabeth 04/11/2008 9 Myrtle Gardens Yatton BRISTOL BS49 4BA **Tel:** 01934833108 w 6261417

O'BOYLE Sharon 26/02/2009 123 Amberton Road LEEDS LS9 6SY **Tel:** 07746146357 w 6439705

O'BOYLE Sinead Clare (see O'NEILL, Mrs)

O'BRIEN Claire (see KELLETT, Mrs)

O'BRIEN Emily Collette 09/05/2008 39 Selwyn Road NEW MALDEN Surrey KT3 5AU w 6379249

Hollie Katherine Rose 06/06/2008 5 Townlands Crescent Wolverton Mill MILTON KEYNES MK12 5GS **Tel:** (07517) 220 367 w 6414614

Melanie Jane (nee Matson) 14/03/2006 The Hart Veterinary Centre Browning Drive Kings Meadow Bicester Oxfordshire OX26 2XL **Tel:** (01869) 323 223 w 6344225

O'BYRNE Evelyn DipAVN(Medical) 18/01/1993 Torrington Orthopaedic Referrals IES House Mission Street Brighouse West Yorkshire HD6 1NQ **Tel:** (01484) 404770 w 6065415

O'CALLAGHAN Mary Catherine 24/08/1989 31-75 29th Street Apt D6 Long Island City New York 11106 USA **Tel:** (001) 718 777 5966 w 6057878

OCKENDEN Gemma Ann (nee Viner) 15/04/2004 Southill Veterinary Group Balsam Fields Wincanton Somerset BA9 9HE **Tel:** (01963) 33226 w 6291579

O'CONNELL Caroline Francesca (nee Bragg) 22/03/2004 16 Plumers Close CLEVEDON Avon BS21 5AW w 6289071

Kerri-Anne 27/05/2009 61 Park Drive Winchmore Hill LONDON N21 2LT **Tel:** 02083609310 w 6455226

O'CONNOR Clare Emily Beatrice (formerly O`Connor) 17/07/2003 161 Wheeler Avenue SWINDON SN2 7HW **Tel:** (07884) 260 136 w 6287630

O'CONNOR Emma Jane (see SWINDALE, Miss)

Lisa Karen 13/07/2004 14 Hatherley Avenue LIVERPOOL L23 0SD w 6264035

O'CONNOR Sharon Theresa (see GASKIN, Mrs)

ODD Joanna Marie (nee Whalley) 03/09/1996 Newnham Court Veterinary Group Bearsted Road Weavering Maidstone Kent ME14 5EL **Tel:** (01622) 734555 w 6100553

ODLE Alison Louise 11/03/2005 63 Hillhouse Road Downend Bristol BS16 5RT **Tel:** (0117) 9562067 w 6300126

O'DOHERTY Caroline Louise 08/11/2006 5 Rowan Glynn Crew Road Maghera County Londonderry BT46 5FG w 6365774

O'DONNELL Clare 10/01/2007 2 Eastfield Farm Cottages Eastfield Morpeth Northumberland NE65 0YE **Tel:** (01665) 712 430 w 6377148

Lisa Elizabeth 18/02/1998 (24/10/2003) 72 Vandeleur Avenue Edinburgh EH7 6UG **Tel:** (0131) 4680430 w 6130555

Toni Ann 17/01/2008 108 Hookfield HARLOW Essex CM18 6QJ w 6293801

O'DRISCOLL Catherine Esther 27/11/2000 (11/11/2003) 6 Garrick Road NORTHAMPTON Northamptonshire NN1 5ND w 6205295

O'DWYER Louise Mary DipAVN(Surgical), DipAVN (Medical) 02/11/1999 52 Kirkstile Crescent Winstanley WIGAN Lancashire WN3 6TE **Tel:** (01942) 200241 w 6186067

Rachel Joanne 28/02/2001 Ashwood Veterinary Clinic 448 Lichfield Road Sutton Coldfield West Midlands B74 4EP **Tel:** (0121) 308 1128 w 6135349

OESTREICH Sophie Ella 08/01/2008 Hayrig Nailsbourne Taunton Somerset TA2 8AG **Tel:** (01823) 451793 w 6358008

O'FARRELL Catriona Juliet 10/06/2009 36 Davey Crescent Great Shelford Cambridge Cambridgeshire CB22 5JF **Tel:** 07732594117 w 6407772

OGDEN Ben James 02/07/2008 Aireworth Vets Aireworth Road Keighley West Yorkshire BD21 4DJ **Tel:** (01535) 602988 m 6402426

OGLE Julie (see HIPKIN, Mrs)

OGLESBY Clare Penelope 24/08/1999 4 Andrew Street Llanelli Carms SA15 3YP w 614028X

O'GRADY Ruth (see COLLETT, Mrs)

O'HALLORAN Lisa 04/07/2007 Church Walk Veterinary Centre Ltd St Mary's Place Church Walk Ulverston Cumbria LA12 7EN **Tel:** (01229) 583675 w 6378171

O'HANRAHAN Siobhain Bridie 05/10/1994 Gortnalon Monaree Nenagh Co Tipperary Ireland **Tel:** (01874) 610776 w 6030492

O'HARA Kathryn Elizabeth 20/03/2009 28 Compton Road London SW19 7QD **Tel:** 02087390926 w 6404439

O'KEEFFE Jennifer Helen 03/05/2005 67 Fuller Way Croxley Green Rickmansworth Hertfordshire WD3 3PL **Tel:** (07939) 372921 w 6300137

OLDFIELD Josephine Margaret (see YATES, Mrs)

OLDMAN Sara Dee (see WOODS, Mrs)

OLDS Clare Louise (see RING, Mrs)

O'LEARY Daniel Michael 09/02/2009 47 Chestnut Drive Hereford Herefordshire HR2 6AY **Tel:** (01432) 263 144 m 6444303

OLEN Sarah Caroline 19/09/2006 70 Mission Road Diss Norfolk IP22 4HX **Tel:** (01379) 651183 w 6374904

OLIVER Inge Louise 29/06/2007 25 Olympia Hill Morpeth Northumberland NE61 1JH **Tel:** 01670516871 w 6377159

Michelle Amy 01/02/2010 101 Mendip Avenue Worle Weston-super-Mare Avon BS22 6HZ **Tel:** (01934) 516494 w 6453213

Nicola Elizabeth 03/10/2008 Eslington Hill Farm Whittingham ALNWICK Northumberland NE66 4UR w 6406210

Tracy Ann (nee Blackburn) 29/05/2003 (08/12/2008) 85 Station Road Healing GRIMSBY South Humberside DN41 7RB **Tel:** (01472) 886811 w 6269975

OLLEY Joanna Claire 11/02/2009 1a Upper High Street CASTLE CARY Somerset BA7 7AR w 6441916

OLLEY Karen Michelle (see MANNING, Mrs)

OLLIER Charlotte Marie 15/02/2002 19 Summerlee Road Finedon WELLINGBOROUGH Northamptonshire NN9 5LJ w 6268446

O'LOUGHLIN Aisling Mary 03/03/2005 Sunset Tinnakilly Aughrim Co Wicklow Ireland **Tel:** (00353) 8776 45098 w 6300247

O'NEIL Genna Margaret 15/11/2005 150 Raeburn Rigg Carmondean Livingston EH54 8PJ w 6278676

O'NEILL Katie 22/02/2007 40 Barlborough Road Ilkeston Derbyshire DE7 8WJ **Tel:** (0115) 973 6151 w 6318089

Kim Annette 03/02/2005 72 Laxey Crescent Leigh Lancashire WN7 5HF **Tel:** (01942) 745 049 w 6275255

Sinead Clare (nee O'Boyle) 19/08/1994 (05/10/2004) 30 Dommetts Lane Frome Somerset BA11 4JD **Tel:** (01373) 463 929 w 602991X

OPENSHAW Michelle Louise (nee Marsh) 14/03/2006 (25/02/2009) 7 Mill Field Close RAYLEIGH Essex SS6 8LX **Tel:** (01268) 775224 w 6247700

OPPERMAN Emma Catherine (nee Jefcoate, formerly Jefcoate) 08/02/1995 (02/11/1999) 1 Oak Villas Church Road North Woodchester STROUD Gloucestershire GL5 5PQ **Tel:** (01453) 872676 w 6035162

ORAM Claire Louise (nee Grey) 24/01/2000 Hook Veterinary Centre Bell Meadow Road Hook Hampshire RG27 9HG **Tel:** (01256) 764771 w 6140698

Elisabeth 24/08/1999 (10/11/2009) Bray Lodge Chittlehampton UMBERLEIGH Devon EX37 9RE **Tel:** (01769) 574485 w 6131628

O'REILLY Julie Louise 18/10/2006 137 Tantallon Road Shawlands GLASGOW G41 3LU **Tel:** (07977) 063692 w 6324645

Karen Elizabeth 25/04/2005 6/22 Wheaton Road Plympton South Australia 5038 Australia w 6304097

Tara Sarah 11/11/2004 228 Painswick Road Gloucester Gloucestershire GL4 4PH **Tel:** (01452) 529480 w 6273352

ORGAN Tracey (nee Haycock) 21/05/2003 Donnington Grove Veterinary Surgery Oxford Road NEWBURY Berkshire RG14 2JB **Tel:** (01635) 47170 w 6275475

ORGLES Melanie Jayne 02/09/2008 Avenue Veterinary Centre 35 Avenue Road Grantham Lincolnshire NG31 6TJ **Tel:** (01476) 563371/564490 w 6437824

ORME Hannah Lucy 16/11/2006 60 Hoveton Close Redditch Worcestershire B98 7HW **Tel:** (07811) 575742 w 6331575

ORMEROD Claire Nicola 06/02/2002 18 Park Avenue Haslingden Rossendale Lancashire BB4 6PP **Tel:** (01706) 222650 w 6271130

Xaria Rachel 04/02/1992 (10/05/2004) Oakmount House Trafalgar Street Burnley Lancashire BB11 1TP **Tel:** (01282) 423640 w 6058099

ORMROD Julie-Anne 28/08/1997 13 Westfield Court Walker Way THORNTON-CLEVELEYS Lancashire FY5 4LG w 6033143

ORMSTON Kate Louise 02/04/2003 Abington Park Veterinary Surgery 427 Wellingborough Road Northampton NN1 4EZ **Tel:** (01604) 628 685 w 6258601

O'ROURKE Andrea (nee Banks) 31/01/1992 21 Harrington Street Clayton le Moors Accrington Lancashire BB5 4DF w 6073517

Jane Louise 05/06/2006 1478 Pollokshaws Road Glasgow G43 1RN **Tel:** (0141) 649 5471 w 6250087

ORPET Hilary Anne DipAVN(Surgical) 30/07/1987 Royal Veterinary College Hawkshead Road North Mymms Hatfield Hertfordshire AL9 7TA w 6058102

ORR Deborah Frances 25/02/2003 Dogs Trust Bolton House 17-26 Wakley Street LONDON EC1V 7RQ **Tel:** (020) 7837 0006 w 6274232

Sarah Maria (nee Duff) 01/03/1984 23 Wests Road BANBRIDGE County Down Ireland BT32 3RR **Tel:** 02840627856 w 6089618

ORSI Gemma Ellen Rosa 22/12/2004 (04/11/2009) 93 Norval Road WEMBLEY Middlesex HA0 3TA **Tel:** (020) 8904 3977 w 6313392

OSBORN Beth Sophie (see DORWARD, Mrs)

Diane Elizabeth 21/08/1985 1 Heol Ffynnon Asa Eglwysbach Colwyn Bay Conwy LL28 5BL **Tel:** (01492) 650578 w 6058124

OSBORNE Clare Louise (see FEENEY, Mrs)

OSBORNE Davina Elizabeth DipAVN(Surgical) (nee Chowdhary) 07/02/1995 76 Station Road Alvechurch BIRMINGHAM B48 7SD w 6033868

Heather Anne (nee Sheppard) 13/12/1991 10 Holly Close HEATHFIELD East Sussex TN21 8AP w 6060596

OSBORNE Jenny (see GORDON, Mrs)

Martin Keith 24/02/2000 Westmoor Veterinary Centre 1 Brook Lane Tavistock Devon PL19 9BA **Tel:** (01822) 612561 m 6190280

Ruth 30/11/2005 Pype Hayes Veterinary Centre 1066 Chester Road Pype Hayes Erdington Birmingham B24 0SA **Tel:** (0121) 350 2303 w 6343829

Wendy Dawn 31/08/1999 348 Franklands Village Haywards Heath West Sussex RH16 3RJ **Tel:** (01444) 455964 w 6134695

O'SHEA Taylor Anthony 16/08/1988 7 Lennox Mews Chapel Road WORTHING Sussex BN11 1GY m 6057936

O'SULLIVAN Melanie Jane (nee Blakesley) 06/09/2001 (04/05/2004) 101 Fairacres Prestwood Great Missenden Buckinghamshire HP16 0LF **Tel:** (01494) 866623 w 6204800

O'SULLIVAN Sara-Jane Marie (see CLARE, Mrs)

O'TOOLE Heidi Rosemary 17/11/2009 28 Green Lane Mossley Hill Liverpool L18 6HB **Tel:** (0151) 724 2664 w 6419971

OUGHTON Siobhan Emelda 16/05/2006 7 Bakehouse Corner East Street Chickerell WEYMOUTH Dorset DT3 4EJ w 6334534

OVER Emma Jane 13/01/2004 3 Pentwyn Avenue Redhill Hereford Herefordshire HR2 7LB **Tel:** (01432) 268133 w 6278962

OVERINGTON Helen Claire 28/10/1998 (05/11/2004) St Anne's Veterinary Group 6 St Anne's Road Eastbourne East Sussex BN21 2DJ **Tel:** (01323) 640011 w 6108891

OWEN Alwen Haf 09/09/2008 Tan y Bryn Gwytherin ABERGELE Clwyd LL22 8UU **Tel:** 01745860585 w 6378710

Anya Dee 13/01/2004 119 Coolidge Gardens Cottenham CAMBRIDGE CB24 8RH **Tel:** (07815) 152403 w 6292140

OWEN Carol-Ann (see HICKS, Mrs)

David Martin 27/09/1999 238 Bute Street Cardiff CF10 5HT **Tel:** (0292) 048 0990 m 6138893

Helen Margaret 23/01/2003 Hillcroft 50A Hall Street Dudley West Midlands DY2 7BT **Tel:** (01384) 252509 w 6276762

Natalie Jane 31/08/2005 23 Lowfield Road Slinfold HORSHAM West Sussex RH13 0SQ **Tel:** (01403) 791843 w 6289962

Nia Moreton 08/03/1999 (24/10/2000) Hafryn Llangynog Oswestry Shropshire SY10 0HE **Tel:** (01691) 860267 w 6139547

Rowena Georgina 15/11/2007 Flat 8a St. Edmunds Avenue HUNSTANTON Norfolk PE36 6AZ w 6381449

Samantha 04/11/2008 Fivelands Veterinary Centre 98 Alcester Road BIRMINGHAM B13 8EG **Tel:** (0121) 449 3716 w 6426230

Samantha Jane 23/08/1999 The Blue Cross Animal Hospital Nelson Street Grimsby South Humberside DN32 7SH **Tel:** (01472) 343278 w 6116392

OWENS Julie 19/03/2007 51 Cae America LLANFAIRFECHAN Gwynedd LL33 0SJ w 6305208

OXFORD Helen Patricia 30/08/1994 15-A Ashcroft Lane Finchdean Rowlands Castle Waterlooville Hampshire PO8 0AX **Tel:** (01243) 377182 w 6029909

OXTOBY Emma Elizabeth (see HARRISON, Mrs)

OYLER Hayley Lynne (nee Bevan) 28/06/2005 West Farm Veterinary Clinic North Road Cowbridge South Glamorgan CF71 7DF **Tel:** (01446) 774016 w 6281459

P

PACE Charlotte Ruth (nee Adrian) 22/03/2004 Queen Mother Hospital for Small Animals Hawkshead Lane North Mymms Hatfield Hertfordshire AL9 7TA **Tel:** (01707) 666366 w 6288829

PACKER Elaine 09/04/2009 28 Clay Hall Place Acton Sudbury Suffolk CO10 0BT **Tel:** 07763136900 w 6401073

PACKHAM Heather Morag (nee Laird, nee Barrett) 27/05/2003 67 Mill Road Cobholm Great Yarmouth NR31 0BA w 6266917

PADDEN-BARR Kirsty Jane 11/12/2001 Palavas 3 Hillview Silver Street Shepton Beauchamp Ilminster Somerset TA19 0JZ w 6270327

PADWICK Elaine 10/10/2005 47a Winchester Road Chandlers Ford Eastleigh Hampshire SO53 2GF **Tel:** (023) 8025 2543 w 6320850

PAGE Gillian Alison (nee Teadley) 11/11/1988 (26/01/2005) Castlethorn Cottage Cathlaw Lane Torphichen EH48 4NN **Tel:** (01506) 652566 w 6061862

Johanna Elizabeth Jayne 09/02/2009 23 Hillview Gardens Felton Bristol Avon BS40 9UH **Tel:** (01275) 474 560 w 6447086

Kelly Louise 09/09/1999 309 The Ridge Hastings East Sussex TN34 2RA **Tel:** (01424) 751595 w 6134505

Kimberley Jane 09/11/2005 12 Priory Road St Neots Cambridgeshire PE19 1AT **Tel:** (07870) 856231 w 6293812

Natasha Melanie 17/08/2005 27 Margaret Avenue Shenfield BRENTWOOD Essex CM15 8RF **Tel:** (01277) 239 785 w 6287707

PAKENHAM Sonya Bridget 23/01/2003 The Brook Veterinary Clinic Rossorry Church Road Enniskillen County Fermanagh BT74 7HB **Tel:** (028) 6632 3335 w 6263001

PALEY Victoria Margaret (see BEASLEY, Mrs)

PALFREY Angela Mary 09/08/1983 Eastbrook Farm Burlescombe Tiverton Devon EX16 7JE **Tel:** (01823) 672700 w 6058215

Emma Jane (nee Reid) 15/03/1999 (05/06/2001) 18 Hidcote Mews Weston Super Mare BS24 7JD **Tel:** (01934) 514165 w 6113369

PALFREYMAN Rachel Louise 13/01/2004 18 Green Lane Freckleton Preston Lancashire PR4 1RN **Tel:** (01772) 632595 w 6290611

Stacey Emma 15/11/2005 608 Veterinary Group 608 Warwick Road Solihull West Midlands B91 1AA **Tel:** (0121) 705 3044 w 6312226

PALIN Caroline 31/10/2003 3 Kensington Avenue Sutton St Helens Merseyside WA9 3TT **Tel:** (01744) 813663 w 6279028

PALLISTER Mary Angela (see RILEY, Miss)

PALLOT Sarah Anne 22/03/2004 63 Ville Du Bocage St Peter Jersey JE3 7YT **Tel:** (01534) 482864 w 6284891

PALMER Amy Louise (see BARFIELD, Mrs)

PALMER Angela 02/09/1997 (24/02/2004) Uplands Way Vets Ltd Uplands Way DISS Norfolk IP22 4DF **Tel:** (01379) 642865 w 6118367

PALMER Carol Elizabeth (see FORD, Mrs)

Claire 02/11/2004 The Veterinary Hospital Colwill Road Estover Plymouth Devon PL6 8RP **Tel:** (01752) 702646 w 6286475

Claire Louise 04/02/2008 71 Somerset Road BRISTOL BS4 2HX **Tel:** 01173005468 w 6390205

Dwynwen Mari 05/02/1996 242 Cricklewood Lane London NW2 2PU **Tel:** (020) 8450 2228 w 6036687

Jane Lesley (nee Wood) 05/03/2002 15 Wood Drive Stevenage Hertfordshire SG2 8NX **Tel:** (01438) 354599 w 6271834

Jennifer Louise 17/01/2008 7a Neighbourhood Centre Culliford Crescent Poole Dorset BH17 9DW **Tel:** (01202) 602766 w 6320146

Joanne Louise 13/07/2007 18 South Drive Warley Brentwood Essex CM14 5DJ **Tel:** (01277) 212238 w 6349439

Laura Margaret 07/05/2009 52 Lakes Lane BEACONSFIELD Buckinghamshire HP9 2LB **Tel:** 01494671574 w 6445975

Matthew Leonard 28/11/2000 15 Manilla Place WESTON-SUPER-MARE Avon BS23 2AB **Tel:** (01934) 637763 m 6202864

Samantha Jayne 14/08/2009 24 Sycamore Avenue Bingley West Yorkshire BD16 1HD **Tel:** (01274) 560923 w 6434876

Shani Yolande 22/03/2004 Martock Veterinary Centre Stapleton Road Martock Somerset TA12 6HH **Tel:** (01935) 825199 w 6300588

PALOS Martine Isabelle 05/02/2008 Ivanhoe 14 Shamrock Way London N14 5RY **Tel:** (02083) 628686 w 6355258

PANTER Elizabeth 27/08/1997 (07/08/2003) 121 Lower Street Pulborough West Sussex RH20 2BP **Tel:** (01798) 872089 w 6112015

PANTON Gillian 17/01/2006 Bishopton Veterinary Group Mill Farm Studley Road Ripon North Yorkshire HG4 2QR **Tel:** (01765) 602396 w 6304834

PAPE Charlotte Emily 22/02/2000 The Coach House Trefrew Road CAMELFORD Cornwall PL32 9TP w 6099987

PARDEN Donna Marie (see CLAY, Mrs)

PARFITT Emma Kathleen 07/12/2005 St. David Veterinary Centre Pentwyn Shopping Precinct Pentwyn Drive Cardiff South Glamorgan CF23 7EY **Tel:** (029) 2073 3111 w 6331300

PARISH Claire Louise (see SIMPSON, Mrs)

PARISH Keri Louise 04/11/2005 39 Butt Lane Blackfordby SWADLINCOTE Derbyshire DE11 8BG w 6337548

Sarah Louise 20/02/2008 15 Brunel Close Micheldever Station WINCHESTER Hampshire SO21 3BX **Tel:** (01962) 774421 w 6402987

PARKER Claire Louise (see LANDSBERG, Mrs)

PARKER Eve 31/10/2006 12 Bromilow Road SKELMERSDALE Lancashire WN8 8TU w 6375586

Georgina Jane 05/11/2008 31 Chyvelah Vale Gloweth Truro Cornwall TR1 3YJ **Tel:** 01872240905 w 6405462

Georgina Marie 15/12/2004 2 North Street Aston BAMPTON Oxfordshire OX18 2DJ **Tel:** (01993) 850973 w 6325305

Grace Angela 27/10/2008 37 Lucerne Road Elmstead COLCHESTER CO7 7YB **Tel:** 01206825116 w 6438594

PARKER Helen (see SANDERS, Mrs)

PARKER Helen Lucy (see COE, Mrs)

Jenna-Kate Louise 09/05/2006 50 Waterloo Road Leyton LONDON E10 7HR **Tel:** (020) 8558 7693 w 6342333

Jennifer Ann 22/05/2009 63 Carrhill Road Roughtown Mossley Lancashire OL5 0SE **Tel:** 07940919626 w 6412997

Jennifer Jane 24/08/2009 28 Windrush Banbury Oxfordshire OX16 1PJ **Tel:** 07771742256 w 6365785

PARKER Rebecca Louise (see THOMPSON, Mrs)

Victoria Charlotte 09/09/2008 35 Ridd Way Wingerworth CHESTERFIELD Derbyshire S42 6UX w 6420939

PARKES Carole Joanne 12/05/2006 22 Maes y Dderwen LLANFYLLIN Powys SY22 5DP w 6353916

PARKES Sarah Jane (see RANCE, Mrs)

PARKIN Tammy Georgina 05/01/2005 26a Tollerdown Road Lanehouse Weymouth Dorset DT4 0SQ **Tel:** (01305) 814138 w 6321994

PARKINSON Debbie Jayne 14/09/2009 1 Bridge Cottage Stakepool PRESTON PR3 6AH **Tel:** (01995) 603349 w 6460990

PARKINSON Rose Ann (see ROCHE, Mrs)

Wendy Ann (nee Lenton) 08/09/2005 Avenue Veterinary Centre 35 Avenue Road Grantham Lincolnshire NG31 6TJ **Tel:** (01476) 563371/564490 w 6346260

PARMENTER Claire Louise (see CAMILLERI, Mrs)

PARMENTER Jodie (see BAYNAM, Mrs)

PARNELL Tracey Louise 25/02/2003 3 Hanford Close Wandsworth London SW18 5AU **Tel:** (020) 88705701 w 6278511

PARREN Jane (nee Cowley) 29/08/1996 The Old Sunday School Millpool BODMIN Cornwall PL30 4HZ **Tel:** (01208) 821369 w 6041857

PARRISH Helen Tracy (nee Parrish, formerly Evans) 22/01/1997 43 Garden Village St. Martins OSWESTRY Shropshire SY11 3AX w 6043435

PARRY Josephine Jeanette DipAVN(Surgical) (nee Scadding) 11/08/1992 25 Cherry Orchard Wotton-under-Edge Gloucestershire GL12 7HT **Tel:** (01453) 842140 w 6008183

Judith Elizabeth DipAVN(Medical) (nee Chell) 23/10/1992 Bryniau Bach Tythe Barn Alton Stoke-on-Trent Staffordshire ST10 4AZ **Tel:** (01538) 703723 w 6008434

Laura Elizabeth 10/04/2007 The Friesian Building 3 + 4 Dairy Business Park Brewer Street Bletchingley RH1 4QP **Tel:** (01883) 741440 w 6374739

Rachel Ann 15/10/2008 Northlands Veterinary Hospital 2 Northampton Road Kettering Northamptonshire NN15 7JU **Tel:** (01536) 485 543 w 6397751

PARRY Sarah (see PERRIN, Mrs)

Scott Lee 12/05/2004 133 Worston Road Highbridge Burnham-on-Sea Somerset TA9 3JX **Tel:** (01278) 792959 m 6251946

PARSONAGE Emma Joy (see SNOWDON, Ms)

PARSONS Dawn Joyce Agnes (see CAMPBELL, Mrs)

PARSONS Debra Jayne 19/10/2008 121 The Hundred ROMSEY Hampshire SO51 8BZ w 6380591

Helen Elizabeth 16/12/2005 83a Field End Road Eastecote PINNER Middlesex HA5 1QG w 6326460

PARSONS Kelly Lorraine (see HAMILTON, Mrs)

PARTON Charlotte Ann 27/02/2006 5 Mill Lane Standon Stafford Staffordshire ST21 6RP **Tel:** (01782) 791 610 w 6328231

PARTON Michelle June (see DUNN, Mrs)

PARTRIDGE Francesca 13/02/1998 59 Grand Drive Herne Bay Kent CT6 8JS w 6118447

Stevie Marie 31/07/2009 23 Queens Crescent Bilston West Midlands WV14 9AQ **Tel:** 01902682084 w 6376708

PARYLO Sharon Suzanne (nee Moore) 22/08/1997 (09/09/2004) College of Animal Welfare My Petstop Pet Resort Topcliffe Close Capital Park Tingley West Yorkshire WF3 1BU **Tel:** (0113) 220 3720 w 6116337

PASHLEY Rachel Laura 19/04/2005 The Veterinary Surgery 23 Mill Hill Road PONTEFRACT West Yorkshire WF8 4HR **Tel:** (01977) 702056 w 6279820

PASK David Thomas John 24/09/2008 739 London Road Grays Essex RM20 3HX **Tel:** 01708863673 m 6355269

PASKELL Leah Marie 01/04/2009 72 Victoria Avenue Margate Kent CT9 2UD **Tel:** 01227749287 w 6409466

PASS Hayley Marie 09/10/2009 281 Nottingham Road Eastwood NOTTINGHAM NG16 2AP w 6466457

PASSINGHAM Caroline Michelle DipAVN(Surgical) 23/01/2003 10 Denburn Place Crail ANSTRUTHER Fife KY10 3WH w 6277697

PASSMORE Fiona Caroline 11/01/1977 University of Bristol Langford House Langford Bristol Avon BS40 5DU **Tel:** (01934) 852022 w 6058408

Jennifer Sarah 23/02/2005 The 1870 Building Jayes Park Courtyard Forest Green Road Ockley Dorking Surrey RH5 5RR **Tel:** (01306) 621269 w 6319585

PATEL Hina Dinesh 02/06/2004 91 Engel Park Mill Hill London NW7 2HN **Tel:** (020) 8349 1920 w 6296463

PATEMAN Karen Julie (see MILLER, Mrs)

PATERSON Joanne Clare 10/05/2007 35 Randolph Drive Farnborough Hampshire GU14 0QQ **Tel:** (01252) 544 783 w 6370603

PATERSON Lynn Janet (see BALLANTYNE, Mrs)

PATERSON Sandra (see MCLEARY, Mrs)

PATIENCE Helen Mary 10/11/2009 Cedar Veterinary Hospital 69 Christchurch Road Ringwood Hampshire BH24 1DH **Tel:** (01425) 473683 w 6437846

PATMORE Simone Michelle 24/11/2004 11 Woodville Crescent Yardley Gobion TOWCESTER Northamptonshire NN12 7UW w 6288499

PATTEN Melanie Rachel DipAVN(Medical) (nee Dumelow) 29/08/1996 30 Field Close Borrowash DERBY DE72 3HJ **Tel:** (01332) 544505 w 6042624

PATTERSON Sarah Louise 06/10/2006 8 Derwent Dale Consett County Durham DH8 0HZ **Tel:** (01207) 591 823 w 6355775

PATTERSON Tracey (see SHILLITO, Mrs)

PATTON Elizabeth Margaret 05/02/1998 11 Black Brook Close Heapey Chorley Lancashire PR6 9AJ **Tel:** (01257) 234649 w 6043708

Sinead Teresa Frances 22/02/2007 Wardtown Ballyshannon Co Donegal Ireland **Tel:** (00353) 71 98 51280 w 6281723

Yvette Michelle 11/08/2008 122 Pepper Lane Standish Wigan Lancashire WN6 0PW w 6406507

PATTULLO Ashley Alice 19/01/2000 20 Forfar Road Southmuir Kirriemuir DD8 5BY **Tel:** (01575) 572643 w 6148992

PAUL Maya Kristina Nadine (see YATES, Mrs)

PAULIN Sarah Jean 27/10/2009 3/11 Coate Avenue Alphington Victoria 3078 Australia **Tel:** (+61) 3 9481 7118 w 6571661

PAULL Christina Marie (see MADEN, Mrs)

PAWLEY Theresa Sophie Lynda 07/02/2007 The Veterinary Hospital 118 Victoria Drive Bognor Regis West Sussex PO21 2EJ **Tel:** (01243) 841111 w 6353146

PAYNE Eloise Layla (see NURSE, Mrs)

PAYNE Hayley Marie 30/01/2009 15 Delage Close Longford COVENTRY CV6 6JP **Tel:** 07890969910 w 6273253

Jenny Yolande (nee Beechey) 05/09/2003 105 Cornwall Road Herne Bay Kent CT6 7SZ w 6258183

PAYNE Laura Gillian (see RICHARDS, Mrs)

Lydia Amy 30/10/2003 5 Croft Street Lower Broughton Salford Lancashire M7 1LR **Tel:** (0161) 7088077 w 6285749

Natasha Louise (nee Southam) 28/09/2005 57 Tucker Road Ottershaw CHERTSEY Surrey KT16 0HD **Tel:** (01932) 248941 w 6329815

Rachel Alice 14/04/2008 Highridge Station Road Gunnislake Cornwall PL18 9DX **Tel:** 07779595811 w 6358844

Stephanie Rose 04/05/2006 5 George Street Stafford Staffordshire ST16 2RJ **Tel:** (01889) 882644 w 6353927

Stewart Ian 18/08/2009 5 Castle Drive HORLEY Surrey RH6 9DB **Tel:** (07789) 006547 m 6347547

PAYTON Sally Joanne 12/08/2003 (21/06/2007) The Farmhouse Kitchen 1 North Street Williton TAUNTON Somerset TA4 4SL w 6276652

PEACE Robin Arthur William 21/05/2009 16 Stubbins Lane Chinley High Peak SK23 6AE **Tel:** 07743904708 m 6405770

PEACOCK Bryony Claire 18/01/2008 17 Browns Square ST. NEOTS Cambridgeshire PE19 1PE **Tel:** (01480) 211451 w 6400105

Caroline Susan 12/04/2002 Guide Dogs Breedinmg Centre Tollgate House Banbury Road Bishops Tachbrook Warwickshire CV33 9QJ **Tel:** (01926) 651226 w 6278302

Dawn Michelle 09/06/2009 109e Balmoral Drive Southport Merseyside PR9 8QH **Tel:** 07920404180 w 6443390

Jennifer Suzanne 13/07/2007 19 Hollywood Way Woodford Green Essex IG8 9LG **Tel:** (0208) 5273106 w 6347558

June Elaine 22/02/1995 36 Henbrook St. Neots Huntingdon Cambridgeshire PE19 2DQ **Tel:** (01480) 354655 w 6031099

Katie Elizabeth 18/11/2009 17 The Laurels New Barn Longfield Kent DA3 7HH w 6451882

Victoria Jane (nee Evans) 31/12/1990 (15/10/2001) Guide Dogs I Quarry Court Lime Quarry Mews Merrow Guildford Surrey GU1 2RD **Tel:** (0845) 3727397 w 6050001

PEAK Alison Roberta (see MCCLENAGHAN, Mrs)

PEAK Sharon (nee Appleton, formerly Port) 18/01/1999 (12/10/2000) 109 Blackburn Road Greenhill Herne Bay Kent CT6 7UT **Tel:** (01227) 375978 (Ex Directory) w 6136841

PEAK Suzi Anna (see CANALE, Mrs)

PEARCE Eloise 16/06/2006 Saveock Hugus TRURO Cornwall TR3 6EQ **Tel:** (01872) 561 456 w 6345534

Kylee Jayne 28/08/2007 Beech House 16 Queens Road Hersham Walton-on-Thames Surrey KT12 5NH **Tel:** (01932) 220768 w 6318122

Larissa Caroline 04/06/2009 6 Peppard Close Southampton Hampshire SO18 6SX **Tel:** 02380445171 w 6407640

Laura 02/03/2007 8 Orchard Road Mortimer Reading Berkshire RG7 3QN **Tel:** (0118) 933 2964 w 6365796

Lisa 13/04/2004 3 Fairfield Close Datchet Berkshire SL3 9NG w 6285738

PEARCE Michelle Julie (see PRINCE, Mrs)

Sally Helen Lillian 20/11/2008 Silva House Veterinary Clinic Silver Street Midsomer Norton Radstock Somerset BA3 2ET **Tel:** (01761) 412223 w 6409488

PEARMAN Zoe Christina 04/08/2003 The Veterinary Centre Wellington New Road Taunton Somerset TA1 5LU **Tel:** (01823) 333722 w 6266004

PEARSALL Lucinda Charlotte (see IRELAND, Mrs)

PEARSON Charlotte Ellen 27/09/1999 (03/08/2001) Flat 2 Mona Villa New Market Street BUXTON Derbyshire SK17 6LP **Tel:** (01298) 23459 w 6186056

Claire-Louise (nee Philpott) 01/04/2003 The Old Golfhouse Veterinary Group The Old Golf House Brandon Road Thetford Norfolk IP24 3ND **Tel:** (01842) 764 244 w 6280216

Debra Marie 11/11/2004 10 Boscawen Way THATCHAM Berkshire RG19 4GA w 6284055

Kirsty Marie 04/06/2008 15 Pond Terrace CARNFORTH Lancashire LA5 9BL w 6396321

Melanie 18/08/2009 40 Temple Mead Roydon HARLOW Essex CM19 5EB **Tel:** 07940447066 w 6373771

Rebecca Amy 04/10/2005 (03/12/2008) 25 Firethorn Crescent Whitnash LEAMINGTON SPA Warwickshire CV31 2RX **Tel:** (07727) 606953 w 6327494

Rosalind Frances 18/04/2005 Flat 2 27 Nightingale Road Southsea Hampshire PO5 3JJ w 6331190

Sarah 15/05/2009 25 Horace Street Coseley Bilston WV14 9HT **Tel:** 01902680459 w 6440805

PEARSON Sarah (see PERCIVAL, Mrs)

Suzanne Alice 22/03/2004 Elizabeth Smith Veterinary Surgeon Ickwell Road Upper Caldecote Biggleswade Bedfordshire SG18 9BS **Tel:** (01767) 627317 w 6296353

PEART Maria Jane 01/04/2003 Dragon Veterinary Centre Prestbury Park New Barn Lane Cheltenham GL52 3LE **Tel:** (01242) 580324 w 6284176

PEDDER Victoria Claire (nee Midgley) 13/08/2004 5 Ladies Walk Caton Road Lancaster Lancashire LA1 3NX **Tel:** (01524) 67777 w 6298718

PEDGE Cathie Lynn 05/09/2008 49 Hendred Way ABINGDON Oxfordshire OX14 2AW w 6429684

PEDLEY Claire Helen (see KEELING, Miss)

PEEDELL Michelle Joy 17/07/2008 17 Miller Road BANBURY Oxfordshire OX16 0QX **Tel:** (01295) 270657 w 6332642

PEEL Elizabeth Mary 02/12/2009 185 Moor Lane Birkenshaw West Yorkshire BD11 2NX **Tel:** (07971) 570 265 w 6387235

Madeline Claire 23/12/2008 Alver Veterinary Group 148 Forton Road Gosport Hampshire PO12 3HG **Tel:** (023) 9258 2991/2 w 6406133

Rebecca Lucy 04/11/2005 33 The Gardens Radford Semele LEAMINGTON SPA Warwickshire CV31 1TH **Tel:** (01926) 335405 w 6325184

PEGRAM Lisa Anne (nee Simpkin) 04/08/2008 Rose Hill Farm Creephedge Lane East Hanningfield CHELMSFORD CM3 8BP w 6410137

PELLOW Rachel Ann (see LEECH, Mrs)

PEMBERTON Amy Louise 31/10/2005 3 High Houses Mill Road Thompson THETFORD Norfolk IP24 1PH **Tel:** (01953) 483125 w 6331586

PEMBERTON Clara Kim (see MACFARLANE, Mrs)

PENALUNA Victoria Lesley 29/06/2007 (03/02/2009) 12 Hedgefield View Dudley CRAMLINGTON Northumberland NE23 7QL **Tel:** (0191) 250 1501 w 6320322

PENDER Christina Patricia 06/03/2008 52 Ballyhosset Road Downpatrick County Down BT30 7ES **Tel:** (028) 44842257 w 6286937

PENDERGAST Chantel 30/01/2009 42 Middlefields Pixton Way Forestdale Surrey CR0 9LF **Tel:** 07909704710 w 6453301

PENNEFATHER Jacqueline (nee Tompkins) 10/02/2004 (20/03/2008) Pinebank Veterinary Surgery 85b London Road MAIDSTONE Kent ME16 0DX **Tel:** (01622) 755098 w 6291568

PENNELL Clare Louise 19/03/2007 Eastfield Veterinary Clinic Ltd Station Road North Thoresby GRIMSBY Lincolnshire DN36 5QU **Tel:** (01472) 840209 w 6371681

PENNICK Joanne 30/05/2007 Claines Veterinary Clinic 238 Ombersley Road Worcester WR3 7HB **Tel:** (01905) 453007 w 6377170

PENNICOTTE-HENRIE Lara Amy (nee Handley) 30/08/1994 (18/02/2009) Manor Cottage 2 Totnes Road SOUTH BRENT Devon TQ10 9BP **Tel:** (01364) 73050 w 6032795

PENNOCK Caroline (see BURN, Mrs)

PENNY Emma Jane 24/09/2001 Ashton Veterinary Surgery 356 Lower Addiscombe Road Croydon CR0 7AF **Tel:** (020) 8654 3887 w 603345X

PENNY Jennifer Marie (see AHEARNE, Mrs)

PENNY Lindsay Patricia (see KNIGHT, Mrs)

Rachel Lynne Wood 07/02/2007 Flat 22, Clifton Manor 352 Clifton Road Aberdeen Aberdeenshire AB24 4DX **Tel:** (01569) 762484 w 6373430

PENROSE Danielle Elizabeth 03/06/2008 30 Northgate HARTLEPOOL Cleveland TS24 0LJ **Tel:** 01429869649 w 6411039

Leanne Dee 01/09/2008 Sunnyhill Stylecroft Road Chalfont St. Giles Buckinghamshire HP8 4HY **Tel:** 01494782001 w 6404230

PENTELOW Tracy Louise 25/09/2007 Brunswick Place Veterinary Clinic Brunswick Place Cranbourne Lane Basingstoke Hampshire RG21 3NN **Tel:** (01256) 473371 w 6377291

PEPLOW Michelle 19/04/2006 27 Fifth Avenue WOLVERHAMPTON WV10 9TE w 6346579

PERCIVAL Davinia 28/06/2005 (05/11/2009) The Kings Arms Main Street Farthingstone TOWCESTER Northamptonshire NN12 8EZ w 6281613

Joanne Christy 01/04/2003 8 Hunts Path Oakley Bedford Bedfordshire MK43 7SR **Tel:** (020) 83010375 w 6280601

Michelle Margaret 05/01/2009 21 Church Row West Rainton HOUGHTON LE SPRING Tyne and Wear DH4 6NR w 6403075

Sarah (nee Pearson) 27/01/2005 Grange Vets Victoria Road Darlington County Durham DL1 5SJ **Tel:** (01325) 465371 w 6325162

PERFECT Alison Jayne 09/05/2006 (09/02/2009) Station Farm London Road Six Mile Bottom Newmarket Suffolk CB8 0UH **Tel:** (01638) 572012 w 6318375

PERKINS Erain Maria 26/07/1993 (12/08/1999) 27 Bulkington Road Shilton Coventry CV7 9JT **Tel:** (024) 76616582 w 6015339

Laura Elizabeth 30/09/2008 3 Mayo Road SHIPSTON-ON-STOUR Warwickshire CV36 4BH w 6434590

PERRATT Kirsty Lianne 19/03/2007 2 Far Field Road Edenthorpe Doncaster South Yorkshire DN3 2NS w 6367105

PERRETT Kate Louise (see TENNISWOOD, Mrs)

PERRIN Sarah (nee Parry) 02/09/1999 (15/08/2005) 4 Dragonfly Road Oakley Park Swindon Wiltshire SN3 4ET w 6128976

PERRIS Victoria Louise (nee McKeown, formerly Beasley) 18/08/1995 98 Wheatmoor Road Sutton Coldfield West Midlands B75 7JS **Tel:** 0121-329-2040 w 6026646

PERRY Deborah Jane 07/03/2008 Twin Pines 12 School Lane Wilbarston MARKET HARBOROUGH Leicestershire LE16 8QN **Tel:** 07946573360 w 6403119

Hannah Clare (nee Izzard) 30/10/2003 71 Partridge Piece Cranfield Bedfordshire MK43 0BL **Tel:** (01234) 752031 w 6296254

PERRY Jessica (see HOWARD, Mrs)

PERRY Karen Joanne (see CHANCELLOR, Mrs)

Nicola Jane (nee Stenson) 30/09/1993 (25/04/2007) The Rochford Veterinary Surgery 19 East Street Rochford Essex SS4 1DB **Tel:** (01702) 545558 w 6064863

PESCOD Susan Elaine 30/06/2003 2 Midley Close MAIDSTONE Kent ME16 0TY **Tel:** (01622) 687637 w 6267676

PESCOTT Kate Donna 28/04/2009 14 Pulborough Way Bognor Regis West Sussex PO22 6QR **Tel:** 07841456707 w 6376565

PESTER Melanie Ann (nee Knowles) 11/01/2005 1 Highfield Close SOMERTON Somerset TA11 6SZ **Tel:** (01458) 273378 w 6331542

PETERS Sophie Arabella 06/10/2006 16 Moonsmead House Tuckers Brook Modbury Ivybridge Devon PL21 0UT **Tel:** (01548) 830249 w 6272450

PETERSEN Eva Alice 02/03/2009 Brook House Veterinary Hospital 12 Landguard Road Southampton Hampshire SO15 5DJ **Tel:** (02380) 228570 w 6437516

PETHER Helen (nee Gowen) 20/11/2002 Wood Green Animal Shelter Kingbush Farm London Road Godmanchester Huntingdon Cambridgeshire PE29 2NH **Tel:** (0844) 2488181 w 6264508

PETRIE Leanne (see MORRISON, Mrs)

PETTS Sally Jennifer Charlotte 21/11/2007 18 Red Oaks Mead Theydon Bois Epping Essex CM16 7LA w 6386553

PEW Rebecca Sarah 16/02/2009 340 Station Road WINSFORD Cheshire CW7 3DG **Tel:** 01606861105 w 6418112

PHELAN Sadie May 28/09/2005 18 Woolvers Way Locking Weston-super-Mare Avon BS24 7DW w 6342223

PHEYSEY Victoria Ann (nee Darby) 17/01/1996 (01/03/2007) 84 Arundel Road Harwood Park BROMSGROVE Worcestershire B60 2HN w 6041890

PHILIPS Jacqueline Louisa Anne (see CAMPUZANO, Mrs)

PHILLIPS Alison Louise (see WILLIAMS, Mrs)

PHILLIPS Amanda (see MOWAT, Mrs)

PHILLIPS Catherine Anne 26/01/1994 10 Frome Valley Way ROSS-ON-WYE Herefordshire HR9 5HU w 606722X

Catherine Emma 06/05/2009 The 1870 Building Jayes Park Courtyard Forest Green Road Ockley Dorking Surrey RH5 5RR **Tel:** (01306) 621269 w 6437032

PHILLIPS Cerys (see KINGDON, Mrs)

Emma Louise 15/02/2002 (10/12/2007) R S P C A Rescue Centre Brent Road Brent Knoll HIGHBRIDGE Somerset TA9 4BL **Tel:** (01278) 782671 w 6269568

Heather Louise 16/10/2009 94 Norbreck Road Thornton-Cleveleys Lancashire FY5 1RP **Tel:** (01253) 357380 w 6459549

PHILLIPS Holly Victoria (see LOYND, Mrs)

PHILLIPS Kay Amanda (see JAMES, Mrs)

Madeleine Emma 26/11/2009 52 Porcher Avenue Glyncoch Ponty Pridd Mid Glam CF37 3DB **Tel:** (07810) 426 973 w 6490404

Michelle 04/01/2006 2 Denny View Portishead Bristol Avon BS20 8BS **Tel:** (01275) 848156 w 6273792

PHILLIPS Rachel (see SMITH, Mrs)

Rebecca Holly Madelaine 11/11/2008 10 Little Brind Road Chesterfield Derbyshire S41 8XW **Tel:** 01246234207 w 6410742

Tracey Ann 26/10/2005 Sunset Bay Farm Burtle Road Burtle Bridgwater Somerset TA7 8NB **Tel:** (01278) 722796 w 6339044

PHILLPOT Joanna 24/02/2004 25 Coppice Gate CHELTENHAM Gloucestershire GL51 9QJ w 6288191

PHILPOT Clare Frances 11/11/2008 9 Haddon Close Grange Park SWINDON SN5 6ER **Tel:** (01793) 877498 w 6292030

PHILPOTT Claire-Louise (see PEARSON, Mrs)

PHILPOTT Tina (see HOLDSWORTH, Miss)

PHIPP Jennifer Sarah 18/01/2010 20 Dryland Road SNODLAND Kent ME6 5HD w 6498588

PHIPPS Aimie 18/10/2005 34 Stafford Road Langley Green Crawley West Sussex RH11 7LQ w 6351397

PHOENIX Rachel Marguerite 25/11/2008 11 Worsley Crescent Marton-in-Cleveland MIDDLESBROUGH Cleveland TS7 8LT w 6366753

PICKARD Rachael (see MCKENZIE, Mrs)

PICKAVANCE Bernadette 23/08/1999 41 Wayfarers Drive Newton Le Willows Warrington Cheshire WA12 8DF **Tel:** (01925) 227648 w 6143972

PICKERING Lucy 11/03/2008 27 Paigle Road Leicester Leicestershire LE2 8HP w 6402525

PICKETT Louisa Mary 14/04/2008 33 Brassey Avenue Broadstairs Kent CT10 2DS **Tel:** (01843) 864289 w 6383693

PICKLES Katherine Lucy 12/06/2008 29 Meadow Way Barrow Bury St. Edmunds Suffolk IP29 5DG **Tel:** (01284) 811799 w 6406221

PIDDINGTON Faye Louise 19/01/1996 Blythwood Veterinary Clinic 500 Uxbridge Road Pinner Middlesex HA5 4SL **Tel:** (020) 8421 0510 w 6033733

PIERCE Christine Jean 10/08/1984 29 Palmerston Road Upton Poole Dorset BH16 5HN **Tel:** (01202) 625815 w 609173X

PIKE Jennifer Susan 01/03/1999 35 Wares Road Ridgewood Uckfield East Sussex TN22 5TP **Tel:** (01825) 763069 w 6129299

Julie Louise 12/05/2004 3 Birds Ln Midgham Reading Berkshire RG7 5UL **Tel:** (0118) 9712720 w 6275497

Katherine (nee Spink) 18/09/2007 4 White Heather Terrace Bovey Tracey Newton Abbot Devon TQ13 9HF **Tel:** (01626) 830 194 w 6373342

Madeline Anne 05/07/2006 27 Downs View Road Westbury Wiltshire BA13 3AQ **Tel:** (01373) 826863 w 6321565

PIKETT Andrea (nee Carrington, formerly Brooks) 10/02/1997 (03/06/2004) 47 Thorne Way Kirton Boston Lincolnshire PE20 1JP **Tel:** (01205) 722032 w 6097582

PILGRIM Dean David Alan 08/11/2006 Briar Cottage 48 West Street Millbrook TORPOINT Cornwall PL10 1AD **Tel:** (07966) 238284 m 6339231

Elizabeth Anne Louise 01/09/2000 4 Garden Street Kendal Cumbria LA9 7EB **Tel:** (01539) 737784 w 6202798

PILLING Helen Mary 30/09/1992 (01/11/2001) 50 Church Street FORDINGBRIDGE Hampshire SP6 1BE w 6008092

PINHEY Bethan Louise 10/06/2009 291 Orphanage Road Sutton Coldfield West Midlands B72 1BH **Tel:** 01213734940 w 6407761

PINKHAM Judith Louisa 03/06/2004 23 Ansell Road Wrexham Clwyd LL13 9NQ **Tel:** (01978) 365791 w 6290204

PINSARD Lyndsay Jane (see MARTIN, Mrs)

PIPE Helen-Marie 22/03/2004 Paws in Daws PO Box 149 EDENBRIDGE Kent TN8 9AY w 6248767

PIPER Anastasia Christina 07/12/2009 Wolverton Woodlands Lane Windlesham GU20 6AQ **Tel:** 07876450326 w 6452025

Donna (nee Stallworthy) 05/09/2003 3 Acre Lane Carshalton Surrey SM5 3AA **Tel:** (0208) 7734369 w 6256335

PIQUE Rachel Louise (see RUSSELL, Mrs)

PIRIE Rachel Claire (see NOCK, Mrs)

PIRNIE Claire Anne (see JONES, Miss)

PITCHER Sarah Michelle 29/01/2010 85 Lord Street DUKINFIELD Cheshire SK16 5JP **Tel:** 07879645358 w 6499710

PITT Mandy Jane 03/09/2004 150 Kingston Road Epsom Surrey KT17 2ET **Tel:** (020) 8393 6049 w 6291788

PITTOCK Victoria Lorraine 28/09/2005 9 Meadow Road Rettendon Common CHELMSFORD Essex CM3 8DT w 6296958

PITTS Celia Marie (nee Bragg) 29/01/2001 40 Station Road Horrabridge Yelverton Devon PL20 7SS **Tel:** (01822) 854255 w 6211411

Natalie Denise 08/01/2008 28 Graham Road Paignton Devon TQ3 1BB **Tel:** (01803) 403131 w 6374112

Nikki Louise Ann 17/01/2008 (17/10/2007) The Animal Hospital Stinchcombe Dursley Gloucestershire GL11 6AJ **Tel:** (01453) 542092 w 6402712

PLANT Tracey Jane 17/08/1990 5 Gordon Avenue Woodston Peterborough PE2 9HS **Tel:** (01733) 311 992 w 6075285

PLATE Rachel Mary (nee White) 19/04/2005 5 High Street Sixpenny Handley SALISBURY SP5 5NR **Tel:** (01725) 552548 w 6314734

PLATT Jacqueline Audrey (formerly White) 06/09/1977 (24/07/2000) 2 Lentran Farm Cottages Lentran INVERNESS IV3 8RL w 6063611

PLAYER Lauren Tanya 04/10/2005 13 Chelmer Road CHELMSFORD Essex CM2 6HN w 6328253

PLAYFOOT Helen Ruth (nee Bowater) 31/01/2000 131 Conway Road SALE Cheshire M33 2TL w 6097742

PLENGE Sasha Kimberly 10/09/2009 56 Coolinge Lane FOLKESTONE Kent CT20 3QE w 6460836

PLIMMER Cheryl Louise (nee Bedford) 25/03/2002 (01/12/2008) 24 Regent Drive Tividale OLDBURY West Midlands B69 1TH **Tel:** (0121533) 0758 w 6270888

PLOWRIGHT Alison Louise 05/04/2005 96 Main Road Barnstone Nottingham Nottinghamshire NG13 9JP w 6304856

PLUMMER Laura Marie 06/05/2009 Davies Veterinary Specialists Manor Farm Business Park Higham Gobion Hertfordshire SG5 3HR **Tel:** (01582) 883950 w 6452784

PLUMRIDGE Rebecca Jayne 06/02/2008 (11/01/2010) 2 The Hig Shrewsbury Shropshire SY1 4TH **Tel:** (01743) 442827 w 6374761

POCKLINGTON Claire Louise (nee Lowton) 28/01/1999 298 The Green Eccleston Chorley Lancashire PR7 5TP **Tel:** (01257) 450156 w 6141385

POCOCK Cheryl Maxine 22/02/2000 Coombefield Veterinary Hospital Coombe Lane Axminster Devon EX13 5AX **Tel:** (01297) 630500 w 6139365

Victoria Samantha 10/04/2003 3 Dunmow Road Hatfield Broad Oak Bishop's Stortford Hertfordshire CM22 7JJ **Tel:** (01992) 575790 w 6276333

PODMORE Julie Ann 27/02/2007 72 Chesterfield Road Wirral Merseyside CH62 8ER **Tel:** (0151) 3276960 w 6358503

POFF Eleanor Joanne 05/07/2006 6 Stowe Road SLOUGH Berkshire SL1 5QF w 6302601

POINTER Sarah 21/07/2008 6 Broxell Close Wedgnock Industrial Estate Warwick CV34 5QF **Tel:** (01926) 400255 w 6415758

POINTON Eleanor Margaret (see BURDGE, Mrs)

POLLARD Emma Lorraine 14/05/2007 89 Clonners Field Stapeley Nantwich Cheshire CW5 7GU **Tel:** (01270) 624530 w 6373320

Rebecca Jane 16/12/2005 9 Chervil Way Great Cambourne CAMBRIDGE CB23 6BA w 6301721

POLLEY Leanne Michelle 22/01/2001 (18/02/2008) The Veterinary Practice Millennium Way Braintree Essex CM7 3GX **Tel:** (01376) 325511 w 6203678

POLLOCK Elaine Marie (nee Lonsdale) 29/12/2003 Grange Vets Victoria Road Darlington County Durham DL1 5SJ **Tel:** (01325) 465371 w 6204635

Hannah (nee Guild) 30/10/2003 1 Rushfield Bungalows High Bar Lane Thakeham PULBOROUGH West Sussex RH20 3EH **Tel:** (01798) 817497 w 6293284

Jacqueline Ann DipAVN(Surgical) 26/01/1998 63 Wilkinson Drive Heritage Gardens Bersham Wrexham Clwyd LL14 4FD w 611644X

POMEROY Anna 10/01/2007 1 Catlings Cottages Sutton Road Four Gotes Tydd WISBECH Cambridgeshire PE13 5PH **Tel:** (01945) 420458 w 6325195

POOK Sharon Margaret (see HARLEY, Mrs)

POOL Cristina Terese 03/03/2005 Clee Veterinary Centre 441-445 Cleethorpe Road Grimsby N.E. Lincs DN31 3BY **Tel:** (01472) 357430 w 6319233

POOLE Laura Helen 01/04/2003 (04/03/2005) 1-5 Hugh Street London SW1V 1QQ **Tel:** (020) 7932 2370 w 6271163

POOLER Rebecca Clare 25/08/1999 204 Bushbury Road Fallings Park Wolverhampton WV10 0NB **Tel:** (01902) 731127 w 614167X

POPE Alison Rachel (see THWAITES, Mrs)

POPE Amber Louise 02/03/2007 216 Lowestoft Road Gorleston Great Yarmouth Norfolk NR31 6JQ **Tel:** (01493) 602 291 w 6371714

Laura Amy 23/07/2009 29 Hatherleigh Road ABERGAVENNY Gwent NP7 7RG **Tel:** (01873) 851426 w 6375597

Lynsey (nee Pope, formerly Turner) 27/02/2002 (20/12/2006) Karma Annexe of the Surfer Green Lane Portreath REDRUTH Cornwall TR16 4NX **Tel:** (01209) 613701 w 6254817

Michelle Louise 21/11/2005 4 Myrtle Terrace TAYPORT Fife DD6 9AQ **Tel:** (07787) 706105 w 6347657

PORT Sharon (see PEAK, Mrs)

PORTER Angela (nee Day) 25/09/1990 (26/06/2001) 114 Kingston Avenue Perdiswell WORCESTER WR3 8PP **Tel:** (01905) 759099 w 6048932

Angela (nee Willaims) 20/01/1997 Bowbridge Surgery Bowbridge Stroud Gloucestershire GL5 2LA **Tel:** (01453) 762350 w 6035107

Jennifer Anne 20/04/2005 35 The Belfry Luton Bedfordshire LU2 7GA **Tel:** (01582) 391629 w 6316461

Jolene Sheila 05/04/2006 12 St. Annes Drive Aylestone LEICESTER LE2 8HT **Tel:** (0116) 2833026 w 6340441

Lisa-Marie 15/10/2009 47 St Dunstans Close Hayes Middlesex UB3 4LU **Tel:** (0208) 561 4698 w 6402162

Natalie Kara 24/11/2008 20 Torland Road Plymouth Devon PL3 5TS **Tel:** 01752787838 w 6410962

Tracey Jane 23/10/2001 (08/05/2003) Heathlands Veterinary Hospital Dorchester Road Winfrith DORCHESTER Dorset DT2 8DD **Tel:** (01929) 462535 w 6271812

PORTMANN Lisa Joanne (nee Reedman) 30/05/2006 Riverside Veterinary Clinic 17 Severnside South Bewdley Worcestershire DY12 2DX **Tel:** (01299) 402960 w 6305890

PORTWAY Stephanie Diane (formerly Tarcsi-Hawkins) 19/02/2001 118 Llangewydd Road BRIDGEND Mid Glamorgan CF31 4JX **Tel:** (07881) 588375 w 6143804

POSNER Samantha Rebecca (nee Davis) 01/08/1988 1 Dean field Bovingdon Hemel Hempstead Hertfordshire HP3 0EW **Tel:** (01442) 832455 w 6058984

POTT Virginia Mabel 09/04/1979 Woodhouse Farm Dalbury Lees Ashbourne Derbyshire DE6 5BS **Tel:** (01332) 824 226 w 6058995

POTTER Claire Louise (see GOUGH, Mrs)

POTTER Hayley 20/03/2008 21 Blair Walk Liverpool Merseyside L26 9XS **Tel:** (0151) 2916676 w 6387246

Julie Ann (nee Thompson) 14/09/1998 (17/06/2002) 22 Crocus Gardens New Bold St Helens Merseyside WA9 4EE w 6018952

Leanne Susan 20/03/2003 Dundas Veterinary Group 99 Dundas Street Edinburgh EH3 6SD **Tel:** (0131) 557 1819 w 6282273

POULTER Clair Marie (see NELSON, Mrs)

POULTER Jessica Helen (see MANSON, Mrs)

POULTNEY Amy Louise 08/07/2003 468 Street Lane Moortown Leeds West Yorkshire LS17 6HA **Tel:** (0113) 236 9030 w 6273715

POULTON Amy Marie 28/11/2008 15 Mitchell Road Havant Hampshire PO9 3QA **Tel:** 02392454602 w 6420785

POULTON Samantha Leigh (see MASSEY, Mrs)

POUND Laura Jane 18/10/2005 7 Orchard Avenue Sonning Common Reading Berkshire RG4 9LT **Tel:** (01189) 722606 w 6301732

Natasha 08/07/2004 10a Courtland Gardens Southampton Hampshire SO16 3PP **Tel:** (023) 8067 6159 w 6369591

POUNTAIN Danielle Michelle 23/07/2007 (12/03/2009) 159 Belt Road Hednesford CANNOCK Staffordshire WS12 4JB **Tel:** (01543) 879 343 w 6292404

POWELL Bethan Sian 30/05/2007 Dan y Deri Pennorth Brecon Powys LD3 7EJ **Tel:** (01874) 658338 w 6351408

Clare Louise 06/12/2004 122 Bedford Road Wootton Bedford Bedfordshire MK43 9JB **Tel:** (01234) 768 400 w 6312072

Lisa Suzanne (nee Powell) 03/09/1999 Shipley Veterinary Centre 91-93 Manor Lane Shipley West Yorkshire BD18 3BS **Tel:** (01274) 531010 w 6143917

POWELL Sharon Jane (see COLING, Mrs)

POWELL-PALMER Kirsty-Jane Charlotte 01/06/2007 Inside Pets at Home, Unit 8 Westmorland Retail Park Cramlington Tyne & Wear NE23 6UY **Tel:** (01670) 715220 w 6349274

POWER Haili Jodi 18/10/2006 5 The Fairstead HOLT Norfolk NR25 6JE **Tel:** (01263) 713 962 w 6330783

POWIS Caroline Angela 06/03/2006 Sabrina 11 Temeside Estate Ludlow Shropshire SY8 1JR w 6349131

POWLES Carolyn Sarah (nee Jasper) 17/08/1992 (15/11/2007) 25 Longleat Road Holcombe RADSTOCK Somerset BA3 5DY w 6007871

POWRIE Laura Jane (see SIMMS, Mrs)

POYSER Carolyn Jane 02/03/2001 11 Sterling Close Worksop Nottinghamshire S81 7NT **Tel:** (01909) 506396 w 6213534

PRANGLEY Rebecca Anne (see MALLARD, Mrs)

PRATT Emma Louise Grace 07/12/2009 Acorn House Veterinary Surgery Linnet Way Bedford MK41 7HN **Tel:** (01234) 261839 w 6449649

Phyllis Jacqueline 12/04/2002 13 Ansdell Grove Marshside Southport Merseyside PR9 9UQ **Tel:** (01704) 229018 w 6274188

Rebecca Jayne 01/09/2008 57 Foxcote Close REDDITCH Worcestershire B98 0PS w 6435778

PRECEY Victoria Emma Louise 17/01/2007 Blue Cross Animals Hospital Argyle Place London W6 0RQ **Tel:** (020) 8748 5150 w 6357458

PRECIOUS Katherine Louise (nee Precious) 09/09/2009 62 Crossways York North Yorkshire YO10 5JQ **Tel:** (07949) 706150 w 6402503

PREECE Anna Margaret Rose 21/04/2009 17 Liswerry Road Newport Gwent NP19 4LB **Tel:** 07932999410 w 6438627

Victoria Elizabeth 12/05/2004 RSPCA Merthyr Tydfil Animal Clinic Abercanaid Industrial Estate Merthyr Tydfil Mid Glamorgan CF48 1YF w 6291007

PREJAC Emily Ruth 26/07/2006 19 Long Meadow Houghton Regis DUNSTABLE Bedfordshire LU5 5RR **Tel:** (01582) 863909 w 6330794

PRENTICE Helen Pritchard (nee Hughes) 06/04/1995 (24/02/2009) 3 Meadow Close Compton Newbury Berkshire RG20 6QQ **Tel:** (01635) 579189 w 6087723

PRESSNELL Kim Lisa 22/09/2008 8 Reading Road DOVER Kent CT17 9NA **Tel:** (01304) 226521 w 6344269

PRESTIDGE Sarah Joy (nee Saville) 30/01/2001 (26/05/2006) 23 Flockton Road Sheffield South Yorkshire S13 9QT **Tel:** (0114) 281 0747 w 6211587

PRESTON Gemma Louise 09/11/2005 28 Kirkstall Drive Barnoldswick Lancashire BB18 6EZ **Tel:** (01282) 421215 w 6284847

Rosalin 02/09/1994 (04/03/2005) 7 Sandpits Road Richmond Surrey TW10 7DU **Tel:** (07973) 338 773 w 6032070

Victoria Sandra 03/04/2008 9 Bridge Road Brompton on Swale RICHMOND North Yorkshire DL10 7HW **Tel:** (01748) 818289 w 6357810

PRETTY Sarah Joanne 09/07/2007 41 First Avenue DURSLEY Gloucestershire GL11 4NW w 6352629

PRICE Elizabeth Sarah 10/01/2007 Abbey Veterinary Centre St Arvans Chambers Hereford Road Abergavenny Monmouthshire NP7 5PR **Tel:** (01873) 852391 w 6331212

Helen Mary 22/02/2007 55 Balfour Road BRIGHTON BN1 6ND w 6378457

Joanne Elizabeth 19/01/2000 20 Lansdowne Way HIGH WYCOMBE Buckinghamshire HP11 1TR **Tel:** (01494) 523541 w 6190148

Julie Ann 24/05/2006 Keeper's Cottage Cwmifor LLANDEILO Carmarthenshire SA19 7AS w 6354730

Kellie 10/10/2000 Barrow Hill House Maidstone Rd Ashford Kent TN24 8TY **Tel:** (01233) 624687 w 6204107

PRICE Maria Louise (see GARDINER, Mrs)

Sarah Jane 23/03/2006 Seadown Veterinary Hospital Frost Lane Hythe Southampton Hampshire SO45 3NG **Tel:** (023) 8084 2237 w 6344280

PRICE Sarah-Jane (see KENWRIGHT, Mrs)

Zoe Louise 25/09/2008 1 Ripple Lodge 16 Lower Howsell Road MALVERN Worcestershire WR14 1EF **Tel:** (01684) 572420 w 6421247

PRIDDLE Lucy 08/08/2005 4 Plemont Close Poole Dorset BH12 4JP **Tel:** 07855019512 w 6329122

PRIEST Miranda Grace 04/01/2006 (31/01/2008) 75 Hellis Wartha HELSTON Cornwall TR13 8WE **Tel:** (07900) 891742 w 6352717

Natalie Jayne 21/02/2000 134 Collis Street Amblecote STOURBRIDGE West Midlands DY8 4EE w 6112875

PRIESTLEY Emma Jane 18/09/1996 Cheadle Hulme Veterinary Hospital 2-4 Queens Road Cheadle Hulme Cheshire SK8 5LU **Tel:** (0161) 485 8444 w 6098633

Victoria Louise (nee Waddoups) 23/08/2000 (11/08/2006) Newnham Court Veterinary Group Bearsted Road Weavering Maidstone Kent ME14 5EL **Tel:** (01622) 734555 w 6184703

PRIESTMAN Carly 17/07/2003 (30/06/2008) Flat 3 Glendale Court King Street Lane Winnersh WOKINGHAM Berkshire RG41 5PW w 6265223

PRINCE Michelle Julie (nee Pearce) 06/06/2008 12 Sunadale Close Deane BOLTON BL3 5RS **Tel:** (01204) 660 540 w 6355280

PRINGLE Shona Elizabeth Thresa 15/09/2009 25 Lime Street Blaydon-on-Tyne Tyne and Wear NE21 5HW **Tel:** ((0191)422) 1652 w 6412414

PRIOR Emily Sian 31/10/2007 Trotters Farm Southend Road Great Wakering SOUTHEND-ON-SEA SS3 0PU **Tel:** (01702) 587183 w 6344291

Emma Claire 18/09/2007 190 Elmsleigh Drive Leigh-on-Sea Essex SS9 4JQ **Tel:** (01702) 475344 w 6373056

PRISK Denise Margaret DipAVN(Surgical) (formerly Bungay) 05/08/1980 Westmayne Mews 17 Martel Close Broadmayne Dorchester Dorset DT2 8PL **Tel:** (01305) 853393 w 6046731

PRITCHARD Fiona Marie 29/12/2008 Penmellyn Veterinary Group Station Road St. Columb Major Cornwall TR9 6BX **Tel:** (01637) 880307 w 6440959

Jessica Leah 15/11/1999 PDSA 1 Dulverton Road Witton Birmingham B 6 7EQ w 6145211

PRITCHARD Louise (see MORRIS, Mrs)

Valerie Anne 29/05/2008 65 Penny Hill Park PENRITH Cumbria CA11 9JW **Tel:** (01768) 865 452 w 6411050

PROBERT Helen Elizabeth 06/03/2006 49 Oakfield WOKING Surrey GU21 3QS **Tel:** (07913) 320 939 w 6419762

PROCTOR Deborah Jayne (see RODEN, Mrs)

PROCTOR Jennifer Ann 21/08/1985 83 Chestnut Drive Congleton Cheshire CW12 4UA **Tel:** (01260) 272474 w 6059139

PROTTY Susan Josephine 16/08/1982 Park Veterinary Clinic 343a Jockey Road Sutton Coldfield West Midlands B73 5XD **Tel:** (0121) 354 4949/2006 w 6059150

PROUD Christopher James 23/08/2005 Cheadle Hulme Veterinary Hospital 2-4 Queens Road Cheadle Hulme Cheshire SK8 5LU **Tel:** (0161) 485 8444 m 6298146

PROUSE Emma Louise (nee Gleave) 02/12/1992 (23/01/2006) 9 Andrew Road Tower View Barnstaple Devon EX31 3AE **Tel:** (01271) 328868 w 6044224

PROVOST Linzi Ann 17/03/2004 47 Derbyshire Avenue West Hallam Ilkeston Derbyshire DE7 6HT w 6274793

PRUDHOE Kelly Anne (nee Prudhoe) 06/09/2000 (22/08/2002) The Conifers North Street Hett DURHAM DH6 5LR **Tel:** (01388) 814419 w 6136874

PRY Bethan Mercedes 29/01/2007 Veterinary Surgery 2 Willen Road Newport Pagnell Buckinghamshire MK16 0DF **Tel:** (01908) 610982 w 6376587

PRYCE Emma 04/11/2005 2075 Paisley Road West Cardonald Glasgow G52 3JH **Tel:** (0141) 883 8118 w 6318562

PRYDE Victoria Lucia 22/09/2008 10 Roberts Road Hythe SOUTHAMPTON SO45 5DJ **Tel:** (02380) 846835 w 6379843

PUDSEY Shelley Anna 21/01/1997 44 Haven Chase Cookridge LEEDS LS16 6SG w 6096487

PUGH Emma Lisa 08/08/2005 12 Brickbarn Close BUCKLEY Clwyd CH7 2GA w 6284044

Fiona Louise 22/03/2004 Luxstowe Veterinary Centre Luxstowe Liskeard Cornwall PL14 3QF **Tel:** (01579) 342120 w 6285265

Rebecca Kate (formerly Pugu) 10/10/2005 36 Clipstone Road West Forest Town Mansfield Nottinghamshire NG19 0BU **Tel:** (01623) 643888 w 6352871

PUGU Rebecca Kate (see PUGH, Miss)

PULFORD Jane (see CLEMENTS, Ms)

PULFORD Lisa Martine 02/08/1989 (16/04/2003) Mahorall Farm Cottage Nash Ludlow Shropshire SY8 3AH **Tel:** (01584) 891 010 w 6059161

PULLAN Annette Gail (formerly Williams) 16/03/2001 11 Broadwas Close Church Hill South Redditch Worcestershire B98 8QB **Tel:** (01527) 69855 w 6137492

PULLEN Natalie Isabel (nee Walters) 15/10/2004 14c Forburg Road Stoke Newington LONDON N16 6HS w 6123752

Sophie France 18/01/1995 Austens Chitcombe Road Broad Oak Brede nr Rye East Sussex TN31 6EU **Tel:** (01424) 882243 w 6038276

PULLEYN Tracy Donna (nee Rampling) 16/07/2001 The Minster Veterinary Practice Salisbury Road York North Yorkshire YO26 4YN **Tel:** (01904) 643997 w 6226294

PUMFREY Victoria Ann 26/10/2005 Arbury Road Veterinary Surgery 32 Arbury Road Cambridge CB4 2JE **Tel:** (01223) 361911 w 6319596

PUNTON Lesley Kathleen 14/03/2006 Ramparts Veterinary Centre Windmill Way West BERWICK-UPON-TWEED TD15 1TB **Tel:** (01289) 330066 w 6348581

PURCHASE Louise Marie 23/01/2003 (04/11/2008) 16 Prestwood Gardens Chapeltown SHEFFIELD S35 1WP w 6281250

PURDIE Suzanne 06/08/2007 37 Greenock Road Largs Ayrshire KA30 8PJ **Tel:** (07833) 731404 w 6349285

PURDY Shona (nee Hoy) 17/01/1995 (29/11/2005) Glenburn Veterinary Surgery 384 Antrim Road

Glengormley Co. Antrim BT36 5EJ **Tel:** (028) 90849350 w 6035504

PURNELL Rebecca Ann 20/03/2008 2 Bridle Avenue OSSETT West Yorkshire WF5 9PS w 6387257

PURSALL Melanie Lisa 03/05/2007 Orchard House Hill Farm Lewis Road Radford Semele LEAMINGTON SPA Warwickshire CV31 1UX w 6297618

PURSSORD Teresa Jane (see LACK, Ms)

PUTTOCK Sarah Louise (see BOOTH, Mrs)

Q

QUANCE Elizabeth Ann 29/01/2007 Stable Flat Blackmore Vale Veterinary Centre Rixon Sturminster Newton Dorset DT10 1BQ **Tel:** (01258) 472293 w 6379271

QUANTRILL Josephine Anne Theresa 22/08/2000 7 Doon East Ballybunion Co Kerry IEire w 6031984

QUARTERMAINE Helen Michaela (nee Horscraft) 22/03/2004 85 Norby Estate Thirsk North Yorkshire YO7 1AH w 6261450

Samantha 09/01/2004 Fielding & Cumber Veterinary Surgeons 176-178 Chickerell Road Weymouth Dorset DT4 0QR **Tel:** (01305) 784197 w 6205823

QUELCH Pamela 09/03/2005 (15/06/2007) 36 Olivet Road Woodseats Sheffield South Yorkshire S8 8QS **Tel:** (0114) 250 7733 w 6319750

QUICK Rachel Leanne 04/10/2007 95 Mill Heath Bettws NEWPORT , Gwent NP20 7RA **Tel:** (01633) 853757 w 6391140

QUIN Susan Alice (formerly Badham) 21/09/1971 (30/07/2007) Church Farm Bungalow East Williamston Tenby Dyfed SA70 8RT **Tel:** (01834) 813158 w 604487X

QUINN Charlotte Anne 26/10/2005 25 Golden Hillock Road Dudley West Midlands DY2 0AG **Tel:** (01384) 637930 w 6334743

Kathleen Emma 15/04/2008 Stonehaven Grove Road Grove WANTAGE Oxfordshire OX12 7PD **Tel:** (07821) 431886 w 6376598

Keira Marie 13/08/2008 16 Osborne Road SOUTHPORT Merseyside PR8 2RJ **Tel:** 01704577675 w 6520577

Paula Mary (nee Muldoon) 05/03/2002 (22/08/2006) 26 Annaghmore Road Cookstown County Tyrone BT80 0JA **Tel:** (028) 867 35749 w 6273297

QUINN Sarah Rebecca (see LANE, Mrs)

QUIRK Fritha Jane (nee Morgan) 20/12/1996 27 Lammack Road BLACKBURN BB1 8JW **Tel:** (01254) 672754 w 6098531

R

RABJOHNS Jennie 03/11/1995 (12/06/2000) Meadow View Quintrell Downs Newquay Cornwall TR8 4PD **Tel:** (01637) 839027 w 6034307

RADBOURNE Lynda Yvonne (nee Sumner) 01/11/1976 (26/06/2001) Riverside Veterinary Centre Pelhams Court London Road Marlborough Wiltshire SN8 2AG **Tel:** (01672) 514875 w 6013353

Stephanie Jane 07/12/2005 Caddsdown Industrial Park Clovelly Road BIDEFORD Devon EX39 3DX **Tel:** (01237) 472075 w 6331597

RAE Jennifer Fiona 28/06/2002 36 Merkland Street Glasgow G11 6DB **Tel:** (0141) 576 0995 w 6271658

RAEBURN Gwendoline Mary Joan 24/01/2006 Little Spring Cottage Fletching Street Mayfield East Sussex TN20 6TN **Tel:** (01435) 872 554 w 6326482

RAINE-ELLERKER Helen Claire 13/10/2000 1 Honleywood Close Castle Grange Hull HU7 4ZP w 6203645

RALPH Amanda Clair 15/11/2006 16 Pierces Lane Haywards Heath West Sussex RH16 4LD w 6344720

Amy Gillian 09/09/2009 C/O Milton Keynes Veterinary Group Veterinary Hospital, Walnut tree Local Centre. Fyfield Barrow Walnut Tree MILTON KEYNES MK7 7AN **Tel:** (01908) 509500 w 6284275

RAMACHANDRA Padma 01/04/2003 The Ann Coleman Centre Ponteland Road Cowgate Newcastle upon Tyne Tyne & Wear NE5 3AL **Tel:** (0191) 214 6800 w 6284220

RAMAGE Fiona Gillian 05/04/2005 Several Farm Drummore Stranraer Wigtownshire DG9 9QW **Tel:** (01776) 840387 w 6318573

RAMAGE Kirstin Eleanor (see GOREY, Mrs)

Mary Forrest 04/11/2005 23 Drummore Avenue Carnbroe COATBRIDGE Lanarkshire ML5 4AW w 6324194

RAMBOANIAINA Phillippe 23/06/2003 14 Chalbury Close Poole Dorset BH17 8BS m 6339165

RAMCHARAN Jennifer Martha 19/03/2007 2 Glen le Side Rushton Spencer Macclesfield Cheshire SK11 0RW **Tel:** (01260) 226 467 w 6357821

RAMPLING Tracy Donna (see PULLEYN, Mrs)

RAMSAY Claire Louise 05/04/2005 11 Kimmerghame Place Edinburgh EH4 2GD w 6323446

Karen Annette 06/10/2006 East Cranberry Glengyre Leswalt STRANRAER Wigtownshire DG9 0RG w 6347239

RAMSIER Daniella Ruth 06/07/2004 15 Manilla Place WESTON-SUPER-MARE Avon BS23 2AB **Tel:** (01934) 637763 w 6300599

RAMSTER Sophie Bowden 30/11/2009 Croft End Wellington Gosforth Cumbria CA20 1BE **Tel:** (07794) 278 374 w 6489326

RAMUS Helen Marie 16/12/2005 3 New Road Forest Green DORKING Surrey RH5 5SA **Tel:** (01306) 621562 w 6327692

RANCE Emma Louise (formerly Kent) 02/11/2004 Pelyn Veterinary Group 8 Kings Avenue St. Austell Cornwall PL25 4TT **Tel:** (01726) 68177 w 6290787

Sarah Jane (nee Parkes) 11/09/1995 (21/07/2008) 7 Portchester Gardens Wakes Meadow NORTHAMPTON NN3 9UP **Tel:** (01604) 416044 w 6036960

RANDALL Rebecca Jane 04/10/2001 19 Oxford Road St. Helier Jersey JE2 4LJ **Tel:** (01534) 872456 w 6229440

RANDLES Nicola Dawn 04/11/2008 73 Sycamore Road ROCHESTER Kent ME2 2PH **Tel:** (07968) 340 968 w 6437978

RANDTOUL Louise Cora (nee Tighe) 10/02/2005 20 Sheepfold Road Guildford Surrey GU2 9TS **Tel:** (01483) 566846 w 6298201

RANGER Helen Louise (see JENKINS, Mrs)

RANKIN Julie Sarah 30/10/2007 Court Two Bronte Road WITHAM Essex CM8 2QQ **Tel:** (01376) 518105 w 6385222

Rachel Louise DipAVN(Surgical) 23/08/2000 Small Animal Teaching Hospital University of Liverpool Leahurst Campus Chester High Road Neston Merseyside CH64 7TE **Tel:** (0151) 795 6100 w 6203238

RANSOM Anne Elizabeth (see ROCK, Mrs)

RANSOME Kelly Louise 19/07/2006 2 Fir Tree Close HEMEL HEMPSTEAD Hertfordshire HP3 8NG **Tel:** (01442) 261162 w 6343180

RANSON Amanda Susan 06/03/2009 Rose Cottage 70 Alstone Lane Cheltenham Gloucestershire GL51 6HJ **Tel:** 07876345159 w 6436515

RAPLEY Jean Sheila (see MARTIN, Mrs)

RAPP Johanna Peggy Maria 16/10/2009 Three Cornered Hat Kintbury Holt NEWBURY Berkshire RG20 0HU w 6452641

RASHLEIGH Anna May 08/11/2006 Garston Veterinary Group Garston House Portway Frome Somerset BA11 1PZ **Tel:** (01373) 451115 w 6356237

RASON Leanne Carly 01/04/2003 20 Gibbons Walk Sheffield South Yorkshire S14 1BR **Tel:** (0114) 2645368 w 6283912

RATCLIFFE Diane 20/01/1999 (26/10/2000) Croft House Veterinary Clinic 378 Soothill Lane Batley West Yorkshire WF17 6EU **Tel:** (01924) 474300 w 6123388

RATTENBURY Kirstin Kathleen 10/10/2005 St Davids Veterinary Hospital St David's Station St David's Exeter Devon EX4 4NT **Tel:** (01392) 271221 w 6343191

RATTRAY Wendy Jacqueline (nee Moncrieff) 06/10/1992 105 Gairn Terrace Aberdeen AB10 6AY w 6012203

RAVEN Emma Elizabeth (nee Raven, formerly Glazebrook) 24/01/2000 Molesey Veterinary Centre 4 Park Road East Molesey Surrey KT8 9LE **Tel:** (020) 8979 1384 w 6100123

Lindsey Marie 17/09/2008 25 Bowes Road Wivenhoe COLCHESTER CO7 9RD w 6434843

RAW Catherine 27/01/1999 10 Avonpark Avonbridge Falkirk Stirlingshire FK1 2LR **Tel:** (01324) 861 063 w 6115559

RAWE Sarah Lynn 18/05/2009 171 Garron Lane SOUTH OCKENDON Essex RM15 5LA **Tel:** 01708403029 w 6440816

RAWLINGS Fiona 29/07/1986 Rock View Veterinary Surgery Tremodrett Road Roche St. Austell Cornwall PL26 8JA **Tel:** (01726) 890 887 w 6092686

RAWLINS Laurie Marie 20/11/2008 615 Wells Road Whitchurch Bristol BS14 9BE **Tel:** (01275) 832410 w 6433446

RAWLINSON Amanda Jane (nee Gibson) 19/10/2000 22 Stoney Lane Whiston Prescot Merseyside L35 2XN **Tel:** (0151) 292 3293 w 609819X

Amy Elizabeth (nee Sturgess) 31/01/2000 18 The Grove Penton Grafton Andover Hampshire SP11 0RS w 6123355

Kayleigh Victoria 11/06/2008 19 Hillhouse Road Edinburgh EH4 3QP **Tel:** (0131) 332 0458 w 6379590

Rebecca Ann 06/08/2008 41a North Street Burwell Cambridge Cambridgeshire CB5 0BA **Tel:** (07887) 854857 w 6409290

RAWNSLEY Gemma Victoria 05/01/2005 62 Anstable Road Morecambe Lancashire LA4 6TH **Tel:** (01524) 409 197 w 6292855

RAY Louise Margaret 31/01/1990 8 Flavian Court Castlefields Avenue North Runcorn Cheshire WA7 2JW **Tel:** (01928) 566076 w 6063702

RAYMOND Catherine Jane (nee Stubbington) 24/11/2009 Kingston House 83-85 Main Street Pembroke Pembrokeshire SA71 4DB **Tel:** (01646) 622943 w 6267500

Victoria Louise 16/06/2004 76 Foredrove Lane Solihull West Midlands B92 9NY **Tel:** (0121) 7113775 w 6288664

RAYNE Anna Susan 31/10/2005 Iona Wanda Chalk Lane Hyde Heath Amersham Buckinghamshire HP6 5SA **Tel:** (01494) 783362 w 6326493

RAYNER Jessica Marie 22/04/2008 30 Brora Close Bletchley Milton Keynes Buckinghamshire MK2 3HD **Tel:** (01234) 266412 w 6390161

READ Katherine Elizabeth 22/12/2004 The Flat, Beaufort Cottage Stables Hight Street Newmarket Suffolk CB8 7NN w 6297332

Samantha Jane 16/05/2006 54 Portway Baughurst Tadley Hampshire RG26 5PE **Tel:** (01189) 820204 w 6352893

Tracey Joy DipAVN(Surgical) (nee Warren) 03/08/1989 120 Oakdale WELWYN GARDEN CITY Hertfordshire AL8 7QX **Tel:** (01707) 892172 w 6063203

READER Cynthia Sze Nga 09/10/2009 Parkwood Veterinary Group 62 Hensington Road Woodstock Oxfordshire OX20 1JL **Tel:** (01993) 811355 w 6466149

READER Jenny Deborah (see LOCKE, Mrs)

Victoria Elizabeth 05/11/2008 19 Stanley Road North RAINHAM Essex RM13 8AX **Tel:** 01708520989 w 6344302

READING Georgina Wendy 04/10/2000 Milford Farm Mill Street Bakewell Derbyshire DE45 1DX **Tel:** (01629) 812035 w 6204932

READMAN Claire Marie (see FLANAGAN, Miss)

REARDON Samantha Debra 23/12/2003 76-77 Maison Dieu Road Dover Kent CT16 1RE **Tel:** (01304) 201617 w 6291931

REDBOND John Christopher James 11/05/2004 10 Allnutt Avenue Eastrop Basingstoke Hampshire RG21 4BW **Tel:** (01256) 352575 m 6290622

REDDING Katherine Sarah 25/02/2003 8 Dorset Rd Bridgewater Somerset TA6 5PP **Tel:** (01278) 459799 w 6269535

REDGE Karen Louise 24/05/2005 Quarry Veterinary Group Brassey Road off Old Potts Way Shrewsbury Shropshire SY3 7FA **Tel:** (01743) 362 556 w 6292877

REDMAN Kirsty Anne 30/01/2009 3 Selsey Avenue Southsea Hampshire PO4 9QL **Tel:** 07854126767 w 6382494

REDMOND Clare 20/11/2008 90 Moor Lane Preston Lancashire PR1 1JQ **Tel:** (01772) 254111 w 6432819

Kerry 06/08/2007 29 Dowar Road Rednal Birmingham West Midlands B45 8RB **Tel:** (0121) 453 2125 w 6373331

REECE Kate Elizabeth 22/09/2006 13 Porthycarne Street Usk Monmouthshire NP15 1RZ **Tel:** (01291) 672637 w 6307210

REED Caroline Margaret 11/12/2001 121-123 Cockfosters Road Cockfosters Barnet Hertfordshire EN4 0DA **Tel:** (020) 8275 0330 w 6258480

Elizabeth Emma 03/12/2003 Chestnut Cottage 16 Panwell Rd Bitterne Southampton Hampshire SO18 6BJ **Tel:** (02380) 433978 w 6281910

Emma Angela (nee Kelly) 31/10/2005 Flat 11 Gainsborough Court Nether Street LONDON N12 8AE w 6343125

Heather Frances 13/08/2004 49 Hazel End Farnham BISHOP'S STORTFORD Hertfordshire CM23 1HG w 6290864

Juliette Edna 18/01/2002 Jamacia House 9 The Crescent Bucklow Hill KNUTSFORD Cheshire WA16 6RQ w 6251704

REED Kay (see SANDERSON, Mrs)

Kelly (nee Boyle) 07/12/2005 (17/09/2009) 4 Adam Close REDCAR Cleveland TS10 4QJ **Tel:** (01642) 477954 w 6346436

Kimberley 16/07/2007 (21/01/2010) Felsenham Main Street Hanworth Middlesex TW13 6SU **Tel:** (020) 8898 0233 w 6301303

Robyn Alice Grace 06/02/2009 13 Farm Avenue Horsham West Sussex RH12 2JY **Tel:** 01403258143 w 6420873

Sallyann (formerly Moulton, nee Moulton) 03/11/2000 25 Bath Crescent Wyton on the Hill Huntingdon Cambridgeshire PE28 2EH w 6205735

Sarah Alison 03/02/2010 2 St. Marys Park Jordanston Milford Haven Dyfed SA73 1HR w 6412755

REEDER Caroline Sophie (nee Deane) 17/02/2000 Stonehenge Veterinary Hospital Larkhill Road Durrington Salisbury Wiltshire SP4 8DP **Tel:** (01980) 654404 w 6191061

REEDMAN Lisa Joanne (see PORTMANN, Mrs)

REENE Clare 29/01/2010 58 Risborough Lane FOLKESTONE Kent CT20 3JT **Tel:** 07739813976 w 6439628

REES Bethan Margaret 05/07/2006 48 The Drive NORTHWOOD Middlesex HA6 1HP **Tel:** (01923) 822004 w 6322005

REES Catherine Amy (see FRASER, Mrs)

Cerys Ann 29/04/2009 Medelfyw Farm Felinfoel Llanelli Dyfed SA14 8NX **Tel:** 01554772844 w 6443764

Michelle Melanie DipAVN(Surgical) 14/09/1989 6 Hareslade Bishopston Swansea SA3 3DU **Tel:** (01792) 234714 w 6059489

Rachel Louise 09/07/2007 The Croeso Veterinary Hospital Ltd 111 Whitchurch Road Cardiff CF14 3JQ **Tel:** (029) 2061 9899 w 6352684

REEVE Suzanne Catherine 29/04/2008 20 Egerton Park Worsley Manchester Lancashire M28 2TR **Tel:** (0161) 9508795 w 6358855

REEVES Michele Diane 27/02/2006 (18/02/2008) Upper Lodge Moredon North Curry TAUNTON Somerset TA3 6HW **Tel:** (01823) 490699 w 6346590

REID Amy Louise (nee Ayre) 11/11/2007 12 Farne Court Ingleby Barwick Stockton-on-Tees Cleveland TS17 0XS **Tel:** (01642) 764869 w 6397817

REID Emma Jane (see PALFREY, Mrs)

Fiona Margaret 10/12/2002 77 Windsor Road Falkirk Stirlingshire FK1 5HB **Tel:** (01324) 883983 w 6282317

Gemma Stephens 07/02/1996 (31/03/2000) Lanwades Park Kentford Newmarket Suffolk CB8 7UU **Tel:** (01638) 552700 w 6043016

REID Julie (see IZARD, Mrs)

Kathryn Elizabeth 13/05/2003 2 Hibbert Street New Mills High Peak Derbyshire SK22 3JJ **Tel:** (01663) 745294 w 6280997

Krisia Elizabeth (nee Jones) 23/12/2003 (26/02/2008) 7 Priory Lane Freefolk WHITCHURCH Hampshire RG28 7NJ **Tel:** (01256) 895930 w 6287300

Lauren (nee Agnew) 10/04/2007 Toachim House Veterinary Surgery Toachim House South Road Faversham Kent ME13 7LR **Tel:** (01795) 531313 w 6338978

Melissa Karen 14/08/2008 15 Faulkner Avenue Laurencekirk Kincardineshire AB30 1GU **Tel:** 01561376290 w 6380349

Selina May 03/12/2003 115 Walker Gardens Hedge End SOUTHAMPTON SO30 2AJ **Tel:** (01489) 692 509 w 6285848

REID-CROUCHER Tristan Mark (formerly Croucher) 24/02/2004 (26/11/2008) 11 Moyes Close Cliffsend RAMSGATE Kent CT12 5HB m 6287982

REILLY Christina Mary 01/09/1997 21 Juniper Close Oxted Surrey RH8 0RX w 6041132

Claire Louise 21/07/2008 20 Gordon Avenue SHOREHAM-BY-SEA West Sussex BN43 6WH w 6406551

Laura Kate 01/02/2010 Meridian Veterinary Practice Ltd 11 Edith Avenue Peacehaven East Sussex BN10 8JB **Tel:** (01273) 585386 w 6494309

REILLY Leeann (see JAMIESON, Mrs)

REIS Vicky 21/03/2001 Greyfriars Farm Hogs Back Guildford Surrey GU3 1AG **Tel:** (01483) 811007 w 6214282

REMBLANCE Stacey Marie 03/09/2009 88 Beccles Road Bungay NR35 1JA **Tel:** 01986896685 w 6452014

RENDELL Michelle DipAVN(Medical) 12/01/2001 76 Chipponds Drive ST. AUSTELL Cornwall PL25 5DE w 6204668

RENGERT Alison 24/06/1999 (08/05/2003) West Double Lodge The Avenue Exton Oakham Rutland LE15 8AH w 6137696

RENNIE Marie Therese Margaret 30/04/2009 15 Shrewsbury Road Beckenham Kent BR3 4DB **Tel:** (020) 8658 4829 w 6372957

RENSHAW Amanda Jane (nee Hatton) 15/12/2004 Veterinary Health Centre Ltd 4 Greeways Lytham St. Annes Lancashire FY8 3LY **Tel:** (01253) 729309 w 6298058

Sharon 16/03/2001 (31/07/2009) 10 Kerrison Close Lidlington BEDFORD MK43 0UW **Tel:** (01525) 403453 w 6214183

RENWICK Clare Emily 11/10/2004 (30/01/2007) 18 Station Mount Bramley Leeds West Yorkshire LS13 3QE **Tel:** (0113) 2575726 w 6299620

Gemma Louise 16/02/2009 106 Dunvegan Drive Southampton Hampshire SO16 8DD **Tel:** 02380734398 w 6412821

Lesley Anne 27/04/2006 Hallowdean Cottage Cavers HAWICK Roxburghshire Scotland TD9 8LL **Tel:** (01450) 374998 w 6345721

RETIEF Louisa Michelle (see SMITH, Mrs)

REVELEY Ellen Elizabeth 11/04/2008 3 Pilgrim Court Pilgrim Drive Bere Alston YELVERTON Devon PL20 7HU **Tel:** (07747) 614655 w 6413393

REVELEY Rosemarie Denise (see BAIGENT, Miss)

REY Natalie Sandrine 05/10/2001 (17/07/2006) 615 Wells Road Whitchurch Bristol BS14 9BE **Tel:** (01275) 832410 w 6229693

REYNOLDS Catherine Carmel 16/12/2005 32 Caxton Road Otley West Yorkshire LS21 3LL **Tel:** (01943) 830748 w 6287322

Heli Lenita 05/10/2009 Peak House Hawksdown Walmer DEAL Kent CT14 7PL w 6440398

Joanna Ellen (nee Morwood) 08/09/2005 82 Spenser Road Bedford Bedfordshire MK40 2BB **Tel:** (01234) 317376 w 6259041

Jodie Marie 15/10/2004 Greenbanks 26a Market Street Dalton-in-Furness Cumbria LA15 8AA **Tel:** (01229) 466295 w 6320168

Kelly Ann 11/07/2007 194 Newington Avenue Southend-on-Sea Essex SS2 4SE **Tel:** (01702) 312760 w 6297640

Kirsty Jane 02/09/2008 24 Anson Drive St. Ives Cambridgeshire PE27 3UZ **Tel:** 01480468994 w 6434821

Linda Jean (nee Williams) 15/01/1998 (09/01/2006) Hawks Nest Farm Moor Lane Whiteparish Salisbury Wiltshire SP5 2QL w 6129798

Sarah-Jane (nee Albrighton) 26/08/1999 Warwickshire College Moreton Morrell Warwick Warwickshire CV35 9BL **Tel:** (01926) 318000 w 6116778

RHODES Christine June 25/01/1995 51 Priory Lane Penwortham Preston PR1 0AS **Tel:** (01772) 465509 w 6037013

RHODES Joanna Elizabeth (see CLUE, Miss)

Kylie Louise 09/02/2009 101 Oak Road Oldham Lancashire OL8 3UL **Tel:** 07810805346 w 6433413

RHODIE Wendy 01/09/2000 25 Milne Crescent Cowdenbeath Fife KY4 9LA **Tel:** (01383) 512691 w 6134436

RICE Catherine Martha (nee Smith) 07/06/2005 6 Windmill Crescent BALLYNAHINCH County Down BT24 8EZ w 6332653

Joanne (nee Holloway) 24/08/1995 (12/11/2001) Bishops Stortford Veterinary Hospital Rye Street Bishop's Stortford Hertfordshire CM23 2HA **Tel:** (01279) 654108 w 6031689

Kathryn Emma 03/06/2004 59 Sidney Road Southport Lancashire PR9 7EX **Tel:** (01704) 212338 w 6293988

RICE Natasha (see BADGER, Mrs)

RICHARDS Amber 08/09/2009 65 Turpins Avenue Holland-on-Sea Essex CO15 5HF **Tel:** (01255) 814261 w 6308266

RICHARDS Anne Louise (see BOUNDS, Mrs)

Beveley Michelle 15/10/2004 Hillside Veterinary Centre 146 Crewe Road Nantwich Cheshire CW5 6NB **Tel:** (01270) 625310 w 6291942

Claire 06/10/2006 5 Greenlees Drive Plymouth Devon PL7 1YW **Tel:** (01752) 347 198 w 6357095

RICHARDS Claire Elizabeth (see KENT, Mrs)

Katy Elizabeth 23/07/2007 Flat 3 67 Highbury Park LONDON N5 1UA w 6381460

Laura Gillian (nee Payne) 03/09/2002 7 Epsom Close Trelai Park Cardiff CF5 5BG **Tel:** (029) 20382211 w 6259063

Lisa Jacqueline 09/09/2004 Maes Glas Veterinary Group Church Acre Brackla Bridgend Mid Glamorgan CF31 2JT **Tel:** (01656) 652 751 w 6250131

Sarah Louise 09/10/2008 55 Trasnagh Drive Newtownards County Down BT23 4PD **Tel:** 02891826982 w 6389886

Zoe Danielle 16/06/2008 North Hall Iddesleigh WINKLEIGH Devon EX19 8BN **Tel:** (01805) 804 695 w 6380855

RICHARDSON Alison Jane (nee Stacey) 19/03/2007 22 Hipkiss Gardens Droitwich Worcestershire WR9 9AT **Tel:** (01905) 827485 w 6328297

Barbara Olivia 04/11/2005 1 Court Farm Road Longwell Green Bristol BS30 9AA **Tel:** (0117) 932 3660 w 6326504

Deborah Jayne 28/08/1996 (21/07/1999) 36 Hunters Way SLOUGH SL1 5UB **Tel:** (01753) 524055 w 6040117

Jamie Louise 09/06/2009 Plane Trees Cottage Plane Trees Wainstalls Halifax West Yorkshire HX2 7UF **Tel:** 01422245030 w 6444314

RICHARDSON Joanne Elizabeth (see MASON, Mrs)

Joanne Marie 08/04/2009 17 Capesthorne Road Wistaston CREWE CW2 8PA w 6439518

Karen Ann 30/10/2001 Caldew Veterinary Hospital Carlisle House Townhead Road Dalston Carlisle Cumbria CA5 7JF **Tel:** (01228) 710208 w 6262660

Karen Jane (formerly Richardson) 29/07/1975 (22/01/2007) High Butterby Farm Shincliffe Durham Co Durham DH1 2TJ **Tel:** (0191) 384 3626 w 6059671

Katharine Louise 05/10/2001 25 Halleys Ridge Hertford Hertfordshire SG14 2TQ **Tel:** (01992) 300798 w 6229627

RICHARDSON Katie Jane (see DINGLE, Mrs)

RICHARDSON Leanne (see DAVIES, Mrs)

Lorna Agnes 21/05/2007 10 House O'Hill Row Blackhall EDINBURGH EH4 2AW **Tel:** (07717) 824186 w 6324656

Michelle Danielle 11/11/2004 48 Northampton Road Market Harborough Leicestershire LE16 9HE **Tel:** (01858) 465668 w 6325052

Michelle Elizabeth 16/08/1988 (16/05/2003) 35 Horsley Hill Road South Shields Tyne and Wear NE33 3ER **Tel:** (0191) 4546542 w 6059660

RICHARDSON Rebecca Alison (see DALE, Mrs)

Samantha Jayne 19/09/2006 9 Stearne Close THETFORD Norfolk IP24 3JF **Tel:** (01842) 751190 w 6329078

Simone Renate 11/11/2008 5 Brierley Close Howden Goole North Humberside DN14 7JB **Tel:** (01430) 431758 w 6433347

RICHENS Jayne Louise (see IGLESIAS, Mrs)

RICHES Hannah Elizabeth (see YOUNG, Mrs)

RICHES Julie Louise (see RICHES-TOMEI, Mrs)

RICHES-TOMEI Julie Louise DipAVN(Medical) (nee Riches) 22/03/1994 (01/03/2007) Davies Veterinary Specialists Manor Farm Business Park Higham Gobion Hertfordshire SG5 3HR **Tel:** (01582) 883950 w 6027901

RICHINGS Dawn Gillian 28/02/2007 T/A Dragon Veterinary Centre Prestbury Park New Barn Lane Cheltenham Gloucestershire GL50 4SH **Tel:** (01242) 580 324 w 6320179

Kay Evelyn 07/11/2008 54 Greet Road Winchcombe Cheltenham Gloucestershire GL54 5JT **Tel:** 07980207693 w 6436361

RICHMOND Jo Clare (see IRESON, Mrs)

RICHMOND Michelle Linda DipAVN(Medical), DipAVN(Surgical) (nee Hales) 16/01/1995 2 Island View Manchester Road Sway Lymington Hampshire SO41 6AS **Tel:** (01590) 682183 w 6032831

RICKARDS Emma Fiona (see RICKARDS-TILLEY, Mrs)

RICKARDS Hannah Louise 18/05/2009 117 Queensfield Upper Stratton Swindon Wiltshire SN2 7SU **Tel:** 01793723772 w 6379931

RICKARDS-TILLEY Emma Fiona (nee Rickards) 27/08/1996 Fairfield House Broomfield Bridgwater Somerset TA5 2EQ **Tel:** (01823) 451731 w 6075999

RICKETT Sally Claire 24/01/2005 Luxstowe Veterinary Centre Luxstowe Liskeard Cornwall PL14 3QF **Tel:** (01579) 342120 w 6291953

RICKETTS Sarah Louise 02/12/2009 9 Coriander Close Stoke Prior BROMSGROVE Worcestershire B60 4ES w 6495717

RICKHUSS Lauren 15/04/2004 86 Coedriglan Drive CARDIFF CF5 4UQ **Tel:** (029) 206 53514 w 6265619

RICKMAN Faye Natasha 09/11/2005 89-93 Park Road Peterborough Cambridgeshire PE1 2TR **Tel:** (01733) 554953 w 6354741

RICKNER Natalie 11/01/2008 Ground Floor Flat 31 Azof Street LONDON SE10 0EG w 6375619

RICKS Amy Elizabeth 17/05/2005 Fernlea Veterinary Clinic Blackhorse Road Kingswood Bristol BS15 8DZ **Tel:** (0117) 960 6145 w 6264024

RIDDELL Jacqueline Margaret (nee Cunningham) 31/08/1999 29 Main Street Kirkliston West Lothian EH29 9AE **Tel:** (0131) 333 3203 w 6143928

RIDGE Tanzi Louise (nee Robinson, nee Dixon) 12/02/1996 Forge Cottage Lower Ashton EXETER EX6 7QN **Tel:** (01647) 253442 w 6043887

RIDGWAY Jane Ann (formerly Scholes) 18/01/1999 8 Arundel Walk Bircotes DONCASTER South Yorkshire DN11 8QZ w 6116472

RIDING Holly Marie 27/11/2009 Close Farm Tockholes Darwen BB3 0LU w 6466688

Katherine Elizabeth (formerly Salisbury, nee Harrison) 14/03/2006 24 Willowfield Road Heysham Morecambe Lancashire LA3 2HF **Tel:** (01524) 852 079 w 6353157

RIDLER Julie Anne 30/03/2006 The Animal Hospital Stinchcombe Dursley Gloucestershire GL11 6AJ **Tel:** (01453) 542092 w 6318870

RIDLEY Kathryn Jane 27/02/2006 14 Bishops Gate Lytham St. Annes Lancashire FY8 4FR **Tel:** (01253) 796706 w 6349769

Teresa Jayne (nee Fennell) 30/03/2006 18 Southdown Close Pembroke Dyfed SA71 5QJ **Tel:** (01646) 687 280 w 6327637

RIGBY Jennah Monique 13/03/2008 184 Brownside Road Burnley Lancashire BB10 3JW **Tel:** (01282) 436794 w 6377214

Olivia Claire 20/03/2008 110 Woodville Drive Marple STOCKPORT Cheshire SK6 7QX **Tel:** (0161) 4279387 w 6406397

RILEY Amy (nee Kemp) 22/03/2004 Northside Veterinary Clinic 1236-1238 Aldridge Road Great Barr Birmingham West Midlands B44 8PE **Tel:** (0121) 360 6010 w 6279666

Amy Laura 11/11/2008 112 Chestnut Drive Congleton Cheshire CW12 4UA **Tel:** 01260272922 w 6439540

Claire Diane 15/04/2004 22 Pine Road Stalybridge Cheshire SK15 1UR w 6262484

Donna Christinna 16/07/2009 89a Watford Way LONDON NW4 4RS **Tel:** 07955364120 w 6560595

Julie Elizabeth 27/01/2005 19 Beechwood Crescent Orrell Wigan WN5 8NL **Tel:** (01942) 621 349 w 6298740

Mary Angela (formerly Pallister) 27/07/1988 3 Grange Cottages Tockwith Road Long Marston YORK YO26 7PL w 6058248

Michaela Marie 24/11/2004 56 Manchester Road Shaw Oldham Lancashire OL2 7DE **Tel:** (01706) 840936 w 6291557

RILSTONE Marie Louise (see BIRD, Mrs)

RIMMINGTON Katie Emma (see KNIGHT, Mrs)

RING Clare Louise (nee Olds) 19/01/2005 5 Chapel Lane HAYLE Cornwall TR27 4LS **Tel:** (01736) 758422 w 6294439

RING Sian Jessica Susan (see ANDERSON, Mrs)

RINGSELL Laura (nee Ringsell) 04/10/2005 19 Heathfield Close Godalming Surrey GU7 1SL **Tel:** (01483) 421710 w 6346601

RIPPIN Helen Rhiain 22/04/2008 Flat 4 12 High Street Abergavenny Gwent NP7 5RY **Tel:** 07788825544 w 6389105

RIST Melanie Alicia 17/02/2009 2 Barley Croft Hertford Hertfordshire SG14 3LN **Tel:** 01992422712 w 6447647

RITCHIE Carole Ann 04/12/2009 2 Purr Wood Godmersham CANTERBURY Kent CT4 7DX **Tel:** (01227) 730567 w 6494111

Emma Louise 10/02/2004 (17/10/2006) 5 Badger Way HATFIELD Hertfordshire AL10 8RY w 6275266

Joanne Elizabeth 23/12/2003 26 Camberley Grove Erdington Birmingham West Midlands B23 6LQ **Tel:** (0121) 6033947 w 6267775

RITCHIE Sandra Dawn (see BANKS, Mrs)

RIVERS Zoe Carol 21/11/2005 The Veterinary Surgery Redmans Hill Blackford Wedmore Somerset BS28 4NG **Tel:** (01934) 712229 w 6351430

RIVETT Melissa (nee Bavister) 10/02/2005 Abington Park Veterinary Surgery 427 Wellingborough Road Northampton NN1 4EZ **Tel:** (01604) 628 685 w 6328396

RIXON Emma Jane 25/09/2009 50 Old Bath Road Charvil READING RG10 9QR **Tel:** (07946) 637161 w 6466831

ROACHE Fleur Louise 10/10/2005 Fenton Veterinary Practice 21 Portfield Haverfordwest Pembrokeshire SA61 1BN **Tel:** (01437) 762806 w 6327703

ROBB Fiona Margaret (nee McKinlay) 23/08/2004 Ayrton Veterinary Centre Burnhouse Industrial Estate Whitburn West Lothian EH47 0LQ **Tel:** (01501) 744736 w 6289940

ROBB Mandy Marie (see TAMBA, Ms)

ROBBIE Emma Jane (see SILCOCK, Mrs)

ROBBINS Allison (see HODGSON, Mrs)

ROBERT Julie Fiona (formerly Oag, nee Fraser) 09/01/2009 13 Gollanfield House Gollanfield INVERNESS IV2 7QP **Tel:** (01333) 451 941 w 6299081

ROBERTS Bridget (formerly Mooney) 19/08/2008 18 Orchis Grove Badgers Dene Grays Essex RM17 5JG **Tel:** 01378406248 w 6294395

Cheryl (nee Evans) 22/07/1993 Ash Veterinary Surgery Aberdare Road Georgetown Merthyr Tydfil Mid Glamorgan CF48 1AT **Tel:** (01685) 385117 w 6066554

Claire Bettina 22/02/2007 Rose Farm Fleckney Lane Fleckney Leicester Leicestershire LE8 8AF **Tel:** (0116) 240 2610 w 6350858

Claire Elizabeth 14/08/2008 11 St. Saviours Street Talke STOKE-ON-TRENT ST7 1LR **Tel:** (01782) 773613 w 6410313

David Stephen 22/04/2002 11 Warbreck Road Orrell Park Liverpool Merseyside L9 8EE **Tel:** (0151) 525 5064 m 6265663

Deborah DipAVN(Surgical) (nee Allen) 02/09/1997 37 Wendover Drive BEDFORD MK41 9QY w 611679X

Emma Louise (nee Hart) 11/03/2009 45 Denham Close Luton Bedfordshire LU3 3TS **Tel:** 01582495031 w 6373034

ROBERTS Gail Susan (see CROSS, Mrs)

ROBERTS Jennifer Ann (see THOMPSON, Ms)

Jessica Ruth 17/11/2009 12 Ledsham Park ST. LEONARDS-ON-SEA East Sussex TN37 7LQ **Tel:** (01424) 752839 w 6459439

ROBERTS Kate (see SLACK, Mrs)

Katie Marie 18/10/2006 178 Furlong Road Goldthorpe Rotherham South Yorkshire S63 9PY **Tel:** (01709) 888092 w 6359185

Katrina 12/05/2004 (27/01/2010) 1 School Road NEATH West Glamorgan SA11 2DR **Tel:** (01639) 630460 w 6262748

Kelly Ann 13/04/2004 16 Tobermory Close Haydock ST. HELENS Merseyside WA11 0YP **Tel:** (01744) 600156 w 6302667

Kerry Anita (nee Gilkes) 14/03/2006 West Bar Veterinary Hospital 19 West Bar Street Banbury Oxfordshire OX16 9SA **Tel:** (01295) 262332/267531 w 6232949

Laura 19/09/2008 24 Rosemary Road WALSALL WS6 7DY **Tel:** 07968440728 w 6366379

Linda Jane DipAVN(Medical) 10/04/2003 Unit 6 Forest Corner Farm Hangersley Hill Hangersley RINGWOOD Hampshire BH24 3JW **Tel:** (01425) 485615 w 6287135

Lindsey Anna Jane 07/11/2008 20 Middleton Close WARMINSTER Wiltshire BA12 8JT **Tel:** (07729) 629 791 w 6400193

Lisa Michelle 14/01/2008 Boness Veterinary Enterprises Ltd 125 Bedford Road Barton le Clay Bedford Bedfordshire MK45 4LP **Tel:** (01582) 612604 w 6386564

Lynda Jo-Ann 26/02/2009 13 Almond Close Feltham Middlesex TW13 4DQ **Tel:** 02088931239 w 6416385

Maria 10/02/2009 147 White Edge Moor SWINDON SN3 6NG **Tel:** 07973791972 w 6374772

Natalie (nee Foord) 09/02/1998 (01/03/2006) The Downwood Veterinary Centre 6-8 High Street Horam Heathfield East Sussex TN21 0EJ **Tel:** (01435) 812 152 w 611273X

Nicola Claire (nee Keay) 29/05/2003 The Coach House 26a Alexandra Grove London N12 8HG **Tel:** (0208) 7234555 w 6277972

Nicola Louise 21/10/2008 30 Willement Road Faversham Kent ME13 7SZ **Tel:** (01795) 535 531 w 6436273

Pippa Louise 13/01/2004 The Animal Hospital Stinchcombe Dursley Gloucestershire GL11 6AJ **Tel:** (01453) 542092 w 6280414

Rachael Louise 13/02/2008 77 High Street Purton Swindon Wiltshire SN5 4AB **Tel:** (01793) 771869 w 6400050

Rachel Lesley 05/11/2007 29 Uphill Road South WESTON-SUPER-MARE Avon BS23 4SG **Tel:** (01934) 425750 w 6380360

Sally-Ann (nee Howe) 19/01/1995 16 Lingfield Stacey Bushes Milton Keynes MK12 6HB **Tel:** (01908) 225420 w 6032558

Sara 08/01/2008 Enchante 11 Wadham Road Liskeard Cornwall PL14 3BD **Tel:** (01579) 340127 w 6411963

Sarah Elizabeth 15/07/2005 Rivendell Waterside Baslow Derbyshire DE45 1RR **Tel:** (01246) 582444 w 6293823

ROBERTS Sarah Jane (see FARRELL, Mrs)

ROBERTS Sarah Louise May (see CLARKE, Mrs)

ROBERTS Tracy Anne (see MAYNE, Mrs)

Victoria Elizabeth 25/08/1998 (27/04/2005) 62 Graburn Road LIVERPOOL L37 3PB **Tel:** (01704) 380251 w 6118684

ROBERTS-BATES Lucy Rachel (nee Warren) 24/01/2005 4 Croft Gardens Alton Hampshire GU34 2EN **Tel:** (01420) 89302 w 6262671

ROBERTS-MORGAN Carla Jane 17/01/2006 Maes Glas Veterinary Group Church Acre Brackla Bridgend Mid Glamorgan CF31 2JT **Tel:** (01656) 652 751 w 6330805

ROBERTSON Alyson Margaret (see DOOLAN, Mrs)

ROBERTSON Julie 23/09/2002 65 Upper Bourtree Drive Rutherglen GLASGOW G73 4EY **Tel:** (0141) 631 2289 w 6260361

Justine 30/05/2003 Unit 6 Forest Corner Farm Hangersley Hill Hangersley RINGWOOD Hampshire BH24 3JW **Tel:** (01425) 485615 w 6281734

Kathryn Louise (formerly Robertson) 08/01/2004 5 Carlton Close Heanor Derbyshire DE75 7YY **Tel:** (01773) 715773 w 6291139

Sarah Jane (nee Shury) 09/09/1996 Moulton College West Street Moulton Northampton NN3 7RR **Tel:** (01604) 491131 w 6100305

ROBESON Leanne Emma (nee Holloway) 08/01/2008 106 Amington Road TAMWORTH Staffordshire B77 3PZ **Tel:** 07717246600 w 6413327

ROBINSON Alison Clare DipAVN(Surgical) (nee Mills, formerly Debnam) 28/09/1998 82 Markwell Wood Harlow Essex CM19 5QZ **Tel:** (01707) 269726 w 6137109

Amanda Jane 08/11/2006 80 Wheatsheaf Drive WARE Hertfordshire SG12 0XR **Tel:** (07957) 345439 w 6331608

Amy 11/10/2004 Old Barn Farm Lodge Lane AXMINSTER Devon EX13 5RT w 6305098

Angela Claire 07/10/2009 3 Ebnal Close LEOMINSTER Herefordshire HR6 8SL w 6435448

Annie Maja Klara 09/12/2009 7 Forstal Road Woolage Village CANTERBURY Kent CT4 6SP **Tel:** 07780642433 w 6491988

Carrie Jane 11/01/2005 399a Green Lanes LONDON N13 4TY **Tel:** (0207) 8541362 w 6329804

Christine Anne 01/08/1979 134 Sherrards Way Barnet Hertfordshire EN5 2BL **Tel:** (0208) 4413225 w 6059795

Danielle Wendy Diana 03/05/2005 9 Young Close CLACTON-ON-SEA Essex CO16 8UQ **Tel:** (01255) 432654 w 6284253

Elisa Nicole (nee Weastell) 04/11/2005 Wear Referrals 5-11 Tenters Street BISHOP AUCKLAND County Durham DL14 7AD **Tel:** (01388) 602707 w 6288235

Emily Claire 17/11/2009 73 Leamoor Avenue Somercotes ALFRETON Derbyshire DE55 1RL **Tel:** (01773) 606387 w 6423975

Emily Louise 09/09/2009 13 Prudden Close Elstow BEDFORD MK42 9EB w 6466391

Emma 01/10/2008 Pwll y Hwyaid Meifod Powys SY22 6XZ **Tel:** 01938500625 w 6378732

Emma Denise (nee Robinson) 15/02/2006 58 The Thatchers St Micheals Mead Bishops Stortford Hertfordshire CM23 4FN w 6324260

Faye 15/05/2009 7 Woodlands Drive Morley LEEDS LS27 9QZ w 6451464

Isla Dawn 15/07/2005 Cambridge Veterinary Group Ltd 89a Cherryhinton Road Cambridge Cambridgeshire CB1 7BS **Tel:** (01223) 249331 w 6296848

Jodie 15/10/2004 33 Ox Hey Drive Biddulph STOKE-ON-TRENT ST8 7EU w 6289566

Laura Janette 03/10/2008 5 Albany Road Capel-le-Ferne FOLKESTONE Kent CT18 7JT w 6437373

Lisa 16/08/1990 The Croft 46 Hook Lane Nyetimber BOGNOR REGIS West Sussex PO21 3PD w 6001552

ROBINSON Lynn (see FARRALL, Mrs)

Melissa Lois 25/09/2009 Avenue Veterinary Surgery 2/4 Park Avenue Redcar Cleveland TS10 3JZ **Tel:** (01642) 490928 w 6451838

Nicola Jayne 25/08/1994 The Vet Commercial Street Rothwell West Yorkshire LS26 0AW **Tel:** (0113) 288 7788 w 6028905

Philippa Helen 03/04/2008 35 Baxter Street Fallin STIRLING FK7 7ET w 6510435

Samantha Leigh (nee Hutton, formerly McCall) 10/04/2003 10 Drumanphy Road Portadown CRAIGAVON County Armagh BT62 1QX w 6280975

Sarah Lindsay 31/10/2003 The Veterinary Centre James Street Louth Lincolnshire LN11 0JW **Tel:** (01507) 602828 w 6291040

Sharon Anne 14/12/2006 11 Streather Drive Corby Northamptonshire NN17 1TN **Tel:** (01536) 394269 w 6284429

Sian Tracy Ann 05/09/2008 Pool House Veterinary Group Fosseway Lane Lichfield Staffordshire WS13 8JY **Tel:** (01543) 262464/ 262433 w 6404450

Sophie Ann 07/02/2006 44 Foxes Way WARWICK Warwickshire CV34 6AY w 6321224

Susan Jane DipAVN(Surgical) 28/01/1998 32 Pealsham Gardens FORDINGBRIDGE Hampshire SP6 1RD w 6041154

ROBINSON Tanzi Louise (see RIDGE, Mrs)

Verity Leejann 16/09/2004 Abbey Veterinary Group 89 Dodworth Road Barnsley South Yorkshire S70 6ED **Tel:** (01226) 242217 w 6291744

ROBOTHAM Sally Anne 24/11/2005 PDSA Petaid Hospital 200 City Gate London Road Derby DE24 8WY **Tel:** (01332) 345771 w 6333445

ROBSON Danielle 20/10/2008 29 North View Whickham NEWCASTLE UPON TYNE NE16 4AY **Tel:** 01914224518 w 6379865

ROBSON Gemma Kate (see COSGROVE, Mrs)

Laura Elizabeth 29/10/2004 13 George Place PEEBLES EH45 8DW **Tel:** 07786022415 w 6318111

ROBSON Nicola Lynne (see STAPLIN, Mrs)

ROBY Emma Jane (nee Darbyshire) 15/09/1998 (18/07/2001) 12 Vicarage Road Orrell Wigan Lancashire WN5 7AX **Tel:** (01942) 222620 w 6098098

ROCHE Rose Ann (nee Parkinson) 18/01/1995 44 Wharfedale Place HARROGATE North Yorkshire HG2 0AY w 6033460

ROCK Anne Elizabeth (nee Ransom) 13/10/2003 (02/03/2007) 5 Edgemond Avenue Erdington Birmingham B24 0QG **Tel:** (0121) 3133016 w 6260702

ROCKALL Helen 22/08/1994 (12/02/2003) Post Office Cottage South The Green Chilgrove Chichester West Sussex PO18 9HU **Tel:** (01243) 519439 w 6037476

ROCKE Hannah Catherine 01/10/2008 81 Fallindale Road BIRMINGHAM B26 3YR **Tel:** 01216054562 w 6437835

ROCKELL Claire Elisabeth 09/09/1994 (20/09/2000) 6 Steppingstone Place LEIGHTON BUZZARD Bedfordshire LU7 3PS **Tel:** 01525384019 w 6032718

RODEN Deborah Jayne (nee Cowap, formerly Proctor) 03/12/2003 29 Lower Appleton Road Widnes Cheshire WA8 6HQ w 6286959

RODGERS Kirstie Jan (see BEDINGHAM, Mrs)

RODWELL Nicola Louise 16/03/2009 23 Croft Down Road Solihull West Midlands B92 9BD **Tel:** 01212463581 w 6278049

ROE Rhiannon Myfanwy 10/12/2009 19 Audnam Wordsley Stourbridge West Midlands DY8 4AJ **Tel:** (01384) 372849 w 6492032

ROEBUCK Jane (nee Kent) 27/12/2001 Sandbed House 2 Wakefield Road Ossett West Yorkshire WF5 9JB **Tel:** (01924) 786688 w 6252188

ROGERS Amber Suzanne 08/01/2008 The Plantation Fiddlers Lane Tutbury B.O.T Staffordshire DE13 9HG **Tel:** (01283) 814557 w 6405671

ROGERS Caroline (see WAINWRIGHT, Mrs)

Claire Edel 03/12/2003 83 Broad Acres HATFIELD Hertfordshire AL10 9LE **Tel:** (01707) 257327 w 6270624

Danielle Joanne 31/08/2000 32 Harbury Close REDDITCH Worcestershire B98 0EF w 6205603

Frances Jane 16/09/2008 Uplands Way Vets Ltd Uplands Way DISS Norfolk IP22 4DF **Tel:** (01379) 642865 w 6429288

ROGERS Joanne Clare (see HIGGINS, Mrs)

Julia Michelle 03/10/2007 29 Megan Street Cwmdu SWANSEA SA5 8LE **Tel:** (01792) 522697 w 6301765

June Ann (nee Davis) 01/09/1977 7 Chestnut Walk Alresford Hampshire SO24 9NA w 6086399

ROGERS Katie (see HAYNES, Mrs)

Louise 16/06/2006 14 Newhall Road Sheffield S9 2QL **Tel:** (0114) 243 3232 w 6306385

Lucy Anne 06/12/2004 Berry House Veterinary Practice 41 Nightingale Road Hitchin Hertfordshire SG5 1RE **Tel:** (01462) 432824 w 6273275

Sarah Ann 06/03/2006 Copthorne Veterinary Clinic 114 Copthorne Road Shrewsbury Shropshire SY3 8NA **Tel:** (01743) 360614 w 6260614

Sarah Jane 28/02/2007 40 Nutfield Court Lower Brown Hill Road Maybush Southampton Hampshire SO16 9QU w 6372407

Sophie Helen 04/04/2008 46 Rosehall Close Redditch Worcestershire B98 7YD **Tel:** (01527) 853304 w 6386575

Vera Catherine (nee Deegan) 22/03/2004 Box No A4 Polonia Manitoba R0J 1R0 Canada w 6282779

ROGERS DEACON Elizabeth Anne 14/01/2000 77 Swifts Hill View Stroud Gloucestershire GL5 1PR **Tel:** (07734) 145 533 w 6129721

ROLF Joanne Theresa 09/11/2009 49 Endless Street Salisbury Wiltshire SP1 3UH **Tel:** (01722) 333 291 w 6453246

ROLFE Rachael Louise 15/07/2005 3a Victoria Road BOURNEMOUTH Dorset BH1 4RT w 6284352

Sara Louise 24/01/2006 Best Friends March 3 Upwell Road MARCH Cambridgeshire PE15 9DT **Tel:** (01354) 653435 w 6268820

Sharon 09/04/2003 26 Worcester Park Road Worcester Park Surrey KT4 0QD w 6333093

Susan Margaret 10/06/2003 10 Linden Way Common Platt Swindon Wiltshire SN5 5DE **Tel:** (01793) 882644 w 6275035

ROLFE JONES Kelly 04/11/2009 Donnington Grove Veterinary Surgery Oxford Road NEWBURY Berkshire RG14 2JB **Tel:** (01635) 47170 w 6490503

ROLLINGS Deborah Jane 02/09/1997 6 Grove Park Avenue Church Lawton Stoke-on-Trent ST7 3EZ **Tel:** (01270) 874782 w 603265X

Jodie Nadine 15/11/2006 Holmer Veterinary Surgery Roman Road Holmer Hereford HR1 1LE **Tel:** (01432) 272468 w 6367149

ROLLINS Caroline Mary (see WILLIAMS, Mrs)

ROLLINSON Alison Margaret (nee Taylor) 19/01/1998 Holden Street Clitheroe Lancashire BB7 1LU **Tel:** (01200) 423763 w 6119087

ROLLITT Claire Evelyn 08/01/2008 35 Hillington Ilfracombe Devon EX34 8LU **Tel:** (01271) 812405 w 6397795

ROLLS Natalie Jayne (formerly Stephens) 18/10/2005 Ash Veterinary Surgery Aberdare Road Georgetown Merthyr Tydfil Mid Glamorgan CF48 1AT **Tel:** (01685) 385117 w 6331630

ROLPH Alison Elizabeth 04/03/2009 Kingfisher Veterinary Practice Tower Hill Road Crewkerne Somerset TA18 8EQ **Tel:** (01460) 77790 w 6436493

RONAN Louise Jane 03/09/1996 Elms Farmhouse Grove Road Grove Wantage Oxfordshire OX12 7PD **Tel:** (01235) 770227 w 6031306

ROOBOTTOM Julie Elizabeth (nee Yates) 05/08/1987 (05/05/2005) 17 New Road Armitage Staffordshire WS15 4AA **Tel:** (01543) 491149 w 6064342

ROOKE Carolyn Mair Feirn 01/07/2003 1 Anthony Way Stallingborough GRIMSBY South Humberside DN41 8BD w 6269062

Georgina Louise 03/04/2009 Sir Harold Harmsworth Memorial Hospital 22 Sonderburg Road London N7 7QD **Tel:** (0870) 753 8081 w 6411589

ROONEY Helen Elizabeth DipAVN(Medical) (nee Crossthwaite) 12/02/1996 (16/03/2005) 10 Jepps Avenue Barton Preston Lancashire PR3 5AS w 6042373

ROPER Victoria 09/07/2007 Cherrytree House Youngwoods Way Alverstone Garden Village SANDOWN Isle of Wight PO36 0HF **Tel:** (01983) 400060 w 6352651

ROPER Zoe Louise (see ATKINSON, Mrs)

ROSA MILHEIRO Dalila 01/02/2008 The Veterinary Centre Queen Annes Road GREAT YARMOUTH Norfolk NR31 0LE **Tel:** (01493) 416700 w 6402173

ROSE Catherine Ann 09/05/2006 Flat 4 Robin Court 72 Wimborne Road BOURNEMOUTH BH3 7AS **Tel:** (01202) 513004 w 6300610

Claire Louise 21/03/2006 12 Hartley Grove Thatto Heath St. Helens Merseyside WA10 3ES **Tel:** (079) 586 13433 w 6333929

ROSE Denise Karen (see TALO, Mrs)

Jillian 15/01/1998 12 Ruskin Square Bishopbriggs Glasgow G64 1QF **Tel:** (0141) 7726801 w 6130577

Katie Elizabeth 27/02/2006 28 South Street Harborne BIRMINGHAM B17 0DB **Tel:** (0121) 427 3545 w 6328275

ROSE Lyony Julie (see WATTS, Mrs)

Nicola 24/11/2004 (05/08/2008) 35 Francis Court Silver End WITHAM Essex CM8 3QW w 6323468

ROSE Sally Elizabeth (see KERRIDGE, Mrs)

Tara Margaret 14/01/2008 Isle Small Animal Veterinary Centre West Fen Road Ely Cambridgeshire CB6 2BZ **Tel:** (01353) 658333 w 6326339

ROSIER Leanne Kimberley 07/12/2009 34 Southwood Gardens RAMSGATE Kent CT11 0BQ **Tel:** 01843596990 w 6466413

ROSS Claire Pauline 21/03/2006 Eton Veterinary Clinic 31 London Road Tonbridge Kent TN10 3AB **Tel:** (01732) 352004 w 6319618

Fiona Marie 29/06/2007 St Clair Veterinary Group 2 Pottery Street Kirkcaldy Fife KY1 3ET **Tel:** (01592) 599500 w 6333962

Gemma Ann 02/09/2008 1 The Drive Bicton East Budleigh Budleigh Salterton Devon EX9 7BH **Tel:** (01395) 568975 w 6379282

ROSS Lindsay (see ATKINSON, Mrs)

ROSS Lyndsey Margaret May (see CIARCIA, Mrs)

ROSSI Nicola Jayne 04/12/2009 Seadown Veterinary Hospital Frost Lane Hythe Southampton Hampshire SO45 3NG **Tel:** (023) 8084 2237 w 6461276

ROSTRON Elizabeth Leander (nee Hammond) 08/09/1994 7 Warwick Road South Old Trafford Manchester M16 0JW **Tel:** (0161) 881 0222 w 6033846

ROTHEN Elizabeth Anne (nee Bromell) 27/08/2004 Rosehill Farm Quarry Lane Mancetter Atherstone Warwickshire CV9 2RB **Tel:** (07881) 553 210 w 6303206

ROUND Laura Jo 23/07/2007 39 Paganel Drive DUDLEY West Midlands DY1 4AZ **Tel:** (01384) 256576 w 6304845

Rachel Louise 04/02/2008 10 Leopold Close Norwich Norfolk NR4 7PR **Tel:** (01603) 456312 w 6401403

ROUSE Cassie Sue 13/04/2004 (23/02/2009) 62 Doveridge Road BIRMINGHAM B28 0LU **Tel:** (0121) 313 1919 w 6268050

ROUTLEDGE Joanne 23/01/2008 Sir Harold Harmsworth Memorial Hospital 22 Sonderburg Road London N7 7QD **Tel:** (0870) 753 8081 w 6259052

ROWE Clare Linda (see WARD, Mrs)

Janice Margaret 15/08/1966 21 Ford Close Herne Bay Kent CT6 8AN **Tel:** (01227) 362602 w 6059999

Janine Laura 21/08/2008 26 Crathie Birtley Chester le Street County Durham DH3 1QJ **Tel:** 01914100288 w 6400765

Jeanette 27/03/1996 25 Bakers Lane SOUTHPORT Merseyside PR9 9RN **Tel:** (01704) 229970 w 6077431

Natalie Jane 15/02/2008 Flat 2 104 Preston Drove BRIGHTON BN1 6EW **Tel:** (07882) 052288 w 6391888

Natalie Jane 05/11/2008 3 Coombers Lane Lindfield HAYWARDS HEATH West Sussex RH16 2SS **Tel:** (01444) 233472 w 6405242

Sophie Jayne 14/09/2004 White Hills Surgery Sibford Road Hook Norton Banbury Oxfordshire OX15 5DG **Tel:** (01608) 730085 w 6287817

ROWELL Jade Laura 22/12/2008 83 Fountains Place Eye PETERBOROUGH PE6 7XX **Tel:** 01733221200 w 6383759

ROWLAND Andrea Rachel (nee Goddard) 10/02/2005 124 Miller Drive FAREHAM Hampshire PO16 7LN w 6265608

Laura Christina 23/02/2005 74 Flat B Upper Grosvenor Road TUNBRIDGE WELLS Kent TN1 2EU **Tel:** (07748) 183 326 w 6305604

ROWLANDS Alma (see BINGHAM, Mrs)

ROWLANDS Anwen Louise 19/07/2004 Cibyn Veterinary Clinic Llanberis Road Caernarfon Gwynedd LL55 2BD **Tel:** (01286) 673026 w 6281965

Elaine Louise 22/01/2008 56 Victory Avenue Waterlooville Hampshire PO8 9PJ **Tel:** 02392596011 w 6382879

Lynne 21/01/1999 32 Caroline Road New Inn Pontypool Gwent NP4 0QL **Tel:** (01495) 759409 w 6112456

ROWLE Lisa Michelle 12/01/2010 533 Battersea Park Road Battersea London SW11 3BL **Tel:** (020) 7924 5350 w 6437879

ROWLES Claire Louise 16/06/2008 94 Malvern Drive BRISTOL BS30 8UZ **Tel:** (07746) 423 372 w 6380877

ROWLEY Danielle 07/10/2009 28 Kingsway Scarborough North Yorkshire YO12 6SG **Tel:** (01723) 370583 w 6420015

ROXBURGH Katie Louise 07/12/2006 (16/11/2009) 8 Poplicans Road Cuxton ROCHESTER Kent ME2 1EH w 6330233

ROY Alison Elizabeth Comerford 24/08/2009 4 Beechwood Road LONDON N8 7NG **Tel:** 07921263017 w 6401029

ROYDEN-HALL Claire Rachael Francis 21/11/2007 2 Bridge House High Street Elsenham Bishop's Stortford Hertfordshire CM22 6DB **Tel:** (01279) 815744 w 6374783

ROYLE Katy Jane 05/11/2007 Pastures Farm Congleton Road Gawsworth MACCLESFIELD Cheshire SK11 9JB **Tel:** (01260) 224783 w 6407442

Rachel Dawn 06/10/2009 16 Riverside NANTWICH Cheshire CW5 5HT w 6461067

RUBBER Lucy Rebecca 12/05/2006 Penmellyn Veterinary Group Station Road St. Columb Major Cornwall TR9 6BX **Tel:** (01637) 880307 w 6240495

RUDD Amy Louise 16/11/2006 30 Alderley Crescent Walsall West Midlands WS3 1TE **Tel:** (07773) 677006 w 6288983

Rebecca Claire 13/07/2007 242 Garth Road Morden Surrey SM4 4NL **Tel:** (0208) 3301215 w 6347569

Shirley 21/01/1999 Ambleside 14 Church View Waltham Grimsby South Humberside DN37 0PH w 6135826

Suzanne DipAVN(Medical) 08/09/1999 The Feline Centre University of Bristol Dept of Clinical Veterinary Science Langford Bristol Avon BS40 5DU w 6148948

RUDGE Jeanette Monika 23/12/2008 C/o Royal College of Veterinary Surgeons 62-64 Horseferry Road LONDON SW1P 2AF w 6533238

Sarah Jeanette 22/08/2008 22 Grantley Crescent Kingswinford West Midlands DY6 9EH **Tel:** 07973322129 w 6421896

RUDGLEY Anna Marie 30/10/2003 Flat 25, Cranbury Court Cranbury Road Sholing Southampton Hampshire SO19 2RT **Tel:** (02380) 441174 w 6280678

RUDLING Lisa Mary Emma (see TAYLOR, Mrs)

RUFFELL Eloise Phillipa Katie 24/07/2003 Sunzway Giddy Green East Burton Wareham Dorset BH20 6EX **Tel:** (01929) 462061 w 6286750

RUFFELL Julie Anne (see WENHAM, Mrs)

RULE Rowena Ann 09/09/2002 Tollgate House Banbury Road Bishops Tachbrook LEAMINGTON SPA Warwickshire CV33 9QJ **Tel:** (01926) 453691 w 6261373

RUMSEY Victoria Louise 29/10/2004 Leadon Vale Veterinary Centre Lower Road Trading Estate Ledbury Herefordshire HR8 2DJ **Tel:** (01531) 632276 w 6282537

RUNDLE Kathryn Joy (see DIXON, Mrs)

RUNDLE Rebecca 02/06/2004 Pelyn Veterinary Group 8 Kings Avenue St. Austell Cornwall PL25 4TT **Tel:** (01726) 68177 w 6274485

RUSDEN Celia Louise (see BROWN, Ms)

RUSHFORD Tracey Patricia 19/09/2006 41 Milliken Drive Kilbarchan JOHNSTONE Renfrewshire PA10 2AW **Tel:** (01505) 706 209 w 6332873

RUSHTON Nicola Elizabeth (see WELLINGS, Mrs)

RUSS Kelly (see DAVIES, Mrs)

RUSSELL Danielle Valerie 19/03/2007 1 Court Farm Road Longwell Green Bristol BS30 9AA **Tel:** (0117) 932 3660 w 6344918

Deborah Elizabeth Jayne 07/04/2006 18 Mounthill Drive Cloughmills BALLYMENA County Antrim BT44 9QX **Tel:** (028) 2588 0641 w 6320190

Emma Agnes 31/05/2001 Overton Towcester Road Maids Moreton Buckingham Buckinghamshire MK18 1RE **Tel:** (01280) 812057 w 6219771

Emma Louise Christina 02/06/2004 Linton Elvaston Road Hexham Northumberland NE46 2HN **Tel:** (01434) 603029 w 6273814

Felicity Mary Lily 26/04/2007 Clent Hills Veterinary Group 34 Stourbridge Road BROMSGROVE Worcestershire B61 0AE **Tel:** (01527) 872488 w 6374134

Geraldine Anne 03/09/2008 Grove Veterinary Centre 231-239 Rawlinson Street Barrow-in-Furness Cumbria LA14 1DW **Tel:** (01229) 820402 w 6367160

Helen Amanda 14/09/2004 56 Gale Moor Avenue Gosport Hampshire PO12 2SJ **Tel:** (023) 926 02079 w 6266587

Jane (nee Meakings) 11/01/1993 (26/08/1999) Straid Veterinary Clinic 121 Station Road Beaconsfield Buckinghamshire HP9 1LH **Tel:** (01494) 673101 w 6065255

Jayne (nee McIntyre) 11/07/2007 80 Fairfield Avenue ROSSENDALE Lancashire BB4 9TH **Tel:** (01706) 222 402 w 6337812

Joanne Sharron (nee Moore) 09/11/1997 (29/01/2008) The Crossings Veterinary Centre Saint John's Way Downham Market Norfolk PE38 0QQ **Tel:** (01366) 382219 w 6118196

RUSSELL June (see BALGOWAN, Mrs)

Kelly Jane 27/02/1997 (01/06/2001) Bell Equine Veterinary Clinic 104 Butchers Lane Mereworth Maidstone Kent ME18 5GS **Tel:** (01622) 813700 w 6100258

Lesley Ann 14/03/2006 12 Burrelton Gardens Dundee Angus DD3 9QT **Tel:** (01382) 827 177 w 6331993

Linsey Tracey 04/03/2009 24 Arran Gardens Hamilton Lanarkshire ML3 7NZ **Tel:** (01698) 459 303 w 6402778

RUSSELL Maria Jayne (see BRAND, Mrs)

Rachel Louise (formerly Pique, nee Holmes) 16/09/1997 104 Morehall Avenue Cheriton Folkestone Kent CT19 4EE **Tel:** (01303) 273448 w 6117782

Romana Jane 01/04/2003 Old School House Church Pulverbatch Shrewsbury Shropshire SY5 8BZ **Tel:** (01743) 718409 w 6280612

Tracey Jane DipAVN(Surgical) 02/02/1998 (09/06/2006) Flat 4 6 Ted Bates Road SOUTHAMPTON SO14 5FH w 6109002

RUSSEN Emmaly (nee Stephens) 07/12/2005 (06/04/2009) The Gables Stocks Hill Bawburgh NORWICH NR9 3LL w 6302161

RUTHERFORD Ellen Elizabeth (see MAKEPEACE, Mrs)

RUTHERFORD Virginia Louise 07/06/2005 (18/08/2009) Kirkley March Farm Kirkley Newcastle upon Tyne Tyne and Wear NE20 0BA **Tel:** (01661) 881287 w 6288257

RUTLAND Clare Victoria 03/12/2003 A120 Veterinary Centre Little Hadham Bishops Stortford Hertfordshire SG11 2DA **Tel:** (01279) 771144 w 6280469

Gary Alan DipAVN(Surgical) 13/05/2003 48 Marconi Road CHELMSFORD Essex CM1 1QD **Tel:** (01245) 607136 m 6271757

RUTLAND Lisa Joanne (see MULHALL, Mrs)

RUTTER Helen Mary 11/11/2008 Green Hill Farm Fenn Lanes Dadlington Nuneaton Warwickshire CV13 6DS **Tel:** (07929) 081944 w 6410841

Maria Louise 03/05/2007 18 Fleetwood Gardens Market Harborough Leicestershire LE16 9LX **Tel:** (01858) 433 785 w 6354004

RYAL Julie Ann (see BREWER, Mrs)

RYALL Helen Margaret 12/05/2004 107 Carisbrooke Road Newport Isle of Wight PO30 1HP **Tel:** (01983) 522822 w 6283692

RYAN Fiona 02/12/2009 1254 Benalla Tatong Road Benalla Victoria 3672 Australia **Tel:** (+61) 403 292 827 w 6574114

Lucy Hannah 29/09/2004 Flat 6 The Old Maltings Skerne Road DRIFFIELD North Humberside YO25 6SP w 6319783

Tara Kathleen 21/03/2007 The Flat 172 Oxford Road KIDLINGTON Oxfordshire OX5 1EA w 6377236

Toni Margaret 18/12/2009 201 St Radigunds Road Dover Kent CT17 0LB **Tel:** (01304) 212113 w 6283582

Victoria Jane 10/02/2004 333 Redditch Road Kings Norton BIRMINGHAM B38 8PP w 6284979

RYDER Megan Louise (nee Nicholas) 04/10/2005 Grove House Holt Road Fakenham Norfolk NR21 8JG **Tel:** (01328) 862137 w 6303756

Michelle Louise 21/04/2005 Streatham Hill Veterinary Surgery 101 Sternhold Avenue London SW2 4PF **Tel:** (020) 8674 3525 w 6264354

Stephanie Louise 28/04/2006 7 Firefly Close Lee-on-the-Solent Hampshire PO13 8FY **Tel:** (02392) 556120 w 6350165

RYDZ Charlotte Sara Louise (nee Blackmore) 13/01/2009 13 Flora Road RAMSGATE Kent CT11 7LN **Tel:** (078431) 69306 w 6407035

RYMELL Claire Leanne (see MATAN, Mrs)

RYNBERK Claire Elizabeth (nee Wilson) 21/09/1984 (19/06/2008) 9 Brimstage Close WIRRAL Merseyside CH60 1YE w 6091853

RZAS Hayley Louisa 25/02/2003 49 West Street Swadlincote Derbyshire DE11 9DN **Tel:** (01283) 213707 w 6281140

S

SADDLETON Karen Susan (nee Martin) 25/08/1993 (14/05/1999) 3 Thompsons Meadow Crowfield Ipswich Suffolk IP6 9SU **Tel:** (01449) 760 334 w 6027730

SADLER Claire (see ALCOCK, Mrs)

SADLER Kirsty Louise 21/07/2008 11 Crawford Close BILLERICAY Essex CM12 0PX **Tel:** (01277) 624332 w 6330816

Naomi Jane (nee Millett) 23/08/2004 63 Norwich Road Wroxham Norwich Norfolk NR12 8RX **Tel:** (01603) 783 920 w 6269282

SADLER Nichola Jane Shirley (see FOWLER, Mrs)

Rachel Louise 20/09/1999 (17/09/2002) 13 Robin Way Chelmsford Essex CM2 8AT **Tel:** (01245) 250 631 w 6145652

Rebecca Elizabeth (nee Brandreth) 08/09/2005 16 Monica Grove Levenshulme Manchester M19 2BN **Tel:** (0161) 2484843 w 6280491

SAFFIN Jennifer Ann 22/05/2009 Fingle Farm Drewsteignton Exeter Devon EX6 6NJ **Tel:** 01647281663 w 6355786

SAGE Miya (nee Willson) 25/06/2004 (19/01/2010) Rose Cottage Cherville Lane Bramling Canterbury Kent CT3 1LZ w 6292492

SAILL Lara Louise (see SCRIVENER, Mrs)

SAINSBURY Melanie May 23/12/2003 Rosedene The Street Stradishall NEWMARKET Suffolk CB8 8YW **Tel:** (01440) 820 933 w 6277070

SALE Kayleigh Jayne 12/12/2005 160 Weston Lane BIRMINGHAM B11 3RX **Tel:** (0121) 624 5422 w 6346029

SALISBURY Katherine Elizabeth (see RIDING, Mrs)

Louise Ann 23/01/2003 163 Seven Star Road Solihull West Midlands B91 2BN **Tel:** (0121) 7055496 w 6272208

SALL Georgina Hannah (see HALL, Mrs)

SALMON Jennifer Louise 30/03/1989 18 Perkins Road Barkinside Ilford Essex IG2 7NJ **Tel:** (0208) 5542573 w 6060166

Sarah Elizabeth 02/06/2004 Glenthorne Veterinary Centre 71 Derby Road Uttoxeter Staffordshire ST14 8EB **Tel:** (01889) 562164 w 6288587

SALT Vivien Jean (see COVE, Mrs)

SALTON Stephanie 18/03/2009 30 Edmonstone Avenue Danderhall Dalkeith Midlothian EH22 1QR **Tel:** (0131) 6542859 w 6349307

SAMPLE Kerry Anne DipAVN(Surgical) (nee Higgins) 28/02/2001 72 Pinemead SHEFFORD Bedfordshire SG17 5BY **Tel:** (01462) 442074 w 6213314

SAMPSON Charlotte Louise May (nee Bradford) 05/04/2005 11-17 The Precinct West Meads Bognor Regis West Sussex PO21 5SB **Tel:** (01243) 842832 w 6320025

Sarah Elisabeth 21/04/2008 4 Drummond Avenue Romford Essex RM7 7EH **Tel:** (07904) 452147 w 6387290

SAMS Daniella Marie 19/07/2006 (23/03/2009) 56 Carnarvon Road GOSPORT Hampshire PO12 3QS w 6349637

Diane Michelle 11/04/2005 5 Crane Avenue Sutton Leach ST. HELENS Merseyside WA9 4HP w 6300621

SAMSON Katie Anne (nee Gooderham) 11/12/2001 (23/05/2005) 34 New Dover Road Canterbury Kent CT1 3DT **Tel:** (01227) 765522 w 6261208

SAMUEL Patricia Rose (see SCORER, Mrs)

SAMUELS Anna 28/09/2005 16 Kecksys SAWBRIDGEWORTH Hertfordshire CM21 9DT w 6318881

SANCHEZ-RODRIGUEZ Lacey May 04/08/2008 21 Tandridge Drive ORPINGTON Kent BR6 8BY **Tel:** (01689) 827660 w 6404340

SANDELLS Jenna Fern 29/10/2007 53 Moore Close Claypole NEWARK Nottinghamshire NG23 5AU **Tel:** (07970) 876 796 w 6368744

SANDERS Amy Rose 10/12/2007 5 Avington Close Maidstone Kent ME15 6SZ **Tel:** (01622) 675210 w 6367776

Carrie-Anne 18/10/2005 Clockhouse Veterinary Hospital Wallbridge Stroud Gloucestershire GL5 3JD **Tel:** (01453) 752555 w 6301171

Helen (nee Parker) 22/08/1997 46 Scargill Avenue Newthorpe Nottingham NG16 2DZ **Tel:** (01773) 716848 w 6113165

Lucy Barbara 02/06/2004 (15/05/2008) Flat 7, Craig y Mor Court 41-43 South Road Sully PENARTH South Glamorgan CF64 5SJ **Tel:** (07967) 809930 w 6280689

Michelle (nee Ford) 17/08/1981 (17/10/2006) 53 Senrab Street London E1 0QF w 6089447

Richard John 24/08/1998 46 Scargill Avenue Newthorpe Nottingham NG16 2DZ **Tel:** (01773) 716848 m 6135316

SANDERSON Kay (nee Reed) 08/01/1993 2 Okehampton Drive The Crofters Newbottle Co Durham DH4 4YA **Tel:** (0191) 5849619 w 6065197

Michelle Lorna 10/08/1984 61 Scott Green Gildersome Leeds West Yorkshire LS27 7AW **Tel:** (0113) 2527158 w 6060202

Nicola Mary 11/08/2009 Grove Veterinary Centre 231-239 Rawlinson Street Barrow-in-Furness Cumbria LA14 1DW **Tel:** (01229) 820402 w 6434337

Samantha Elizabeth 16/04/2007 35 Springfield Road RETFORD Nottinghamshire DN22 6QR **Tel:** (01777) 702209 w 6349802

SANDRY Joanne (see MASTERS, Mrs)

SANGER Judith Karen Linda 18/04/2005 1 Midland Road Hemel Hempstead Hertfordshire HP2 5BH **Tel:** (01442) 389951 w 6276212

SANSOM Sandra Christina 28/02/2001 55 Blumfield Crescent Slough SL1 6NL **Tel:** (01628) 543973 w 6213347

SANTINI Sian Eve 26/09/2006 15 Brachdy Close Rumney Cardiff South Glamorgan CF3 3AU **Tel:** (029) 2031 8017 w 6371725

SARGANT Emma Louise 27/02/2006 11 Fleetwood Way South Oxhey WATFORD hertfordshire WD19 6NB **Tel:** (020) 8421 0966 w 6345061

SARGEANT Lisa Carol 11/07/2005 18 Plumian Way Balsham Cambridgeshire CB1 6EG **Tel:** (01223) 290 709 w 6286497

SARGENT Anna Louise 08/01/2009 18 Lychfield Drive Rochester Kent ME2 3LY **Tel:** (01634) 295105 w 6416759

SARGENT Michelle Lorraine (see WILSON, Mrs)

SATTERTHWAITE Amy Louise 10/09/2008 117 Swift Close Letchworth Garden City Hertfordshire SG6 4LH **Tel:** (01462) 626488 w 6404087

SAUNBY Kelly Marie 06/08/2007 Field Street Boston Lincolnshire PE21 6TR **Tel:** (01205) 363073 w 6382791

SAUNDERS Carrie Louise 07/12/2000 39 Greenside Mangotsfield BRISTOL BS16 9EE **Tel:** (07515) 726 239 w 6205416

Claire Helen 17/07/2008 1 Heol Dderwen Tonteg PONTYPRIDD Mid Glamorgan CF38 1TD **Tel:** 07796460067 w 6414515

Donna (nee Smart) 23/12/2003 Medivet Veterinary Group 237 St Albans Road WATFORD WD24 5BP **Tel:** (01923) 243429 w 6292250

Hayley Sarah 09/03/2005 120 Scarf Road Canford Heath Poole Dorset BH17 8QL **Tel:** (01202) 683 103 w 6274441

Kate Jane 01/09/1999 48 Valbourne Road Kings Heath BIRMINGHAM B14 6NE **Tel:** (01527) 873125 w 6149089

SAUNDERS Lesley Fiona (see DEAN, Mrs)

Marie Jean 03/05/2007 (28/08/2009) 6 Hazel Drive Martham GREAT YARMOUTH Norfolk NR29 4QL **Tel:** (07818) 451285 w 6377247

Rebecca Aimee (formerly Harvey, nee Harvey) 17/05/2005 Downwood Veterinary Centre 4 High Street Horam Heathfield East Sussex TN21 0EJ **Tel:** (01453) 812152 w 6308211

SAVAGE Elizabeth Claire 07/10/1999 (25/09/2007) Plumpton College Ditching Road Plumpton Lesws East Sussex BN7 3AE **Tel:** (01273) 890454 w 6185847

Jane Elizabeth 06/03/2006 The Stable Flat 89 Middlecave Road MALTON North Yorkshire YO17 7NQ **Tel:** (01653) 692 242 w 6345545

Rachel 18/05/2009 12 John Street Earby Barnoldswick Lancashire BB18 6XH **Tel:** 07963168122 w 6396299

SAVELL Victoria Ann (see FIELDSON, Mrs)

SAVILE Mary Helen (see STEELE, Mrs)

SAVILLE Sarah Joy (see PRESTIDGE, Mrs)

SAVORY Angela Lesley 28/07/1987 (31/10/2000) 19 Highfield Close Thorpe St. Andrew Norwich NR7 0RQ **Tel:** (01603) 436819 w 6048524

SAWYER Elaine 22/01/1991 210 Hesketh Lane Tarleton PRESTON PR4 6AT w 6060279

Helen Louise 15/11/2001 30 Holden Corner TUNBRIDGE WELLS Kent TN4 0LP **Tel:** (01892) 547 458 w 6251825

SAXBY Lorrayne (see STRETTON, Mrs)

SAYERS Jennifer Ann (see CHANDLER, Mrs)

SAYLES Tiffany Catherine 21/05/2003 48 Curlew Drive Crossgates Scarborough North Yorkshire YO12 4TP **Tel:** ((0115)) 9373842 w 6233015

SAYNOR Nicole Gemma 30/09/2008 12 Heywood Avenue MAIDENHEAD Berkshire SL6 3JA w 6413305

SCADDING Josephine Jeanette (see PARRY, Mrs)

SCAIFE Catherine Anne 10/04/2007 Fivelands Veterinary Centre 98 Alcester Road BIRMINGHAM B13 8EG **Tel:** (0121) 449 3716 w 6365829

SCALES Carol Avril 09/09/1970 Coco Markus House Nelson street Grimsby North East Lincolnshire DN32 7SH **Tel:** (01472) 343278 w 6060315

Nichola Suzanne 01/04/2003 The Blue Cross Animal Hospital Nelson Street Grimsby South Humberside DN32 7SH w 6279149

SCANTLEBURY Clare Avis 05/04/2005 21 Cordelia Close Dibden Southampton Hampshire SO45 5UD **Tel:** (023) 8084 4940 w 6311401

SCARR Joanna 19/09/2006 14 St. Cuthberts Green Barton Richmond North Yorkshire DL10 6LR **Tel:** (02392) 525796 w 6330321

SCARSBROOK Lindsey Marie (see GAYLARD, Mrs)

SCATES-PROUD Victoria 07/06/2005 Cheadle Hulme Veterinary Hospital 2-4 Queens Road Cheadle Hulme Cheshire SK8 5LU **Tel:** (0161) 485 8444 w 6316472

SCHILLER Amy Louise 01/09/2000 174 Moreton Park Road Bideford Devon EX39 3HB **Tel:** (01237) 420805 w 6203271

SCHNEIDAU Deana Louise 13/01/2004 21 Gestridge Road Kingsteignton Newton Abbot Devon TQ12 3EZ **Tel:** (01626) 354260 w 6288323

SCHOFIELD Kelly Louise 01/04/2003 50 Lawnswood Houghton Le Spring Tyne & Wear DH5 8JA **Tel:** (0191) 5846311 w 6287773

Lindsey Jane 20/11/2002 298 Sinfin Avenue Shelton Lock Derby DE24 9QX **Tel:** (01332) 605269 w 6283153

Vanessa 01/09/2008 Apple Tree Cottage 1 Highfields Burntwood Staffordshire WS7 9DB **Tel:** (01543) 683528 w 6407068

SCHOLES Jane Ann (see RIDGWAY, Miss)

SCHOLES Rachael Elizabeth 07/02/2007 80 Housesteads Road Carlisle Cumbria CA2 7XG **Tel:** (01228) 536359 w 6379524

Sarah Amanda (nee Nelson) 22/03/2004 28 Beechdale Road Liverpool Merseyside L18 5EL **Tel:** (0151) 733 5755 w 6275387

SCHOLEY Angela Louise 03/09/2002 (05/02/2010) 1 Holborn Avenue Dronfield Derbyshire S18 2NA **Tel:** (01246) 415270 w 6270063

SCHOLEY Claire Karen (see BIRD, Mrs)

SCHREINER Alison Jane 20/01/1997 104 Congreve Road Worthing West Sussex BN14 8EW **Tel:** (01903) 234674 w 610027X

SCHULZ Amanda Grace 19/10/2007 93 Cornwall Avenue Blackpool Lancashire FY2 9QP **Tel:** (01253) 500 118 w 6401414

SCOBBIE Sharon (see KLIMAS, Miss)

SCOLLICK Michelle (nee Honour) 23/08/2004 42 Daneacre Road RADSTOCK BA3 3JS **Tel:** (01761) 435 229 w 6301116

SCORER Patricia Rose (nee Samuel) 24/08/1998 The Annex Abbots Court Farm Deerhurst Gloucestershire GL19 4BX **Tel:** (01684) 290632 w 6131242

SCOTT Amy Elizabeth 08/11/2006 Thrums Vet Group (Flat) Black Brae Blairgowrie Perth Perthshire PH10 6NW **Tel:** (01738) 551709 w 6347327

SCOTT Claire Anne (see GOULD, Miss)

Clare Elizabeth 24/06/2004 25 Moneyer Road ANDOVER Hampshire SP10 4NG w 6280733

Clare Louise 15/11/2001 54 Dorset Rd St Annes Lancashire FY8 2EB **Tel:** (01253) 726895 w 6276278

Joanna Elizabeth 21/08/1985 5 Littlefield Lane Sixpenny Handley Salisbury SP5 5NP **Tel:** (01725) 552946 w 6060359

SCOTT Judith Mary (see LUMB, Mrs)

Julie Ann 24/02/2009 1 Breach Down Cottages Valley Road Barham Canterbury Kent CT4 6LL **Tel:** 01227831051 w 6435866

Kathryn Elizabeth 10/03/2008 12 Pinetrees Westdn favell NORTHAMPTON NN3 3ET w 6386179

Louise 15/05/2009 14 Grenville Way THAME Oxfordshire OX9 3YW **Tel:** 01844213167 w 6439815

Melanie (nee Charlton) 06/09/1994 (27/03/2001) Jimal Ulgham Morpeth Northumberland NE61 3AX **Tel:** (01670) 790 813 w 6034806

Rachel Ann 13/12/2001 169 Branksome Ave Stanford-le-Hope Essex SS17 8DD **Tel:** (01375) 402685 w 6270316

Sarah Jayne 02/09/1999 45 Kipling Road Kettering Northamptonshire NN16 9JZ **Tel:** (01536) 712519 w 6141421

Susan Jane (nee Nelson) 04/11/1992 (10/06/2003) 68 Moorgate Road Hindringham FAKENHAM Norfolk NR21 0PT **Tel:** (01328) 878277 w 6012043

Victoria Louise 31/10/2006 Runnymede Hill Veterinary Hospital Tite Hill Egham Surrey TW20 0NB **Tel:** (01784) 436 367 w 6368755

Wendy Louise 03/05/2005 6c Johnston Avenue Cornton Stirling FK9 5BW **Tel:** (01786) 473398 w 6291447

SCOTT-BURGE Samantha 17/09/2007 41 Harwood Avenue Tamerton Foliot Plymouth Devon PL5 4NX **Tel:** (01752) 789173 w 6331223

SCOULAR Frances Teresa (nee Towneley) 16/10/1997 20 Aldgate Ketton STAMFORD Rutland PE9 3TD w 6118673

SCOURFIELD Paula Jane 13/11/2009 Fenton Veterinary Practice 21 Portfield Haverfordwest Pembrokeshire SA61 1BN **Tel:** (01437) 762806 w 6453257

SCRIBBINS Natalie Louise (see KINGDON, Mrs)

SCRIVENER Lara Louise (nee Saill) 16/01/1995 East Grinstead Veterinary Hospital Maypole Road East Grinstead West Sussex RH19 1HL **Tel:** (01342) 323072 w 6036803

SCUFFHAM Debra Kay 07/06/2005 109 Standhill Crescent BARNSLEY South Yorkshire S71 1SS **Tel:** (01226) 299018 w 6319629

SCULLARD Kirsty Sarah (see GRANT, Mrs)

SEABROOK Dawn Victoria 01/04/2003 5 Chevers Pawen Basildon Essex SS13 3EJ **Tel:** (01375) 641288 w 6283835

Kerry 24/12/2002 46 Wordsworth Close Popley Basingstoke Hampshire RG24 9DF **Tel:** (01256) 412521 w 6279061

SEAGROVE Sharon Alexandra 22/04/2002 2 Mill Hill Close Lilliput Poole Dorset BH14 8RL **Tel:** (01202) 733826 w 6274815

SEALEY Nicola Jane (see MANN, Mrs)

SEANEY Emma Jane (see ANDERSON, Mrs)

SEARLE Dianne Lorraine Theresa (nee Blackett) 17/07/2003 228 Hunters Hall Rd Dagenham Essex RM10 8HU **Tel:** (020) 8595 4635 w 6269513

SEARS Andrea Julie 23/03/2007 24 Hillylaid Road Thornton-Cleveleys Lancashire FY5 4DZ **Tel:** (01253) 860346 w 6358514

SEDGWICK Alison (see CONN, Mrs)

SEDGWICK Claire 20/05/2003 10 St. Lukes Terrace BRIGHTON BN2 9ZE **Tel:** (0208) 984 0316 w 6284132

SEED Kathryn Emma 21/05/2009 25 Harper Terrace Yeadon Leeds LS19 7RP **Tel:** (01132) 505522 w 6445271

SEGEV Marianne Angela 06/10/2006 RSPCA Putney Animal Hospital 6 Clarendon Drive London SW15 1AA **Tel:** (0300) 123 0716 w 6358866

SEGHINI Nicola (see GREEN, Mrs)

SELBY Clare Frances Rosy 18/10/2006 (06/11/2008) 242 Cricklewood Lane London NW2 2PU **Tel:** (020) 8450 2228 w 6351441

SELLECK Ruth Elizabeth (see LEGG, Mrs)

SELLERS Allison Louise 08/04/2005 12 Oat Close AYLESBURY Buckinghamshire HP21 9LN **Tel:** (01296) 428594 w 6290226

Emma Jane 21/04/2008 20 Station Road Owston Ferry Doncaster South Yorkshire DN9 1AW **Tel:** (01427) 728215 w 6389369

Megan Holly Anne 24/04/2009 153 Mercer Way Romsey SO51 7PN **Tel:** 07828165152 w 6452003

SEMMLER Vicky Jane 14/12/2006 5 Wessex Gardens ROMSEY Hampshire SO51 5RD **Tel:** 07786620124 w 6358019

SEMPLE Cheryl 07/01/2004 111 Market Street Musselburgh East Lothian EH21 6PZ **Tel:** (0131) 665 2124 w 6299642

Olive Frances (nee McKinley) 23/09/2002 Fron Farm Glan Conwy COLWYN BAY Clwyd LL28 5PL **Tel:** (01492) 573116 w 6263914

SESSIONS Amy Victoria Louise 10/11/2009 13 Ramsay Road WINCHESTER Hampshire SO23 7PW **Tel:** 01962881734 w 6465324

SEVERS Nicola 23/03/2009 1 Bury Road Tottington Bury Lancashire BL8 3HD **Tel:** (01204) 886655 w 6448175

SEWARD Andrea Jane 15/04/2009 12 Aldergate Grove Ashton-under-Lyne Lancashire OL6 8YE **Tel:** (0161) 3300544 w 6272747

SEWELL Anne-Marie (see FRODSHAM, Mrs)

SEWELL Dawn (nee Sewell, formerly Sewell-Huggins) 01/09/1995 Blenheim Veterinary Centre Blenheim Road Airfield Industrial Estate Ashbourne Derbyshire DE6 1HA **Tel:** (01335) 342111 w 6039429

SEWELL Rebecca Elizabeth (see LOCK, Ms)

Tina Mary Jane 28/02/2001 Oakham Veterinary Hospital Ashwell Road Oakham Rutland LE15 7QH **Tel:** (01572) 722646 w 6142924

SEWELL-HUGGINS Dawn (see SEWELL, Miss)

SEXTON Gemma Jane (nee Beales) 09/05/2005 21 Claxtons Close Mileham KING'S LYNN Norfolk PE32 2RU **Tel:** (01328) 701148 w 6291612

SEXTON Louise Frances Michelle (see HEARNE, Mrs)

SEYMOUR Carly Georgina 26/10/2005 Puddyphats Cottage Puddyphats Lane Markyate ST. ALBANS Hertfordshire AL3 8AZ w 6347613

SHALA Gillian Ann Catherine (formerly Finegan) 01/04/2003 34 Raheen Park Tallaght Dublin 24 Ireland **Tel:** (00353) 14520991 w 6263243

SHALE Elizabeth Mary 17/11/2009 19 Church Street Southport Merseyside PR9 0QT **Tel:** (01704) 533602 w 6438330

SHAND Allison Malcolm 05/04/2005 142 Ruthrieston Circle ABERDEEN AB10 7LU **Tel:** (01224) 503733 w 6291458

Samantha Jane 14/09/2009 32 Springfield Estate Scopwick LINCOLN LN4 3NP **Tel:** (01526) 322059 w 6453356

SHANLEY Joanne Margaret 02/03/2007 3 Eastlands Court St Peters Road Rugby Warwickshire CV21 3QP **Tel:** (01788) 575300 w 6377258

SHANNON Katherine (see BICHARD, Mrs)

SHAPIRO Lisa Hayley 30/11/2006 Arden House Animal Hospital 56 Pembroke Road Ruislip Middlesex HA4 8NF **Tel:** (01895) 633600 w 6346623

SHARMA Rachel Marianne (nee Lindsay) 08/04/2005 Seadown Veterinary Hospital Frost Lane Hythe Southampton Hampshire SO45 3NG **Tel:** (023) 8084 2237 w 6311390

SHARMAN Katie (nee Haynes) 05/09/2008 48 Simons Walk Pattishall Towcester Northamptonshire NN12 8NX **Tel:** (01327) 830671 w 6280843

Ria Kathryn 16/09/2009 7 Kestral Close Beckrow Bury St Edmunds Suffolk IP28 8EP **Tel:** 07885672303 w 6366390

SHARP Louise 27/03/2008 8 Barrie Road Stenhousemuir Larbert Stirlingshire FK5 4LF **Tel:** (01324) 557 557 w 6405121

Simone 09/05/2005 Moorcroft Veterinary Practice 223 Dorchester Road Weymouth Dorset DT3 5EQ **Tel:** (01305) 776686 w 6331234

SHARPE Karen (see GORDON, Mrs)

SHARPLES Catherine Ruth (nee Heal) 31/03/2003 54 Railway Terrace Great Harwood Blackburn Lancashire BB6 7EH **Tel:** (01254) 877 840 w 6281514

SHARPLES Lisa (see MARSHALL, Mrs)

SHATFORD Deborah Tracey 30/07/1987 27 Ash Rise Kingsthorpe Northampton NN2 8SB **Tel:** (01604) 845371 w 6060530

SHAUGHNESSY Lorna Jane 19/01/2005 Kilclooney Mill Town Tuam County Galway Ireland w 6286948

SHAW Carol (nee Sheppard) 01/02/2000 Veterinary Health Centre Ltd 4 Greeways Lytham St. Annes Lancashire FY8 3LY **Tel:** (01253) 729309 w 6145426

Christopher Shaun 22/10/2004 42 Ewe Lamb Lane Beeston NOTTINGHAM NG9 3JZ **Tel:** (07762) 343994 m 6323699

Emma Louise 09/09/2008 39 Lancaster Road Carnforth Lancashire LA5 9LD **Tel:** (01524) 720002 w 6437703

SHAW Helen Christine (see STEER, Mrs)

Linda Joanne 06/03/2008 61 Temple Grove Bakers Lane West Hanningfield CHELMSFORD CM2 8LH **Tel:** (01277) 841211 w 6324678

Lisa Jane 01/02/2008 28 Hurworth Road Billingham Cleveland TS23 3LU **Tel:** 07759477215 w 6404241

Nicola (formerly Barrenetxea) 10/02/2009 P D S A Hepton Court Leeds West Yorkshire LS9 6PW **Tel:** (0113) 2408818 w 6445304

Nicola Jane 04/12/2003 8 Ashford Road CHELMSFORD Essex CM1 2ST **Tel:** (01245) 265540 w 6278456

Yvonne Munro (nee Goldie) 21/05/2003 (10/07/2007) 14 Gareloch Avenue AIRDRIE Lanarkshire ML6 6SH **Tel:** (01236) 604362 w 6263628

SHAWLEY Joanne 02/02/1996 26 West Crescent PETERLEE County Durham SR8 3HQ **Tel:** (0191) 438 3338 w 6040605

SHEA Elizabeth Michaela 05/07/2006 8 Brushwood Road Chesham Buckinghamshire HP5 3DW **Tel:** 07766333811 w 6324689

SHEARD Becky 10/09/2009 17 Albany Road WICKFORD Essex SS12 9BP w 6466105

SHEARLAW Claire Corina 22/09/2004 Ramparts Veterinary Centre Windmill Way West BERWICK-UPON-TWEED TD15 1TB **Tel:** (01289) 330066 w 6266653

SHEARS Victoria Louise (nee Bartholomew) 26/10/2005 5 Saunders Close UCKFIELD East Sussex TN22 2BX w 6316725

SHEEN Alison Fiona (see CHURCH, Mrs)

SHELDON Laura Katy 12/09/2008 Headingley View Church Street Bonsall MATLOCK Derbyshire DE4 2AE w 6437065

Nicola Carolyn 10/04/2003 The Veterinary Hospital Cannock Road Penkridge Stafford ST19 5RY **Tel:** (01785) 712235 w 6272538

SHELLIM Claire Vanessa DipAVN(Surgical) 13/09/2000 11 Badshot Park Badshot Lea FARNHAM Surrey GU9 9JU w 6204173

SHELTON Jennifer 30/01/2008 28 Salisbury Drive New Ferry Wirral CH64 1BD **Tel:** (0151) 644 7398 w 6400754

SHENSTON Crian Rebecca (nee Williams) 19/01/1996 (19/08/2002) 24 Barley Meadows LLANYMYNECH Powys SY22 6JX **Tel:** (01691) 831908 w 6037272

SHEPARD Ruth (see GIBBONS, Mrs)

SHEPHERD Julie Lisa 31/12/2003 58 Long Walk EPSOM Surrey KT18 5TW **Tel:** (01737) 359976 w 6268710

Rachael Ann 11/01/1993 (05/06/2001) P D S A Woolfall Heath Avenue Liverpool Merseyside L36 3YD **Tel:** (0151) 480 2288 w 6065313

SHEPPARD Angela Louise DipAVN(Surgical) (nee Huntley) 29/09/2000 Davies Veterinary Specialists Manor Farm Business Park Higham Gobion Hertfordshire SG5 3HR **Tel:** (01582) 883950 w 6203722

SHEPPARD Carol (see SHAW, Mrs)

Hazel Anne (nee Bourne) 13/02/1995 St Anne's Veterinary Group 6 St Anne's Road Eastbourne East Sussex BN21 2DJ **Tel:** (01323) 640011 w 6035490

SHEPPARD Heather Anne (see OSBORNE, Mrs)

Kathryn Margaret 27/05/2003 87 Watford Road Cotteridge Birmingham B30 1NP **Tel:** (0121) 459 4333 w 6271449

SHERIFF Alice Caroline (see BUGG, Mrs)

SHERLOCK Rebecca Louise 10/02/2004 31 Tymeinwr Avenue Pontycymer Bridgend Mid Glamorgan CF32 8NE **Tel:** (01656) 766181 w 6261131

SHERRATT Fern Susan 13/04/2004 (27/02/2009) The Bungalow Ferndale Court Barrows Close BIRCHINGTON Kent CT7 0DB **Tel:** (01843) 845198 w 6282020

SHERRY Annette Marie 10/12/2008 53 Wrexham Road LONDON E3 2TJ **Tel:** 07943102428 w 6435954

Natalie Victoria 20/02/2009 3 Webster Croft Old Whittington CHESTERFIELD Derbyshire S41 9NX **Tel:** 07806819624 w 6438682

SHERWOOD Alison Karen (nee Thomson) 24/06/2004 41 Burton Bank Road BARNSLEY South Yorkshire S71 2AB w 6298179

SHERWOOD Faye (see ALDRIDGE, Mrs)

Jonathan Christopher 24/06/2004 41 Burton Bank Road BARNSLEY South Yorkshire S71 2AB **Tel:** (01226) 217974 m 6298157

SHIELD Kirstie May DipAVN(Surgical) 26/08/1999 42 Christopher Drive CHIPPENHAM Wiltshire SN15 3UT w 6141374

SHIELDS Gemma Victoria 12/02/2009 20 Manor Fields Rawcliffe GOOLE North Humberside DN14 8TN w 6444083

SHIELDS Julia Margaret (see WITHERS, Mrs)

SHILLING Lydia Andrea 10/10/2005 The Barn Animal Hospital Great Binfields Road Old Basing BASINGSTOKE Hampshire RG24 8AD **Tel:** (01256) 329522 w 6290237

SHILLITO Tracey (nee Patterson) 18/10/2006 12 Swannington Road Broughton Astley Leicester LE9 6TU **Tel:** (01455) 282512 w 6293867

SHINE Katie Leigh 11/11/2008 16 Cordwell Road London SE13 5QX **Tel:** 07908213734 w 6373804

SHINN Sarah Louise (see KENYON, Mrs)

SHIPLEY Sarah-Jane Anne 10/09/2009 27 Wilsley Pound Kents Hill MILTON KEYNES MK7 6DT **Tel:** (01908) 232072 w 6251979

SHOOTER Hannah Leanne 03/05/2007 Stocton Veterinary Centre Stocton Close Woodbridge Road Guildford Surrey GU1 1HR **Tel:** (01483) 575155 w 6372484

SHOOTER Karen Michelle (see SMITH, Mrs)

SHOREMAN Ian 10/05/2007 20 Ellenhall Close Manchester Lancashire M9 5XG **Tel:** (01612) 024515 m 6353949

SHORT Katie Louise 11/11/2004 The Veterinary Practice Millennium Way Braintree Essex CM7 3GX **Tel:** (01376) 325511 w 6325316

Rachel Elizabeth 24/02/2004 Victoria Veterinary Centre Ltd 25 Victoria Street Glossop Derbyshire SK13 8HT **Tel:** (01457) 852367 w 6293856

Sophie Louise 29/01/2010 9 Hill View Close TADWORTH Surrey KT20 5QA **Tel:** 07727181954 w 6410830

SHORTHOUSE Anna Lubinka 24/09/2001 16 Station Road Cuxton Rochester Kent ME2 1AB **Tel:** (01233) 624687 w 6228648

SHOTT Rebekah Mary 18/10/2006 7 St. Johns Cottages Weston Road Totnes Devon TQ9 5AW **Tel:** (01803) 865 002 w 6375201

SHOULT Nicola Jane 01/04/2003 68 North Way Lewes East Sussex BN7 1DJ w 6278467

SHURY Sarah Jane (see ROBERTSON, Mrs)

SIDDALL Paula 24/05/2005 108 Carr Road Fleetwood Lancashire FY7 6QQ w 6325822

SIER Gemma Clare (nee Cater) 22/03/2004 35 Queen Street Warley BRENTWOOD Essex CM14 5JZ **Tel:** (01277) 220826 w 6291634

SIKKINK Katherine Jean 29/09/2008 11 Acacia Terrace ASHINGTON Northumberland NE63 0AQ **Tel:** 07756117636 w 6334754

SILCOCK Emma Jane (nee Robbie) 08/04/2005 6 Rufford Close Eastleigh Hampshire SO50 4RU **Tel:** (02380) 617646 w 6142629

SILLITOE Domini Karen 20/02/1985 PDSA PAH Tuxford Close Wolverhampton WV10 0JQ **Tel:** (01902) 451519 w 6060643

SILVANI Anja 06/03/2008 St Mary's Cottage 56 Church Lane Oxted Surrey RH8 9NB **Tel:** (01883) 714595 w 6400083

SILVER Sarah Helen DipAVN(Surgical) (nee Lidster) 05/09/2000 (06/11/2008) 25 Calthorpe Close BURY ST. EDMUNDS Suffolk IP32 7LQ **Tel:** (01284) 701267 w 6204492

SILVEY Michelle Louise (see WILLIAMS, Mrs)

SIM Donna-Marie Allison (formerly Sim) 31/08/2005 37 Penton Way BASINGSTOKE Hampshire RG24 9RT w 6288521

Donna-Marie Allison (formerly Sim) 31/08/2005 37 Penton Way BASINGSTOKE Hampshire RG24 9RT w 6288521

SIMCOCK Emma Dee (see FOREMAN, Mrs)

SIME Emma Louise 19/07/2006 North Highland College Ormlie Road THURSO Caithness KW14 7DR w 6324700

SIMKIN Jennifer (see ZORLUTUNA, Mrs)

SIMM Laura Emily 03/10/2007 The Veterinary Hospital 221 Beccles Road Gorleston Great Yarmouth Norfolk NR31 8BZ **Tel:** (01493) 661833 w 6366852

SIMMONDS Jennifer Mary 19/03/2007 22 Rosehill Drive Bransgore Christchurch Dorset BH23 8NW **Tel:** 01425673133 w 6372418

Natalie Jane Leader 22/04/2002 147 Maidenhead Road Windsor Berkshire SL4 5EZ **Tel:** (01753) 869477 w 6261065

SIMMONS Emma Jean 04/11/2008 215a Perry Street Billericay Essex CM12 0NZ **Tel:** (01277) 654425 w 6409092

Emma Kate 22/10/2004 34 Kinfauns Ave Hornchurch Essex RM11 2AN **Tel:** (01708) 479653 w 6279776

Jackie Louise 29/06/2007 1 Willow Cottages Nobold Lane Nobold SHREWSBURY SY5 8NN **Tel:** (01743) 365958 w 6328286

SIMMONS Karen Liza (see WEBB, Mrs)

SIMMS Laura Jane (nee Powrie) 20/03/2001 11 Storey Close Helmsley YORK YO62 5DP **Tel:** (01439) 771532 w 6205339

SIMON Kirsty Samantha 06/03/2006 2 Home Lawn The Homend Ledbury Herefordshire HR8 1DA **Tel:** (07973) 223005 w 6334765

SIMPKIN Andrea Gail 29/01/2007 18 Caspian Way Wheaton Aston STAFFORD ST19 9PR **Tel:** (01785) 840740 w 6266136

SIMPKIN Lisa Anne (see PEGRAM, Mrs)

SIMPKINS Emma Jeanne (see JOHNSON, Mrs)

SIMPSON Claire Louise (nee Parish) 06/10/2006 Willow Brook 20 Lonewood Way Hadlow TONBRIDGE Kent TN11 0JB w 6318364

SIMPSON Donna (see SLATER, Mrs)

Hannah Jane 01/06/2007 64 West End Road Bitterne Southampton Hampshire SO18 6TG **Tel:** (02380) 447797 w 6372968

Helen Mary 18/06/2008 The Minster Veterinary Practice Salisbury Road York North Yorkshire YO26 4YN **Tel:** (01904) 643997 w 6400732

SIMPSON Jemma (see JOHNSON, Mrs)

Jessica Claire 29/07/2005 1 Carthona Drive Avon Dale Fleet Hampshire GU52 7SF w 6277411

Joanna Elizabeth 20/09/2006 41 Chantrey Road Sheffield South Yorkshire S8 8QU **Tel:** (0114) 281 7951 w 6333467

SIMPSON Lana Helen (see BARCLAY, Mrs)

Laura Jean 16/11/2006 18 St. Oswalds Road Catterick Garrison North Yorkshire DL9 4TD **Tel:** (07763) 331997 w 6351452

Rachel Claire 09/11/2008 6 Willow Court Cleveland Drive FAREHAM Hampshire PO14 1TD **Tel:** (07825) 916106 w 6377786

Sally (nee Jones, formerly Jones) 24/01/2006 (05/01/2010) 122 Brown Lees Road Brown Lees STOKE-ON-TRENT Staffordshire ST8 6PW w 6328990

Sarah Elizabeth 16/05/2006 Quarteracre 12 Stonehill Road Headley Down Bordon Hampshire GU35 8JJ **Tel:** (01428) 714 056 w 6319640

Shirley DipAVN(Surgical) (nee Burke) 21/07/1993 9 Burnbank Grove Straiton LOANHEAD Midlothian EH20 9NX w 6015011

SIMPSON-EYRE Ian Charles 12/04/2001 166 Nottingham Road Eastwood Nottingham NG16 3GG **Tel:** (01773) 769298 m 6205856

SIMPSON-FOORD Cassey 17/01/2008 Sunset View Pett Level Road Winchelsea Beach Winchelsea East Sussex TN36 4ND **Tel:** 07715860042 w 6386608

SIMS Bernadette (formerly Cooper) 19/01/1998 Parvins Cottage South-End Damerham Fordingbridge Hampshire SP6 3HW w 6117159

Sharon Joanne (nee Levett) 27/08/1999 (24/07/2001) Sparrowbush Farm House Thornicombe Blandford Dorset DT11 9AQ **Tel:** (01258) 453275 w 6186232

SINCLAIR Emma Elizabeth 06/04/2001 24 Buckerills BASILDON Essex SS13 3EP **Tel:** (01268) 556464 w 6035515

Jennifer Nicola 11/03/2005 125 Main Street Coaltown Glenrothes Fife KY7 6HZ **Tel:** (01592) 77 9174 w 6288620

Kirsty Jean 23/01/2003 (27/04/2005) Moray Coast Veterinary Group West Road Greshop Estate Forres Morayshire IV36 2GW **Tel:** (01309) 672243 w 6271669

SINES Daniella 04/06/2009 68 Ballards Way South Croydon Surrey CR2 7JN **Tel:** 07590840881 w 6407750

SINEY Rebecca Helen 06/08/2008 17 Bayfield Avenue Frimley Camberley Surrey GU16 8TT **Tel:** (07754) 655 808 w 6387312

SINGLETON Helen Jane 16/12/2009 7 Milner Road Long Eaton NOTTINGHAM NG10 1LB **Tel:** 07709825415 w 6436724

Isabelle 03/12/2003 Cliffe Veterinary Group 21 Cliffe High Street Lewes East Sussex BN7 2AH **Tel:** (01273) 473232 w 6280227

Rachel Lucy (nee Beauchamp) 24/11/2005 Rocky Peak Froggatt Edge Calver HOPE VALLEY Derbyshire S32 3ZB w 6333742

SIRRELL Fiona Elizabeth (nee McGregor) 03/05/2007 20 Pretoria Court Coalburn Lanark Lanarkshire ML11 0DY **Tel:** (01555) 820616 w 6377742

SITCH Natalie Elaine (see WARD, Mrs)

SIVELL Rebecca Elizabeth Ann 29/05/2008 40 Primrose Way Kidderminster Worcestershire DY10 1NG **Tel:** (01562) 827746 w 6352849

SIVYER Samantha (nee Sivyer, formerly Honeywill) 13/08/2003 69 Compton Crescent Chessington Surrey KT9 2HD **Tel:** (020) 8287 6129 w 6282031

SKATES Gemma Louise (see BARKER, Mrs)

SKEET Holly Elizabeth 14/01/2008 31 Kite Farm WHITSTABLE Kent CT5 2PA **Tel:** (01227) 791933 w 6383704

SKELTON Alison Jean DipAVN(Surgical) 01/08/1986 27 Hunters Lane Leavesden Hertfordshire WD25 7BA **Tel:** (01923) 678797 w 6045272

SKEOCH Cheryl Linda (see MURRAY, Mrs)

SKIDMORE Kathryn 22/02/2007 2 Mallowdale Nunthorpe Middlesbrough Cleveland TS7 0QA **Tel:** (01642) 276 933 w 6358877

SKILLEN Nicola Susan 15/01/2008 36 Bassant Road London SE18 2NP **Tel:** (0208) 8553101 w 6378886

SKILLING Caroline Christina 19/03/2007 125 Millhouse Lane Moreton Wirral Merseyside CH46 6EF **Tel:** (0151) 522 0834 w 6376609

SKINGLE Janine Fay (see HOUGHTON, Mrs)

SKINNER Kerry Marie DipAVN(Surgical) 06/03/2001 Ivel Cottage Tingeys Corner Lower Caldecote Bedfordshire SG18 9BE **Tel:** (01767) 313502 w 6205724

Pamela Jayne 27/09/1999 19 Summerfields Dalston Carlisle Cumbria CA5 7NW **Tel:** (01228) 712230 w 6144295

SKIPSEY Helen (see BLAMIRES, Ms)

SKIRROW Emma Elizabeth 07/04/2008 Troutbeck Horebeech Lane Horam HEATHFIELD East Sussex TN21 0HR w 6378897

SLACK Julie Margaret (see KELSALL, Mrs)

SLACK Kate (nee Roberts) 04/09/1997 40 Lambert Court Kingswinford West Midlands DY6 7RA w 6131661

SLADE Lisa Jane 30/09/2008 27 Wades Road Bristol Avon BS34 7EA **Tel:** (07775) 518 835 w 6439727

Louisa Marion 09/06/2009 98 Deepfield Road Bracknell Berkshire RG12 2NX **Tel:** 01344483685 w 6449121

SLADEN Joanne Marie 25/08/2009 Drybridge Veterinary Clinic 2a Wonastow Road Monmouth Gwent NP25 5AH **Tel:** (01600) 712206 w 6447119

SLATER Donna (nee Simpson) 26/10/2006 5 Friary Court 25 Lower Port View Saltash Cornwall PL12 4BZ **Tel:** (01752) 844909 w 6344929

SLATER Elaine (see MOIR, Mrs)

SLATER Victoria Louise (see MORRIS, Mrs)

SLATTER Claire Louise (nee Longshaw) 22/04/2003 University of Cambridge Madingley Road Cambridge Cambridgeshire CB3 0ES **Tel:** (01223) 337621 w 6278434

SLEE Heather 18/02/2009 Flat 37 Scotney Gardens Riverside Crescent St. Peters Street MAIDSTONE Kent ME16 0GR w 6441828

SLEIGH Lisa 16/06/2006 36 Clipstone Road West Forest Town Mansfield Nottinghamshire NG19 0BU **Tel:** (01623) 643888 w 6354752

SLINGER Laura 27/03/2009 8 Jacklin Close Branston BURTON-ON-TRENT Staffordshire DE14 3HH w 6288994

SLOANE Julie Anne 24/12/2002 The Green Main Road Dibden SOUTHAMPTON SO45 5TE **Tel:** (023) 8084 2292 w 6277334

SMALL Claire Angela 27/04/2005 Three Gables Heath Close Homer Green High Wycombe Buckinghamshire HP15 6UB **Tel:** (01494) 713773 w 6279886

Deborah Louise 15/11/2005 6 The Fairway ST. LEONARDS-ON-SEA East Sussex TN38 0UT **Tel:** (01424) 426357 w 6346040

Suzanne 15/12/2004 (05/03/2009) 32 Rylands Road Whitecross Dunblane Perthshire FK15 0HN **Tel:** (01786) 825 023 w 6291480

SMALLEY Joanne Emma 13/05/2003 Glenthorne Moss House Lane Much Hoole Preston Lancashire PR4 4TD **Tel:** (01772) 614982 w 6281074

SMART Donna (see SAUNDERS, Mrs)

SMART Michelle Louise 29/04/2009 Barton Lodge Veterinary Centre 1 Midland Road Hemel Hempstead Hertfordshire HP2 5BH **Tel:** (01442) 216048 w 6431818

Naomi Alice 04/07/2007 Barn Lodge Veterinary Hospital 54A Southport Road Ormskirk Lancashire L39 1LX **Tel:** (01695) 572837 w 6355896

SMEATH Michelle Louise (nee Bailey) 29/01/2001 Pelyn Veterinary Group 8 Kings Avenue St. Austell Cornwall PL25 4TT **Tel:** (01726) 68177 w 6143939

SMEE Rebecca Anne 05/12/2008 18 Somerset Walk Tilehurst Reading Berkshire RG31 5NG **Tel:** (0118) 9412895 w 6378908

SMILLIE Diane Irene (nee MacLean) 04/08/1981 (21/10/2003) 44 MacFarlane Road Bearsden Glasgow Lanarkshire G61 2HN **Tel:** 01419428694 w 6089356

SMIT Pauline Marije 07/02/2006 511 Wilbraham Road Manchester M21 0UB **Tel:** (0161) 881 3329 w 6417947

SMITH Adrian Eric 18/09/2008 Paws by the Park Vets 122 Glenthorne Road Hammersmith London W6 0LP m 6378919

Amanda Jane (nee Clayton) 02/08/1988 82 Wellington Road Ashton-under-Lyne Lancashire OL6 6DP **Tel:** (0161) 330 2514/4839 w 6047735

SMITH Amanda Louise (see WARMAN, Mrs)

Amy Jane 18/05/2009 68 Greenway Lane Chippenham Wiltshire SN15 1AF **Tel:** (07814) 880 383 w 6437967

SMITH Beverley Denise (see ANDREWS, Ms)

Carla Louise 11/11/2009 32 Howberry Green Arlesey Bedfordshire SG15 6ZA **Tel:** 01462834629 w 6445579

Carly Rebecca 19/03/2007 7 Woodfield Road Dursley Gloucestershire GL11 6HA **Tel:** (01453) 548 815 w 6359757

SMITH Catherine Martha (see RICE, Mrs)

Cathy 03/05/2007 1 Picton Drive Winsford Cheshire CW7 2JB **Tel:** (01606) 863 630 w 6377797

Claire Joy (nee Trebble) 29/08/2007 City Vets 101 Buddle Lane St Thomas Exeter EX4 1QS **Tel:** (01392) 250000 w 6305351

Claire Rachel 21/07/2008 22 West Road Ormesby GREAT YARMOUTH Norfolk NR29 3RP **Tel:** 07816969849 w 6376158

Clare Agnes (nee Morgan) 09/09/1996 (26/01/2004) 17 Argyle Street Rothesay ISLE OF BUTE PA20 0AU **Tel:** (01700) 503017 w 603564X

Clare Jayne (nee Stockton) 13/04/2004 42 Newport Grove Mitchells Wood Chesterton Newcastle Staffordshire ST5 7QL **Tel:** (01782) 564129 w 6277906

SMITH Clare Louise (see ESPLEY, Mrs)

Dawn Elizabeth 23/08/2000 (07/04/2005) 15 Westfields Little Harrowden WELLINGBOROUGH Northamptonshire NN9 5BQ w 6203073

Debbie Anne 27/01/2005 The Veterinary Surgery Hollybush Road Bridgnorth Shropshire WV16 4AR **Tel:** (01746) 763 998 w 6272472

Deborah 04/04/2008 86 Farneworth Road Mickleover Derby Derbyshire DE3 0ES w 6351463

Deborah Ann 08/11/2006 8 Laverock Lea Fareham Hampshire PO16 8DA **Tel:** (023) 9271 9509 w 6378259

Debra Kay (nee Leigh) 30/07/2002 38 Dunlin Drive Washington Tyne and Wear NE38 0EB **Tel:** (0191) 4170898 w 6269084

Donna Lorraine 03/03/2005 43 Empingham Road STAMFORD Lincolnshire PE9 2RJ **Tel:** (07943) 838916 w 6319189

Donna Maria 09/09/2004 New Era Veterinary Hospital Victoria Road St Saviour Jersey JE2 7QG **Tel:** (01534) 730521 w 6292041

Eilidh Gail Hunter 23/02/2005 50/6 Manor Place EDINBURGH EH3 7EH w 6271152

Eleanor Elizabeth 09/09/2004 36 Cae Onan Morda OSWESTRY Shropshire SY10 9PX **Tel:** (01691) 670037 w 6290655

Elise Rachel 05/07/2006 88-92 Merton High Street Merton London SW19 1BD **Tel:** (020) 8254 1400 w 6322027

Emma Charlotte 16/07/2007 5 Hood Walk Romford Essex RM7 8NU **Tel:** (01708) 721275 w 6381933

Emma Louise 09/12/2009 5 South View Hipsburn Alnwick Northumberland NE66 3PZ **Tel:** 01665830718 w 6489348

Erin Laura 29/05/2009 Saratoga Castledyke Bank Gipsey Bridge BOSTON Lincolnshire PE22 7BW **Tel:** 07921088253 w 6417595

Estelle Frances (nee Kilb) 03/02/2005 97 River Meads Stanstead Abbotts WARE Hertfordshire SG12 8EL w 6320938

SMITH Esther Jayne (see JONES, Mrs)

Gayle Wendy 06/03/2009 Apple Croft Aberchirder HUNTLY Aberdeenshire AB54 7QD w 6446844

Gemma 07/04/2006 Castle Veterinary Surgeons Montalbo Road Barnard Castle County Durham DL12 8ED **Tel:** (01833) 695695 w 6350781

Gemma Louise 04/04/2008 16 Mayenne Place Devizes Wiltshire SN10 1QJ **Tel:** (01380) 722 178 w 6403691

Haley Joanne 07/02/2006 Greenhedges East Grinstead Road North Chailey LEWES East Sussex BN8 4HX **Tel:** (01825) 724421 w 6333731

Hannah Katie Jean 11/01/2005 14 Teddington Close EPSOM Surrey KT19 9DW w 6301182

Helen Elizabeth 24/11/2004 52 Kemp Street Fleetwood Lancashire FY7 6DY **Tel:** (01253) 872860 w 6287355

Holly Elaine 29/06/2007 73 Woods Avenue Hatfield Hertfordshire AL10 8QF **Tel:** (01707) 260064 w 6384914

Holly Suzanne DipAVN(Surgical) 03/08/1992 (01/03/2002) Queen Mother Hospital for Small Animals Hawkshead Lane North Mymms Hatfield Hertfordshire AL9 7TA **Tel:** (01707) 666366 w 6007736

Jacqueline Mary (nee Allen, formerly Bishop) 01/08/1972 7 Fox Close Saddington Grange Fleckney Leicester LE8 8DE **Tel:** (01162) 402468 w 6045658

Janet 27/02/2002 20 Archer Street Ilkeston Derbyshire DE7 8JX w 6269678

Jemma 25/09/2009 2 Castle Close Noak Hill Romford Essex RM3 7LN **Tel:** 01708341238 w 6488985

Jennifer DipAVN(Surgical) 09/08/1983 (06/12/1999) University of Nottingham Sutton Bonington Campus LOUGHBOROUGH Leicestershire LE12 5RD **Tel:** (0115) 9516464 w 6060869

SMITH Jennifer Joanne (see BETTERIDGE, Mrs)

Jennifer Louise 06/05/2009 54a Main Road Portskewett Caldicot Gwent NP26 5SA **Tel:** 01291422255 w 6411930

SMITH Jessica Fay (see DEACON, Mrs)

Joanna 11/09/2009 32 Exning Road NEWMARKET Suffolk CB8 0AB **Tel:** (01638) 601142 w 6249889

Julia Catherine 02/06/2004 c/o Christine Smith 60 The Manor Drive Worcester Park Surrey KT4 7LJ **Tel:** (07817) 763 806 w 6302678

Julia Michelle (nee Ford) 24/09/1987 Glenthorne Veterinary Centre 71 Derby Road Uttoxeter Staffordshire ST14 8EB **Tel:** (01889) 562164 w 6050555

Julie Elizabeth 29/05/2009 14 Abbotswood Close Winyates Green REDDITCH Worcestershire B98 0QD **Tel:** (07843) 482809 w 6445238

SMITH Justine (see THORNE, Mrs)

Karen Michelle (nee Shooter) 30/11/2006 53 The Green Rawcliffe GOOLE North Humberside DN14 8QF **Tel:** (01405) 831 096 w 6267511

Katie Jane 01/04/2003 (16/06/2009) Cats Protection National Cat Centre Veterinary Clinic Chelwood Gate Haywards Heath West Sussex RH17 7TT **Tel:** (01825) 741991 w 6282097

SMITH Katrina Joanne (see JOHNSON, Mrs)

Kelly Jayne 10/10/2005 The Veterinary Centre Queen Annes Road GREAT YARMOUTH Norfolk NR31 0LE **Tel:** (01493) 416700 w 6322038

Kelly Marie 16/11/2006 Dogs Trust Hillhouse Lane Sadberge DARLINGTON County Durham DL2 1SL **Tel:** (01325) 333114 w 6355797

Kirstie Eileen 22/03/2004 128 Hazeldene Road Northampton Northamptonshire NN2 7NB **Tel:** (01604) 720560 w 6271031

Kirsty 27/01/2010 80 Willoughby Road Bourne Lincolnshire PE10 0DQ w 6489744

Laura Amy 12/10/2007 The Mewes Veterinary Clinic 4 Haywards Road Haywards Heath West Sussex RH16 4HT **Tel:** (01444) 456886 w 6356303

Laura Catherine (nee Cox) 13/07/2004 Eastfield Veterinary Clinic Ltd Station Road North Thoresby GRIMSBY Lincolnshire DN36 5QU **Tel:** (01472) 840209 w 6284539

Laura Dawn 17/01/2008 6 Queens Close Ludgershall ANDOVER Hampshire SP11 9SN **Tel:** (07515) 664 226 w 6386190

Laura Jane 04/05/2006 26 Marine Court Torpoint Cornwall PL11 2RB **Tel:** (07812) 114069 w 6301809

Laura Madeline 02/07/2008 59 March Road Wimblington March Cambridgeshire PE15 0RW **Tel:** 07949568647 w 6376631

Lesley Louise 05/04/2005 1-5 Hugh Street London SW1V 1QQ **Tel:** (020) 7932 2370 w 6322390

Lisa 21/06/2005 9 Admiral Way Berkhamsted Hertfordshire HP4 1TE **Tel:** (01442) 862 573 w 6291810

Louisa Michelle (nee Retief) 24/01/2003 (18/03/2009) 8 Rothesay Avenue LONDON SW20 8JU w 6328814

Lucy Alison 04/02/2002 68 Ratcliffe Court Sweetman Place BRISTOL BS2 0FB w 6254586

Michelle Lesley 31/10/2003 (08/01/2009) 3 Borden Lane Sittingbourne Kent ME10 1BT **Tel:** (01795) 423227 w 6268864

Michelle Louise 15/11/2005 (08/02/2008) 12 Highfield Drive Longridge Preston Lancashire PR3 3SN **Tel:** (01772) 783688 w 6325844

SMITH Michelle Louise (see BRISTOW, Mrs)

Natalie Angela 22/12/2009 14 Cubert Road Croxteth LIVERPOOL L11 0BU w 6494474

Natasha Emma 26/08/2009 65 The Copse Hertford Hertfordshire SG13 7TX **Tel:** (01992) 628 574 w 6445282

Neil Leslie John 01/04/2003 (12/01/2009) 57 Manton Villas WORKSOP Nottinghamshire S80 2QJ m 6268963

Penelope Frances Hilton 27/02/2006 (11/02/2009) 73 Gainsborough Drive Selsey Chichester West Sussex PO20 0HH **Tel:** (01442) 212560 w 6349142

Philomena Helen 26/10/2005 2 Ellen House Clarendon Road HOVE East Sussex BN3 3WX w 6350198

Rachel (nee Phillips) 01/04/2003 (21/07/2006) 3 Pool Lane Brocton Stafford Staffordshire ST17 0TR w 6285815

Rachel Elizabeth 04/09/1998 Winning Park West Sleekburn Bedlington Northumberland NE22 7BY **Tel:** (01670) 828451 w 6098713

Rachel Lee 13/05/2003 29 Forsythia Close Northfield BIRMINGHAM B31 1XN **Tel:** (01527) 853570 w 6272197

Rebecca Clare 27/02/2007 51 Doubleday Drive Bapchild Sittingbourne Kent ME9 9PJ **Tel:** (07810) 552902 w 6352882

Rebecca Louise 21/05/2003 Wilton House Veterinary Clinic Wilton Lane Guisborough Cleveland TS14 6JA **Tel:** (01287) 637470 w 6260306

Rebecca Louise 06/06/2003 4 Battersea Park Road Battersea London SW8 4AA **Tel:** (020) 7627 9256 w 6273616

Sally Marie 15/04/2004 (20/05/2009) 1 Gamekeepers Drive WORCESTER WR4 9SN w 6299653

Samantha Jane 25/01/1994 Bridge Veterinary Surgery 205 Fir Tree Road Epsom Surrey KT17 3LB **Tel:** (01737) 351482 w 6066190

Sarah Elizabeth 29/12/2009 Avonvale Veterinary Centres Ltd 88 Coventry Street Southam Warwickshire CV47 0EA **Tel:** (01926) 812826 w 6495849

Sarah Louise (nee Tatford) 17/11/2004 Vale Veterinary Group 28 Birmingham Road Kidderminster Worcestershire DY10 2DA **Tel:** (01562) 822692 w 6273044

SMITH Selena Jane (see BURROUGHS, Mrs)

Sharon 18/09/2000 183 The Loaning Motherwell Lanarkshire ML1 3LN **Tel:** (01698) 275990 w 6138408

Shelley Anne 06/12/2004 81 Hoveton Close REDDITCH Worcestershire B98 7HW **Tel:** (07800) 743037 w 6327527

Sheree Angela 31/07/2009 134 Arlescote Road SOLIHULL West Midlands B92 9HZ w 6561750

SMITH Tracey Jayne (see TRIPICCHIO, Mrs)

SMITH Valerie Ann (see BELBIN, Mrs)

Victoria Elizabeth 04/10/2005 Chapelfield Veterinary Partnership Wellesley Road Tharston Industrial Estate Long Stratton Norfolk NR15 2PD **Tel:** (01508) 530686 w 6300643

SMITH Victoria Joyce (see ANDREWS, Mrs)

Victoria Lillian 05/07/2006 32 Annalee Gardens South Ockendon Essex RM15 5DF **Tel:** (0208) 507 3904 w 6321620

Vivien Nellie 05/02/1992 (06/11/2000) March Wall Kings Drive North Caldy Wirral Merseyside CH48 1LL **Tel:** (0151) 625 2320 w 6002217

Wendy Louise DipAVN(Surgical) (nee Waller) 09/01/1990 (07/08/2009) 54 King Arthur Drive Glen Waverley Victoria 3150 Australia w 6063021

SMITH-CRESSWELL Perdita (see WELSH, Mrs)

SMITH-GILLARD Wayne Russell 21/10/1999 NKR Veterinary Specialists Warren Road Bluebell Hill Chatham Kent ME5 9RD **Tel:** (01634) 666655 m 6152557

SMYTH Brian Christopher 08/02/2000 (07/12/2001) Attimore Veterinary Hospital Ridgeway Welwyn Garden City Hertfordshire AL7 2AD **Tel:** (01707) 331693 m 611839X

Marie 20/11/2009 53 The Swallows WELWYN GARDEN CITY Hertfordshire AL7 1BX **Tel:** 01707328179 w 6437802

SNAITH Clare Elizabeth 10/12/2007 Valley View Farm Marefield Lane Tilton on the Hill Leicester Leicestershire LE7 9LJ **Tel:** 01162597715 w 6377577

SNART Toni Melanie (see MIDDLETON, Mrs)

SNEDDEN Lauren Carolyn 03/10/2007 195 Renfrew Rd Paisley Renfrewshire PA3 4JJ **Tel:** (0141) 5697458 w 6276905

SNELGROVE Victoria Jayne (see JERMEY, Mrs)

SNELL Victoria Elizabeth 25/04/2008 3 Dowlaw Farm Cottages Coldingham EYEMOUTH Berwickshire TD14 5TY w 6385728

SNOW Lisa Julie Elizabeth 14/03/2006 10 Catherine Street Avonmouth Bristol Avon BS11 9LG **Tel:** (0117) 9828 388 w 6350209

SNOWDEN Lynda Amy 20/07/2009 6 Osterley Close Botley Southampton Hampshire SO30 2EX **Tel:** (01489) 691012 w 6378930

SNOWDON Emma Joy (nee Snowdon, formerly Parsonage) 02/02/1999 56 Brackenhill Close Brayton Selby North Yorkshire YO8 9RZ **Tel:** (01757) 708805 w 6026941

SOAR Kylie Louise 28/01/2009 62 Ravenswood Hill Coleshill BIRMINGHAM B46 1BW **Tel:** 07795154164 w 6436955

SOFFE Natalie Charlotte 18/03/2008 178 Locks Road Locks Heath Southampton Hampshire SO31 6LE **Tel:** (01489) 607001 w 6351991

SOFTLEY Beverley 26/04/1973 1 Ashendene Road Bayford Hertford SG13 8PX **Tel:** (01992) 511254 w 6061046

SOLEY Dawn Allison 23/11/2000 Adelaide Veterinary Centre Long Lane Bursledon Southampton Hampshire SO31 8DA **Tel:** (023) 8040 6215 w 6132585

SOLOMAN-KRETAY Jennifer Karen 01/03/2001 207 Valley Way Stevenage Hertfordshire SG2 9BU **Tel:** (01438) 357548 w 6204404

SOMERFIELD Jodie Selina 06/11/2007 35 Church Road Pelsall WALSALL WS3 4QW **Tel:** (01922) 684918 w 6378743

SOMMERFELD Sandra Katrina 03/08/1993 19a Hillside Avenue Frindsbury ROCHESTER Kent ME2 3DB **Tel:** (01634) 310 964 w 6024478

SONLEY Sarah Kathleen (nee Gifford) 15/08/1991 1 St. Marks Close Newington SITTINGBOURNE Kent ME9 7JQ **Tel:** (01795) 843085 w 6000752

SOUTHALL Anna 04/12/2003 'Dene Bank' Racecourse Lane Stourbridge West Midlands DY8 2RF **Tel:** (01562) 833621 or 01527 872488 w 6277785

Miranda Jane 15/04/2004 135d Cemetery Road Stourbridge West Midlands DY9 8AL w 6277389

SOUTHAM Natasha Louise (see PAYNE, Mrs)

SOUTHGATE Emma Jane 22/12/2004 21 Dukes Farm Road Billericay Essex CM12 0QA **Tel:** (01277) 651989 w 6316846

SOUTHWORTH Sarah May 07/12/2007 89 Shakespeare Road Gillingham Kent ME7 5QJ **Tel:** (01634) 853783 w 6383715

SOUTRY Lucinda Caroline (see THUILLIEZ, Mrs)

SOUTTAR Kim (nee Grieve) 16/07/2002 Dept Veterinary Basic Sciences Royal Veterinary College Royal College Street London NW1 0TU **Tel:** (0207) 4685260 w 6261978

SOWERBY Alison Elizabeth 08/09/1998 95 High Street Stonebroom ALFRETON Derbyshire DE55 6JY **Tel:** (01773) 874315 w 6136739

SPARKERS Rachel (see SPARKES, Mrs)

SPARKES Rachel (formerly Sparkers) 06/08/2008 14 Sudbrook Close Wickford Essex SS12 9BN **Tel:** (01268) 471517 w 6298168

SPARKS Leanne Claire 18/01/2008 1 Harmony Place Mountain Queensbury Bradford West Yorkshire BD13 1LD **Tel:** (01274) 818 424 w 6409378

Sophie Elizabeth 25/06/2004 (05/06/2006) 314 Ball Road RD2 Patea South Taranaki 4598 New Zealand w 6273121

SPARKSMAN Kate Patricia 04/06/2009 First Floor Flat 10 Bellevue Clifton BRISTOL Avon BS8 1DA **Tel:** 07939321621 w 6426538

SPARLING Clare Marie 24/01/2000 141 St. Austell Way SWINDON SN2 2DF w 6190489

SPARROWHAWK Sinead May 25/02/1999 6 Stoneleigh Road OXTED Surrey RH8 0TR **Tel:** (01883) 717734 w 612911X

SPEAKES Karen Elizabeth 05/08/1992 36 Brookwater Close Tottington Bury Lancashire BL8 3LD **Tel:** (01204) 882486 w 6005466

SPEAR Amanda 03/12/2003 187 Pellon Lane Halifax West Yorkshire HX1 5RJ **Tel:** (01422) 354542 w 6284803

Katherine Victoria 09/12/2008 The Chase Harlyn Bay PADSTOW Cornwall PL28 8SB w 6439694

Lesley Ann 26/10/2005 17 Rutland Drive MORDEN Surrey SM4 5QD **Tel:** (020) 8648 4273 w 6334787

SPECHT Anna Elizabeth (nee Comber) 05/06/2006 The Meopham Veterinary Surgery Wrotham Road Meopham Gravesend Kent DA13 0QG **Tel:** (01474) 815333 w 6345424

SPENCE Katherine Anne (see ALEXANDER, Mrs)

SPENCE Kierann Louise 07/11/2008 18 Cranleigh Drive CHEADLE Cheshire SK8 2DJ w 6419982

SPENCELEY Alexandra Gentle (nee Lewins) 24/10/2008 24 Tiberius Road ANDOVER Hampshire SP10 5JX **Tel:** (0779) 1014366 w 6412810

SPENCER Bethan Sian (nee Cook) 21/01/2008 10 Taliesin Close Pencoed Bridgend Mid Glamorgan CF35 6JR **Tel:** 01656-865-320 w 6337592

Helen 24/09/1999 66 Holly Avenue Breaston DERBY DE72 3BG **Tel:** (07930) 692243 w 6185220

Jodi Diane 07/12/2006 Apartment 10 4 Rea Place Digbeth BIRMINGHAM B12 0NP **Tel:** (07977) 239374 w 6351804

SPENCER Louise Catherine (see HUMPHREYS, Mrs)

Sarah Elizabeth Joan 18/02/2008 37 Rock Avenue Nailsea BRISTOL BS48 2AN **Tel:** (07769) 844 981 w 6411391

Sarah Jane 10/02/2000 11 Hurstville Drive WATERLOOVILLE Hampshire PO7 7NB w 6191402

SPERRING Lucy Joanne 10/01/2007 4 Elm Court Keynsham Bristol Avon BS31 2RB **Tel:** (0117) 9865217 w 6371747

SPIERS Laura Ann 08/01/2008 2 Whitworth Mews Hucclecote Gloucester Gloucestershire GL3 3TN **Tel:** (01452) 612499 w 6404021

SPILLER Kerry Louise (see GULLIVER, Mrs)

SPILLETT Abigail Louise 22/10/2004 39 Dover Way Pitsea Basildon Essex SS13 3RJ **Tel:** (01268) 417 042 w 6297343

SPINK Katherine (see PIKE, Mrs)

SPINKS Clare 21/06/2005 35 Sawkins Gardens CHELMSFORD CM2 9SD **Tel:** (01953) 454945 w 6276619

SPITZMAUL Katie Dawn 10/02/2005 7 Quantock Close Hereford Herefordshire HR4 0TD **Tel:** (01432) 265744 w 6323501

SPOONER Elyse 29/08/1995 (27/11/2000) Flat 2 HollyBank Southampton Road RINGWOOD Hampshire BH24 3HL **Tel:** (07809) 372217 w 6038196

SPRINGALL Jessica Laura 15/06/2009 8 Poynton Close Grappenhall Warrington Cheshire WA4 2NG **Tel:** 01925269045 w 6407618

SPRING-GAY Cassandra Jane 02/06/2004 7 Kipling Drive Larkfield Aylesford Kent ME20 6UJ **Tel:** (01732) 847986 w 6293504

SPRY Joanne Lesley (see KERR, Mrs)

SPURR Katherine Anne 19/10/2009 Crossways 4 Coolinge Lane Folkestone Kent CT20 3RE **Tel:** 07854363394 w 6440431

SQUIRE Sally Jane (nee Webber) 20/11/2002 92 Carlton Avenue WESTCLIFF-ON-SEA Essex SS0 0QL **Tel:** (01702) 430796 w 6268226

SQUIRRELL Joanne Victoria 09/05/2008 11 Parkhurst Road Bexley Kent DA5 1AX **Tel:** (01322) 523523 w 6290248

Zoe Anne 05/01/2005 (11/05/2009) 65 Claremont Road SWANLEY Kent BR8 7QS **Tel:** (01322) 664563 w 6293042

SRAMKO Olga Aleksandrovna 02/06/2004 Flat 65, Harold Gibbons Court Victoria Way London SE7 7LY w 6333478

SRIH Sarah 17/01/1995 4 Jubalton Close Allenton Derby Derbyshire DE24 9BN w 603767X

SROWE Charlene Jemima (see STOWE, Miss)

ST CLAIR TISDALL Sophie Diana 06/05/2008 Kings Apartments 13/13 Valleyfield Street EDINBURGH EH3 9LP w 6377544

ST JOHN Tracey Jane 31/10/2003 (27/06/2005) 26 Keward Avenue Wells Somerset BA5 1TS **Tel:** (01749) 679528 w 6259217

ST JOHN-SMITH Estelle (nee Barber) 10/04/2003 12 Sandford Leaze Avening Tetbury Gloucestershire GL8 8PB **Tel:** (01666) 505209 w 6269480

ST PIERRE Nicole Marie 05/10/2001 (13/08/2009) 5 Bassant Road Plumstead LONDON SE18 2NP w 6135804

STACEY Alison Jane (see RICHARDSON, Mrs)

STACEY Nicola 18/01/1996 (02/10/2001) RSPCA Wildlife Hospital West Hatch Taunton Somerset TA3 5RT **Tel:** (01823) 278420 w 6036064

STACKHOUSE Elizabeth Grace (nee Lancaster) 27/02/2006 Dale View Bilsborrow Lane Bilsborrow Preston Lancashire PR3 0RN **Tel:** (01995) 640 297 w 6304064

STAFFORD Karen Louise 09/05/2006 Bond Street Veterinary Clinic 1 Ryles Park Road Macclesfield Cheshire SK11 8AH **Tel:** (01625) 425637 w 6351474

Sara Dawn 25/01/1999 Avenue Veterinary Centre Pendennis Avenue Staple Hill Bristol BS16 5DW **Tel:** (0117) 956 9038 w 6131311

STAFFORD Sarah Louise (see BANNING, Mrs)

Sharon 04/10/2005 74 Hambleton Avenue THIRSK North Yorkshire YO7 1EG w 6346051

STAGGS-O'GRADY Kira 17/11/2009 71 Surrey Road IPSWICH IP1 2LF **Tel:** (01473) 210115 w 6573157

STAHL Natalie Clare (nee Tree) 21/06/2005 The Lodge R S P C A West Hatch Taunton Somerset TA3 5RT **Tel:** (01823) 480156 w 6293515

STALKER Amanda Jane 08/09/2009 2 Highfield Cottages Wingfield Road ALFRETON Derbyshire DE55 7AP **Tel:** 01773835465 w 6448395

STALLON Emma Louise 09/04/2003 70 Trinity Road Stamford Lincolnshire PE9 1BP **Tel:** (01780) 751493 w 6278104

STALLWORTHY Donna (see PIPER, Mrs)

STAMPER Elizabeth Amy 11/04/2005 3 Arnold Road Manchester Lancashire M16 8NQ **Tel:** (0161) 881 4578 w 6307947

STANDFORD Jennifer Merenda (see STANFORD, Miss)

STANFIELD Karen Anne 27/10/2009 Craigend Albert Street NAIRN IV12 4HF **Tel:** (01667) 453289 w 6407970

STANFIELD Laura Linda (see MCALLISTER, Mrs)

STANFORD Ann Elizabeth 05/07/2006 Steep Side Cross Lane Findon Worthing West Sussex BN14 0UG **Tel:** (07762) 156989 w 6321631

Jennifer Merenda (formerly Standford) 07/06/2005 Steepside Cross Lane Findon West Sussex BN14 0UG **Tel:** (0779) 322 8521 w 6326537

Kimberlee Hannah 16/04/2007 Northdale Veterinary Surgery 48 Victoria Road Worthing West Sussex BN11 1XE **Tel:** (01903) 202474 w 6367193

STANGER Louise Jane 24/07/2003 24 Ash Crescent Nuthall NOTTINGHAM NG16 1EY w 6276586

Michelle Louise 23/03/2007 4 Park View Burnopfield Newcastle upon Tyne Tyne and Wear NE16 6QE **Tel:** (01207) 271 801 w 6381944

STANHOPE Victoria Jayne 04/11/2008 53 Kent Street FLEETWOOD Lancashire FY7 6AS **Tel:** (07762) 811 712 w 6411028

STANIER Karen Louise (nee Bailey) 02/03/1994 10 Fitz Crescent MACCLESFIELD Cheshire SK10 2HX **Tel:** (01625) 619988 w 6033121

STANISLAS Kirstie Louise (nee Morris) 03/12/2003 56 Holmesland Drive Botley Southampton Hampshire SO30 2SH **Tel:** (07900) 252166 w 6266840

STANLEY Claire Lorraine (nee Mundy) 06/10/1999 Daventry Veterinary Clinic Stephenson Close Drayton Fields Daventry Northamptonshire NN11 8RF **Tel:** (01327) 877767 w 6186034

STANLEY Hannah Marie (see JONES, Mrs)

STANLEY Jennine Marie (see IREDALE, Mrs)

Lisa 17/01/2007 (06/04/2009) 37 Luton Road Chalton Bedfordshire LU4 9UJ **Tel:** (01525) 872152 w 6296870

STANSMORE-HALL Amy Louise 19/09/2006 11 Uplands Avenue WORTHING West Sussex BN13 3AA **Tel:** (01903) 265641 w 6340452

STANTIFORD Emma Kate 15/11/2001 Honeysuckle Veterinary Surgery Tunnel Road Beaminster Dorset DT8 3HB **Tel:** (01308) 862312 w 6205746

STANTON Cheryl Dawn (see HOLE, Mrs)

STANTON Lyndsey Ann 02/11/2004 14 Summerdale BILLERICAY Essex CM12 9EL **Tel:** (01277) 227462 w 6311412

STAPLIN Nicola Lynne (nee Robson) 24/01/1996 Hare & Hounds Veterinary Centre Sunderland

Road Gilesgate DURHAM DH1 2LG **Tel:** (0191) 386 4477 w 6033824

STARKEY Helen Elizabeth 20/11/2002 31 Tintagel Gardens Rochester Kent ME2 2RD **Tel:** (01634) 726377 w 6277664

Naomi Ruth (nee Gooding) 03/06/2004 6 Windsor Drive Brinscall Chorley Lancashire PR6 8PX **Tel:** (01772) 743933 w 6292756

STARKIE Hannah Jane 04/02/2000 22 Medlars Mead Hatfield Broad Oak Bishop's Stortford Hertfordshire CM22 7JB **Tel:** (01279) 718 447 w 6190665

STARLING Erica Carla 31/10/2003 28 Station Road Walmer Deal Kent CT14 7QS **Tel:** (01304) 365846 w 6285441

STARSMORE Amanda Helen 02/06/2004 6 Hillside Walk Yaxley Peterborough Cambridgeshire PE7 3ES **Tel:** (01832) 273342 w 6288213

START Donna Michelle (see HERON, Mrs)

START Victoria Jane 18/10/2005 99 Dunster Road Newthorpe Nottingham Nottinghamshire NG16 2DW **Tel:** (01773) 763283 w 6332004

STATHAM Katie Louise 16/09/2009 41 Underhill Lane Underhill Wolverhampton WV10 8NT **Tel:** (01902) 685219 w 6435360

STEAD Lisa Jayne (see COLLINS, Mrs)

STEADMAN Hayley Suzanne 24/02/2009 77 Old Road Hyde Manchester Cheshire SK14 4SP **Tel:** (07897) 444 299 w 6449143

Maria Daniella Collette 31/12/2008 Grange Farm Platts Lane Bucknall Woodhall Spa Lincolnshire LN10 5DY **Tel:** 01526388662 w 6398246

Sarah Maureen 21/08/1998 48 Albert Road St Philips Bristol BS2 0XA **Tel:** (0117) 972 4567 w 6131333

STEANS Gemma Katie 11/12/2009 6 Heol y Bryn Synod Inn LLANDYSUL Dyfed SA44 6JQ **Tel:** 07792357920 w 6433523

STEBBING Margaret Anne 06/11/1972 28 Ash Grove Melbourn Royston Hertfordshire SG8 6BJ **Tel:** (01763) 261956 w 6061217

STEEL Kathryn Tammy (see WHITTLE, Mrs)

STEELE Katie Danielle 06/10/2006 38 Cleeve Close Churchill Redditch Worcestershire B98 9HR **Tel:** (01527) 63011 w 6272230

Mary Helen (nee Savile) 03/03/2005 3 Whydown Cottages Whydown Road Bexhill-on-Sea East Sussex TN39 4RD **Tel:** (01424) 842 097 w 6317726

STEER Helen Christine (nee Shaw) 13/05/1999 Flat 6, Burns Court Broad Street Modbury Ivybridge Devon PL21 0PY **Tel:** (01548) 830857 w 6134651

Vanessa Marie 02/12/1999 Corner House Veterinary Practice Ltd 84 Withycombe Village Road Exmouth Devon EX8 3AG **Tel:** (01395) 277775 w 6186320

STEERS Zoe 18/04/2005 90 Hamsterly Park Southfields Northampton Northamptonshire NN3 5DX **Tel:** (079) 670 99835 w 6296375

STELL Caroline Frances 14/09/2001 85 Northbourne Street Gateshead Tyne and Wear NE8 4AE **Tel:** (0191) 4787810 w 6228296

STENHOUSE Emma Elizabeth 04/12/2003 8 Viewforth Gardens Edinburgh EH10 4EU **Tel:** (0131) 228 1741 w 6282339

STENSON Nicola Jane (see PERRY, Mrs)

STEPHANIE JAYNE Derry (see DERRY, Miss)

STEPHENS Amy Louise 26/10/2005 16 Eskdale Road Ashton-in-Makerfield WIGAN Lancashire WN4 8QT **Tel:** (01942) 202059 w 6325855

STEPHENS Clare Louise (see VALENTINE, Mrs)

Danielle Zoe 18/09/2003 27 Fairmeads Pyrles Lane Loughton Essex IG10 2NE **Tel:** (020) 8539 3538 w 6271372

STEPHENS Emmaly (see RUSSEN, Mrs)

Leanne 30/11/2006 115 Leigh Road WIMBORNE Dorset BH21 2AB **Tel:** (01202) 888465 w 6344940

STEPHENS Natalie Jayne (see ROLLS, Ms)

Samantha Christine 03/12/2003 The Veterinary Surgery Harleigh Road Bodmin Cornwall PL31 1AQ **Tel:** (01208) 72323 w 6280293

Theresa Jane 28/10/2008 159 Nutbeem Road Eastleigh Hampshire SO50 5JS **Tel:** (07766) 691715 w 6356314

STEPHENSON Helen (see MCHUGH, Mrs)

STEPHENSON Louise (nee Taylor) 13/01/2004 Calcot House Winterton Road Scunthorpe North Lincolnshire DN15 6AH **Tel:** (01724) 860045 w 6289731

Mary-Ellen (nee Graham) 08/04/2005 Drapers Cottage The Lane Creeting St Peter Ipswich Suffolk IP6 8QR **Tel:** (01449) 678686 w 6293889

Victoria Elizabeth 13/11/2007 18 Comer Terrace Cockfield Bishop Auckland County Durham DL13 5DN **Tel:** (01388) 710976 w 6404901

STERRY-JONES Caroline Marie 02/09/1999 5 Cotton Terrace St. Helens Merseyside WA9 3GG **Tel:** (01744) 21723 w 6185682

STEVEN Angela Karine 26/07/2006 The Old Smith Straiton Ayrshire KA19 7NF w 6348713

STEVENS Anne Marie (see WARD, Ms)

STEVENS Elizabeth Mary 17/01/2006 41 Fotherby Court MAIDENHEAD Berkshire SL6 1SU w 6287278

Elvina 22/07/2008 238 Pampisford Road South Croydon Surrey CR2 6DB **Tel:** (020) 8686 6070 w 6519840

Hannah Jayne 29/07/2005 (26/02/2008) Manor Veterinary Centre 113-119 Kent Road Halesowen West Midlands B62 8PB **Tel:** (0121) 422 5411 w 6265531

Jo-Anne (nee Graham) 15/08/2003 2 Lavender Row GATESHEAD Tyne and Wear NE9 6GA **Tel:** (0191) 4383338 w 6279017

Katherine Jane (nee Van Rooyen) 30/11/2006 Waingate Corston Malmesbury Wiltshire SN16 0HD w 6350693

Katie 16/06/2004 31 The Rowans Broughton CHESTER CH4 0TD w 6284033

Lisa Marie 23/08/2004 46 Lower Elmstone Drive Tilehurst READING RG31 5EB w 6289005

Naomi Jane 02/12/2009 Avon Lodge Veterinary Group 21 Stratford Road Salisbury SP1 3JN **Tel:** (01722) 412211 w 6465390

Natalie Ann 05/09/2008 13 Ridgeway Hurst Green ETCHINGHAM East Sussex TN19 7PJ **Tel:** 07968782624 w 6419916

Susan Jane 01/02/1995 26 Beverstone Tetbury Gloucestershire GL8 8TT **Tel:** (01666) 504 346 w 6034384

Zoe Elizabeth 23/02/2005 w 6285397

STEVENSON Amanda Kay 21/05/2007 468 Street Lane Moortown Leeds West Yorkshire LS17 6HA **Tel:** (0113) 236 9030 w 6375685

Caroline 29/01/2009 24 Madin Street New Tupton Chesterfield Derbyshire S42 6EH **Tel:** 01246251035 w 6390414

Hayley Michelle 27/02/2002 44 Barbers Hill Werrington PETERBOROUGH PE4 5ED w 6271383

Jan (formerly Harwood) 17/09/1973 (02/08/1999) 6 Highwell Lane BROMYARD Herefordshire HR7 4DG **Tel:** (01885) 482538 w 6052494

Janet Alexandra 07/02/1989 (06/05/2008) 16 View Road NAIRN IV12 5AH w 6061283

STEVENSON Jayne Margaret (see MANLEY, Mrs)

STEVENSON Michelle Mary (see MEGAW, Mrs)

Sarah Rose 29/06/2007 2 Duncryne Place Bishopbriggs Glasgow G64 2DP **Tel:** (0141) 772 1019 w 6349318

STEWARDSON Gemma 23/08/2004 23 Young Street West Bromwich West Midlands B70 9TU w 6275464

STEWART Anne Marie 23/10/2000 (06/12/2006) 8F Lancaster Crescent Glasgow Lanarkshire G12 0RR **Tel:** (0141) 561 6829 w 6096567

Brenda Ann 06/10/2006 Loriston Cottage Hillside Portlethen ABERDEEN AB12 4RB w 6318892

Debbie 21/07/2008 43 Blackcraigs Kirkcaldy Fife KY2 6TL **Tel:** (01592) 205660 w 6389303

Donna 09/09/2002 Cuando Densole Lane Densole FOLKESTONE Kent CT18 7BL w 6270877

STEWART Felicity Megan (see NEWMAN, Mrs)

Gemma 12/05/2004 25 Society Road SOUTH QUEENSFERRY West Lothian EH30 9XP w 6292261

Jane 11/04/2008 3 Birch View Barrow Clitheroe Lancashire BB7 9BB **Tel:** (01254) 822509 w 6323512

STEWART Johanna Clare (see IRESON, Mrs)

Lindsay Jane Diana 19/09/2006 27 Maxwell Avenue Bearsden GLASGOW G61 1PA **Tel:** (0141) 945 2892 w 6330255

Louise 15/01/2009 16 The Castings Dunfermline Fife KY12 9AU **Tel:** (01383) 732696 w 6408014

Nicola 04/12/2008 23 Mount Merrion Drive Belfast County Antrim BT6 0FX **Tel:** (07811) 971960 w 6353168

STIBBS Emily Catherine 14/08/2008 12 Neville Road Hillborough HERNE BAY Kent CT6 6NZ w 6409048

STILLMAN Terri Ann 11/05/2009 Darwin Veterinary Centre Ltd 2 Haig Road Biggin Hill Kent TN16 3LJ **Tel:** (01959) 541153 w 6418123

STIMPSON Lucy Jane 13/11/2009 Spring Corner Veterinary Centre 4 Knyveton Road Bournemouth BH1 3QN w 6451475

STIMPSON Sarah Louise (see BRADLEY, Mrs)

STITTLE Emma Elizabeth 11/04/2005 Grove House Holt Road Fakenham Norfolk NR21 8JG **Tel:** (01328) 862137 w 6244796

STOCK Elizabeth Mae 17/07/2003 (12/05/2006) 84 New Wanstead Wanstead London E11 2SY **Tel:** (020) 8989 7744 w 6281602

Emma Jayne 28/02/2005 44 Eden Road Dundonald Belfast County Antrim BT16 1XF w 6289181

STOCKINGS Natalie 17/01/2007 222 Victoria Road Ruislip Middlesex HA4 0BN **Tel:** (01895) 677 918 w 6363343

STOCKS Esther Jayne (see JONES, Mrs)

STOCKTON Clare Jayne (see SMITH, Mrs)

Emma Marie 19/02/2001 Nantwich Veterinary Hospital Crewe Road End Nantwich Cheshire CW5 5SF **Tel:** (01270) 610349 w 6212478

STOCKWELL Marie Elaine (see GORDON, Mrs)

STOKES Louise Michelle 24/09/2009 15 Hawthorne Rise Awsworth NOTTINGHAM NG16 2RG w 6466039

STOLLERY Alison Joanne 31/10/2003 Units 5 & 6, 19 - 21 Elmshott Lane Cippenham Slough Berkshire SL1 5QS **Tel:** (01628) 600586 w 6271900

STONE Angela Marie 25/04/2005 58 New Lane Penwortham Preston Lancashire PR1 9JJ **Tel:** (01772) 743933 w 6302172

Carly Louise 04/10/2005 67 Shelson Avenue FELTHAM Middlesex TW13 4QS w 6321147

STONE Caroline May (see CROSS, Mrs)

Kelly Louise DipAVN(Surgical) 25/02/2003 2 Yew Tree Cottage Dishwell Lane Harthill SHEFFIELD S26 7XJ w 6284143

STONE Leigh Crawford (see DALY, Mrs)

STONEHAM Kathryn Anne 24/05/2006 53-55 Maidstone Road Footscray SIDCUP Kent DA14 5HB **Tel:** (020) 8300 8111 w 6343158

STONEMAN Rhian Mary 01/09/2000 118 Gower Road Sketty Swansea SA2 9BT **Tel:** (01792) 201688 w 6203975

STONER Belinda Jane DipAVN(Surgical) (nee Apps) 15/08/1989 (30/04/1999) MYF Training Hippodrome House Station Road Aldershot Hampshire GU11 1LZ w 6044701

STONES Emma Louise 23/12/2003 Eastfield Veterinary Clinic Ltd Station Road North Thoresby GRIMSBY Lincolnshire DN36 5QU **Tel:** (01472) 840209 w 6287146

STOPPS Sarah Louise 25/02/2003 Castle Park Chiseldon Lane Brixham Devon TQ5 9QS **Tel:** (01803) 854500 w 6263089

STORER Charlotte Louise (nee Weyman) 30/08/1994 (08/11/2001) 107 East Barnet Road New Barnet Barnet Hertfordshire EN4 8RF **Tel:** (020) 8440 5742 w 6033380

STORES Gemma 27/02/2006 Lowland Cottage Newcastle Road SUNDERLAND SR5 1RP **Tel:** (0191) 5369766 w 6329100

STOREY Carol Elizabeth (nee Thomas) 19/09/1988 (19/11/2007) 15 East Woodyates SALISBURY Wiltshire SP5 5QZ **Tel:** (01725) 516915 w 6001847

Sally Ann 10/03/2008 46 Morland Road Aldershot Hampshire GU11 3SF **Tel:** 01252321739 w 6410401

STORMONT Kathryn Elizabeth 15/02/2002 72/2 Lochend Road South Edinburgh Midlothian EH7 6DE **Tel:** (0131) 6202211 w 6271680

STOTT Laura Jayne 25/08/2009 32 Turnberry Way Carlisle Cumbria CA3 0QL **Tel:** (077) 37812071 w 6414482

Michelle 07/12/2005 10 Mountain Ash Rooleymoor Rochdale Lancashire OL12 7JE **Tel:** (07751) 709360 w 6354048

STOWE Charlene Jemima (formerly Srowe) 14/05/2008 Silver Birch High Street March Cambridgeshire PE15 9LQ **Tel:** (07854) 905403 w 6406243

STRADLING Amy Elizabeth 11/07/2005 (25/06/2008) Upper Ley Farm Ley Westbury-on-Severn Gloucestershire GL14 1PR **Tel:** (01452) 750321 w 6283780

STRAIN Irene Margaret (see WATSON, Mrs)

STRAND Carole Lynda (see HARVEY, Mrs)

STRANGWOOD Hayley Jane 03/10/2007 28 Arbour Close Mickleton CHIPPING CAMPDEN Gloucestershire GL55 6RR **Tel:** (01386) 438 747 w 6303316

STRATFORD Holly Anne 30/12/2008 Pilgrims Hatch Glebe Road Ramsden Bellhouse BILLERICAY Essex CM11 1RL **Tel:** 07773006548 w 6342245

STRATTON Lesley Alison 21/09/1987 (27/09/1999) 18a Bedford Avenue BEXHILL-ON-SEA East Sussex TN40 1NG w 6061410

STRAUGHTON Amanda Jayne (nee Worrall) 25/08/1998 2 St. Hughs Drive Langworth LINCOLN LN3 5DB w 6131730

STRAWBRIDGE Nadine Joanne 17/08/2005 Veterinary Hospital Fyfield Barrow Walnut Tree Local Centre Milton Keynes Buckinghamshire MK7 7AN **Tel:** (01908) 397777 w 6317264

STREET Katy Lisa 02/10/2009 10 Lodge Crescent Orpington Kent BR6 0QF **Tel:** (01689) 874436 w 6488941

Nichola Dawn 03/05/2007 11 Midland Road Baildon SHIPLEY West Yorkshire BD17 6AT **Tel:** (01274) 591 212 w 6267335

STRETTON Lorrayne (nee Saxby) 16/08/1982 15 Sandalwood Drive St Nicholas at Wade Kent CT7 0PE w 606028X

STRETTON-DOWNES Lesley Anne 16/09/2004 Buttercross Veterinary Centre Ltd Long Acre Bingham Nottingham NG13 8AF **Tel:** (01949) 837571 w 6283648

STREVENS Annette Tracy (see EASTWICK, Mrs)

STRIBLEY Kelly Dawn 05/10/2001 Ferlys House Overton Park Road Cheltenham Gloucestershire GL50 3BP **Tel:** (01242) 522 429 w 6229704

STRICK Jacqueline Anne 12/12/2005 P O Box 29922 Sharjah United Arab Emirates w 6414933

STRIDE Kelly 25/01/2000 Priory Veterinary Hospital 59 Purewell Christchurch Dorset BH23 1EN **Tel:** (01202) 484466 w 6190819

STRINGER Anna Marie (nee Cooke) 29/01/2001 Hykeham Green Lincoln Road North Hykeham Lincoln Lincolnshire LN6 8NH **Tel:** (01522) 683300 w 6211367

Joanne Karen 16/02/1998 Beechwood Veterinary Group Ltd 132 Austhorpe Road Leeds LS15 8EJ **Tel:** (01132) 645422 w 6108268

Katherine Ann 09/03/2005 Linkscroft Olney Road Weston Underwood Buckinghamshire MK46 5JZ **Tel:** (01234) 712991 w 6301842

STRONG Joanne Karen 09/03/2005 37 Montreal Street Carlisle Cumbria CA2 4EE **Tel:** (01228) 545825 w 6304119

STRONGE Laura Jane 14/01/2008 34 Hartley Meadows WHITCHURCH Hampshire RG28 7BW **Tel:** (07786) 673813 w 6388709

STROUD Katy Elizabeth 18/10/2006 Oakfield Veterinary Group The Old Library Hockley Road Wilnecote Tamworth Staffordshire B77 5EF **Tel:** (01827) 281284 w 6355192

Zoe Louise 02/09/2009 39 Westfield Walk HIGH WYCOMBE Buckinghamshire HP12 3JN **Tel:** (0773) 603 3225 w 6445964

STUBBINGTON Catherine Jane (see RAYMOND, Mrs)

STUBBINGTON Dawn Angela 21/04/2009 4 St. Marys Close Great Plumstead Norwich Norfolk NR13 5EY **Tel:** (01603) 715643 w 6437725

STUBBS Clare Diana (nee Waller) 26/08/2003 Davies Veterinary Specialists Manor Farm Business Park Higham Gobion Hertfordshire SG5 3HR **Tel:** (01582) 883950 w 6280524

Kerry Sandra Jean 29/09/1999 84 Bredhurst Road GILLINGHAM Kent ME8 0QT w 6186298

Lauren Anne 09/10/2009 117 Maple Way Burnham-on-Crouch Essex CM0 8TS **Tel:** (01621) 786034 w 6447075

Nicola 27/04/2009 24 St. Brides Way Bothwell GLASGOW G71 8QQ w 6330838

STUNDON Rhiannon 06/01/2009 Maindee House Veterinary Surgeon Mount Pleasant Road Pontnewydd Cwmbran Gwent NP44 1AN **Tel:** (01633) 483208 w 6266477

STURCH Angela Nicola 09/09/2009 25 Ashworth Road BIRMINGHAM B42 2RB w 6460891

STURGESS Amy Elizabeth (see RAWLINSON, Mrs)

STURROCK Marion Jane 11/09/2009 16 North Lane Norham Berwick-upon-Tweed Northumberland TD15 2LG **Tel:** (01289) 382653 w 6407211

STYLES Mandy Kim 23/02/2005 9 Turners Field Downley HIGH WYCOMBE Buckinghamshire HP13 5YZ **Tel:** (01494) 436258 w 6280799

SUCKLING Heidi Anne 26/05/2005 Grove House Holt Road Fakenham Norfolk NR21 8JG **Tel:** (01328) 862137 w 6307958

SULEYMAN Ashley 24/10/2008 9 Blanchard Close London SE9 4TZ **Tel:** (0208) 2936580 w 6415230

SULLIVAN Kimberley Michelle 26/10/2006 Icknield Veterinary Group 1 Brook Street Luton LU3 1DS **Tel:** (01582) 727571 w 6342773

SULLIVAN Lucy Jayne (see FLYNN, Mrs)

SULLIVAN Paula June (see BEADLE, Mrs)

SUMMERELL Beverley Jane 09/08/1983 (07/06/2000) The Veterinary Surgery 44 Rodney Road Backwell BRISTOL BS48 3HW **Tel:** (01275) 462691 w 6061512

SUMMERFIELD Nicola Dawn (nee Hartley) 27/04/2006 76 Fackley Road Stanton Hill Sutton-in-Ashfield Nottinghamshire NG17 3HG **Tel:** (01623) 556599 w 6342597

SUMMERHAYES Gemma Susan 08/09/2009 College Road CULLOMPTON Devon EX15 1TG **Tel:** (01884) 32228 w 6492802

SUMMERHILL Julie Elizabeth (see MORRIS, Mrs)

SUMMERS Deborah Kay 27/08/1997 71 Queensway Shelley Ongar Essex CM5 0BP **Tel:** (01277) 365950 w 6118651

Helen Elisabeth 05/10/2004 37 Victoria Street DALTON-IN-FURNESS Cumbria LA15 8HJ **Tel:** (0775) 220 27 20 w 6314690

Zoe Louise (nee Howard) 25/02/2003 35 Fairfield Way STEVENAGE Hertfordshire SG1 6BG w 6272901

SUMNAL Nicola Claire 21/09/2009 6 Ffordd Trefaldwyn Wrexham Clwyd LL11 2LB **Tel:** (01978) 366250 w 6368777

SUMNER Lynda Yvonne (see RADBOURNE, Mrs)

SUNDHOO Geeta 20/11/2002 34 Killowen Ave Northolt Middlesex UB5 4QT **Tel:** (0208) 8647373 w 6279974

SUTER Joanne Lesley (see MITCHELL, Mrs)

SUTHERLAND Joanna Elizabeth 13/01/2004 Zoological Society of London Veterinary Department Welcome Building Regents Park LONDON NW1 4RY **Tel:** (020) 7449 6675 w 6263155

SUTTON Annica Maria 05/04/2005 (05/06/2007) 26 Ashford Rise BELPER Derbyshire DE56 1TJ w 6329199

Clare Margaret (nee Hosie) 20/09/1996 38 Middlewich Road Northwich Cheshire CW9 7BG **Tel:** (01606) 44530 w 6064499

Ruth Mary 10/02/2004 Bray House Veterinary Practice 36 Asfordby Road Melton Mowbray Leicestershire LE13 0HR **Tel:** (01664) 562054 w 6282944

Susan Elaine (nee Goode) 20/05/2002 15 Hailes Park Edinburgh EH13 0NG **Tel:** (0131) 4411393 w 6273396

SWAIN Karen Yvette (see LINDLEY, Mrs)

SWAIN Sarah Karen (see WHITE, Mrs)

Tamsin Juliet 29/09/2004 73 Raymonds Plain WELWYN GARDEN CITY Hertfordshire AL7 4TE **Tel:** (01707) 894173 w 6322104

SWAINE Lesley Jayne (see LATHAM, Mrs)

SWALLOW Laura (nee Watson) 17/01/2008 146 Brooklands Road Spring Bank West HULL HU5 5AG **Tel:** (07971) 464041 w 6386586

SWAN Helena Elizabeth (see BAZLEY, Mrs)

SWAN Ruth 26/07/1993 (18/01/1999) Veterinary Health Centre Daisy Street Blackburn BB1 5EW **Tel:** (01254) 53622 w 6044348

SWANKIE Angela Doreen 29/11/2007 24 St. Margaret Street Dunfermline Fife KY12 7PE **Tel:** (01383) 732897 w 6322566

SWANN Sharon Jayne (see BROWN, Mrs)

SWANNELL Michael John 21/06/2005 67 Station Road Woburn Sands Milton Keynes Buckinghamshire MK17 8SH **Tel:** (01908) 282101 m 6296881

SWANNICK Rachel Jayne 09/09/1998 (27/01/2009) Willow Barn Plox Green Minsterley SHREWSBURY SY5 0HT **Tel:** (01743) 792064 w 6112773

SWANSON Charlotte Rebecca (nee Hart) 23/12/2003 (26/02/2009) Oakwood House Fuller Road Harleston Norfolk IP20 9EA **Tel:** (01379) 852146 w 6269843

SWEENEY Elizabeth Helen 02/06/2004 (08/02/2008) 12 Mill Bank Brymbo WREXHAM Clwyd LL11 5FJ w 6265245

SWEET Catherine Joy 03/05/2005 North Shore Augusta Road Ryde Isle of Wight PO33 3AU w 6300170

SWEETING Alison Rachel 13/03/2002 University of Bristol Division of Companion Animal Studies Langford House Langford Bristol Avon BS40 5DU **Tel:** (0117) 928 9280 w 6265311

SWEETLOVE Rebecca Louise 24/07/2009 4 Wilsheres Road BIGGLESWADE Bedfordshire SG18 0BU **Tel:** (01767) 600948 w 6331256

SWETTENHAM Claire Catherine 04/11/2005 77 Redbreast Road Bournemouth Dorset BH9 3AN **Tel:** (01202) 533654 w 6348768

SWIFT Tanya Louise Jane (see MILNER, Mrs)

SWIFT Whilmari (see WORROW, Mrs)

SWINDALE Emma Jane (nee Swindale, formerly O'Connor) 11/01/2005 47 Nelson Street Tredworth GLOUCESTER GL1 4QX **Tel:** (01452) 412505 w 6301853

SWINDELLS Julie 21/03/2007 9 Daisy Hill Road Mossley Ashton-under-Lyne Lancashire OL5 9ET **Tel:** (01457) 838541 w 6375212

Rebecca Clare (nee Denton) 03/09/1996 74 Moor Pool Avenue Birmingham West Midlands B17 9DT **Tel:** (01522) 822749 w 6098101

SWORDER Anna 27/02/2006 18 Westland Road Knebworth Hertfordshire SG3 6AS **Tel:** (01438) 811307 w 6294483

SYCAMORE Hayley Denise (see HYGATE, Mrs)

SYCKELMOORE Katherine Ann (see LIMEBEAR, Mrs)

SYMON Denise 04/08/1988 80 Peockland Gardens Johnstone Renfrewshire PA5 8AZ **Tel:** (01505) 344925 w 6061614

SYMONDS Susan Margaret (nee Hatfield) 08/04/2005 18 Waresley Court Road Hartlebury KIDDERMINSTER Worcestershire DY11 7TQ w 6302535

SYMONDSON Georgiana Rowan Theadora 03/06/2009 765 Burnage Lane Manchester Lancashire M19 1RW **Tel:** (0161) 431 9547 w 6311445

SZARAT Victoria 09/04/2009 192 Wimborne Road Poole Dorset BH15 2EJ **Tel:** 01202202563 w 6381361

T

TABBERER Rebecca Louise 06/04/2009 63 Peel Street BIRMINGHAM B18 7DX **Tel:** 01215517347 w 6257479

TACK Sarah Louise (nee Brook) 22/09/2004 309 Ugg Mere Court Road Ramsey Heights Ramsey Huntingdon Cambridgeshire PE26 2RJ **Tel:** (01487) 812998 w 6291623

TADD Victoria Louise 29/10/2009 82 Westcroft Gardens Morden Surrey SM4 4DL **Tel:** (0208) 5422184 w 6398279

TALBOYS Maria 24/11/2009 Woodside South View Amen Corner Binfield Nr Bracknell Berkshire RG12 8SZ w 6243971

TALO Denise Karen (nee Rose) 14/08/1987 17 Pippin Avenue Homer Hill Halesowen West Midlands B63 2PW **Tel:** (01384) 837 012 w 6061669

TAMBA Mandy Marie (formerly Robb) 02/09/1997 Sparsholt College Sparsholt Winchester Hampshire SO21 2NT **Tel:** (01962) 797 388 w 6118662

TAN KUM HUA Patricia Wendy 04/07/2007 Woodland Veterinary Centre Grange Road Midhurst West Sussex GU29 9LT **Tel:** (01730) 814321 w 6329826

TANDY Rebecca Lorainne Joanne (see JONES, Miss)

TANNAHILL Rebecca Louise (see LEWIS, Mrs)

TANNER Faye Elizabeth 17/07/2008 Haven Veterinary Practice 35 Holland Road Clacton-on-Sea Essex CO15 6EH **Tel:** (01255) 422150 w 6378270

Philippa Jane 06/08/2008 42 Meadow Road SALISBURY SP2 7BN **Tel:** 07890061494 w 6414460

TANSLEY Jennifer Louise 26/10/2009 Fir Tree Farm Church Lane Papworth Everard Cambridge Cambridgeshire CB3 8QN **Tel:** (01480) 830964 w 6375663

TARCSI-HAWKINS Stephanie Diane (see PORTWAY, Mrs)

TARRAN-JONES Suzanne Meryl (see HAYES, Mrs)

TARRANT Claire Elizabeth (nee Willcocks) 13/05/2003 224 Winchester Road Shirley Southampton SO16 6TL **Tel:** (023) 8077 9388 w 6283285

TART Katie Louise (see MORLEY, Mrs)

TATE David 01/09/1998 (11/09/2008) 77 Beacon Glade SOUTH SHIELDS Tyne and Wear NE34 7QU m 6108519

Janet Elizabeth (nee Dover) 14/03/1986 31 Farlea Drive Bradford West Yorkshire BD2 3RJ **Tel:** (01274) 788782 w 6049335

TATFORD Sarah Louise (see SMITH, Mrs)

TAYLOR Adela Marie Anne 21/10/2008 181 Galahad Close ANDOVER Hampshire SP10 4BP w 6434909

TAYLOR Alison Margaret (see ROLLINSON, Mrs)

Beth 27/10/2008 1 Edwards Terrace Bedlinog TREHARRIS Mid Glamorgan CF46 6RN w 6421643

Claire Louise 22/10/2008 2 Top Cottages Woodnook Grantham Lincolnshire NG33 5AD **Tel:** (01780) 764333 w 6417056

Claire Louise (nee Frazer) 07/02/2005 4 Whitefriars Drive Cawston Rugby Warwickshire CV22 7GD **Tel:** (01788) 521919 w 6327043

Elizabeth Ann 17/01/2006 6 Chelsham Road Warlingham Surrey CR6 9EQ w 6353971

TAYLOR Emily Carole (see ANGELL-PARSONS, Mrs)

Emma Louise 13/01/2004 14 Park Street Neath West Glamorgan SA11 3DF **Tel:** (01639) 776478 w 6264552

Gabrielle Lauren 06/08/2008 22 Oakley Close Guisborough Cleveland TS14 7NF **Tel:** (01287) 610056 w 6389050

Gemma 26/09/2006 Abbeymoor Veterinary Centres 110-116 Halifax Road Sheffield S6 1LH **Tel:** (0114) 233 4673 w 6366863

Gemma Kirsty 14/01/2008 8 Station Road Cuffley Potters Bar Hertfordshire EN6 4HT **Tel:** (01707) 875588 w 6343840

TAYLOR Gemma Verity Paula (see FOX, Mrs)

Hannah Elizabeth 07/12/2006 13 Mumbles Head Park Pembrey Burry Port Dyfed SA16 0DJ **Tel:** (01554) 832 852 w 6368843

Helen Joyce 19/09/2006 c/o 41 Oakleigh Drive Orton Longueville PETERBOROUGH PE2 7BB w 6372440

Helen Louise 24/11/2004 33 Aintree Road Tean STOKE-ON-TRENT ST10 4EU **Tel:** (01538) 722617 w 6319662

Isabel 17/08/2005 39 Larksfield Englefield Green Egham Surrey TW20 0RB **Tel:** (020) 7587 1128 w 6320223

Jane (nee Hall) 27/08/1997 35 Gold Close Nuneaton Warwickshire CV11 4XZ **Tel:** (024) 7644 1982 w 6099386

TAYLOR Jane Anouska (see JAMES, Mrs)

Janice 29/08/1997 (22/01/2007) Sagar Lane Farm Kebs Road Todmorden Lancashire OL14 8SB **Tel:** (01706) 818789 w 6113471

Jennie Louise 24/11/2009 Rowcliffe House Crown Square Penrith Cumbria CA11 7AB **Tel:** (01768) 865661 w 6465049

TAYLOR Judith Mary (see MONTGOMERY, Mrs)

Julie Carol 06/02/2002 10 Glamorgan Close ST. HELENS Merseyside WA10 3XT **Tel:** (01744) 23250 w 6272791

TAYLOR Karen Louise (see LEWENDON, Mrs)

Katherine Tamara 08/01/2004 41 Southlands Road Denham Uxbridge Middlesex UB9 4MD w 6287784

Katy Rebecca (nee Hobson) 22/03/2004 166 Nottingham Road Eastwood Nottingham NG16 3GG **Tel:** (01773) 769298 w 6292151

Lee 16/08/2006 (20/05/2009) 60 Tynemouth Drive Enfield Middlesex EN1 4LS **Tel:** (0208) 482 2906 m 6349659

Lisa Mary Emma (nee Rudling) 05/03/1997 (18/11/2008) 37 De Havilland Road DEREHAM Norfolk NR19 2XN **Tel:** (01362) 854663 w 6100247

TAYLOR Louise (see STEPHENSON, Mrs)

Lucy Anne 16/08/2007 Severn Veterinary Centre Tybridge House Tybridge Street Worcester Worcestershire WR2 5BA **Tel:** (01905) 421296 w 6353179

Lynn Catherine 15/01/1988 (07/04/2005) The Laurels Veterinary Centre 4 Ryelands Street Hereford HR4 0LA **Tel:** (01432) 354433 w 6061793

Melissa Kirsty 21/08/1998 8 Rupert Street Redfield BRISTOL BS5 9SA w 6042657

Melissa Nina (nee Billington) 15/04/2004 480 Manchester Road Bury Greater Manchester BL9 9NY **Tel:** (0161) 763 6333 w 6258513

Michelle Joanne (nee Davies) 05/03/1993 (02/12/1999) 1 Mayfield Ridge Hatch Warren BASINGSTOKE Hampshire RG22 4RS **Tel:** (01256) 476024 w 6014685

Philippa Gemma 10/02/2005 18 Pound Road CHATTERIS Cambridgeshire PE16 6RL w 6320234

Rachel Diane 10/01/2007 55 Illingworth Road Halifax West Yorkshire HX2 9EN **Tel:** (01422) 252 037 w 6359768

Rebecca Louise (nee Coleridge Simpson) 11/11/2004 3 Callon Close Barleyfields Worthing West Sussex BN13 3SP **Tel:** (01903) 537 956 w 6320861

Robyn Kathleen 14/10/2008 2 New Cottages Hawkshead Lane North Mymms HATFIELD Hertfordshire AL9 7TF w 6527122

Rosemary 04/01/2006 1 Caton Drive Atherton MANCHESTER M46 0NY **Tel:** (07745) 535807 w 6343851

TAYLOR Ruth (see UNSWORTH, Mrs)

Sandra 23/02/2005 (05/02/2007) 31 Roomlin Gardens Kirkcaldy Fife KY1 3BQ **Tel:** (01592) 650094 w 6325327

Sascha Madeleine 12/07/2006 8 Twisell Thorne Zebon Copse Church Crookham FLEET Hampshire GU52 0YT w 6346062

Sonia Catherine (nee Taylor, formerly Marsh) 13/05/2003 9 Cottage Fields Eaves Green CHORLEY Lancashire PR7 3QE w 6275794

Tracey Ann 17/05/1991 6 Station Terrace Ramshaw Bishop Auckland County Durham DL14 0NH **Tel:** (01388) 833142 w 6061840

Victoria Katherine O'Mara 19/03/2007 Donnington Grove Veterinary Surgery Oxford Road NEWBURY Berkshire RG14 2JB **Tel:** (01635) 47170 w 6340463

TEADLEY Gillian Alison (see PAGE, Mrs)

TEAGLE Claire Marie 07/02/2005 Arg Beiyn Veterinary Practice Unit 9 Onchan Precinct Onchan Isle of Man IM3 4EA **Tel:** (01624) 622259 w 6293911

TEBBLE Claire Rebecca (see ALLEN, Mrs)

TEBBUTT Alison Jane (see WELCH, Mrs)

TECKMAN Minnie (formerly Minney) 29/12/2003 89 St Matthews Parade Kingsley Northamptonshire NN2 7HD w 6259547

TEDSTONE Nicola Emma 06/02/1997 (11/09/2007) 24 Maesygarn Road Oakdale Blackwood Gwent NP12 0NA **Tel:** (01495) 228784 w 6040580

TEMPLE Kirsty Louise 11/11/2008 28a Raynes Road Lee-On-The-Solent Hampshire PO13 9AL w 6433138

TEMPLETON Karen Elizabeth 03/02/1995 (01/04/2004) Pets A & E 78 Stanley Street Kinning Park Glasgow Lanarkshire G41 1JH w 6035526

TENNISWOOD Kate Louise (nee Perrett) 01/10/1982 (05/11/1999) 44 Brewer Mead Chippenham Wiltshire SN15 3FB **Tel:** (01249) 654029 w 6065073

TERRY Jade Louise 31/10/2006 61 Wordsworth Place Horsham West Sussex RH12 5PS **Tel:** (01403) 756 668 w 6343862

Justine Amie 29/01/2009 24 Fairview Road Basildon Essex SS14 1PW **Tel:** 01268206147 w 6435536

TESH Kirsty Marie 24/11/2004 Bridge Farm Sweffling SAXMUNDHAM Suffolk IP17 2BA w 6293196

TESSYMAN Craig Rodney 03/05/2007 35 Brynn Street ST. HELENS Merseyside WA10 1JB **Tel:** (07870) 125336 m 6298762

TETT Felicity Christine 29/06/2007 Torrington Orthopaedic Referrals IES House Mission Street Brighouse West Yorkshire HD6 1NQ **Tel:** (01484) 404770 w 6375322

THACKER Angela Rose 30/07/2004 65 Rose Walk West Wickham Kent BR4 0SB **Tel:** (020) 8777 6163 w 6292426

THACKER Jane (see HARPER, Mrs)

THAIN Kate Rebecca (nee Wilcox, nee Wilcox) 05/09/2000 Wards Veterinary Centre New Elgin Road Elgin Morayshire IV30 6BA **Tel:** (01343) 544811 w 6134072

THEOBALD Michelle Josephine 31/10/2006 51 West Park Avenue Ashton-on-Ribble Preston Lancashire PR2 1UH **Tel:** (01772) 736 487 w 6376719

Susan Elizabeth 08/09/1998 Taylor & Lees Catley Cross Equine Clinic Halstead Essex CO9 2PE **Tel:** (01787) 269 006 w 6137200

THEYSE Isabelle Anne Elizabeth Agnes 18/07/2005 24 Pochin Drive MARKET HARBOROUGH Leicestershire LE16 7LP **Tel:** (07984) 673036 w 6295594

THIEL Dawn Anne 14/03/2006 83 Whitby Road RUISLIP Middlesex HA4 9DU **Tel:** (01895) 632 079 w 6321642

THOMAS Annika Helen 02/09/2009 Tresi Aur Trelech CARMARTHEN Dyfed SA33 6RU **Tel:** (01994) 484554 w 6367732

Bridie Kate 25/03/2009 Woods Cottage Woodham Road Battlesbridge Wickford Essex SS11 7QU **Tel:** (01245) 321879 w 6386201

THOMAS Carol Elizabeth (see STOREY, Mrs)

Ceri Samantha 20/10/2008 36 Cardonnel Road Skewen NEATH West Glamorgan SA10 6DD w 6421852

Charlotte Victoria 09/06/2008 5 Nasmith Close GOSPORT Hampshire PO12 2ST **Tel:** (02392) 587258 w 6402481

Claire Louise (nee Girling) 04/09/1997 (22/03/2004) Highcliff Veterinary Practice 93 Cliff Lane Ipswich Suffolk IP3 0PQ **Tel:** (01473) 828846 w 6099262

Claire Nicola 03/09/1998 The Wylie Veterinary Centre 196 Hall Lane Upminster Essex RM14 1TD **Tel:** (01708) 251200 w 6138656

Deborah Ann 06/03/2006 White Hills Surgery Sibford Road Hook Norton Banbury Oxfordshire OX15 5DG **Tel:** (01608) 730085 w 6352013

Deborah Elaine (nee Harvey) 03/06/2004 (26/02/2008) 6 Edna Street South Elmsall Pontefract West Yorkshire WF9 2RZ **Tel:** (07943) 835999 w 6290754

Harriet Luella 20/11/2002 Coswarth Newquay Cornwall TR8 4LZ **Tel:** (01726) 860322 w 6276828

Hayley Marie 18/10/2006 53 Curlew Way Sleaford Lincolnshire NG34 7UD **Tel:** (01529) 410 774 w 6347360

Heidi Pollyanna 15/12/2004 201 High Street Great Wakering Southend-on-Sea Essex SS3 0EA **Tel:** (01702) 218656 w 6285155

Jacqueline Barbara 21/08/1974 National Animal Welfare Trust Tylers Way WATFORD WD25 8WT **Tel:** (0208) 9500177 w 6084595

Jane Alison DipAVN(Surgical) 12/08/1991 56 Cherrybrook Drive Penkridge STAFFORD ST19 5EB **Tel:** (01785) 715 258 w 6095654

Janine Veronica 27/04/2006 (19/06/2008) Brookpark Veterinary Clinic The Old Railway Station Dunmanway Co.Cork Ireland **Tel:** (00353) 2345 777 w 6346645

Julia Ann 01/08/1988 Morn Cottage 2 Holland Close Holland Close Broadstairs Kent CT10 3QJ **Tel:** (01843) 861016 w 6061953

Lorna Elaine 05/10/2009 14 Rossendale Close CHESTERFIELD Derbyshire S40 3EL **Tel:** (01246) 206991 w 6464301

Michelle Rose (nee Lewis) 21/07/2004 Fairwater Veterinary Surgery Fairwater Square Cwmbran Gwent NP44 4TA **Tel:** (01633) 869300 w 6289170

Nia 14/05/2007 Priory Veterinary Ltd Gwalia Gardens Pwllhai CARDIGAN Dyfed SA43 1DB **Tel:** (01239) 612479 w 6344324

Nina Louise 15/05/2008 1a Spring Walk WHITSTABLE Kent CT5 4PP **Tel:** 07845247417 w 6401425

Rebecca Leanne 08/06/2006 412 Liverpool Road Newcastle Staffordshire ST5 9DY **Tel:** (01782) 860 428 w 6358888

Sara Doreen 19/02/2009 Greenside Farm St. Boswells MELROSE Roxburghshire TD6 0AJ **Tel:** (01835) 823257 w 6443104

Sarah Louise (nee Donald) 29/08/2002 Afon Veterinary Centre Lletty Nedd Pen Y Dre Neath West Glamorgan SA11 3HH **Tel:** (01639) 642739 w 6257677

THOMAS Susan Elizabeth (see ATKINSON, Mrs)

THOMAS Teresa Elizabeth (see HORSPOOL, Mrs)

THOMASON Julia Mary (see COX, Mrs)

Melanie Anne 31/08/1994 33 St. Andrews Close Sutton ELY Cambridgeshire CB6 2QU w 6027049

THOMPSETT Lydia Frances (nee Barton) 08/04/2005 (26/01/2010) 27 Church Road Kirkcolm Stranraer Wigtownshire DG9 0NW **Tel:** (01776) 853548 w 6320828

THOMPSON Alex 10/01/2003 242 Cricklewood Lane London NW2 2PU **Tel:** (020) 8450 2228 m 6258095

Angel Lise 14/01/2008 9 Pendrick Close Coton CAMBRIDGE CB23 7GZ w 6390447

Anna Elizabeth 20/01/2000 2 Haldene Villas Duck Street Pilling Preston Lancashire PR3 6HN **Tel:** (01253) 790431 w 6191215

Carol DipAVN(Surgical) 23/11/1987 31 Otley Close Cramlington Northumberland NE23 2YP **Tel:** (01670) 731500 w 6062028

THOMPSON Davine Marie (see HEATH, Mrs)

Debbie Karen (nee Trenaman) 18/01/2008 31 Main Road Pinhoe Exeter EX4 9EY **Tel:** (01392) 460300 w 6350242

Jennifer DipAVN(Surgical) 19/10/1999 27 Don St SHEFFIELD S36 6HA **Tel:** (01226) 370579 w 6152331

Jennifer Ann (nee Roberts) 08/09/2003 12 Brunswick Drive Brookwood Woking Surrey GU24 0NR **Tel:** (01483) 481085 w 6284583

THOMPSON Julie Ann (see POTTER, Mrs)

Katherine Elizabeth (nee Haydon) 27/09/2006 Cromwell Veterinary Hospital 36-36a St. Johns Street HUNTINGDON Cambridgeshire PE29 3DG **Tel:** (01480) 52601/52222 w 6374607

THOMPSON Katherine Mary (see DORRICOTT, Mrs)

Kathryn Alison DipAVN(Surgical) 23/01/1995 9 Malvern Road Frenchwood Preston Lancashire PR1 4PQ **Tel:** (01772) 250567 w 6037115

Lesley-Anne Catherine 13/05/2003 33 Primrose Place Eliburn LIVINGSTON West Lothian EH54 6RN **Tel:** 01506202460 w 6277081

Lisa Michelle DipAVN(Surgical) 01/12/2000 Torrington Orthopaedic Referrals IES House Mission Street Brighouse West Yorkshire HD6 1NQ **Tel:** (01484) 404770 w 6205669

THOMPSON Melissa Jane (see EWING, Mrs)

THOMPSON Michaela Ann (see BRICKLES, Mrs)

Michelle (nee Anstiss) 12/12/2005 Goddard Veterinary Group 96 Roding Road Loughton Essex IG10 3EJ **Tel:** (020) 8508 3340 w 6279468

Natalie Alison 06/10/2009 85 Aspen Drive Burnley Lancashire BB10 3FB **Tel:** (01282) 830015 w 6443423

Nicola Jayne 13/05/2003 5 Thames Road ST. HELENS Merseyside WA9 4HB w 6261230

Nicola Samantha Jayne 30/01/2001 Jubilee Veterinary Centre 3 Jubilee Road Newtownards County Down BT23 4YH **Tel:** (02891) 812226 w 6211598

Rachel Elizabeth 08/10/2008 2 Thyme Court GUILDFORD Surrey GU4 7BZ w 6442037

Rebecca Louise 22/10/2008 8 Avenue Nozay Broughton Brigg South Humberside DN20 0TR **Tel:** 01724860045 w 6437527

Rebecca Louise (nee Parker) 03/05/2005 10 Highfield Court Winchester Road Bishops Waltham SOUTHAMPTON SO32 1PJ **Tel:** (07742) 670950 w 6300148

Samantha Helen (nee Gill) 05/10/2004 Bloxwich Veterinary Centre 18 Wallington Heath Bloxwich Walsall WS3 3NP **Tel:** (01922) 405200 w 6319134

THOMPSON Sarah Louise (see BEANEY, Mrs)

THOMPSON Sherene Laura Marie (see LONG, Mrs)

Tiffany Abigail Edana 29/11/2007 Starnes Gatward Blowey & Wood Fairfield House New Town Uckfield East Sussex TN22 5DG **Tel:** (01825) 764268 w 6407112

THOMSON Alison Catherine 04/10/2005 4 Long Hale Pitstone LEIGHTON BUZZARD Bedfordshire LU7 9GF w 6407453

THOMSON Alison Karen (see SHERWOOD, Mrs)

THOMSON Angela (see FERRIER, Mrs)

Erica Lynn 01/10/2008 54 Simeon Way STONE Staffordshire ST15 8FJ w 6417100

Joyce Iris 15/10/2008 Ashgrove Veterinary Centre Ltd 10 Belmont Road Aberdeen AB25 3SR **Tel:** (01224) 486444 w 6379535

Louise Elizabeth 29/07/2005 232 Richmond Road Kingston Surrey KT2 5HG **Tel:** (0208) 5463569 w 6290457

THORNBORROW Amy Elizabeth 11/11/2009 4 Broughton Mews SKIPTON North Yorkshire BD23 1TW **Tel:** 07702731781 w 6445843

Caroline (nee Leaver) 23/08/1990 7 Wensleydale Avenue Skipton North Yorkshire BD23 2TS **Tel:** (01756) 797923 w 6054979

THORNBORROW Carrie Ann (see WISHART, Miss)

THORNDYCRAFT-HUGGETT Jenny 10/02/2005 The Paddock 53 Cherrydown West Basildon Essex SS16 5AW **Tel:** (01268) 533636 w 6313370

THORNE Amy 29/12/2003 (26/02/2008) 2 Ingram Close Larkfield AYLESFORD Kent ME20 7GP **Tel:** (01634) 666655 w 6274969

Justine (nee Mears, formerly Smith) 30/07/1992 (01/02/2002) The Veterinary Hospital 230 Prince Avenue WESTCLIFF-ON-SEA Essex SS0 0NN **Tel:** (01702) 322222 w 600478X

Shelly Marie (formerly Lawley) 24/08/1995 The Cottage 135c Grange Road Ramsgate Kent CT11 9PT w 6040139

THORNHILL Danielle Louise 26/08/2008 Groomlake House 154 Drove Road BIGGLESWADE Bedfordshire SG18 0HP w 6420895

Karen 10/04/2007 Flat 8 Chaucer Court 2 Glebe Avenue RUISLIP Middlesex HA4 6QZ w 6453125

THORNHILL Natalie Jill (see MCLENNAN, Mrs)

THORNLEY Amy Leanne 25/02/2009 6 Silver Close Dukinfield Cheshire SK16 4XD **Tel:** 01613308866 w 6449176

THORNTON Jenny Louise 30/09/2008 3 The Downlands WARMINSTER Wiltshire BA12 0BD w 6412656

Lucy Louise (nee Byrne) 09/01/2004 105 Greenside BOREHAMWOOD Hertfordshire WD6 4JD **Tel:** (0208) 207 5734 w 6293350

Sharon Rachel 29/04/2008 4a Clarence Street Cleckheaton West Yorkshire BD19 5HJ **Tel:** ((01274)) 876 278 w 6411985

THORNYCROFT Lynn Dorothy (see BYFORD, Mrs)

THOROGOOD Jemma Claire 10/01/2003 (19/05/2006) PDSA Pet Aid Hospital 7 Warwick Road Manchester M16 0JW **Tel:** (0161) 881 0222 w 6263694

THORP Alexander Gordon 24/05/2006 64 Pennymead HARLOW Essex CM20 3HY **Tel:** (01279) 424216 m 6325360

THORPE Helen Claire 27/12/2001 The Mews Chilworth Manor Halfpenny Lane Chilworth GUILDFORD Surrey GU4 8NN w 6203887

Julie Anne 13/03/2008 40 Barrington Road Altrincham Cheshire WA14 1HJ **Tel:** (0161) 9288367 w 6334710

Leana (nee Findlay) 06/07/2004 (21/01/2010) Equipet Veterinary Hospital 24 Nicol Street Kirkcaldy Fife KY1 1NY **Tel:** (01592) 641333 w 6290083

THORRINGTON Donna Lynn 02/03/2004 25 All Saints Road Ipswich Suffolk IP1 4DG **Tel:** (01473) 256307 w 6204657

THOSEBY Rebecca 09/05/2006 38 Kenmore Road CLECKHEATON West Yorkshire BD19 3YB w 6346172

THRELFALL Lysbeth Jane (see FOWLER, Mrs)

THUILLIEZ Lucinda Caroline (nee Soutry) 18/01/1996 5 Church Lane Dalham NEWMARKET Suffolk CB8 8TE **Tel:** (01342) 833374 w 6038265

THWAITES Alison Rachel (nee Pope) 15/12/2004 Stirling Lodge Clinic 2 Stirling Road CHICHESTER West Sussex PO19 7DJ **Tel:** (01243) 786101 w 6308255

TIBBETTS Samantha Mary 13/04/2004 Sunnybank 5 Bridgnorth Road Stourton Stourbridge West Midlands DY7 6RP **Tel:** (01384) 873395 w 6271361

TIDBALL Emma Jane 30/07/2004 Lynwood Veterinary Group Station Road Wimborne Dorset BH21 1RQ **Tel:** (01202) 882101 w 6293922

TIDBY Deborah Margaret (nee Tidby) 28/01/1991 (04/04/2006) 5 Durley Avenue Cowplain Portsmoth Hampshire PO8 8XF **Tel:** (023) 92263152 w 6062210

TIDD Catherine Louise (nee Gibson) 29/01/2007 63 Norwich Road Wroxham Norwich Norfolk NR12 8RX **Tel:** (01603) 783 920 w 6372847

TIERNEY Nicola Jane (see MARSHALL, Mrs)

TIFFNEY Lianne (nee Davis) 16/09/2004 PO Box 72 C/o Sawley Marina Long Eaton Nottingham NG10 3AE w 6312149

TIGHE Louise Cora (see RANDTOUL, Mrs)

TIGHE Stacey Jayne 06/03/2006 Fivelands Veterinary Centre 98 Alcester Road BIRMINGHAM B13 8EG **Tel:** (0121) 449 3716 w 6345567

TILDESLEY Amy (see BOWCOTT, Mrs)

TILLEY Michele Clair 15/08/1988 (10/03/2004) 5 Pilgrims Close Chandler's Ford Eastleigh Hampshire SO53 4ST **Tel:** (023) 8026 8001 w 6062221

Rebecca Louise 23/09/2009 Woodlands Gunby Road Orby Spilsby Lincolnshire PE23 5SW **Tel:** (01754) 890044 w 6449583

TILSTONE Emma Louise 07/12/2005 Belmont House Veterinary Surgery Salisbury Road Business Park Salisbury Road Pewsey Wiltshire SN9 5PZ **Tel:** (01672) 563413 w 6291975

TIMMS Kelly Lorraine (formerly Wardle) 13/12/2001 Perryway Cottage Perryway Frampton on Severn GLOUCESTER GL2 7HS **Tel:** (07917) 155704 w 6263760

TINDALL Lynsey Anne DipAVN(Medical) (nee Warwick) 09/02/2001 New Priory Veterinary Practice The Deneway London Rd Brighton East Sussex BN1 8QR **Tel:** (01273) 540430 w 6203656

TINLIN Claire 03/09/1998 22 Orchard Road Barnstaple Devon EX32 9JQ w 6129754

TIPPING Michelle Jane (see COATSWORTH, Mrs)

TISDALE Hayley (see FORDYCE, Mrs)

TISSIMAN Victoria Kate 16/02/2009 North Hall Cottage Houghton Sancton York North Yorkshire YO43 4RE w 6383726

TITLEY Laila Julie 21/06/2005 65 Sirdar Road London N22 6QS **Tel:** (020) 88813601 w 6298773

Lauren Christina 07/04/2006 (20/01/2010) 25 Clos Rheidol Caldicot Gwent NP26 4JD **Tel:** (01291) 420000 w 6346744

TOBIN Laura Louise 05/04/2005 (29/05/2007) 21 Bourne Road Farncombe GODALMING Surrey GU7 3NL w 6300181

TODD Alison Heather 09/06/2008 158 Clewer Hill Road Windsor Berkshire SL4 4DB **Tel:** (01753) 770948 w 6389314

Bethany Kate 01/09/1998 78 Sycamore Road Brookhouse LANCASTER LA2 9PE **Tel:** (01362) 668659 w 6138907

Catherine Mary 24/06/2004 Woodbrow Cottage 35 York Road Malton Yorkshire YO17 6AX w 6284462

TODD Yvette Helen (see HUTCHINGS, Mrs)

TOKLEY Kayleigh Anita 06/05/2008 35 Moneypiece Close Haverhill Suffolk CB9 9NP **Tel:** (01440) 704177 w 6401964

TOLFREE Lisa Victoria 06/02/1992 Episode Three Hobbs Wall Farmborough Bath BA2 0BJ **Tel:** (01761) 472919 w 6062301

TOMKINS Lucinda Jane 13/01/2004 (17/10/2006) 2 Harsfold Cottages Harsfold Lane Wisborough Green BILLINGSHURST West Sussex RH14 0BD w 6281283

Samantha Jane 14/09/2009 12 Ashfield Road Thurmaston LEICESTER LE4 8GZ **Tel:** (0116) 2692234 w 6464972

TOMKINSON Zoe Anne 21/05/2009 83 Southgate Urmston Manchester Lancashire M41 9EQ **Tel:** 01565632253 w 6394308

TOMLIN Lucy Hannah Elizabeth (nee Collinson) 05/07/2007 207 Daventry Road Coventry West Midlands CV3 5HH **Tel:** (02476) 503000 w 6381130

Tracy Karen 06/03/2006 11 Magenta Close Bletchley Milton Keynes MK2 3NE **Tel:** (01908) 375806 w 6301193

TOMLINSON Caroline Elizabeth (see HOLMES, Ms)

TOMLINSON Sarah Louise DipAVN(Surgical) 01/08/1988 142 Derby Road Long Eaton Nottingham NG10 4ER **Tel:** (0115) 972 7050 w 6001891

TOMPKINS Jacqueline (see PENNEFATHER, Mrs)

TONES Darren 05/07/2006 18 Hillcrest Drive HEXHAM Northumberland NE46 1ED **Tel:** (07535) 618704 m 6432313

TONKIN Helen 17/01/2000 (17/03/2008) Quarrington Veterinary Surgery London Road Sleaford Lincolnshire NG34 8NX **Tel:** (01529) 307878 w 6190808

TONKINSON Wenda Jayne (nee Tonkinson) 12/02/2004 Rase Veterinary Centre Gallamore Lane Industrial Estate MARKET RASEN Lincolnshire LN8 3RX **Tel:** (01673) 842448 w 6289445

TONKS Victoria Jacqueline 22/03/2004 Dogs Trust Ltd Woodlands Farm York Road Leeds West Yorkshire LS15 4NL **Tel:** (0113) 281 4920 w 6289016

TOOGOOD Helen Nicol 05/10/2004 23 Dover Street SOUTHAMPTON SO14 6GG w 6307430

TOOLEY Sarah Lesley (see BUSCOMBE, Mrs)

TOOP Samantha Jayne 22/12/2004 78 Tramway Hirwaun Aberdare RCT South Wales CF44 9NY **Tel:** (01685) 813224 w 6276322

TOPHAM Laura Kirsty 28/07/2008 130 Waveney Drive Chelmsford Essex CM1 7QB **Tel:** (01245) 265 240 w 6404153

TOSSELL Lesley Allison 27/01/2010 21 Ruskin Way BROUGH North Humberside HU15 1GW **Tel:** 07792336002 w 6411567

TOWART Lisa Ann (nee Money) 30/06/2003 12 Whitton Place Seaton Delaval WHITLEY BAY Tyne and Wear NE25 0BJ **Tel:** (0191) 237 5218 w 6259074

TOWLE Michelle Louise 04/01/2006 Chase Veterinary Group Acacia Villas 357 Seaside Eastbourne East Sussex BN22 7RP **Tel:** (01323) 412673 w 6350814

TOWNELEY Frances Teresa (see SCOULAR, Mrs)

TOWNSEND Heather Bell 29/05/2003 264 Paisley Road West Ibrox Glasgow Lanarkshire G51 1BN **Tel:** (0141) 427 0848 w 6266576

Louise Marie 26/07/2004 2 Hibbert Street New Mills High Peak Derbyshire SK22 3JJ **Tel:** (01663) 745294 w 6289599

Sharon Elaine 03/09/2004 39 Brassey Avenue Eastbourne East Sussex BN22 9QD **Tel:** (01323) 500199 w 6295638

TOWNSHEND Charlotte Anne 07/11/2008 Bay Tree House 50 Station Road Tiptree COLCHESTER CO5 0BB w 6435701

TOWNSON Jill (see HALL, Mrs)

TOWSE Louise 11/11/2008 38 Warwick Road REDCAR Cleveland TS10 2HB **Tel:** 01642480480 w 6411017

TRAMONTIN Amanda Nadine 15/12/2004 Castlewood Otterbourne Place East Grinstead West Sussex RH19 1RQ **Tel:** (01342) 313560 w 6287520

TRAVERS Julie Ann 01/08/1979 Strathmore Veterinary Clinic 6 London Road Andover Hampshire SP10 2PH **Tel:** (01264) 352 323 w 6062414

TRAVIS Lyndsey Jane 22/03/2004 1 Mill Cottages Old Mill Lane Knowsley Merseyside Liverpool L34 8HF **Tel:** (0151) 549 1004 w 6275728

TREACHER Clare Joan 24/11/2005 Passey Veterinary Surgery 24 Passey Place Eltham London SE9 5DQ **Tel:** (020) 8850 3206 w 6330288

TREAGUST Michael Jonathan 25/02/2009 32 Burlish Avenue SOLIHULL West Midlands B92 8BF **Tel:** (0121) 704 2022 m 6429662

TREBBLE Claire Joy (see SMITH, Mrs)

TREDGETT Adele Louise 08/01/1986 (08/03/2002) Clarendon House Veterinary Group Ltd Bexfields Farm Galleywood Road Chelmsford Essex CM2 8BY **Tel:** (01245) 353741 w 6062425

TREE Natalie Clare (see STAHL, Mrs)

TREGASKES Karenza 16/12/2008 88a Fore Street BODMIN Cornwall PL31 2HR **Tel:** 07843105596 w 6109126

TREGIDGO Kelly Jane 26/01/2009 3 Broad Park St. Keyne Liskeard Cornwall PL14 4RH **Tel:** 01579349053 w 6358371

TRELOAR Kimberley Sue 03/05/2007 5 Heron Close Knutsford Cheshire WA16 8HL **Tel:** (01565) 653688 w 6340474

TRENAMAN Debbie Karen (see THOMPSON, Mrs)

TRETTON Rachel Victoria 11/10/2004 13 Bewdley Close Chellaston Derby DE73 6PT **Tel:** (01332) 705 873 w 6284671

TREVASKIS Claire Elizabeth 08/01/2010 94 Caldbeck Road WHITEHAVEN Cumbria CA28 6XQ **Tel:** 07793730988 w 6445634

TREVETHAN Jacqueline (see BROWNING, Mrs)

TREVOR Melanie Jayne 27/02/2008 78 Bedford Way Norman by Grange SCUNTHORPE South Humberside DN15 8GF **Tel:** (07828) 554 693 w 6351606

TREVORROW Nicola Claire 30/05/2008 3 Kings Court 29a Saxonbury Road BOURNEMOUTH BH6 5NB **Tel:** (01202) 425845 w 6416418

TRICKETT Rachel Anne (see BURRILL, Mrs)

TRIGG Michelle Patricia (see CORBETT, Mrs)

Nicola Angelica 23/05/2008 10 Rays Avenue Windsor Berkshire SL4 5HG **Tel:** (01628) 77 66 99 w 6372814

TRIM Julie 14/01/2008 38 Wildern Lane Hedge End Southampton SO30 4EH **Tel:** (01489) 782317 w 6328319

TRIPICCHIO Tracey Jayne (formerly Smith) 25/02/2003 203 Newbury Lane Oldbury West Midlands B69 1JQ **Tel:** (0121) 5332136 w 6271262

TRIPP Diana Mary (see LEGGO, Mrs)

TRIPP Emma Claire (see BAYLISS, Mrs)

TROMAN Elizabeth Clare 03/09/1996 Royal College of Veterinary Surgeons Veterinary Nursing Department Belgravia House 62/64 Horseferry Road London SW1P 2AF **Tel:** (020) 7222 2001 w 6100484

TROMANS Catherine Clare 18/07/2005 19 Brooke Grove Ely Cambridgeshire CB6 3WT **Tel:** (01353) 654101 w 6297178

TROOP Kerry Danielle 01/06/2007 30 Twycross Road Burbage Hinckley Leicestershire LE10 2SG **Tel:** (01455) 634713 w 6381185

TROTT Zoe (see WESTERN, Mrs)

TROTTER Sara 10/03/2009 18 Cramber Close Roborough PLYMOUTH PL6 7AZ **Tel:** 01752777194 w 6407156

TRUE Sarah Louise (formerly True) 16/01/2008 3 Oak Road Charlton Down DORCHESTER Dorset DT2 9UR **Tel:** (01305) 250 988 w 6389831

TRUELOVE Claire Louise 04/08/2009 17 Ennerdale Crescent Slough Berkshire SL1 6EH **Tel:** (01628) 605845 w 6389072

TRUNDELL Gemma Tracey Louise Yvonne 15/07/2005 Chestnut Veterinary Group 1 Hoe Lane Ware Hertfordshire SG12 9LS **Tel:** (01920) 468874 w 6297376

TRYE Hannah Louise (nee Chapman) 08/06/2006 (23/04/2009) 2 Nursery Close Potton SANDY Bedfordshire SG19 2QE w 6326834

TRYHORN Sarah Louise 07/02/2007 Southill Veterinary Group Balsam Fields Wincanton Somerset BA9 9HE **Tel:** (01963) 33226 w 6354774

TUBB Helen Elizabeth 03/08/2006 45 Tiverton Street Liverpool Merseyside L15 4LR **Tel:** (0151) 475 2111 w 6355313

TUCK Samantha Louise 07/10/2009 2 South View Down Ampney CIRENCESTER Gloucestershire GL7 5QS w 6372462

TUCKER Helen Ann 22/02/2007 4 Whelan Way Amesbury Salisbury Wiltshire SP4 7TS **Tel:** (01980) 676 259 w 6277466

Joanna Margaret (nee Crane) 15/08/2003 65 Oakley Road Caversham Reading Berkshire RG4 7RN **Tel:** (0118) 947 9298 w 6278445

Karen Jane 22/03/2004 Pinewood Lodge 16 Clayhill Road Burghfield Common READING RG7 3HE w 6293526

Karen Louise 28/03/2008 225 Kings Tamerton Road Plymouth Devon PL5 2BS **Tel:** (01752) 367 147 w 6357106

Katherine Marion 27/05/2003 33 Greenfinches Hempstead Gillingham Kent ME7 3PN **Tel:** (01634) 313619 w 6276729

Lianne Melanie 16/08/2007 (19/11/2009) 51 Front Street Slip End Luton Bedfordshire LU1 4BP **Tel:** (01582) 727 725 w 6283824

TUCKER Yolanda Jane Louise (see JONES, Mrs)

TUDHOPE Amanda Jane 01/02/1994 21 Hereford Way Banbury Oxfordshire OX16 1FT **Tel:** (01295) 273768 w 6067707

TUDOR Lynn Margaret (nee Hyland) 10/04/2003 57 Graham Road HALESOWEN West Midlands B62 8LJ **Tel:** 07973270236 w 6287663

Nina Rachael (nee Blower) 14/09/1998 Sutton Farm Veterinary Surgery Tilstock Crescent Sutton Farm Shrewsbury Shropshire SY2 6HW **Tel:** (01743) 352274 w 6133986

TUFFEY Danielle Olivia 30/05/2003 15 Aspen Gardens ASHFORD Middlesex TW15 1ED **Tel:** (01784) 240243 w 6283725

TUGWELL Victoria (formerly Williams) 15/08/1990 5 River Mount Walton-on-Thames Surrey KT12 2PW **Tel:** (01932) 224 684 w 6063950

TULLY Victoria Frances 09/09/2008 61 Spring Road Ettingshall Wolverhampton West Midlands WV4 6LQ **Tel:** 01902405314 w 6405473

TUNNICLIFFE Lisa (see WILLSHER, Mrs)

TURLEY Louise Ann 30/05/2006 35 Sandringham Road STOURBRIDGE West Midlands DY8 5HN **Tel:** (01384) 838235 w 6345083

TURNBULL Lindsey 27/07/2004 16 Ashling Park Road Denmead Waterlooville Hampshire PO7 6EH w 6273968

TURNBULL Melanie Anne (see GOLDIE, Mrs)

Sarah 24/11/1988 22 Grange Road Shilbottle Alnwick Northumberland NE66 2XN **Tel:** (01665) 575 877 w 6062527

TURNER Anne Margaret 02/09/1997 39 Hawkins Road Shoreham-by-Sea West Sussex BN43 6TH **Tel:** (01273) 591790 w 6032026

Anne-Marie 13/08/2003 43 Fern Grove Bradley Stoke BRISTOL BS32 8DS **Tel:** (07791) 912975 w 6273429

TURNER Claire Louise (see HALLAS, Mrs)

Clare Michelle (nee Turner) 31/07/2009 73 Peveril Bank Dawley Bank TELFORD Shropshire TF4 2BZ w 6289280

Gemma Margaret 14/11/2008 4 St. Mary's Court LANARK ML11 7EN **Tel:** 07933528763 w 6404758

TURNER Helen (see GRIFFITH, Mrs)

Helen Rachel 11/03/2005 Admirals Rest Bellingdon CHESHAM Buckinghamshire HP5 2XU **Tel:** (01494) 758220 w 6308277

Helen Sarah 12/01/1987 (25/06/1998) Cat & Rabbit Care Clinic 1 Limehurst Square NORTHAMPTON NN5 6LP **Tel:** (01604) 478888 w 606255X

Jean Margaret 10/11/1971 Greenway 1 Eastcote Lane Northolt Village Middlesex UB5 5RE **Tel:** (020) 8841 5517 w 6062560

TURNER Jody Marie (see BLYTH-TANCOCK, Mrs)

TURNER Julia Suzanne (see BUTLER, Mrs)

Kelly Ann 16/12/2005 106 Hendford Hill Yeovil Somerset BA20 2RF **Tel:** (01935) 474690 w 6319200

Laura Ellen 22/12/2004 (21/04/2009) Spinney Hill Veterinary Centre 136 Spinney Hill Addlestone Surrey KT15 1BB **Tel:** (01932) 853991 w 6263551

Louise 06/11/2009 8 Boniface Close Totton Southampton SO40 3SJ **Tel:** 02380869234 w 6452036

Lucy Ann (nee Meadows) 17/07/2003 5 Chestnut Close Tean STOKE-ON-TRENT ST10 4JD **Tel:** (01538) 724 630 w 6252584

TURNER Lynsey (see POPE, Ms)

Ruth 14/01/1991 Les Frenes La Rue Militaire St. John JERSEY JE3 4DP **Tel:** (07812) 715688 w 6001880

Susan Alice 08/02/1999 (11/10/2000) Ark Veterinary Centre 14 Church Lane Lexden Colchester Essex CO3 4AF **Tel:** (01206) 572410 w 6137448

TURPIE Charlotte Jane 12/01/2009 33 Green Lane Chinley High Peak Derbyshire SK23 6ET **Tel:** 01663750833 w 6438671

TURRALL Carolyn Jane 16/12/2005 16 Ramparts Close Great Horkesley COLCHESTER CO6 4AZ **Tel:** (01206) 271105 w 6332367

TURRINGTON Ann Hazel 27/03/2001 12 Sidney Gardens Haslingfield Cambridge CB3 7NA **Tel:** (01223) 870526 w 6204987

TURTON Christine June 27/01/1992 39 Lordswood Road Harborne BIRMINGHAM B17 9QT **Tel:** (0121) 426 4343 w 6062571

Tina 19/01/2005 (01/02/2007) Calweton Veterinary Centre 79 Tavistock Road Callington Cornwall PL17 7RD **Tel:** (01579) 383231 w 6294494

TUTT Amy Louise 06/08/2008 1 Bellhanger Cottages Station Road Bentworth Alton Hampshire GU34 5QZ **Tel:** (01420) 563020 w 6409356

TWEEDIE Hilary 26/10/2005 9 Buchanan Place Torrance GLASGOW G64 4HW **Tel:** (01360) 622158 w 6318606

TWEEDLE Katie 04/01/2001 Ormiston 93 Eastham Village Road Eastham Cheshire CH62 0AW **Tel:** (0151) 327 5120 w 6205790

TWELLS Amanda Marie 28/08/1997 142 Derby Road Long Eaton Nottingham NG10 4ER **Tel:** (0115) 972 7050 w 6098790

TWEMLOW Victoria Jayne (see VASS, Mrs)

TWOMEY Joan Mary 31/08/2005 4 Sedbergh Crescent CHESTERFIELD Derbyshire S41 8DY w 6242343

TWYMAN Lianne Frances (see MIDSON, Mrs)

TYLER Lynne Barbara 29/01/2009 Flat 2 Parker House Parkers Road CHIPPING NORTON Oxfordshire OX7 5LQ **Tel:** 01608642547 w 6436031

Sally Linda 04/08/1987 (01/03/2002) 39 Uplands Road Saltford BRISTOL BS31 3JQ w 6062607

TYRRELL Julie 05/07/2006 Ashgrove Veterinary Centre Ltd 10 Belmont Road Aberdeen AB25 3SR **Tel:** (01224) 486444 w 6329837

TYRRELL-ASPREY Elizabeth Jane 01/09/2004 13 Longfield Mells FROME Somerset BA11 3PY **Tel:** 07900817171 w 6346073

TYSON Gemma Victoria Jane 02/06/2004 The Veterinary Centre Queen Annes Road GREAT YARMOUTH Norfolk NR31 0LE **Tel:** (01493) 416700 w 6283769

TYSON Maria May (see CORCORAN, Mrs)

U

UBYSZ Paula Jane 29/08/1997 Ty Capel Moelfre Abergele Clwyd LL22 9RF **Tel:** (01745) 823572 w 6118764

UDALE Christina 24/05/2006 41 Manor Road UTTOXETER Staffordshire ST14 7JL w 6342784

UEBERSAX Stephanie Ann (see UEBERSAX'-BLINCOE, Mrs)

UEBERSAX'BLINCOE Stephanie Ann (nee Uebersax) 31/10/2003 12 Station Road Clifton Upon Dunsmore Rugby Warwickshire CV23 0BT w 6289621

UMNEY Elizabeth Rachel 10/11/2009 Farleigh Beech Lane Jordans BEACONSFIELD Buckinghamshire HP9 2SZ **Tel:** 01494873106 w 6321785

UNDERDOWN Amy Louise 06/10/2006 46 Beech Avenue Alvaston DERBY DE24 0DZ w 6365840

UNDERHILL Kimberley Ann 06/06/2008 127 Chelmsley Road BIRMINGHAM B37 7SJ w 6350264

UNDERWOOD Emma Jane 18/10/2006 Swanspool Veterinary Clinic 1 London Road Wellingborough Northamptonshire NN8 2BT **Tel:** (01933) 222145 w 6357117

UNSWORTH Ruth (nee Taylor) 10/02/2004 32 Bradley Fold Cottages Bolton Lancashire BL2 6RN **Tel:** (01204) 532 782 w 6283516

UPTON Kirsty Jayne 20/11/2008 87 Longmead Avenue Hazel Grove Stockport Cheshire SK7 5PJ w 6438583

URQUHART Catherine Anne 15/08/1991 63 Upper Albert Road Sheffield South Yorkshire S8 9HT w 601315X

Melissa Anne 21/03/2007 28 The Farthings Crowborough East Sussex TN6 2TW **Tel:** (01892) 663037 w 6367787

Sharon Jean 26/09/1994 18b Gateside Street West Kilbride Ayrshire KA23 9BA **Tel:** (01294) 829675 w 602545X

URWIN Danielle Louise (nee Cooper) 19/01/2005 24 Montsale Pitsea BASILDON Essex SS13 1JL **Tel:** (01268) 4589113 w 6303228

USHER SMITH Rosemary Kate 01/04/2003 3 Station Road Haddington East Lothian EH41 3NU w 6282416

UWINS Alison Kate 03/05/2007 12 Calais Dene Bampton Oxfordshire OX18 2NR **Tel:** (01993) 851107 w 6373045

V

VAITES Wendy Susan 26/06/1998 27 Kirkham Drive Beeston Nottingham NG9 6HG **Tel:** (0115) 9176109 w 6076857

VALE Trudie Anne (nee Granville) 02/09/1999 86 Horton Drive Middleton Cheney BANBURY Oxfordshire OX17 2LL **Tel:** (01295) 713814 w 6033030

VALENTINE Clare Louise (nee Stephens) 25/01/1994 Rivendell Tir Griffin Garth Llangollen Wrexham LL20 7UR **Tel:** (01978) 812113 w 6066204

Jane 17/09/2007 83 Sandersons Croft LEIGH Lancashire WN7 2BB **Tel:** (01942) 201901 w 6351507

Lisa Joanne 02/09/1997 (24/10/2002) Davies Veterinary Specialists Manor Farm Business Park Higham Gobion Hertfordshire SG5 3HR **Tel:** (01582) 883950 w 6110856

VAN DER MERWE Tracy-Shelagh 27/02/2006 37 Grasvenor Avenue BARNET Hertfordshire EN5 2BY **Tel:** (0777) 357 7376 w 6419377

VAN EEDEN Helene Elizabeth 18/05/2009 21 Wild Flower Way Ditchingham BUNGAY Suffolk NR35 2SF **Tel:** 07833025842 w 6550926

VAN HAGHT Sarah Lynne 10/02/2004 18 Sutton Road Soudley Cinderford Gloucestershire GL14 2TX **Tel:** (01594) 826397 w 6356138

VAN ROOYEN Katherine Jane (see STEVENS, Mrs)

VAN WEZEL Fiona (nee Mitchell) 18/10/2006 88-92 Merton High Street Merton London SW19 1BD **Tel:** (020) 8254 1400 w 6375575

VAN ZOMEREN Leandra Gerdina Marlena (formerly Zomerem Van) 24/01/2005 The Marlowes Veterinary Surgery 59 Marlowes Hemel Hempstead Hertfordshire HP1 1LE w 6386058

VANCE Gemma Ashleigh 29/01/2007 125 The Stables Minorca Drive Carrickfergus County Antrim BT38 8WS **Tel:** (07739) 561500 w 6344335

VANCOEVORDEN Laura Claire 09/07/2009 15 Byfield LEIGH-ON-SEA Essex SS9 5TG **Tel:** (01702) 529346 w 6305615

VAN-DE-VYVER Tracey Elizabeth (see NETHERTON, Mrs)

VANGEN Maia Liv 20/01/1998 Alder Veterinary Hospital 284 Brodie Avenue Liverpool Merseyside L19 7NQ **Tel:** (0151) 291 9393 w 6116621

VANNER Victoria Mary (nee Horswell) 31/10/2003 Milehouse Clinic 28 Outland Road Milehouse Plymouth Devon PL2 3DF **Tel:** (01752) 567567 w 6264750

VANSTON Gillian Louise 07/12/2006 46 Landseer Avenue Warrington Cheshire WA4 6DJ **Tel:** (01925) 636425 w 6372990

VANSTONE Kate Marie 27/01/2005 Penbode Veterinary Group Penbode North Road Holsworthy Devon EX22 6HB **Tel:** (01409) 253418 w 6300214

VANT Jessica (see HUTCHINGS, Mrs)

VARGA Charlotte Anna 26/02/2003 14 Billing Road Coventry West Midlands CV5 8EU **Tel:** (02476) 468986 w 6264860

VARLOW Margaret Hilary DipAVN(Surgical) 22/12/1994 10 Shepherds Leaze Wotton under Edge Gloucestershire GL12 7LQ **Tel:** (01453) 521850 w 6034817

VARNAM Heather 15/10/2004 44 Charolais Crescent Lightwood Stoke-on-Trent ST3 4TE w 6283043

VARNEY Alison Sarah (see DONALD, Ms)

VASS Victoria Jayne (nee Twemlow) 04/12/2003 Johnson & Farrell Victoria Road Tain Ross-Shire IV19 1AU **Tel:** (01862) 894223 w 6289203

VEAL Susan 12/12/1997 Holmfield Norwood End Fyfield Essex CM5 0RW **Tel:** (01277) 899684 w 6100520

VENABLES Katrina Laura (nee Bond) 03/05/2005 19 Argosy Road Benson Wallingford Oxfordshire OX10 6DG **Tel:** (07866) 517842 w 6319970

VENN Marie Louise 06/08/2007 77 Loxton Road WESTON-SUPER-MARE Avon BS23 4RW w 6374816

VENNI Jennifer May 26/10/2000 Hall Farm Church Lane Roydon King's Lynn Norfolk PE32 1AR **Tel:** (01485) 600022 w 6205075

VENNING Katherine Elizabeth (see KEENE, Mrs)

VENTOUR Lisa Caroline 28/06/2002 18 Oakdale Avenue PETERBOROUGH PE2 8TA w 6314602

VENTURI ROSE Joy (nee Weingartner) 05/08/1976 Leospring The Keepe Conford Liphook Hampshire GU30 7QN **Tel:** (01428) 751125 w 6014095

VENUS Cassie 10/11/2009 43 Hillside Avenue GRAVESEND Kent DA12 5QN **Tel:** 01474566214 w 6465280

VERNAU Antony James 30/07/2004 Colne Valley Veterinary Practice Off Maudlyn Road Colchester CO1 2GU **Tel:** (01206) 794695 m 6299114

VERNON Caroline Anna 12/02/2008 208 Whiteway Road Bath BA2 2RJ **Tel:** (01225) 442280 w 6381438

VERNOUM Georgina Suzanne (nee Archbold) 18/01/2001 The Shepton Veterinary Group Allyn Saxon Drive Shepton Mallet Somerset BA4 5QH **Tel:** (01749) 343955 w 6210740

VERRECCHIA Zara Marie 07/01/2010 76 Addison Road CATERHAM Surrey CR3 5LR w 6405319

VICKERY Clare Louise 18/04/2005 25 Walmesley Chase Hilperton TROWBRIDGE Wiltshire BA14 7HX **Tel:** (01225) 350022 w 6282504

VILLIERS Stacey Marie 21/04/2008 Swanspool Veterinary Clinic 1 London Road Wellingborough Northamptonshire NN8 2BT **Tel:** (01933) 222145 w 6357887

VINCENT Carrie Anne (see WARD, Mrs)

VINCENT Clare Susan 05/09/2000 Beaulieu Thornhill Road Stalbridge Sturminster Newton Dorset DT10 2PS **Tel:** (01963) 350307 w 6134629

Julie Clare 05/07/2006 16 Treetops Brentwood Essex CM15 9DE **Tel:** (01277) 214313 w 6267214

Kate Martha 04/02/2009 65 Bexhill Road Ingol Preston Lancashire PR2 3SY **Tel:** 01772727491 w 6436471

Kelly Louise 29/08/2000 Filham Park Veterinary Clinic Goodwell Lane Ivybridge Devon PL21 0LE **Tel:** (01752) 892700 w 6134673

Kim 07/12/2005 Grove Dene Veterinary Clinic The Forum Abbey Manor Park Yeovil Somerset BA21 3TL **Tel:** (01935) 421177 w 6328330

Louise Nicola 29/08/2000 Hurleyford Farm Shepherds Lane Hurley Maidenhead Berkshire SL6 5NG **Tel:** (01628) 829000 w 6122180

VINER Gemma Ann (see OCKENDEN, Mrs)

VINER Hayley-Marie Jayne 03/10/2008 108 Bradstock Road Stoneleigh Epsom Surrey KT19 2LG **Tel:** 07825743128 w 6412447

VIRRILL Laura June 03/12/2003 18 The Spinney Calmore SOUTHAMPTON Hampshire SO40 2WB w 6286772

VISAGIE Gillian Margaret 10/05/2007 23 Newland Mews Culcheth Warrington Cheshire WA3 4EN **Tel:** 07817867024 w 6376950

VISZKED Rebecca 24/11/2009 11 Martin Close BUCKINGHAM MK18 7HB **Tel:** (01280) 813562 w 6465291

VIVEASH Fiona Mary 13/05/2008 473 Ferndale Road Swindon Wiltshire SN2 1DF **Tel:** (01793) 694082 w 6391877

VOIGT Julia Carola 17/07/2003 348 South Lambeth Road Stockwell London SW8 1UQ **Tel:** (020) 7498 6363 w 6281217

VOSE Dawn Alison (nee Cowling) 15/10/1996 Houseboat Luisa 5 Ryepeck Moorings Ryepeck Meadow Chertsey Road Shepperton Middlesex TW17 9NU w 6098994

VOSPER Samantha 04/11/2008 11 Franks Court Gillingham Kent ME8 6JA **Tel:** 01634231297 w 6441102

VOSSER Gemma Marie (see VOSSER-SMITH, Mrs)

VOSSER-SMITH Gemma Marie (nee Vosser) 23/12/2003 24 Prince Charles Crescent FARNBOROUGH Hampshire GU14 8DJ **Tel:** (01252) 375384 w 6290897

VYAS Krishma Serita 11/02/2008 4 Oak Road Bursledon SOUTHAMPTON SO31 8DU **Tel:** (07950) 264972 w 6351518

VYSE Joanne (see VYSE-KILLA, Mrs)

VYSE-KILLA Joanne (nee Vyse) 09/11/2005 28 Parc Starling Johnstown Carmarthen Dyfed SA31 3HX **Tel:** (01267) 222396 w 6351540

W

WADDOUPS Victoria Louise (see PRIESTLEY, Mrs)

WADE Gemma 16/09/2008 Elands Veterinary Clinic Station Road Dunton Green Sevenoaks Kent TN13 2XA **Tel:** (01732) 452333 w 6436988

Lauren Ann Edith (nee Gerrard) 05/06/2006 (03/12/2009) Flat 41 Coleman Court Kimber Road LONDON SW18 4PA **Tel:** (020) 8874 4339 w 6427902

WADHAM-SMITH Julia Claire (see GRIFFIN, Mrs)

WADMORE Danielle Simone 26/01/2000 Highcroft Veterinary Group 25 London Road Hailsham East Sussex BN27 3BN **Tel:** (01323) 841666 w 6190621

WAGER Catherine Jane 03/10/2008 Oakdene High Road Great Finborough Stowmarket Suffolk IP14 3AP **Tel:** 07790842432 w 6433435

Rachel (nee Allen) 17/09/1998 Myerscough College Bilsborrow Preston Lancashire PR3 0RY **Tel:** (01995) 642222 w 6134389

WAGG Amy Lorraine 22/03/2004 15 Border Crescent Alvaston Derby DE24 0HU **Tel:** (01332) 753656 w 6289027

WAGSTAFF Sarah Susan 24/08/1998 1 Alexander Cottage Brampton Lane Chapel Brampton Northampton NN6 8BE **Tel:** (01604) 847977 w 6121799

WAINWRIGHT Caroline (formerly Rogers) 23/07/2007 84 Cardiff Place Bassingbourn ROYSTON Hertfordshire SG8 5LR w 6355412

Dawn Elizabeth 21/11/2005 32-34 Market Place Ashbourne Derbyshire DE6 1ES **Tel:** (01335) 342227 w 6346656

Eran 01/04/2003 30 Whiteside Road Haydock ST. HELENS Merseyside WA11 0XN **Tel:** (01744) 27662 w 6273154

Hailey Marie 27/05/2008 The Willows The Street Wramplingham Wymondham Norfolk NR18 0RU **Tel:** (01603) 757887 w 6350825

WAISTELL Caroline Mari 02/06/2006 4 Arden Road Bulkington Bedworth Warwickshire CV12 9JJ **Tel:** (024) 7631 3376 w 6355808

WAITE Victoria Jainie 01/03/2000 (02/03/2009) 93 Mountview Crescent St. Lawrence SOUTHMINSTER Essex CM0 7NR **Tel:** (01621) 778436 w 6191028

WAKE Emma Louise 29/07/2005 37 Skeaping Close NEWMARKET Suffolk CB8 0GP **Tel:** (01638) 717871 w 6289984

WAKE Paula Lisa (see BRZENCZEK, Mrs)

WAKEFIELD Karen DipAVN(Medical) (nee Jameson) 04/02/2002 (07/01/2010) 132 Mowbray Road South Shields Tyne and Wear NE33 3AZ **Tel:** (0191) 454 8293 w 6266609

WAKELING Michelle Nina 03/06/2003 12 Southwood Road DUNSTABLE Bedfordshire LU5 4EA w 6266422

WAKELY Jessica Frances 11/05/2004 4 Battersea Park Road Battersea London SW8 4AA **Tel:** (020) 7627 9256 w 6274265

WAKERELL Naomi Claire 24/10/2008 1 Briarsleigh Stafford Staffordshire ST17 4QP **Tel:** (077199) 62109 w 6410753

WALDIE Katherine Jane (see JAMESON, Mrs)

WALFORD Sarah Alethea 31/08/1999 Ashtead Veterinary Centre 12 Craddocks Parade Ashtead Surrey KT21 1QL **Tel:** (01372) 276262 w 6135338

WALKER Catherine Ellen 24/01/2000 69 Waverley Avenue NUNEATON Warwickshire CV11 4RS **Tel:** (02476) 345970 w 6140235

Charlotte Emily 07/11/2008 53-55 Maidstone Road Footscray SIDCUP Kent DA14 5HB **Tel:** (020) 8300 8111 w 6396057

Claire Donn 24/11/2005 Cascella Brough Hempriggs WICK Caithness KW1 5TP w 6272912

Dawn Syrita 15/02/2008 7 Fenton Street BARROW-IN-FURNESS Cumbria LA14 1DE **Tel:** (07825) 237 256 w 6359207

Deborah 23/01/2003 (13/03/2009) 26 Shepley Road Audenshaw MANCHESTER M34 5DJ **Tel:** (0161) 3350387 w 6249757

Elizabeth Anne 02/09/1999 224 Mitcham Road Tooting London SW17 9NN **Tel:** (020) 8672 8322 w 6141556

Emma Jayne 14/03/2008 36 Boston Road Kirton Boston Lincolnshire PE20 1DS **Tel:** (01205) 722696 w 6272978

Helen Claire 19/02/1997 Seadown Veterinary Hospital Frost Lane Hythe Southampton Hampshire SO45 3NG **Tel:** (023) 8084 2237 w 6100531

WALKER Helen Elizabeth (see CLARKE, Mrs)

Jennifer Lyndsey 20/10/2008 18 Argyll Road Marton-in-Cleveland MIDDLESBROUGH Cleveland TS7 8JJ **Tel:** 07951213301 w 6288730

Karen Jean 15/07/2008 Braefoot Cottage Crossroads Hurlford Kilmarnock Ayrshire KA1 5JQ **Tel:** (01563) 884394 w 6377555

Karen Mabel 07/10/1991 L.I.T.E. Ltd 3a Church Street St. Helens Merseyside WA10 1BA **Tel:** (01744) 24062 w 6002035

Katie Teresa 15/08/2003 (19/06/2008) 3 Davies Drive St. Annes Park BRISTOL BS4 4HJ **Tel:** (01179) 041478 w 6264442

Laura Jane 29/10/2004 Chimneys Hailsham Road Heathfield East Sussex TN21 8AD **Tel:** (01435) 864422 w 6284264

Leanne Carole 18/02/2008 3 Bradley Street Burton-on-Trent Staffordshire DE15 9LJ **Tel:** (01283) 534 682 w 6401920

Lucy 04/03/2008 54b South Road HAILSHAM East Sussex BN27 3JQ **Tel:** (07976) 229090 w 6402833

Michelle (nee Brown) 20/08/2002 Brunswick Place Veterinary Clinic Brunswick Place Cranbourne Lane Basingstoke Hampshire RG21 3NN **Tel:** (01256) 473371 w 6262880

Patricia Lawrie 11/01/1991 24 St. Margaret Street Dunfermline Fife KY12 7PE **Tel:** (01383) 732897 w 6062957

Ruth Karen 17/01/2000 75 Bunns Lane Dudley West Midlands DY2 7RG **Tel:** (01384) 254252 w 6128342

Sarah Louise (formerly Foster) 02/08/1988 8 Pinfold Close Osbournby Sleaford Lincolnshire NG34 0DJ **Tel:** (01529) 455359 w 6050668

Suzanne 10/02/2004 53 Pearson Park HULL HU5 2TG **Tel:** (01377) 255353 w 6269579

Victoria Alanda Elizabeth 21/01/1999 37 Canterbury Street Chaddesden Derby DE21 4LF **Tel:** (01332) 349862 w 6135098

WALKER Victoria Louise (see WALKER-PARLANE, Mrs)

WALKER-BOYCE Emma Jayne 26/08/2008 31 Ormiston Avenue Glasgow Lanarkshire G14 9EE **Tel:** (077991) 68452 w 6350253

WALKER-PARLANE Victoria Louise (nee Walker) 31/10/2003 84 Lower Lichfield Street Willenhall West Midlands WV13 1QE **Tel:** (01902) 605080 w 6288433

WALL Gemma 05/07/2007 201 Pilch Lane Liverpool Merseyside L14 0LD **Tel:** (0151) 228 8299 w 6387873

Jennifer Sarah 10/07/2009 Ranelagh Farm Crouch Lane Winkfield WINDSOR Berkshire SL4 4TN **Tel:** 07719734799 w 6560452

Karen Louise 30/11/2005 The Annex Kingsnorth Veterinary Centre Ashford Road Kingsnorth ASHFORD Kent TN23 3EA **Tel:** (07790) 924670 w 6345578

WALLACE Clare Rachel 18/05/2009 The Ardmore Veterinary Group 57 Cornard Road Sudbury Suffolk CO10 2XB **Tel:** (01787) 372588 w 6385288

WALLACE Kerry Margaret (see NICHOLSON, Mrs)

Linsey 05/04/2005 17 Burnside Road Rutherglen Glasgow Lanarkshire G73 4RL **Tel:** (0141) 569 2465 w 6318617

Ruth Pauline 05/09/1996 16 Dalsholm Place GLASGOW G20 0UH w 6036814

Sharon Louise 09/09/1998 The Maisonette 5 Broad Street Bromyard Herefordshire HR7 4BS **Tel:** (07967) 750 576 w 6098826

WALLER Clare Diana (see STUBBS, Mrs)

WALLER Rosalie Kim 05/09/2008 The Coach House 10 Russell Place Edinburgh Midlothian EH5 3HH **Tel:** (0131) 551 3792 w 6379601

WALLER Wendy Louise (see SMITH, Mrs)

WALLIS Catherine Ann 29/06/2007 89 Weston Road Lichfield Staffordshire WS13 7PA **Tel:** 07910529291 w 6351551

WALMSLEY Jill Christine (see BAXTER, Mrs)

WALSH Emma Louise 31/12/2008 48 Woodgrange Avenue London N12 0PS **Tel:** 07779252482 w 6384925

Mark Nicholas Stephen 01/06/2007 Wood Street Veterinary Hospital 74 Wood Street Barnet Hertfordshire EN5 4BW **Tel:** (020) 8449 0074 m 6376642

Michael Allan 05/04/2005 25 Harper Terrace Yeadon Leeds LS19 7RP **Tel:** (01132) 505522 m 6313414

Sinead Lillian 23/08/2005 18 Lansdell Road MITCHAM Surrey CR4 2JE **Tel:** (0208) 6406475 w 6307441

Vicky 22/11/2001 48 Lower Chestnut Street Worcester Worcestershire WR1 1PD **Tel:** (01905) 613 570 w 6265135

WALTER Emma Elizabeth 10/09/2009 Regency House Bow Street Langport Somerset TA10 9PS **Tel:** (01458) 250459 w 6434766

Wendy Louise 14/04/2008 65 Marsh Lane Misterton Doncaster South Yorkshire DN10 4DL **Tel:** (01427) 890415 w 6327538

WALTERS Amanda Jane 25/09/2000 Cobb Cottage Thornicombe BLANDFORD FORUM Dorset DT11 9AE **Tel:** (01258) 450736 w 6203590

Hayley Myfanwy 27/09/1999 The Old Barn Cottage Manchester Road Tideswell Buxton Derbyshire SK17 8LL **Tel:** (01298) 872 294 w 6185374

Laura Kate (nee Frith) 03/02/1997 (02/11/2009) 12 Albion Street KENILWORTH Warwickshire CV8 2FW w 6038618

Lisa Helen 16/06/2008 34 Chalice Way GLASTONBURY Somerset BA6 8EX **Tel:** (01458) 834 205 w 6380888

WALTERS Louise Marie (see DAVIES, Mrs)

WALTERS Natalie Isabel (see PULLEN, Mrs)

Stacey Christine 04/08/2008 55 Kings Road Biggin Hill WESTERHAM Kent TN16 3XY w 6403460

WALTON Amy Suzanne 05/03/2009 42 Longden Coleham Shrewsbury Shropshire SY3 7DQ **Tel:** 07956902697 w 6446063

Chloe Louise 22/04/2008 Lynwood Veterinary Group Station Road Wimborne Dorset BH21 1RQ **Tel:** (01202) 882101 w 6389325

WALTON Jane (see FRANCIS, Mrs)

Jennifer Louise 04/01/2008 13 Essex Grove SUNDERLAND SR3 1BG w 6376961

Julia Kim (nee Wilkie) 05/09/1996 62 Wiltshire Avenue Burton-upon-Stather SCUNTHORPE South Humberside DN15 9ER **Tel:** (01724) 720809 w 6038185

WALTON Julie (see FORREST, Mrs)

Zoe Ellen Crichton (nee Fisher) 12/03/2002 (20/01/2010) 5 Cherry Tree Walk Stretford Manchester M32 9AT w 6271394

WANNELL Clare Louise 02/04/2000 Inside Pets at Home Unit 213 Rydon Lane Retail Park Exeter Devon EX2 7HX **Tel:** (01392) 266860 w 6191424

WANT Mary Louise (nee Barron) 01/11/1992 Feldon Veterinary Centre 1 Guy Street Leamington Spa Warwickshire CV32 4RX **Tel:** (01926) 423161 w 6045115

Sarah Margaret (nee Harbage) 02/02/2001 713-715 Chester Road Kingshurst Birmingham B36 0LN **Tel:** (0121) 770 4966 w 6211917

WARD Anne Marie DipAVN(Surgical) (nee Ward, formerly Stevens) 04/09/1995 Barony College Parkgate Dumfries DG1 3NE **Tel:** (01387) 860251 w 6028009

Beverly Davina 11/01/2005 Artfinney House 23 Glen Road Hillsborough Co Down BT26 6ES **Tel:** (028) 92682037 w 6300654

Carrie Anne (nee Vincent) 10/05/2007 (03/07/2009) Flat 67, Brentwood Court Lowther Road Prestwich Manchester Lancashire M25 9PX **Tel:** (0161) 798 6152 w 6383264

Catherine Jennifer 22/11/2001 Birchmere South Road Hythe Kent CT21 6AT **Tel:** (01303) 260295 w 6259536

Clare Linda (nee Rowe) 29/08/2000 Parkside Veterinary Centre 61 Ruskin Road Carshalton Surrey SM5 3DD **Tel:** (020) 8395 8222 w 6202622

Donna Michelle 28/09/2001 (12/07/2007) Sparsholt College Sparsholt WINCHESTER Hampshire SO21 2NF **Tel:** (01962) 797477 w 6190522

Gemma Claire 07/04/2008 Windy Ridge Walesby Road Market Rasen Lincolnshire LN8 3EY **Tel:** (01673) 842132 w 6406034

Gemma Louise 21/03/2006 57-59 Broadleys Clay Cross Chesterfield Derbyshire S45 9JN **Tel:** (01246) 862266 w 6344346

Juliet 18/02/2009 48 Badgers Brook Road Drayton Norwich Norfolk NR8 6EY **Tel:** 01603869276 w 6437769

Karen Louise (nee Arents) 10/04/2003 31 Zander Road CALNE Wiltshire SN11 9QS w 6252397

Laura Alison 26/01/1999 Willow Veterinary Surgery 323 Drayton High Road Norwich NR6 5AA **Tel:** (01603) 411520 w 612890X

Michelle Jane (nee Ward, formerly Chacksfield) 31/03/2003 34 Kings Way Burgess Hill West Sussex RH15 0TP **Tel:** (01444) 233947 w 6278324

Natalie Elaine (nee Sitch) 31/08/1999 Grange Hill Veterinary Centre Grange Lane LICHFIELD Staffordshire WS13 8HX **Tel:** (01543) 416246 w 6185286

Nicola Jane 17/07/2008 Ardene House Veterinary Hospital Kingswells Aberdeen AB15 8PJ **Tel:** (01224) 740700 w 6414559

Nicola Jane (nee Bell) 21/01/2008 15 Ennerdale Road Stockton-on-Tees Cleveland TS18 4ND **Tel:** (01642) 652196 w 6257413

Rebecca Jane 08/01/2008 81 Epsom Road Guildford Surrey GU1 3PA **Tel:** (01483) 566322 w 6367798

Rebecca Julia DipAVN(Medical) 24/08/1999 7 Burnsall Close Pendeford Wolverhampton WV9 5RU **Tel:** (01902) 780086 w 6141669

Sarah Louise 13/01/2004 Lanwades Park Kentford Newmarket Suffolk CB8 7UU **Tel:** (01638) 552700 w 6254047

WARDLE Dawn (see FRATER, Mrs)

WARDLE Kelly Lorraine (see TIMMS, Miss)

WARD-MUNDIN Sarah Ann 27/03/2008 72 Ashburnham Road Northampton Northamptonshire NN1 4RA **Tel:** (01604) 468320 w 6407178

WARDROP Rhona Elizabeth 27/02/2007 37 Temple Grove Park Bakers Lane West Hanningfield CHELMSFORD CM2 8LQ w 6337581

WARE Sharon Tracey 16/01/1991 (06/08/2002) 33 Phoenix Way Cardiff South Glamorgan CF14 4PR w 6063134

WARFORD Karen Elizabeth 24/11/2004 9 Thirston Close Nottingham Nottinghamshire NG6 7FR **Tel:** (0115) 877 3384 w 6316505

WARING Nicola Gail (nee Brown) 03/12/2003 5 Dales Avenue Whitefield MANCHESTER M45 7RN w 6281019

WARMAN Amanda Louise (nee Smith) 04/10/2005 Silva House Veterinary Clinic Silver Street Midsomer Norton Radstock Somerset BA3 2ET **Tel:** (01761) 412223 w 6277037

WARNER Carol 15/09/1980 37 Ophelia Drive Heathcote Warwick CV34 6XJ **Tel:** (01926) 313459 w 6063167

Jill Diana Murrell 09/08/1983 (16/11/1998) Well Cottage Norleaze Heywood WESTBURY BA13 4LQ **Tel:** (01373) 826322 w 6002068

Juliet Ruth Alice 13/05/2003 Rahern Coombe Hill Langton Matravers Swanage Dorset BH19 3EU w 6276476

Sarah Louise 26/08/2008 4 Stoney Bank GILLINGHAM Kent ME7 3AG **Tel:** (01795) 476411 w 6421731

WARREN Katherine Anne 24/01/2006 Godalming Veterinary Surgery The Old Auction Mart Station Approach Godalming Surrey GU7 1EU **Tel:** (01483) 422644 w 6281976

WARREN Lucy Rachel (see ROBERTS-BATES, Mrs)

Nicola Jayne (nee Bretton) 23/12/1992 (01/06/2001) The Horse Clinic and The Pet Clinic at Blackmore Rookery Road Blackmore Ingatestone Essex CM4 0LE **Tel:** (01277) 823858 w 6044097

WARREN Tracey Joy (see READ, Mrs)

Vanessa Clare 18/10/2005 15 Catchpole Close CORBY Northamptonshire NN18 8DE **Tel:** (01536) 747549 w 6346667

WARRINGTON Dawn Angela 06/07/2004 6 Speers Road LEICESTER LE3 6QY w 6269656

Kerry Michelle 19/09/2006 22 Goodlake Avenue Faringdon Oxfordshire SN7 7AT **Tel:** (01367) 240 004 w 6329848

Samantha Jane 11/07/2007 (27/02/2009) 5 Bloxham Road CRANLEIGH Surrey GU6 7EY **Tel:** (01483) 274 067 w 6328341

WARWICK Lynsey Anne (see TINDALL, Mrs)

WARWICK Michelle Jane 29/07/2005 (07/07/2009) 15 Primrose Close CANVEY ISLAND Essex SS8 9YW w 6321158

WASHINGTON Becky Kuiama (nee Jackson) 13/05/2003 54 Cressett Avenue Brierley Hill West Midlands DY5 3XY **Tel:** (01384) 865803 w 6279490

WATE Layla Frances (see MACKIE, Mrs)

WATERFIELD Lucy Victoria (see WHARMBY, Mrs)

WATERS Catherine 18/09/2003 6 Wishaw Rise NEWCASTLE UPON TYNE NE15 7LL w 6253398

Tamsyn Rachel 30/01/2009 Rose Cottage Monmouth Road Usk Gwent NP15 1QY **Tel:** 01291673803 w 6400094

WATKINS Andrea Danielle 24/02/2004 The Bungalow Powkesmore Farm Ditton Priors Bridgnorth Shropshire WV16 6TW **Tel:** (01746) 712293 w 6275145

Bryony (nee Fletcher) 09/02/2009 55 Pines Road PAIGNTON Devon TQ3 3PF **Tel:** 07891124484 w 6429244

Fleur Martine 05/10/2004 (24/03/2006) 357 Hollins Lane Hollins Bury Lancashire BL9 8BD **Tel:** (0161) 767 9968 w 6291986

WATLING Emma Elizabeth 07/06/2005 12 Fundrey Road WISBECH Cambridgeshire PE13 3TP **Tel:** (01945) 587411 w 6295649

WATSON Amy Margaret 21/12/2007 1 Sycamore Street Haltwhistle Northumberland NE49 0AQ **Tel:** 07729303664 w 6376972

Chloe May 17/08/2005 Longlands Farm Mickleton CHIPPING CAMPDEN Gloucestershire GL55 6LL w 6301908

Clare Louise 05/04/2006 6 Wavell Drive Rosehill Industrial Estate Carlisle CA1 2ST **Tel:** (01228) 521393 w 6316516

Debra Louise 10/04/2003 Top Floor Flat 34 Knowle Road Totterdown Bristol Somerset BS4 2ED **Tel:** (0117) 9085969 w 6280953

Fiona Jean (nee Lumsden) 13/05/2003 175 Portobello High Street Edinburgh EH15 1EU **Tel:** (0131) 669 3790 w 6282383

Gillian Lena 12/02/2008 Flat 17 37 Chatsworth Road LONDON NW2 4BL w 6503120

Hayley Louise 04/11/2008 77 Bedford Road HESSLE North Humberside HU13 9DG w 6404989

Irene Margaret (nee Strain) 11/09/2003 The Veterinary Hospital 175 Newport Lincoln Lincolnshire LN1 3DZ **Tel:** (01522) 800333 w 6281811

Joanna Hilary 16/06/2008 Wessex House Calcraft Road Corfe Castle WAREHAM Dorset BH20 5EL **Tel:** (07973) 933 298 w 6380899

WATSON Laura (see SWALLOW, Mrs)

Lisa Jane 28/08/1996 61 School Hill NUNEATON Warwickshire CV10 0NF **Tel:** (024) 76396645 w 6098848

Nicola Jane (nee MacKinnon) 26/01/1996 33 Sunnyside Avenue Drumoak Banchory Kincardineshire AB31 5EF **Tel:** (01330) 811665 w 6038006

WATSON Nicola Jane (see EWERS, Mrs)

Rachel Hannah 08/12/2008 73 Chelmer Road BRAINTREE Essex CM7 3PX w 6434623

Rebecca Anne 14/10/1996 (23/04/2008) Corryvreckan Brownstown Road Curragh Co Kildare Ireland **Tel:** (00353) 87613 9698 w 6096534

WATSON Samantha Jane Lisa (see KENYON, Mrs)

Sophie Ann 27/04/2009 1-2 Lightwoods Road Smethwick West Midlands B67 5AY **Tel:** (0121) 429 1400 w 6350847

Vicki 17/11/2004 Crindle Cottage Mendlesham Green STOWMARKET Suffolk IP14 5RG w 6233312

Victoria Christine 09/03/2005 39 Dickinson Avenue Croxley Green Rickmansworth Hertfordshire WD3 3EU **Tel:** (01923) 223321 w 6277917

WATT Rebecca Jayne 08/09/2009 Alnorthumbria Veterinary Practice Ltd Fairmoor Morpeth Northumberland NE61 3JN **Tel:** (01670) 505321 w 6449550

WATTS Deborah (nee Ives) 16/01/1990 (27/10/2006) Moonfleet Bere Road Coldharbour Wareham Dorset BH20 7PA **Tel:** (01929) 555060 w 6053691

Joanne 11/01/2008 62 Pine Road Brentry BRISTOL BS10 6RU **Tel:** (0117) 949 0371 w 6392449

Joanne Carole (nee Nightingale) 13/12/1984 (25/04/2007) 39 Lordswood Road Harborne BIRMINGHAM B17 9QT **Tel:** (0121) 426 4343 w 6013331

Lyony Julie (nee Rose) 12/05/2004 6 Ealing Close Lordswood Chatham Kent ME5 8YJ w 6288708

Melanie Kay 04/09/1997 Mill House Veterinary Surgery & Hospital 20 Tennyson Avenue King's Lynn Norfolk PE30 2QG **Tel:** (01553) 771457 w 6039735

Rebecca Louise 15/10/2009 17 Fairglen HAYLE Cornwall TR27 4DL **Tel:** (01736) 752981 w 6463828

Rowena Jo 03/10/2007 (23/02/2009) The Wheel House Veterinary Centre Amersham Road Chesham Buckinghamshire HP5 1NQ **Tel:** (01494) 782001 w 6373001

WAUDBY Janine 11/08/2008 113 Goddard Avenue Hull North Humberside HU5 2AW w 6339253

WAUGH Angela Kay (nee Worthy) 01/09/1998 35 Roker Park Road Roker Sunderland SR6 9PL **Tel:** (0191) 516 0056 w 6132574

Jessica 29/01/2007 87 Bournemouth Road Parkstone Poole Dorset BH14 0ER **Tel:** (01202) 739484 w 6359218

WAYLEN Helen Claire (nee Morse) 18/01/2002 Crossways Farm Ashton Common Trowbridge Wiltshire BA14 6DX **Tel:** 01380-870310 w 6260834

WEASTELL Elisa Nicole (see ROBINSON, Mrs)

WEAVER Heather Ruth 13/03/1995 (25/11/2003) 64 Mill Street Ottery St. Mary Devon EX11 1AF **Tel:** (01404) 814322 w 6026260

WEAVER Helen Felicity (see CROFTS, Mrs)

Kelly Ann 10/02/2005 The Byre Manor Road Chedzoy Bridgwater Somerset TA7 8QZ **Tel:** (01278) 453532 w 6275618

WEBB Alys Rebecca 01/09/1998 13 The Causeway Quedgeley Gloucester GL2 4LD **Tel:** (07837) 207319 w 6076008

Charlotte- Anne 10/09/2009 9 Gilian Road Llandaff Cardiff CF5 2PZ **Tel:** 07816065085 w 6490393

Helen Lorraine (nee Whitaker) 08/04/2005 46 Hillbrow LETCHWORTH GARDEN CITY

Hertfordshire SG6 3RE **Tel:** (07740) 355580 w 6325261

Karen Liza (nee Simmons) 28/08/1998 16 Denver Road Fforestfach Swansea SA5 4DA **Tel:** (01792) 524859 w 6108494

Laura Elisabeth 05/10/2004 Nantwich Veterinary Hospital Crewe Road End Nantwich Cheshire CW5 5SF **Tel:** (01270) 610349 w 6292701

Lorraine (nee Clark) 16/08/1982 (20/03/2000) 47a Winchester Road Chandlers Ford Eastleigh Hampshire SO53 2GF **Tel:** (023) 8025 2543 w 6091172

Louise Natalie 08/09/2005 5 Peitley Cottages Trowley Bottom Flamstead ST. ALBANS Hertfordshire AL3 8DU w 6330266

Sarah Anne Louise 01/04/2003 (03/03/2009) Pets at Home Seamer Road Retail Park Seamer Road Scarborough Yorkshire YO12 4DH **Tel:** (01723) 503144 w 6282603

Suzanne Michelle 03/03/2005 Castle Vets Pet Healthcare Centre 1 Tilehurst Road Reading Berkshire RG1 7TW **Tel:** (0118) 957 4488 w 6319244

WEBBER Alexandra Colette 23/12/2008 6 Brookside Close Preston Weymouth Dorset DT3 6DW **Tel:** (01305) 834 453 w 6436449

Clare 30/11/2006 NKR Veterinary Specialists Warren Road Bluebell Hill Chatham Kent ME5 9RD **Tel:** (01634) 666655 w 6353201

WEBBER Sally Jane (see SQUIRE, Mrs)

WEBDELL Victoria Jayne 16/12/2005 46 Longworth Avenue Chesterton CAMBRIDGE CB4 1GU w 6337845

WEBSTER Francesca Maria 25/02/2003 37 Oakworth Drive Wirral Merseyside CH62 1HL **Tel:** (0151) 512 6959 w 6282878

Hannah Michelle 11/05/2009 4a Seaview Road GILLINGHAM Kent ME7 4NL **Tel:** 07809367656 w 6392416

Julie Fiona (nee Campbell) 13/04/2004 4 Threipmuir Avenue Balerno Edinburgh EH14 7EY w 6291315

WEDD Cindy Ann DipAVN(Medical) 06/04/2001 (26/04/2005) Hillview House Handcross Road Plummers Plain Horsham West Sussex RH13 6NU **Tel:** (01403) 891282 w 6215129

WEDDERBURN Marion Tait (nee Wedderburn, formerly Liddle) 23/02/1994 The Ann Coleman Centre Ponteland Road Cowgate Newcastle upon Tyne Tyne & Wear NE5 3AL **Tel:** (0191) 214 6800 w 6068303

WEEKES Clare Joanne DipAVN(Surgical) (nee Harrison) 14/09/2001 2 Parker Street Briercliffe Burnley Lancashire BB10 2HH **Tel:** (01282) 421 352 w 6029341

WEEKLEY Anita Jane 27/02/2007 3 Leyland View Wellingborough Northamptonshire NN8 1LA **Tel:** (01933) 227 164 w 6375234

WEIGHT Laura Ellen (see WILLIAMS, Mrs)

WEINGARTNER Joy (see VENTURI ROSE, Mrs)

WEIR Joanne Jane 04/03/1987 Quarry House Veterinary Centre 148 Teignmouth Road Torquay TQ1 4RY **Tel:** (01803) 324341 w 6003516

WELCH Alison Jane (nee Tebbutt) 31/05/2001 50 Canterbury Road Werrington Peterborough PE4 6PD **Tel:** (01733) 706238 w 6219760

Shelley Marie 04/02/1999 27 Heron Close Calne Wiltshire SN11 8PJ **Tel:** (01249) 812113 w 6133126

WELLARD Gemma Elizabeth 02/03/2009 38 Argyle Avenue Margate Kent CT9 5RN **Tel:** 01843228619 w 6304141

Laura Elizabeth 01/04/2003 3 Borden Lane Sittingbourne Kent ME10 1BT **Tel:** (01795) 423227 w 6281745

WELLER Claire Louise 05/08/2003 Inside Pets at Home Unit 4 White Lion Retail Park Luton Road DUNSTABLE Bedfordshire LU5 4RF **Tel:** (01582) 691504 w 6276993

Jennifer Elizabeth 15/04/2009 365 Upper Elmers End Road BECKENHAM Kent BR3 3DA **Tel:** (020) 8658 32346 w 6293416

WELLER Liza Jane (see LEIGHTON, Mrs)

WELLINGS Nicola Elizabeth (nee Rushton) 23/12/2003 39 St. Michaels Close Penkridge STAFFORD ST19 5AD **Tel:** (01785) 716180 w 6286299

WELLS Amy Emily (see HORNSEY, Mrs)

WELLS Karen Deborah (see MALONE, Mrs)

Maxine Helen (formerly Brookes) 02/11/2004 Alfreton Park Veterinary Hospital 216 King Street Alfreton Derbyshire DE55 7DF **Tel:** (01773) 832218 w 6319486

Rachel Louisa 03/12/2003 21 Springfiled Crescent Oakham Dudley DY2 7EX **Tel:** (01384) 357047 w 6296397

Samantha 24/11/2005 27 Cromer Road Hevingham Norwich Norfolk NR10 5QX **Tel:** (01603) 755180 w 6304438

WELSBY Joanna Frances (nee Welsby, formerly Hoaksey) 27/07/1993 (06/03/2007) 37 Railway Street Hadfield Glossop SK13 2AA **Tel:** (01457) 866344 w 6019082

WELSH Adele 27/02/2009 1 Swain Mount Bradford West Yorkshire BD2 1HJ **Tel:** 01274770760 w 6448472

Gillian Margaret 11/11/1996 P D S A Veterinary Centre 2b Hutchison Crossway 7 Slateford Road Edinburgh EH14 1RR **Tel:** (0131) 443 6180 w 6109181

Kathryn Natalie 21/10/2008 48b Fermor Road Tarleton PRESTON PR4 6AP **Tel:** 01772814458 w 6378963

WELSH Lesley Elizabeth (see WOJNAROWICZ, Mrs)

Marianne 01/03/2004 3 Sandgate Hill Sandgate Folkestone Kent CT20 2JF **Tel:** (01303) 248501 w 6292954

WELSH Nicola (see MANSON, Mrs)

Perdita DipAVN(Surgical) (nee Smith-Cresswell) 09/08/1991 18 Carnarvon Road BARNET Hertfordshire EN5 4LU **Tel:** (02084) 416171 w 6060993

WEMPLE Ashley 21/02/2008 5 St. James Court Felling GATESHEAD Tyne and Wear NE10 0AW **Tel:** (07905) 014 888 w 6503153

WENBAN Shelley Louise (see FOOTE, Mrs)

WENHAM Julie Anne (nee Ruffell) 30/11/2006 7a Neighbourhood Centre Culliford Crescent Poole Dorset BH17 9DW **Tel:** (01202) 602766 w 6370636

WENN Letitia Louise Marie 19/12/2006 61 Harecroft Road WISBECH Cambridgeshire PE13 1RL w 6375245

WENT Rebecca Claire (nee Willie) 12/09/2008 Flat 7 Mountfield House 24 Newtown UCKFIELD East Sussex TN22 5DD w 6436427

WEST Claire Louise 24/02/2009 28 Austin Way BRACKNELL Berkshire RG12 9HN **Tel:** (07515) 737187 w 6386091

Claire Rebecca 08/09/2005 94 Castle Road BEDFORD MK40 3PS **Tel:** (01234) 211875 w 6322401

Emma Victoria 01/04/2003 Flat 3 Springfield Highland Avenue BRENTWOOD Essex CM15 9DD w 6283758

WEST Hayley Nicole (see KELLY, Mrs)

Laura Joanne 10/04/2007 The Spinney Crow Trees Farm Thornton le Beans NORTHALLERTON DL6 3SX **Tel:** 07968293072 w 6379403

WEST Sarah Morgan (see HAINEY, Mrs)

Stacey Louise 07/12/2007 49 Vicarage Square West Street GRAYS Essex RM17 6JJ **Tel:** (01708) 556508 w 6382813

Tracey Louise 07/04/2008 15 Ravens Avenue Halstead Essex CO10 7NG **Tel:** (07739) 715661 w 6390183

WEST Zillah May (see COXON, Mrs)

WESTCOTT Kerry Jane (see WICKENS, Mrs)

WESTCOTT Lucy Ruth 05/04/2005 The Hart Veterinary Centre Browning Drive Kings Meadow Bicester Oxfordshire OX26 2XL **Tel:** (01869) 323 223 w 6303800

WESTERN Kelly Marie 09/01/2008 46 Wedlands Taunton Somerset TA2 7AE **Tel:** 01823336895 w 6392405

Zoe (nee Trott) 22/02/2007 Sparrows Brightstone Lane Lower Farringdon ALTON Hampshire GU34 3DG w 6371769

WESTLAKE Julie Rose 11/09/2003 (01/02/2010) 511 Wilbraham Road Manchester M21 0UB **Tel:** (0161) 881 3329 w 6230397

WESTLAKE Lisa Michelle (see BUNSTON, Mrs)

Michelle Emma 11/12/2001 New Priory Veterinary Practice The Deneway London Rd Brighton East Sussex BN1 8QR **Tel:** (01273) 540430 w 6270679

WESTMORE Sharon Louise 04/02/2009 31 Celandine Way CHIPPENHAM Wiltshire SN14 6XH **Tel:** 07825651088 w 6395903

WESTON Joanne Rachel 24/01/2006 54 Culver Road Basingstoke Hampshire RG21 3LT **Tel:** (01256) 355314 w 6349648

Leanne 26/11/2009 60 Brecon Road Abergavenny Gwent NP7 7RB **Tel:** (01873) 857544 w 6494155

WESTWOOD Diane 12/05/1989 (19/06/2002) 21 The Alley Dudley West Midlands DY3 2UL **Tel:** (01902) 238543 w 6063451

Joanne Lee 16/09/2004 9 The Courtyard Pontefract West Yorkshire WF8 2UY **Tel:** (01977) 709 127 w 6281239

Julie Christine 01/10/1999 Abbey Lodge Veterinary Surgery 118 Sea Street Herne Bay Kent CT6 8QZ **Tel:** (01227) 364084 w 6186287

Vanessa Jane 11/05/2004 2 Doctors Hill Bournheath Bromsgrove Worcestershire B61 9JE **Tel:** (01527) 877753 w 6301226

WEYMAN Charlotte Louise (see STORER, Mrs)

WEYMAN Hazel Louise 13/10/2008 The Veterinary Surgery Redmans Hill Blackford Wedmore Somerset BS28 4NG **Tel:** (01934) 712229 w 6411314

WHALE Elaine Sharon (nee Evans) 03/12/2003 38 Pinetree Walk Creekmoor Poole Dorset BH17 7EH **Tel:** (01202) 771232 w 6292118

WHALLEY Joanna Marie (see ODD, Mrs)

WHARMBY Lucy Victoria (nee Waterfield) 23/02/2005 20 Penwithick Road Penwithick ST. AUSTELL Cornwall PL26 8UQ **Tel:** (01726) 851 867 w 6282009

WHATLEY Juliet Mary 09/08/1978 (20/01/1999) Knapp Barn Aston Ingham ROSS-ON-WYE Herefordshire HR9 7LS w 6063484

Toni Leigh 04/06/2009 16 Valley Gardens Voguebeloth REDRUTH Cornwall TR16 4EE **Tel:** (01209) 213689 w 6415263

WHATLING Caroline (nee Ingham) 08/09/1998 4 Station Road Long Sutton Spalding Lincolnshire PE12 9BP **Tel:** (01406) 364708 w 6043945

WHATMORE Holly Anne 10/10/2008 105 Cooling Road ROCHESTER Kent ME2 4RT w 6412678

WHEAT Christine 11/03/2008 Oak House 9 Eaves Lane Cheadle Stoke-on-Trent Staffordshire ST10 ITL **Tel:** (01538) 750121 w 6406474

WHEATLEY Alison Sonia 08/01/2008 5 Popeley Rise Gomersal Cleckheaton West Yorkshire BD19 4QT **Tel:** (01274) 855352 w 6373353

Nicola 08/10/1999 (29/07/2003) Spring Lodge Farm Powers Hall End Witham Essex CM8 2HG **Tel:** (01376) 513247 w 6118935

WHEELDON Victoria Jane 27/10/2008 Manor House Upper Leigh Leigh Stoke-on-Trent Staffordshire ST10 4NU **Tel:** (07966) 415 379 w 6435459

WHEELER Erin 02/09/2009 87 Rivermead CULLOMPTON Devon EX15 1LH **Tel:** (01884) 34275 w 6492868

Philippa Lucy 22/02/2007 24 Suffolk Close SLOUGH Berkshire SL1 6JN **Tel:** 07888703206 w 6344951

WHEELER Victoria Louise (see COLEMAN, Mrs)

WHEELER-LYNGSO Deborah Susan (formerly Wingfield) 14/08/1990 20 Star Lane Margate Kent CT9 4EE **Tel:** (01843) 871454 w 6095042

WHELAN Danielle Leonora 02/03/2007 19 Frensham Walk Farnham Common Slough Berkshire SL2 3QF **Tel:** (01753) 644 023 w 6342267

Emma-Marie 19/11/2007 Hollybarn Cottage Drumkeen Claremorris County Mayo Republic of Ireland **Tel:** (00) 353 0877 823 957 w 6502735

Pamela Marie 06/04/1995 51 Bawtry Road Bessacarr Doncaster South Yorkshire DN4 7AA **Tel:** (01302) 534999 w 6095665

WHELDRICK Sheryl 07/01/2010 Calder Veterinary Group/Calder Vets 69 Westgate End Wakefield West Yorkshire WF2 9RL **Tel:** (01924) 372017 w 6489029

WHELLAMS Clare Deirdre 30/10/2001 9 Marshfield Way Fairfield Park Bath BA1 6HA **Tel:** (01225) 420293 w 6264486

WHERLOCK Rachel Evelyn 08/09/2009 9 Orlebar Gardens Lawrence Weston Bristol BS11 0SG **Tel:** (01179) 380203 w 6430003

WHIPPS Nicola 23/03/2006 14 Spire Road Laindon Basildon Essex SS15 5GF **Tel:** (01268) 451 371 w 6324733

Tanya Nadine 26/11/2009 Ashdale Veterinary Centre 4 Edward Street GLOSSOP Derbyshire SK13 7AF **Tel:** (01457) 867884 w 6403152

WHITAKER Helen Lorraine (see WEBB, Mrs)

WHITAKER Joanne Susan (see MCNICHOL, Mrs)

WHITE Beverley Jane 04/08/1981 Abbey House Veterinary Hospital Commercial Street Morley Leeds West Yorkshire LS27 8AG **Tel:** (0113) 252 5818 w 6063575

Caroline Louise 07/02/2006 15 Beaconsfield Road Weston-super-Mare North Somerset BS23 1YE **Tel:** (01934) 624608 w 6350275

David John 12/09/2008 41 Hardy Crescent WIMBORNE Dorset BH21 2AR **Tel:** (01202) 882 101 m 6396024

Deborah Ann 01/04/1982 (28/01/2000) 23 Whitebarns Furneux Pelham Buntingford Hertfordshire SG9 0JH **Tel:** (01279) 777 645 w 6063597

Diana Anneliese Sylvia 17/01/2006 205 Elm Drive HOVE East Sussex BN3 7JD **Tel:** (07817) 586656 w 6342278

Emma Jane 16/06/2006 11a Oakroyd Crescent WISBECH Cambridgeshire PE13 3AR **Tel:** (07879) 656895 w 6343213

Fiona Jane 04/01/2006 The Chymes Westbrook Gillingham Dorset SP8 5DT **Tel:** (01747) 822832 w 6295660

Gemma Louise 05/04/2005 12 Columbine Road Walton Cardiff Tewkesbury Gloucestershire GL20 7SP **Tel:** (01684) 290088 w 6301897

Gemma Louise (nee Neiles) 30/11/2005 4 Glenfield Road DOVER Kent CT16 2AL **Tel:** (07793) 712223 w 6284110

WHITE Jacqueline Audrey (see PLATT, Mrs)

Jennie Alexandra 29/08/2008 143 Corringham Road Stanford-le-Hope Essex SS17 0BA **Tel:** (01375) 674 158 w 6417562

Laura Jane (nee Cartmel) 02/09/1999 (27/03/2001) Claremont Veterinary Group Ltd 8 Wainwright Road Bexhill-on-Sea East Sussex TN39 3UR **Tel:** (01424) 222835 w 6135520

Lisa Claire 27/08/1996 (03/04/2002) The Veterinary Centre 10A Colomendy Industrial Estate DENBIGH Clwyd LL16 5TA **Tel:** (01745) 812047 w 6043956

Lisa Jane (nee Young) 13/03/2002 41 Warwick Crescent HAYES Middlesex UB4 8RF **Tel:** (020) 8561 7482 w 6260427

Lisa Marie 09/05/2005 26 Elmbank Avenue Englefield Green EGHAM Surrey TW20 0TJ w 6323567

Margaret Mary 18/08/1977 Royston Veterinary Centre Newmarket Road Royston Hertfordshire SG8 9GH **Tel:** (01763) 242221 w 6086592

Natalie Louise 22/09/2006 Flat 11, Staburn Court Burnt Oak Broadway Edgware Middlesex HA8 5JT **Tel:** (079) 856 15846 w 6346711

Natalie Susan 10/12/2002 13 Laurel Avenue BLACKPOOL FY1 6QX **Tel:** (01253) 315690 w 6281085

Natasha Diana Frances 29/06/2007 1 Chylds Court Allesley Park COVENTRY CV5 9LP **Tel:** (07877) 908810 w 6351815

Rachel 20/10/2008 3 Sydney Cottage Drive BRIDGNORTH Shropshire WV16 4PW **Tel:** 01746765024 w 6437747

Rachel Anne 14/01/2008 Hill's Lea Winchester Road Alresford Hampshire SO24 9EZ **Tel:** (01962) 733554 w 6383902

WHITE Rachel Mary (see PLATE, Mrs)

Sally Marie 03/03/2005 127 Wennington Road Southport Merseyside PR9 7AH **Tel:** (01704) 214460 w 6303789

Sarah Karen (nee Swain, formerly Moore) 29/01/1997 Castle Veterinary Clinic 624 Dorchester Road Weymouth Dorset DT3 5LH **Tel:** (01305) 813303 w 6035446

Sean Josef 29/01/2007 Belmont House Veterinary Surgery Salisbury Road Business Park Salisbury Road Pewsey Wiltshire SN9 5PZ **Tel:** (01672) 563413 m 6299664

Sheila Elizabeth 20/09/2005 21 Benton Road Watford Hertfordshire WD19 6XD **Tel:** (0208) 3867497 w 6328374

Sophie Louise 26/10/2006 44 Princes Terrace Brighton East Sussex BN2 5JS **Tel:** (01273) 690805 w 6374893

WHITEFOOT Michelle Louise 23/10/2001 9 Barn Close Epsom Surrey KT18 7HQ **Tel:** (0208) 3933577 w 6254267

WHITEFORD Jane 04/11/2008 Moulandale Fetternear Inverurie Aberdeenshire AB51 5JU **Tel:** 01467621429 w 6437956

WHITEHEAD Megan Angharad 08/09/2009 Dail na Coille Garden Cottage 21 West Moulin Road PITLOCHRY Perthshire PH16 5EA w 6565050

WHITEHEAD Nicola Jane (see EASTWOOD, Miss)

Nicola Louise 14/09/2005 31 Heaton Close Romford Essex RM3 7HP **Tel:** (01708) 379465 w 6289643

Shelly Margaret 06/05/2008 37 Coppice Farm Park Tring Hertfordshire HP23 6LG **Tel:** (01296) 625045 w 6381955

WHITEHOUSE Jennifer Jayne 17/07/2008 6 Red House Avenue Wednesbury West Midlands WS10 0QL **Tel:** (0121) 5569872 w 6375740

WHITELEY Charlotte Louise 15/04/2004 5 Knowl Bank Golcar Huddersfield West Yorkshire HD7 4BJ **Tel:** (01422) 376702 w 6290270

WHITEWAY Jacqueline Sandra 27/01/1999 Flat 10 Malcolm Court Lower Vauxhall Wolverhampton WV1 4SS **Tel:** (01902) 428237 w 6135859

WHITEWOOD Kerrie Louise 29/10/2009 12 North Stroud Lane Petersfield Hampshire GU32 3PP **Tel:** (01730) 231525 w 6491867

WHITFIELD Catherine Elizabeth 29/01/2010 The Bridge Veterinary Hospital Victoria Street Middlesbrough Cleveland TS1 5QZ **Tel:** (01642) 242338 w 6466886

WHITFORD Katherine Molly 18/10/2005 Cibyn Veterinary Clinic Llanberis Road Caernarfon Gwynedd LL55 2BD **Tel:** (01286) 673026 w 6329111

WHITING Christine Anne 03/09/1998 31 Farrow Road Whaplode Drove Spalding Lincolnshire PE12 0TS **Tel:** (01406) 330379 w 6136003

Sandra Samantha DipAVN(Surgical) 19/01/1998 Flat 4 111 Station Road Lower Stondon HENLOW Bedfordshire SG16 6JJ **Tel:** (01462) 816383 w 6131424

Teresa Jane 10/08/2009 14 Stanhope Road Littlehampton West Sussex BN17 6AQ **Tel:** (01903) 730257 w 6255730

WHITLOCK Emma Louise (nee Maddocks) 15/04/2004 Hartpury College Hartpury House Hartpury GLOUCESTER GL19 3BE **Tel:** (01452) 700283 w 6288356

WHITNEY Susan Gail 03/08/2006 Hannam House Lamberts Lane Midhurst West Sussex GU29 9EA **Tel:** (01730) 816833 w 6342795

WHITTAKER Rachel Claire 22/04/2003 Farthings Veterinary Group Farthings Hill Guildford Road HORSHAM West Sussex RH12 1TS **Tel:** (01403) 252900 w 6246248

Sarah Diane 10/04/2003 Eye Veterinary Clinic Marlbrook Leominster Herefordshire HR6 0PH **Tel:** (01568) 616616 w 6283989

Zoe Claire Louise 12/02/2009 139 Middlecliff Lane Little Houghton Barnsley South Yorkshire S72 0HW **Tel:** 01226756532 w 6437351

WHITTALL Caroline Anne 19/01/1983 Synod Isaf Cross Inn Llandysul Dyfed SA44 6LY **Tel:** (01545) 580352 w 6063724

WHITTINGHAM Carly 14/10/2008 10 Walshaw Lane BURNLEY Lancashire BB10 2DL **Tel:** 01282831662 w 6350286

WHITTINGHAM Louise (see CHALLICE, Mrs)

Sarah Anne (nee Woodward) 15/12/2004 (04/09/2008) Gorsefield Cottage 20 East Terrace Milford BELPER Derbyshire DE56 0RF **Tel:** (01773) 820 323 w 6279985

WHITTINGHAM Sarah Louise (see NEWINGTON, Mrs)

WHITTLE Elaine Ann 13/01/2009 91 Bitton Park Road Teignmouth Devon TQ14 9BZ **Tel:** 01626778034 w 6385299

Kathryn Tammy (nee Steel) 02/02/1995 19 Washington Road Sunderland Tyne and Wear SR5 3LA **Tel:** (0191) 552 9539 w 6032172

WHORDLEY Jean Ann (see GREEN, Mrs)

WHORDLEY Lisa Jayne (nee Woolman) 13/05/2003 Fairfield Veterinary Centre 51 Leicester Road Hinckley Leicestershire LE10 1LW **Tel:** (01455) 637642 w 6279875

WHYLES Gemma Louise 23/12/2003 Wildbore Veterinary Group 5 Newcastle Street Worksop Nottinghamshire S80 2AS **Tel:** (01909) 472059 w 6292448

WHYTE Brenda MacKintosh 04/08/1993 The Granary Bunstead Barns Poles Lane Hursley Winchester Hampshire SO21 2LL **Tel:** (01962) 767920 w 6029851

Fiona Louise (nee McIntyre) 05/07/2006 11 The Crescent Coagh Cookstown County Tyrone BT80 0BE w 6351320

Laura Ann 24/11/2008 107 Bicker Road Donington Spalding Lincolnshire PE11 4XR **Tel:** 01775822860 w 6435547

WICKENS Carina Sarah 13/01/2004 23 Broughton Road Otford SEVENOAKS Kent TN14 5LY w 6291766

Kerry Jane (nee Westcott) 29/10/2004 Westwick House Woodford Williton TAUNTON Somerset TA4 4HR w 6300225

WICKS Tanya Leigh 10/01/2008 83 Fieldend Road Eastcote Pinner Middlesex HA5 1QG **Tel:** (020) 8866 1842 w 6279380

WICKSTEAD Leanne 10/02/2004 Inside Pets at Home Unit 1 Didsbury Road STOCKPORT Cheshire SK4 2LQ **Tel:** (0161) 475 5720 w 6259404

WIDDISON Amy Sarah 24/01/2008 41 Cardale Road Pleasley Mansfield Nottinghamshire NG19 7RW **Tel:** 01623489267 w 6375256

WIGGINS Rebecca Louise 03/05/2007 30 Beldham Road Wrecclesham FARNHAM Surrey GU9 8TP w 6387334

WIGHT Nicola Caroline (formerly Groves-Hambidge) 04/08/1987 (15/10/2001) 92 Pulens Lane PETERSFIELD Hampshire GU31 4DF **Tel:** (01730) 816867 w 6051934

WIGLEY Helen Rebecca 04/11/2008 2 The Tannery Horn Street Winslow BUCKINGHAM MK18 3AL **Tel:** 01296713136 w 6413481

WIGNALL Stephanie Ann 26/02/2009 16 Mond Road Liverpool Merseyside L10 7LJ **Tel:** 01512802787 w 6444105

WILCOX Kate Rebecca (see THAIN, Mrs)

WILCOX Katy Louise 29/01/2007 2 Pen-y-Lan Ebbw Vale Gwent NP23 5LS **Tel:** (01495) 303 802 w 6374827

Sara-Jane 20/01/1999 2 Hobbs Close Beckley Rye East Sussex TN31 6TP **Tel:** (01797) 260844 w 6118979

Susan Elizabeth 13/02/1995 (17/01/2003) 608 Veterinary Group 608 Warwick Road Solihull West Midlands B91 1AA **Tel:** (0121) 705 3044 w 6026657

WILCOX-WOOD Elizabeth Victoria (nee Kenyon) 18/10/2006 26 Farrington Road Bacup Lancashire OL13 9TE w 6339143

WILD Christine (see FAIRBAIRN, Mrs)

Helen Laura Elizabeth 06/02/2002 Inside Pets at Home Ventura Shopping Centre Ventura Park Road Bonehill Tamworth Staffordshire B78 3HB **Tel:** (01827) 317524 w 6270140

Joanne 22/01/2010 15 Abbey Place Renishaw Sheffield South Yorkshire S21 3TY **Tel:** 01246434480 w 6416462

Laura Jane 01/06/2007 Pet Doctors Bagshot Road Knaphill Woking Surrey GU21 2SE **Tel:** (01483) 488008 w 6290666

WILDE Joanne (see FINDLAY, Mrs)

WILDE Simone Sharon DipAVN(Surgical), DipAVN (Medical) 22/07/1993 8 Collier Street GLOSSOP Derbyshire SK13 8LS **Tel:** (01457) 865003 w 6066587

WILDER Emma Louise 13/08/2003 36 Olivet Road Woodseats Sheffield South Yorkshire S8 8QS **Tel:** (0114) 250 7733 w 6286794

WILDING Amanda Jane 10/02/2004 197 Willowfield Woodside Telford Shropshire TF7 5NY w 6275508

WILDISH Maria-Teresa (see CHITTENDEN, Mrs)

WILDMAN Lyndsey Ann 04/02/2002 (13/06/2007) 1 Dairy Cottages Lower Barnsley WIMBORNE Dorset BH21 4JA w 6254025

Suzanne Marie (nee Mace) 23/08/1994 (13/10/2000) 82 Cloverdale Stoke Prior Bromsgrove Worcestershire B60 4NF **Tel:** (01527) 878361 w 6026500

WILES Karen Denise 05/08/1977 25 Oakley Road Bocking Braintree Essex CM7 5QS **Tel:** (01376) 324 386 w 606378X

WILKES Zoe Vanessa 02/11/2004 Leadon Vale Veterinary Centre Lower Road Trading Estate Ledbury Herefordshire HR8 2DJ **Tel:** (01531) 632276 w 6267093

WILKIE Julia Kim (see WALTON, Mrs)

WILKINS Ammee Jane 07/02/2008 Acorn House Veterinary Surgery Linnet Way Bedford MK41 7HN **Tel:** (01234) 261839 w 6389842

Rebecca Leanne 16/06/2006 4 Jupiter Gate STEVENAGE Hertfordshire SG2 7ST w 6324315

WILKINSON Ashley 01/02/2010 13 Scalby Grove Fairfield Stockton on Tees TS19 7RP **Tel:** (01642) 640473 w 6498632

Claire Anne Patricia 09/06/2008 (04/01/2010) 55 Parknasilla Way Aghagallon CRAIGAVON County Armagh BT67 0AU **Tel:** (02892) 650 937 w 6326570

Claire Louise 09/05/2005 Alfreton Park Veterinary Hospital 216 King Street Alfreton Derbyshire DE55 7DF **Tel:** (01773) 832218 w 6323644

Clare Louise 31/03/2000 63 Mill Hayes Road Stoke-on-Trent Staffordshire ST6 4JB **Tel:** (01782) 824702 w 6191149

Heather Barbara 28/02/2005 37 Fairfield Drive CLITHEROE Lancashire BB7 2PE w 6323611

WILKINSON Jane (see COTTRELL, Mrs)

Jane Lesley 20/01/1999 (01/03/2006) 50 Dekker Road LONDON SE21 7DJ **Tel:** (07768) 690168 w 6136069

WILKINSON Joanne Claire (see BENTLEY, Mrs)

Kathryn Ruth 25/02/2003 46 Craiglea Stirling Stirlingshire FK9 5EE **Tel:** (01786) 823309 w 6274628

WILKINSON Kay Marie (see BROAD, Mrs)

Layla Susan 28/09/2009 Station House Vets 157B Ashley Road Hale ALTRINCHAM Cheshire WA14 2UZ **Tel:** 01619414760 w 6465852

Mandy 31/08/2005 232 Allerton Road Allerton Bradford West Yorkshire BD15 7AA **Tel:** (01274) 480031 w 6326086

Monique Irene 08/07/2003 Queen Mother Hospital for Small Animals Hawkshead Lane North Mymms Hatfield Hertfordshire AL9 7TA **Tel:** (01707) 666366 w 6273660

Natalie Ann 06/03/2009 91 Brazley Avenue Horwich Bolton Lancashire BL6 6LT **Tel:** 07946166402 w 6385244

Nicola Jane 06/02/2002 Grange Hill Veterinary Centre Grange Lane LICHFIELD Staffordshire WS13 8HX **Tel:** (01543) 416246 w 6266642

Samantha Louise 19/03/2007 Higher End Farm Coal Pit Lane Bickerstaffe Ormskirk Lancashire L39 0HH **Tel:** (01695) 727 244 w 6373859

WILKS Kimberley Heather Alison 07/02/2007 The Flat The Veterinary Centre Carleton Penrith Cumbria CA11 8TZ **Tel:** (01768) 862 454 w 6371802

Lauren Gemma 28/09/2005 53 Parvis Road Byfleet Surrey KT14 7AA **Tel:** (01932) 349690 w 6293537

Sarah 01/04/2003 2 Upright Villas Braunton Devon EX33 2AL **Tel:** (01271) 815557 w 6271878

WILL Katie Louise (nee Coleman) 05/04/2005 130 Shaftesbury Road CARSHALTON Surrey SM5 1HL w 6263892

WILLAIMS Angela (see PORTER, Mrs)

WILLCOCKS Claire Elizabeth (see TARRANT, Mrs)

WILLCOCKS Louise Ann 24/10/2008 35 Holland Road OXTED Surrey RH8 9AU **Tel:** (07887) 727 173 w 6436295

WILLCOX Sarah Elizabeth 11/04/2005 Flat 4 The Granary Tewin Hill Tewin WELWYN Hertfordshire AL6 0LL w 6282515

WILLEMS Carola 07/03/2008 3 Slate Cottages The Green Matching Tye HARLOW Essex CM17 0QS w 6503692

WILLEY Carla May 27/10/2008 219 Eastwick Road Taunton Somerset TA2 7HQ **Tel:** (01823) 276959 w 6439507

WILLEY Heather Frances (see LEDBURY, Mrs)

WILLEY Patricia Ann (see BROWN, Mrs)

WILLIAMS Alison Grace (nee Clark) 18/12/2000 37 Place Crescent Purbrook WATERLOOVILLE Hampshire PO7 5UP w 6205306

Alison Jayne 17/07/2008 6 Bro Pedr Llandyfaelog Kidwelly Dyfed SA17 5PA **Tel:** (01267) 267391 w 6378765

Alison Louise (nee Phillips) 01/06/1992 Hesp Alyn Farm Pantymwyn Road Cilcain MOLD Clwyd CH7 5NL **Tel:** (01352) 742117 w 6058703

Amanda Jane Connan 03/05/2005 19 Church Road Wavertree Liverpool L15 9EA **Tel:** (0151) 733 5755 w 6305252

Amy Louise 10/02/2004 30 Seventh Row Ashington Northumberland NE63 8HX **Tel:** (01670) 857440 w 6293262

WILLIAMS Angela Dawn (see HART, Mrs)

WILLIAMS Annette Gail (see PULLAN, Mrs)

WILLIAMS Bonnie (see CUTLER, Mrs)

Caroline Mary (formerly Rollins) 02/02/1998 19 Lindisfarne Avenue Stanney Oaks Ellesmere Port Cheshire CH65 9JF w 6040423

WILLIAMS Ceri (see LAND, Mrs)

Charlotte Elizabeth (nee Harrison) 20/02/2008 33 Hopper Vale Easthampstead BRACKNELL Berkshire RG12 7GH w 6385255

Claire Louise 26/10/2005 Avon Lodge Veterinary Group 283 Wells Road Bristol BS4 2PP **Tel:** (0117) 977 3230 w 6346117

Clare Louise 20/11/2009 73 Alton Park Road CLACTON-ON-SEA Essex CO15 1EA **Tel:** (01255) 862441 w 6299092

WILLIAMS Crian Rebecca (see SHENSTON, Mrs)

WILLIAMS Dawn Pauline (see GREENAWAY, Mrs)

Deborah Wilhelmina (nee Cowin) 12/06/2008 22 Churchill Crescent ST. ANDREWS Fife KY16 8EF w 6404912

Emma 11/02/2008 Hall Farm Felbrigg Norwich Norfolk NR11 8PR **Tel:** (01263) 837250 w 6408344

Emma Louise 10/02/2004 The Wylie Veterinary Centre 196 Hall Lane Upminster Essex RM14 1TD **Tel:** (01708) 251200 w 6289214

Gillian Claire 07/06/2001 22 Weaver Avenue Simonswood Liverpool Merseyside L33 4YU **Tel:** (0151) 548 3012 w 6221762

Hannah 19/01/2000 3 Lion Mews Newbury Street Lambourn HUNGERFORD Berkshire RG17 8YY w 6190709

Hayley Emma 07/02/2006 (08/01/2009) 6 Essex Road HODDESDON Hertfordshire EN11 0AA **Tel:** (01992) 411244 w 6270833

Helen Margaret 25/02/2003 59 Beckingham Orton Goldhay PETERBOROUGH PE2 5TL **Tel:** (01773) 390161 w 6282075

Jane Bryony Siobhan 24/05/2005 3 Lower Terrace Bradworthy Holsworthy Devon EX22 7TE **Tel:** (07786) 934429 w 6305934

Jenny Marie 04/10/2005 2 Golden Hay Main Street Dumbleton EVESHAM Worcestershire WR11 7TY **Tel:** (01386) 881084 w 6305626

Joanna Rachel 18/09/2007 7 Royal Way Starcross EXETER EX6 8EQ w 6288631

Joanne Louise (nee Campbell) 04/09/1997 42 Chadderton Drive BURY Lancashire BL9 8NR **Tel:** (0161) 2802460 w 6115719

Karen Ann 05/09/2000 Mountain View Tredilion Llantilio Pertholey Abergavenny Monmouthshire NP7 8BB **Tel:** (07802) 182691 w 6203953

WILLIAMS Karen Laura (see JONES, Mrs)

Laura Asherly 11/11/2008 12 Pen y Pentre Sychdyn Mold Clwyd CH7 6EZ **Tel:** (0798) 3619347 w 6352860

Laura Ellen (nee Weight) 14/01/2008 2 Cross's Grange Hartwell NORTHAMPTON NN7 2FD **Tel:** (07901) 882552 w 6403724

Laura Jane 29/01/2009 51 Silverdale Barton on Sea NEW MILTON Hampshire BH25 7DE **Tel:** 07742881064 w 6367699

Laura Jane 11/03/2008 Spring Lodge Farm Powers Hall End Witham Essex CM8 2HG **Tel:** (01376) 513247 w 6381383

Lauren Kate 13/03/2002 7 Higham Station Avenue Chingford London E4 9AY **Tel:** (020) 8531 5045 w 6270470

Lauren Stephanie 09/06/2009 10 Quernmore Road Caton Lancaster Lancashire LA2 9QA **Tel:** 01524771450 w 6443368

Leanne 18/10/2006 14 Hollybrook Gardens Locks Heath Southampton Hampshire SO31 6WJ **Tel:** (01489) 482955 w 6370669

WILLIAMS Linda Jean (see REYNOLDS, Mrs)

Lisa 20/09/1988 (11/03/2002) 1 Celia Street Kirkdale Liverpool Merseyside L20 2BG **Tel:** (0151) 2608064 w 6063928

Louise 11/12/2008 Afon Veterinary Centre Lletty Nedd Pen Y Dre Neath West Glamorgan SA11 3HH **Tel:** (01639) 642739 w 6434678

WILLIAMS Lowri Wynne (see FROST, Mrs)

Lucy Jane 20/11/2009 The Cobbies Barn End Lane Dartford Kent DA2 7PP **Tel:** (01322) 287851 w 6351562

WILLIAMS Lydia Claire (see MORGAN, Mrs)

Lynette 26/10/2009 12 Pasture Drive Garstang Preston Lancashire PR3 1TH **Tel:** (01995) 600167 w 6406353

Lynsey Ann 17/07/2008 6 Bechin Close Church Crookham FLEET Hampshire GU52 6DJ **Tel:** 07900624629 w 6319805

Maria 04/11/2008 15 Pearson Avenue WARRINGTON WA4 2RN **Tel:** (079504) 61862 w 6429090

Maria Ann 14/12/2006 Witten Lodge Heywood Road Northam Bideford Devon EX39 3QB **Tel:** (01237) 473278 w 6346128

Melanie Dawn 14/12/2009 49 Nursery Road Great Cornard Sudbury Suffolk CO10 0NJ **Tel:** 01787373638 w 6451915

Michelle Louise (nee Silvey) 13/05/2008 102 Headlands Fenstanton Huntingdon Cambridgeshire PE28 9LW **Tel:** (01480) 468898 w 6401898

Nicola (nee Hewes) 16/02/1990 Ashfield Cottage The Ridgeway Mill Hill London NW7 1AY **Tel:** (0208) 9061024 w 6052803

Rachael Sarah (nee Martin) 16/12/1997 (19/12/2002) Blue Dolphins Tregos Road Carbis Bay St. Ives Cornwall TR26 2QU **Tel:** (01736) 794 837 w 6029002

Rachel 04/12/2003 Abbey Veterinary Centre St Arvans Chambers Hereford Road Abergavenny Monmouthshire NP7 5PR **Tel:** (01873) 852391 w 6282812

Rachel 01/04/2003 Bridge Farm Kennels Moss Bridge Farm Parkers Road Leighton CREWE CW1 4RZ w 6283714

Rebecca Louise 10/04/2007 30 Skillman Drive THATCHAM Berkshire RG19 4GG **Tel:** (01635) 861293 w 6329155

Rebecca Lucy (nee Bowen) 13/11/2006 Steffan Veterinary Services Ltd 5 High Street Lampeter Ceredigion SA48 7BA **Tel:** (01570) 422322 w 6270349

WILLIAMS Sally Rachael (see HENDRY, Mrs)

Sara Elizabeth 30/05/2003 56 Uplands Road Dudley West Midlands DY2 8BD w 6263606

Sarah Bridget 26/09/2006 41 Tunnel Hill Worcester Worcestershire WR4 9RP **Tel:** (01905) 29788 w 6269491

Selina 11/11/2009 9 Kinmel Terrace Nantlle CAERNARFON Gwynedd LL54 6BN **Tel:** (01286) 882339 w 6289995

Stacey 10/03/2008 8 Langland Road Cleobury Mortimer Kidderminster Worcestershire DY14 8EH **Tel:** (01299) 271035 w 6397740

Stacey Victoria 30/08/2006 (05/05/2009) Pines Veterinary Clinic 146a Bath Road Maidenhead Berkshire SL6 4LB **Tel:** (01628) 776699 w 6347635

Stephanie DipAVN(Surgical) 09/08/1990 14 Black Horse Lane Swainby Northallerton North Yorkshire DL6 3EW **Tel:** (01642) 825 793 w 606394X

Susan 25/11/2008 42 Pilgrim Drive Bere Alston Yelverton Devon PL20 7DB **Tel:** 07901674037 w 6445425

WILLIAMS Victoria (see TUGWELL, Mrs)

Victoria Rachel 12/04/2002 20-24 Alexandra Road Clevedon North Somerset BS21 7QH **Tel:** (01275) 343457 w 6263100

Zoe Marie 15/04/2004 34 Heather Way Rise Park Romford Essex RM1 4TA w 6286805

WILLIAMSON Beverley Ann (nee Evans) 20/02/2001 50 Richmond Close Calmore Southampton Hampshire SO40 2TH **Tel:** (07747) 045217 w 6212599

Christine Eileen (nee Nestor) 17/11/2000 The Mews Veterinary Centre Preseland Road LIVERPOOL Merseyside L23 5TE **Tel:** (0151) 924 2025 w 6205713

Emma Louise 05/04/2006 65 Leysholme Crescent Leeds West Yorkshire LS12 4HH **Tel:** (0113) 279 2428 w 6344357

WILLIAMSON Helen Mary (see BLAGG, Mrs)

Nicole Josephine 05/01/2005 Uplands Way Vets Ltd Uplands Way DISS Norfolk IP22 4DF **Tel:** (01379) 642865 w 6326636

Pamela 18/09/2007 51/4 Comely Bank Avenue EDINBURGH EH4 1ES w 6372473

Pamela Mary 16/09/2008 Lunna Farm Lunna Vidlin Shetland ZE2 9QF **Tel:** 01806577287 w 6416781

Sarah Alice 13/08/2008 10 Bennett Close Welwyn Garden City Hertfordshire AL7 4JA **Tel:** 01707375767 w 6409037

Sarah Helen (formerly Williamson-Howes) 24/07/2003 2 Lions Way East Road Sleaford Lincolnshire NG34 8GN **Tel:** (01529) 303 344 w 6286530

WILLIAMSON-HOWES Sarah Helen (see WILLIAMSON, Mrs)

WILLIE Rebecca Claire (see WENT, Mrs)

WILLINGALE Victoria Elizabeth 28/04/2009 179 Hillyfields LOUGHTON Essex IG10 2PW **Tel:** (07595) 935456 w 6428969

WILLIS Amy Joanne 29/07/2005 Russett House Capel Road Bentley IPSWICH IP9 2BL **Tel:** (01473) 311484 w 6321169

Emily Charlotte 22/06/2009 11 Oak Road Southwater West Sussex RH13 9ED w 6321180

Kathryn Louise 14/04/2008 24 Dene Crescent CARLISLE CA3 9TA **Tel:** (01228) 540314 w 6348735

Natalie Anne 13/11/2009 Flat 2 263 Park Lane MACCLESFIELD Cheshire SK11 8AE **Tel:** 07845660351 w 6374838

WILLISON Donna Margaret 29/07/2005 3 Queen Street TAYPORT Fife DD6 9JY **Tel:** (07789) 725873 w 6292008

WILLMORE Anna Elizabeth 27/09/2000 Bredy Veterinary Centre Sea Road North Bridport Dorset DT6 4RR **Tel:** (01308) 456 771 w 6017835

WILLMOTT Verity Lee (nee Willmott, formerly Box) 06/07/2004 Mimram Veterinary Centre 31 Church Street Welwyn Hertfordshire AL6 9LW **Tel:** (01438) 712300 w 6301237

WILLS Christina Samantha 15/05/2008 35a Lower Stoke Limpley Stoke BATH BA2 7FR **Tel:** (07944) 338773 w 6386905

Donna Anne 22/03/2004 28 Pewsey Vale Forest Park Winkfield Bracknell Berkshire RG12 9YA **Tel:** (0777) 618 2911 w 6285166

Laura 09/06/2009 5 Ballymacash Drive Lisburn County Antrim BT28 3EU **Tel:** 02892660820 w 6443456

WILLSHER Lisa (nee Tunnicliffe, formerly Jukes) 04/01/1993 22 Bush Drive RUGELEY Staffordshire WS15 2AQ w 6065142

WILLSON Anne Marie (nee Moody) 30/10/2003 39 Kithill Crewkerne Somerset TA18 8HY **Tel:** (01460) 76587 w 6292283

WILLSON Miya (see SAGE, Mrs)

WILMAN Heidi Joanne (see ZOUROUDIS, Mrs)

WILMER Katherine Ann 30/03/2006 12 Mandeville Close Manfield Grange Northamptonshire NN3 6QE **Tel:** (01604) 583233 w 6342289

WILMOT Rachel Diana 23/02/2005 (03/02/2010) Roach Valley Veterinary Centre 92 Main Road Hockley Essex SS5 4RL **Tel:** (01702) 200300 w 6299125

WILMOTT Carli Jayne (formerly Wilmott) 19/05/2008 20 Mountfields BRIGHTON BN1 7BT **Tel:** (01273) 240915 w 611361X

WILMSHURST Susanna Maria (see WILMSHURST-CLARK, Mrs)

WILMSHURST-CLARK Susanna Maria (nee Wilmshurst) 04/08/2003 21 Chapel Lane Milford Godalming Surrey GU8 5HB **Tel:** (07879) 817667 w 6276938

WILSDON Sarah Harcourt (see DAGGER, Mrs)

WILSHER Jennifer Anne (see BOYD, Mrs)

WILSON Amie Judith (see BRITTON, Mrs)

WILSON Ann Kathleen 20/09/2005 Lodge Farm Upper Heyford NORTHAMPTON NN7 3NF **Tel:** (01604) 830337 w 6332378

Beth Romayne 19/03/2007 Ambleside Whimple EXETER Devon EX5 2TS **Tel:** (01404) 822744 w 6305362

Chantal 24/05/2005 15 Sycamore Close LITTLEBOROUGH Lancashire OL15 8RN **Tel:** (01706) 372636 w 6321675

Claire (nee Etherington) 11/04/2005 4 St. Laud Close Bristol Avon BS9 1DJ **Tel:** (0117) 9505 888 w 6326867

WILSON Claire Elizabeth (see RYNBERK, Mrs)

Claire Louise 06/09/1995 263 Birchover Way Allestree Derby Derbyshire DE22 2RS w 6034497

Diana Elizabeth Joyce 07/10/2009 Hale House 19 Langley Road Chippenham Wiltshire SN15 1BS **Tel:** (01249) 653561 w 6330860

Helen Mary 26/08/1999 55 Cherry Park Brandon Durham DH7 8TN **Tel:** (0191) 3712924 w 6184989

Jasmine Pearl 03/09/2002 6 Milton Close Ramsey HUNTINGDON Cambridgeshire PE26 1LU **Tel:** (07751) 666266 w 6254036

WILSON Jessica Jane (see CRUMP, Mrs)

Julie Ann (nee Bradley) 09/01/2004 Westwood House 106 High Street Boston Spa Wetherby West Yorkshire LS23 6DR **Tel:** (01937) 842210 w 6263045

WILSON Karen (see BANKS, Mrs)

Kathryn Vicki 31/01/1992 (07/02/2002) 38 Brandon Way Kingswood HULL HU7 3EL w 6064014

Kerry Jane 30/05/2008 15 Lairs Crescent Snainton Scarborough North Yorkshire YO13 9BQ **Tel:** (01723) 859 354 w 6415208

Lisa Anne 29/06/2007 47 Kittys Road Kilkeel Newry County Down BT34 4EJ **Tel:** (028) 417 64487 w 6379326

Lisa Jane (nee Brown) 24/02/2004 High Street Veterinary Hospital 169-170 High Street Lowestoft Suffolk NR32 1HU **Tel:** (01502) 572141 w 6289654

Lucy Anne 16/06/2008 11 The Dicklands Rodmell LEWES East Sussex BN7 3HT **Tel:** (07917) 154 757 w 6380921

Mark Steven 21/07/2008 2 Corinna Gardens Dibden Southampton Hampshire SO45 5UB **Tel:** 02380849646 m 6376202

Megan Jane 03/12/2007 Ardvreck 3 Braeport Dunblane Perthshire FK15 0AT **Tel:** 07841658440 w 6381394

Melissa Jayne 06/08/2008 2 Northdown Road St Peters BROADSTAIRS Kent CT10 2UL **Tel:** (01843) 861514 w 6404846

WILSON Michelle Ann (see MERRETT, Mrs)

Michelle Lorraine (nee Wilson, formerly Sargent) 18/02/2000 (09/08/2004) The Horse Clinic and The Pet Clinic at Blackmore Rookery Road Blackmore Ingatestone Essex CM4 0LE **Tel:** (01277) 823858 w 611900X

Miriam Joy 26/03/2002 (05/02/2008) 8 Violet Street Haworth KEIGHLEY West Yorkshire BD22 8AU w 6270085

Natalie 14/12/2006 Huntworth Farm Giggleswick SETTLE BD24 0DJ w 6337856

Paula Jean 29/12/2003 26 Birley Street Bury Lancashire BL9 5DT **Tel:** (07835) 810904 w 6291073

Pauline Anne 24/05/2006 11 Gladstone Street Featherstone PONTEFRACT West Yorkshire WF7 6LU w 6353212

WILSON Rachel Helen (see HEWSON, Mrs)

WILSON Sandra Dawn (see MCKEATING, Mrs)

Sara Louise 10/12/2009 The Brook Veterinary Clinic Rossorry Church Road Enniskillen County Fermanagh BT74 7HB **Tel:** (028) 6632 3335 w 6492274

Stacey Ellen 14/10/2009 55 Aultone Way SUTTON Surrey SM1 3LD **Tel:** 07944491608 w 6450056

Tracy Ann 11/11/2004 Springfield Veterinary Group 39 Moorgate Road Rotherham South Yorkshire S60 2AD **Tel:** (01709) 377241 w 6292019

Tracy Elizabeth 02/06/2004 The Veterinary Surgery 100 Cathedral Road Armagh City Co Armagh BT61 8AE **Tel:** (028) 3752 6777 w 6293944

Vanessa Leigh 05/04/2005 10 Drumlanrig Square Hawick Roxburghshire TD9 0AS **Tel:** (01450) 372038 w 6311731

WILTSHEAR Claire Elizabeth 29/06/2007 Lavender Cottage Westhorpe STOWMARKET Suffolk IP14 4SU **Tel:** 07814036949 w 6381405

WILTSHIRE Amy Louise Victoria 04/06/2009 37 Court Farm Road Longwell Green BRISTOL BS30 9AA **Tel:** (0117) 9323156 w 6415384

Clare Elizabeth 12/05/2004 The Firs Veterinary Surgery 21 The Firs Combe Down Bath BA2 5ED **Tel:** (01225) 832521 w 6298795

Sian Marie Anne (nee Evans) 24/01/1997 (12/01/2009) 17 Garson Road Abbey Meads Swindon Wiltshire SN25 4XD **Tel:** (01793) 726418 w 604268X

WINDEATT Nicola (see LANE, Mrs)

WINDER Joanne Christine 04/11/2008 25 St. Andrews Road Gosport Hampshire PO12 1QA **Tel:** 01392786459 w 6409422

WINDIATE Clare 11/09/1998 (07/10/2005) Greyfriars Small Animal Clinic Hogs Back Puttenham Guildford Surrey GU3 1AG **Tel:** (01483) 812100 w 6136852

WINDLE Christina Jayne 21/03/2007 Springfield Veterinary Group 451 Richmond Road Sheffield South Yorkshire S13 8LW **Tel:** (0114) 264 8913 w 6376664

Laura Jane 18/10/2006 4 Mowson Drive Worrall Sheffield South Yorkshire S35 0AH **Tel:** (0114) 286235 w 6354785

Lindsey Maria 19/03/2009 33 Ayot Path Borehamwood Hertfordshire WD6 5BL **Tel:** (0208) 952 4881 w 6437329

WINDLER Tracy Annette 12/08/2008 121 Sundorne Road Sundorne SHREWSBURY SY1 4RP **Tel:** (01743) 344566 w 6367215

WINGFIELD Deborah Susan (see WHEELER-LYNGSO, Mrs)

WINKLE Lisa Maria 13/11/2009 14 Uttoxeter Road Lower Tean STOKE-ON-TRENT ST10 4LJ **Tel:** 07870469320 w 6495057

WINKLER Lisa 20/04/2005 34 Rosewall Road Maybush SOUTHAMPTON Hampshire SO16 5DW w 6311423

WINSOR Gemma Louise 19/09/2008 5 The Kilns Frith End Bordon Hampshire GU35 0QN **Tel:** 01420475877 w 6397828

WINSTON Georgina Rose 21/07/2008 74 Lodge Hill WELLING Kent DA16 1BW **Tel:** (0208) 311 9316 w 6376213

WINSTONE Sarah Louise 09/06/2009 24 Church View Ollerton Newark Nottinghamshire NG22 9BH **Tel:** 07973934466 w 6443445

WINTER Lisa Marie (nee Little) 17/08/2005 (08/05/2008) Welenuk Cottam House Farm Cottam DRIFFIELD North Humberside YO25 3BY w 6268336

Rebecca Louise Ramsey (nee Boag) 17/01/2008 Rainsbrook Veterinary Group 1 Craven Road Rugby Warwickshire CV21 3JX **Tel:** (01788) 562844 w 6385585

Stephanie Caroline (nee Forster) 22/12/2004 Birdsong Pound Hill Landford Salisbury Wiltshire SP5 2AA **Tel:** (01794) 39 829 w 6316791

Tracy Jane 12/09/2000 Penmans Littlewood Lane Buxted East Sussex TN22 4LW **Tel:** (01825) 732460 w 6040365

WINTERTON Annabelle Victoria 25/02/2003 (26/01/2005) 18 Field Street Shepshed Loughborough Leicestershire LE12 9AL **Tel:** (01509) 503850 w 6276894

WINTHROP Claire 24/08/1998 (17/05/2004) 3 Dalrymple Court Townhead Kirkintilloch Glasgow G66 3AA **Tel:** (0141) 775 2503 w 6115592

WINWOOD Susan (nee Muir) 10/02/2004 Clifton Lodge Veterinary Group 24 Stockton Road Hartlepool Cleveland TS25 1RL **Tel:** (01429) 272435 w 6205449

WISBEY Katherine Jayne 04/02/2009 47 Lanes End Heath and Reach LEIGHTON BUZZARD Bedfordshire LU7 0AE **Tel:** 01525237686 w 6449044

WISHART Carrie Ann (nee Wishart, formerly Thornborrow) 29/12/2003 Easter Bush Veterinary Centre University of Edinburgh Easter Bush Roslin Midlothian EH25 9RG **Tel:** (0131) 650 7650 w 6286541

WITCHELL Holly Rebecca 24/10/2008 30 The Brambles Lichfield Staffordshire WS14 9SE **Tel:** (01543) 301 539 w 6401865

WITCOMB Lucy 18/10/2005 10 Henrys Way LYME REGIS Dorset DT7 3BW w 6305945

WITHERS Heidi Annke Sara 27/02/2007 Vaughan Jones Veterinary Practice Ltd 17-18 Dean Street Aberdare Mid Glamorgan CF44 7BN **Tel:** (016) 8587 4675 w 6314701

Julia Margaret DipAVN(Surgical) (nee Shields) 03/08/1993 56 Spring Close Sherborne St John Nr Basingstoke Hampshire RG24 9JF **Tel:** (01256) 850369 w 602908X

WITHEYMAN Louise Frances 12/02/2009 31 Rokeby Crescent Strathaven Lanarkshire ML10 6EG **Tel:** 01357520073 w 6412425

WITHYCOMBE Kim Louise 24/01/2000 The Sidings Veterinary Surgery Sheep Street Cirencester Gloucestershire GL7 1QW **Tel:** (01285) 643146 w 6190654

WITT Bernadette Elisabeth (see BATES, Mrs)

WITTON Joanne Marie 16/05/2001 (30/01/2003) 3 The Laurels New Forest Village Leeds LS10 4FJ w 6205702

WIXEY Amanda Jane 21/11/2007 Oakville Veterinary Surgery Station Road Lawley Bank Telford Shropshire TF4 2LP **Tel:** (01952) 506360 w 6321686

WOJNAROWICZ Lesley Elizabeth (nee Welsh) 03/03/1998 77 Long Lane COALVILLE Leicestershire LE67 4EJ w 6043719

WOLF Alice Cecilia (see JONES, Mrs)

WOLFE Elizabeth Ann 16/08/1995 8 South Barrwood Road Kilsyth Glasgow G65 0EZ **Tel:** (01236) 821356 w 6039531

WOMERSLEY Hannah Jane 11/11/2008 Church Lane Tibberton Worcestershire w 6435514

WONFOR Rebecca Madeleine 10/01/2007 Green Pastures Veterinary Centre Green Pastures Moor Lane Weston-super-Mare Somerset BS24 7LA **Tel:** (01934) 622022 w 6365851

WONG Christina Chun Yee 15/09/2009 Barnfield House Veterinary Centre 405 Pinner Road Harrow Middlesex HA1 4HN **Tel:** (020) 8427 7360 w 6380657

WONG Man Sheung (see YEUNG, Mrs)

WOOD Ann Marie 15/11/2001 Ashwood Veterinary Clinic 448 Lichfield Road Sutton Coldfield West Midlands B74 4EP **Tel:** (0121) 308 1128 w 6240462

Bonnie 11/08/2008 6 Middlesex Drive Bletchley Milton Keynes Buckinghamshire MK3 7JD **Tel:** 01908374014 w 6378776

Charlotte Anne 11/02/1997 (27/02/2003) 1334/6 Uxbridge Road Hayes End Middlesex UB4 8JG **Tel:** (020) 8561 2123 w 6109206

Charlotte Lucy 11/01/2008 2 The Croft Bretton Wakefield West Yorkshire WF4 4LH **Tel:** 07725551261 w 6366401

Claire Louise 10/04/2007 11 Braywood Road London SE9 2RH **Tel:** (0208) 850 0737 w 6389853

Gemma Enid DipAVN(Medical) 17/07/2003 3 Little Oxley Leybourne West Malling Kent ME19 5QU **Tel:** (01732) 874343 w 6279908

Hayley Rebecca (nee Johnson) 08/04/2005 (13/11/2007) 16 Holm View WATCHET Somerset TA23 0AF **Tel:** (01984) 634007 w 6324337

Jane 05/09/1995 9 Holborn Court WIDNES Cheshire WA8 9UG **Tel:** (0151) 257 8200 w 6042023

WOOD Jane Lesley (see PALMER, Mrs)

Jane Victoria 10/03/1995 (27/02/2008) 19 Manors Way Silver End WITHAM Essex CM8 3QR w 6028847

Joanna Mary 15/04/2008 85 Brimfield Road Purfleet Essex RM19 1RQ **Tel:** (01708) 864328 w 6405638

Joanne Louise 09/03/2005 Sandbed House 2 Wakefield Road Ossett West Yorkshire WF5 9JB **Tel:** (01924) 786688 w 6325338

WOOD Karen Jayne (see DAVIDSON, Mrs)

WOOD Karen Mary (see HIBELL, Mrs)

Laura Suzanne 04/12/2003 Clayhill Veterinary Centre 351 Clay Hill Road Basildon Essex SS16 4HA **Tel:** (01268) 284281 w 6270184

Lucy Jane 25/06/2004 2 Sandalwood Close Clanfield Waterlooville Hampshire PO8 0QH **Tel:** (02392) 599905 w 6283406

Rebecca Louise 17/07/2008 14 Heswall Road STOCKPORT Cheshire SK5 6SN **Tel:** 07896533103 w 6343906

Rebecca Samantha (nee Mountier) 09/04/2008 4 Goddards Close Farnborough Hampshire GU14 9GU **Tel:** (01252) 371244 w 6289511

Robert Karl 18/10/2007 57 Forest Lane Worksop Nottinghamshire S80 2QQ **Tel:** (01909) 474937 m 6239175

WOOD Sally Ann (see BOND, Mrs)

Samantha Leigh 21/07/2008 5 Kemperleye Way Bradley Stoke BRISTOL BS32 8EB **Tel:** 01179798303 w 6376224

Suzanne Claire 18/07/2005 Flat 20 Thackeray House Herbrand Street LONDON WC1N 1HN **Tel:** (07841) 525 505 w 6296914

Suzanne Denise (nee Cox) 15/11/2001 8 Leopold Road BEXHILL-ON-SEA East Sussex TN39 3PF **Tel:** (01424) 222149 w 6260130

Tessa Louise 06/08/2008 14 Doctors Close Impington Cambridge Cambridgeshire CB4 9ND **Tel:** (07731) 918132 w 6353256

Wendy (nee Flook) 22/12/2004 The Veterinary Surgery 169 Luton Road Harpenden Hertfordshire AL5 3BN **Tel:** (01582) 462323 w 6326097

WOODBURN Lucy Elizabeth 05/10/1992 Three Rivers Veterinary Group Veterinary Clinic London Road Beccles Suffolk NR34 9YU **Tel:** (01502) 712169 w 6012032

WOODCOCK Julie Liane 25/02/2003 22 Lowry Close Willenhall West Midlands WV13 3BD **Tel:** (01902) 368021 w 6260229

WOODCOCK Sharon Patricia (see CARTER, Mrs)

WOODFIELD Lois Michelle 10/10/2007 58 Madingley Birch Hill BRACKNELL Berkshire RG12 7TF w 6319222

WOODHALL Elizabeth Anne 08/08/2005 828 Kingstanding Road Kingstanding Birmingham B44 9RT **Tel:** (0121) 355 3305 w 6291282

WOODHEAD Helen Clare 03/02/2005 8 Brackenborough Brixworth Northampton Northamptonshire NN6 9JW **Tel:** (01604) 515 485 w 6254443

WOODINGTON Louise Ann 12/02/1997 Oakview Cottage Herberts Way Oldcroft LYDNEY Gloucestershire GL15 4NN **Tel:** (07980) 667097 w 6025380

WOODLANDS Cathy Anne 04/06/2009 4 Crowthers Avenue Yate BRISTOL BS37 5SZ **Tel:** (01454) 316213 w 6415406

WOODLEY Rachael Lucy DipAVN(Surgical) 11/02/1999 C/o Royal College of Veterinary Surgeons 62-64 Horseferry Road LONDON SW1P 2AF w 6146157

WOODMAN Georgina Diane 05/02/2009 112 Northall Road BEXLEYHEATH Kent DA7 6JE w 6415516

WOODS Sara Dee DipAVN(Surgical) (nee Oldman) 24/12/2002 The Veterinary Hospital 221 Beccles Road Gorleston Great Yarmouth Norfolk NR31 8BZ w 6275530

WOODSBY Louise (nee Egmore) 04/02/1998 Amical Veterinary Centre Ltd 90 High Street March Cambridgeshire PE15 9LQ **Tel:** (01354) 652246 w 6117374

WOODTHORPE Tirzah Lucy 18/10/2006 The Veterinary Hospital 175 Newport Lincoln Lincolnshire LN1 3DZ **Tel:** (01522) 800333 w 6328385

WOODVINE Sarah 18/10/2006 The Old Rectory Jacobstowe Okehampton Devon EX20 3RQ w 6357370

WOODWARD Hannah Louise (see COLBORNE, Mrs)

WOODWARD Joanne Sally (nee Woodward) 24/01/1992 (12/07/2001) Alma Veterinary Surgery 11 Alma Square Scarborough North Yorkshire YO11 1JR **Tel:** (01723) 360484 w 6064251

Melissa Catherine 28/08/2008 15 Nell Gwynn Crescent Arnold NOTTINGHAM NG5 8NQ **Tel:** 01159196896 w 6376983

WOODWARD Sarah Anne (see WHITTINGHAM, Mrs)

WOOLFORD Claire Louise 08/05/2001 The Granary Bunstead Barns Poles Lane Hursley Winchester Hampshire SO21 2LL **Tel:** (01962) 767920 w 6216988

WOOLGER Victoria Eileen 21/08/2008 5 Cumberland Road LONDON SE25 4RE w 6326592

WOOLLACOTT Vanessa Annis 03/10/2007 Newnham Court Veterinary Group Bearsted Road Weavering Maidstone Kent ME14 5EL **Tel:** (01622) 734555 w 6252639

WOOLLARD Laura Megan 29/08/2008 60a Station Road SHERINGHAM Norfolk NR26 8RG **Tel:** (07900) 563118 w 6419443

WOOLLASTON Georgina Clare 22/02/2000 70 Doxey STAFFORD Staffordshire ST16 1EE w 6128477

WOOLMAN Lisa Jayne (see WHORDLEY, Mrs)

WOOLSTON Clare Elizabeth 07/12/2006 The Veterinary Centre Queen Annes Road GREAT YARMOUTH Norfolk NR31 0LE **Tel:** (01493) 416700 w 6367248

WOON Meii-Pheng 03/10/2007 (11/03/2009) Celia Hammond Animal Trust 151-153 Barking Road LONDON E16 4HQ **Tel:** (020) 7474 8811 w 6492098

WOOTEN Michelle Susan 05/04/2005 13 Moore Avenue Derbyshire Hill St Helens Merseyside WA9 2PP **Tel:** (01744) 601087 w 6271108

WOOTTEN Michelle (see HOLMES, Mrs)

WOOTTON Ellen Margaret 08/02/2008 24 Polisken Way St. Erme TRURO Cornwall TR4 9RB **Tel:** (01872) 270 899 w 6388203

WORDSWORTH Nicola Marie 02/12/2009 Springfield Veterinary Group 39 Moorgate Road Rotherham South Yorkshire S60 2AD **Tel:** (01709) 377241 w 6452696

WORRALL Amanda Jayne (see STRAUGHTON, Mrs)

WORRALL Beth Louise 29/06/2007 Unit A1 Priestley Road Wardley Business Park Worsley Manchester M28 2LY **Tel:** (0161) 794 4999 w 6382472

WORRELL Natalie Joy 06/08/2008 4 Rowlands Square PETERSFIELD Hampshire GU32 3QJ **Tel:** (01730) 262101 w 6347371

WORROW Whilmari (nee Swift) 14/04/2004 68 Ipswich Road Colchester Essex CO1 2YE w 6359119

WORSLEY Stephanie Elizabeth 04/06/2003 26 Hampden Road BIRKENHEAD Merseyside CH42 5LH w 6274892

WORTHINGTON Lynne 26/04/2007 15 New Park Walk Farsley PUDSEY West Yorkshire LS28 5UF **Tel:** (0113) 2194855 w 6326031

WORTHY Angela Kay (see WAUGH, Mrs)

WORWOOD Catherine Anne 18/03/2008 186 Manchester Road Westhoughton Bolton Lancashire BL5 3LA **Tel:** (01942) 815276 w 6305120

WRATE Bilitis June 04/12/2009 4 Olympus Close Little Stoke BRISTOL BS34 6HZ w 6464378

WRATHALL Emma Jane (nee Heap) 03/09/1998 (06/11/2008) 5 Ladies Walk Caton Road Lancaster Lancashire LA1 3NX **Tel:** (01524) 67777 w 6132097

WRATTEN Kirsty Ann (formerly Wratton) 09/01/2008 2 Ardmory Lane Toryglen GLASGOW G42 0BX **Tel:** (0141) 563 4788 w 6347382

WRATTON Kirsty Ann (see WRATTEN, Ms)

WRENNALL Emma Victoria 01/05/2009 59 Princess Way Euxton Chorley Lancashire PR7 6PL **Tel:** 01257262398 w 6446976

WRIDE Terri Ann 27/09/2004 (17/12/2008) 36 Burnt House Road BATH BA2 2AQ w 6293317

WRIGHT Adam Neil 21/07/2008 20 Cameron Avenue RUNCORN Cheshire WA7 4BN **Tel:** (01928) 590796 m 6377819

Amy Elizabeth 02/06/2008 8 Pattons Cottages Stoke St. Mary Taunton Somerset TA3 5DB **Tel:** (01823) 442656 w 6374849

Anna Elizabeth 06/08/2007 107 Haymeads Welwyn Garden City Hertfordshire AL8 7AD **Tel:** 07887942782 w 6358525

Emma Sarah 16/08/2006 Palmerston Veterinary Hospital 93 Palmerston Road Buckhurst Hill Essex IG9 5NH **Tel:** (020) 8505 1435 w 6343873

Gemma Samantha 15/05/2009 37 Wyndham Avenue Huyton LIVERPOOL L14 6TD **Tel:** (0151) 290 0185 w 6405231

Holly Susan 10/09/2008 88 Larchcroft Road Ipswich Suffolk IP1 6PF **Tel:** 01473412571 w 6434227

WRIGHT Joanna Louise (see HOBBS, Mrs)

WRIGHT Kirstie Jan (see BEDINGHAM, Mrs)

WRIGHT Kirsty Anne (see FURNIVAL, Mrs)

Laura Jayne 02/03/2007 1 Churchside Cottages Cerney Wick Cirencester Gloucestershire GL7 5QL w 6332917

Leanne Marie 21/09/2009 Cromwell Veterinary Hospital 36-36a St. Johns Street HUNTINGDON Cambridgeshire PE29 3DG **Tel:** (01480) 52601/52222 w 6453334

Lucy Margaret 21/07/2008 The Two Cottages The Street West Somerton Great Yarmouth Norfolk NR29 4EA **Tel:** (01493) 393898 w 6376235

Paula Jayne 27/10/2008 (26/01/2010) 40 Victoria Avenue Cheadle Hulme CHEADLE Cheshire SK8 5DL **Tel:** (01614) 853578 w 6418519

Rebecca Linda 03/05/2007 38 Cumberland Road Wigston Leicestershire LE18 4XL **Tel:** (0116) 278 3404 w 6376994

WRIGHT Vanessa Helen (see GRANGE, Mrs)

Victoria Wendy 28/01/2010 Three Rivers Veterinary Group Veterinary Clinic London Road Beccles Suffolk NR34 9YU **Tel:** (01502) 712169 w 6491977

WRIGLEY Claire Michelle 10/09/2008 33 Tudor Street GLOUCESTER GL1 5HP **Tel:** 07976267037 w 6435800

Kathryne Belinda 18/10/2005 58 Station Road Hugglescote COALVILLE Leicestershire LE67 2GB **Tel:** (01530) 814885 w 6342806

WRITER Gemma Rebecca 19/12/2006 11 Oakfield Road Frome Somerset BA11 4JE **Tel:** (07731) 506629 w 6355357

WRONSKA Ewa 24/11/2009 81 Arborfield Close Slough SL1 2JP **Tel:** (0782) 109 2283 w 6494408

WYARD Pebbles Edith Jane 18/09/2007 106 Lymington Road Dagenham Essex RM8 1RS w 6381416

WYATT Leanne Jane 21/03/2006 22 Pippin Court Illingworth HALIFAX West Yorkshire HX2 8BG **Tel:** (07786) 574714 w 6342674

Sarah Peggy (nee Lewis) 20/09/2005 9 Speedwell Close Trowbridge Wiltshire BA14 0YA **Tel:** (01225) 341802 w 6332598

WYER Emma Louise 28/03/2008 11 Fairford Road Tilehurst Reading Berkshire RG31 6PY **Tel:** (01189) 414505 w 6382901

Maria Anne (nee Evans) 23/08/2004 Taverham Veterinary Practice Ltd Fir Covert Road Taverham Norwich Norfolk NR8 6HT **Tel:** (01603) 867330 w 6262528

WYLDE Gemma Jane Hazel 01/06/2009 Waverley Church Lane Whittington Worcester Worcestershire WR5 2RQ **Tel:** 07809724942 w 6405077

WYLIE Andrea Toni 03/10/2008 1 East Brizlee Hulne Park ALNWICK Northumberland NE66 3JD w 6437813

Claire Rose 21/07/2008 185 Townhill Road Portglenone Ballymena County Antrim BT44 8AW w 6376246

Samantha 05/03/2009 Equipet Veterinary Hospital 24 Nicol Street Kirkcaldy Fife KY1 1NY **Tel:** (01592) 641333 w 6421280

WYNN Diane (nee Leach) 31/08/2005 The Veterinary Clinic 893 Manchester Road Castleton Rochdale Lancashire OL11 2ST **Tel:** (01706) 521117 w 6244708

Joanne Elizabeth (nee Burton) 11/09/1995 Hollycroft 66 Roston Drive Hinckley Leicestershire LE10 0XP **Tel:** (01455) 616012 w 6039633

WYNNE Martina Antoinette 03/11/2000 Urbal Ballinaglera Co Leitrim Ireland **Tel:** (00353) 719 6430 26 w 6202754

Paula (nee Galvin) 23/01/1998 473 Hoylake Road Wirral Merseyside CH46 6DQ w 603548X

Y

YAKERSON Michal 25/01/2010 Wood Street Veterinary Hospital 74 Wood Street Barnet Hertfordshire EN5 4BW **Tel:** (020) 8449 0074 w 6504550

YALLAND Kate 01/07/2003 30 Ringway Waverton Chester Cheshire CH3 7NP **Tel:** (01244) 332630 w 6275233

YALLOP Elizabeth 01/09/2008 Pine House 47 Flitwick Road Ampthill BEDFORD MK45 2NS **Tel:** 07970331057 w 6437494

YARDLEY Michelle (nee Halsey) 26/01/1994 28 Chaul End Road Caddington Luton LU1 4AS **Tel:** (01582) 482424 w 6066747

YATES Adam James 08/11/2006 15 Summerheath Road Hailsham East Sussex BN27 3DS **Tel:** (01323) 846 910 m 6368854

YATES Alison Ruth (see CARTY, Mrs)

Gemma 31/12/2008 25 Kingsway Park Urmston MANCHESTER M41 7EB **Tel:** (0161) 747 4816 w 6349670

Hannah 05/08/1993 (24/11/2006) Priory Veterinary Surgeons Limited 10 Evesham Road Reigate Surrey RH2 9DF **Tel:** (01737) 242190 w 6026872

Jacqueline Elizabeth 25/01/2010 116 Lent Rise Road Burnham Berkshire SL6 7BH w 6465368

Josephine Margaret DipAVN(Surgical) (formerly Oldfield) 25/10/1978 26 Main Street Breedon-on-the-Hill Derbyshire DE73 8AN **Tel:** (01332) 862159 w 6058022

YATES Julie Elizabeth (see ROOBOTTOM, Mrs)

Laura 21/11/2005 371/373 Hagley Road Edgbaston Birmingham West Midlands B17 8DL **Tel:** (0121) 429 3833 w 6330871

Maya Kristina Nadine (formerly Paul, formerly Daniel) 31/10/2006 56 Horsley Road Kilburn BELPER Derbyshire DE56 0NE w 6378479

YATES Nicola Jane (see EARNSHAW, Mrs)

YEARBY Rachel 28/01/2000 19 Alderbrook Drive Nuneaton Warwickshire CV11 6PL **Tel:** (024) 76329224 w 6190302

YEOMANS Rebecca Louise 03/02/2005 14c Whitehouse Street BILSTON West Midlands WV14 8HE w 6281954

YESIL Zoie Marie (nee Brown) 03/12/2003 23 Spring Grove Farncombe Godalming Surrey GU7 3SS **Tel:** (01483) 428427 w 6279391

YEUNG Man Sheung (nee Wong) 18/10/2006 2 Sandstone Grove Hermitage Thatcham Reading Berkshire RG18 9WS **Tel:** (07887) 504455 w 6352024

YORK Claire Louise 11/05/2009 75 Beech Grove Whitley Bay Tyne and Wear NE26 3PL **Tel:** 01912891121 w 6423986

YOUELL Lisa Jayne 20/05/2008 5 Weymouth Close Clacton-on-Sea Essex CO15 1BS **Tel:** (07966) 415 687 w 6325921

YOUNG Alison Jane 15/01/1988 (23/10/2002) 79 Brookfield Road Grimsby South Humberside DN33 3JN **Tel:** (01472) 594704 w 6064400

Alison Sarah DipAVN(Surgical) (nee Godfrey) 26/10/2000 Queen Mother Hospital for Small Animals Hawkshead Lane North Mymms Hatfield Hertfordshire AL9 7TA **Tel:** (01707) 666366 w 6203876

Christine Elizabeth Barnbrook 25/02/2003 Three Counties Equine Hospital Stratford Bridge Ripple Tewkesbury Gloucestershire GL20 6HE **Tel:** (01684) 592099 w 6281195

Diane Louise 27/04/2001 (06/09/2007) Earlswood Veterinary Hospital 193 Belmont Road Belfast BT4 2AE **Tel:** (028) 9047 1361 w 6134367

Eleanor 19/01/1998 130a Streatham Vale LONDON SW16 5TB **Tel:** 02088931366 w 6038902

Gillian 20/03/2008 19 Spoutwells Drive Scone Perth Perthshire PH2 6RR **Tel:** (01738) 553269 w 6357469

Gillian Dawn 09/08/1983 (22/04/2004) Stonehenge Veterinary Hospital Larkhill Road Durrington Salisbury Wiltshire SP4 8DP **Tel:** (01980) 654404 w 6064422

Hannah Elizabeth (nee Riches) 19/01/1998 (22/08/2006) Argyll Veterinary Clinic Unit 4 Brannam Crescent Roundswell Business Park Barnstaple Devon EX31 3TD **Tel:** (01271) 375356 w 604217X

Hannah Louise 04/11/2008 40 Green Lane Broadstairs Kent CT10 2RR **Tel:** (01843) 868024 w 6383913

Hayley Anne 17/08/2005 PDSA Pet Aid Hospital Campus Way Gillingham Business Park Gillingham Kent ME8 0RR **Tel:** (01634) 376347 w 6327098

Janette Boyd (nee Donaldson) 06/10/2009 2/2 480 Tollcross Road Glasgow Lanarkshire G31 4XX w 6419454

Joanne Marie 04/09/1997 Ashcroft Road Surgery 2a Ashcroft Road Ipswich IP1 6AA **Tel:** (01473) 743460 w 6042078

Kathleen Teresa 24/08/1998 P D S A Veterinary Centre 2b Hutchison Crossway 7 Slateford Road Edinburgh EH14 1RR **Tel:** (0131) 443 6178 w 6133636

Katie Louise 20/11/2008 36 Murton Garth Murton YORK YO19 5UL w 6403163

Kerrie Louise 29/05/2008 The Regent Veterinary Group 147 Binley Road Coventry CV3 1HX **Tel:** (024) 7645 7778 w 6356721

Lesley Anne 18/09/2007 15 Lighthouse Close Happisburgh Norwich Norfolk NR12 0QE **Tel:** (01692) 650317 w 6375267

YOUNG Lisa Jane (see WHITE, Mrs)

Melissa Emma 23/03/2007 4 Battersea Park Road Battersea London SW8 4AA **Tel:** (020) 7627 9256 w 6378215

Nicola Jane 13/07/2007 21 Chigwell View Romford Essex RM5 2JH **Tel:** (01708) 746201 w 6349450

Pamela June 12/02/1981 26 Ffrwdgrech Estate Ffrwdgrech Road Brecon Powys LD3 8LA **Tel:** (01874) 611811 w 6002104

Rachel Elizabeth 06/10/2006 Silva House Veterinary Clinic Silver Street Midsomer Norton Radstock Somerset BA3 2ET **Tel:** (01761) 412223 w 6288334

Sarah Dawn 15/02/2008 45 Pimpern Close POOLE Dorset BH17 9EB **Tel:** (01202) 603 807 w 6383803

YOUNG Terri-Ann Coral (see CORBETT, Mrs)

YOUNGER Victoria Louise 11/05/2009 6 Skelgillside Nenthead Road Alston Cumbria CA9 3TR **Tel:** (01434) 381792 w 6410093

YUILL Kirsteen Edwards 13/07/2004 No 3 Cairnbaan Cottages Cairnbaan Lochgilphead Argyll PA31 8SJ **Tel:** (01546) 606219 w 6292976

Z

ZABEK Lynne 28/01/1999 Luing Cottage Keltybridge KELTY Fife KY4 0JH w 6139412

ZALIDIS Katrina 23/06/2009 140 Powerscroft Road London E5 0PR **Tel:** 02089869479 w 6407728

ZDYBAL Carly 18/10/2006 10 Earl Road Ramsbottom Bury Lancashire BL0 9EF **Tel:** (01706) 826285 w 6370647

ZEBEIRI Nadia Jayne 08/01/2008 Maes Glas Veterinary Group Church Acre Brackla Bridgend Mid Glamorgan CF31 2JT **Tel:** (01656) 652 751 w 6414526

ZOMEREM VAN Leandra Gerdina Marlena (see VAN ZOMEREN, Miss)

ZORLUTUNA Jennifer (nee Simkin, nee Zorlutuna) 20/09/1999 158-160 Chorley New Road Horwich Bolton BL6 5QW **Tel:** (01204) 694004 w 6184681

ZOUROUDIS Heidi Joanne (nee Wilman) 23/12/2003 2 Grand Drive Raynes Park London SW20 0JT **Tel:** (020) 8542 4524 w 6297387

Register of Equine Veterinary Nurses 2010

Notes:

1. The current Schedule 3 of the Veterinary Surgeons Act 1966 permits those Veterinary Nurses whose names are on the Register (incorporated as part of the List) of Veterinary Nurses, maintained by the Royal College of Veterinary Surgeons, to carry out any medical treatment or minor surgery (not involving entry into a body cavity) to an animal providing the guidance given in Section 4 of this List, incorporating the Register of Veterinary Nurses, is complied with.

2. The first date after a veterinary nurse's name is the date of initial qualification. The date in brackets (if any) is the date of the last restoration to the Register or List, should a nurse's name have lapsed/been removed from the Register or List at any time. These dates are not intended to indicate the periods for which a name has been on the Register or List. Should information be required as to the full period or total periods a name has been on the Register or List, a request should be made to the Registration Department.

3. Equine Veterinary Nurses whose names are on the Register are entitled to use the postnominal letters "REVN" whilst their name is maintained on the Register.

A

ASTON Sarah Ruth 28/01/2009 9 Bell Close Cassington Witney Oxfordshire OX29 4EP **Tel:** 01865880757 w 6401777

ATKINS Elisabeth Jane Byard 19/08/2008 The Liphook Equine Hospital Forest Mere Liphook Hampshire GU30 7JG **Tel:** (01428) 723594 w 6418288

B

BARRIFF Jillian Louise 07/10/2008 6 Downsview Avenue Storrington PULBOROUGH West Sussex RH20 4PS **Tel:** 01903745658 w 6389391

BARROW Lucy Catherine 29/09/2008 17 Ashmead Gloucester Gloucestershire GL2 9RU **Tel:** 01452527252 w 6433556

BEALES Raymond Jack 29/06/2007 Manor Farm Dereham Road Litcham King's Lynn Norfolk PE32 2RW **Tel:** (01328) 701734 m 6355841

BENT Natalie Karla 13/03/2008 Rossdales Equine Hospital Cotton End Road Exning Newmarket Suffolk CB8 7NN **Tel:** (01638) 577 754 w 6414977

BREINGAN Julie Ann 28/08/1996 13 Nightingale Close Mildenhall Bury St. Edmunds Suffolk IP28 7HQ **Tel:** (01638) 510154 w 6097800

BROOKS Elizabeth Charlotte 01/06/2007 White House Station Road Bentworth Alton Hampshire GU34 5QT **Tel:** (01420) 560 093 w 6374915

BROWN Heidi Elizabeth 30/05/2007 Cotts Farm Robeston Wathen Narberth Pembrokeshire SA67 8EY **Tel:** (01834) 860871 w 6356732

C

CHAPPELL Heidi Marie 09/02/1995 Beaufort Cottage Equine Hospital Cotton End Road Exning Newmarket Suffolk CB8 7NN **Tel:** (01638) 577 754 w 6033562

COX Helen Louise 04/09/1997 (25/05/2005) Tremain Veterinary Practice Ltd 1 Farm Mill Lane WITNEY Oxfordshire OX28 4BJ **Tel:** (01993) 703146 w 6117192

CUTLER Victoria (see MILNE, Mrs)

D

DALTON Emma Louise 09/05/2006 7 Hallefield Road Macclesfield Cheshire SK11 7BH **Tel:** (07748) 580148 w 6356325

DAY Anita Jane 05/07/2007 15 Telegraph Hill Higham ROCHESTER Kent ME3 7NW w 6347789

E

ELLEFSEN Tina Charlotte 24/11/2008 Fetveien 159d Leil 407 2007 Kjeller Norway **Tel:** (0047) 94196307 w 6439826

F

FORSTER Sarah Louise 12/11/2009 12 Falcon Close WINSFORD Cheshire CW7 1SG w 6496916

G

GAPP Joanna Inga 19/03/2007 Frith Farm Frith Way Great Moulton Norwich Norfolk NR15 2AS **Tel:** (01379) 677 693 w 6354807

GATHERER Mary Elizabeth 18/01/1995 4 Milliken Drive Kilbarchan Renfrewshire PA10 2AW **Tel:** (01505) 706253 w 6036009

GEORGE Linda Traill 03/12/2008 Weipers Centre for Equine Welfare University of Glasgow Veterinary School Bearsden Road Bearsden Glasgow Lanarkshire G61 1QH **Tel:** 01413305999 w 6352090

GIDDENS Sophie Marie 03/09/2008 5 Belvoir Drive Leicester Leicestershire LE2 8PB **Tel:** 07739800351 w 6423634

GREENSLADE Heather Julie 19/08/1976 (17/01/2002) Newhill Farm Whitnage Uplowman TIVERTON Devon EX16 7EZ **Tel:** (01884) 821699 w 6051796

GREGORY Joanne 10/04/2008 6 The Haydens Tonbridge Kent TN9 1NS **Tel:** 07977297191 w 6368865

Victoria Jennifer 17/01/2008 35 Cotton End Road Exning NEWMARKET Suffolk CB8 7NW **Tel:** (07917) 364 996 w 6356743

GRIEVE Elizabeth Louise 24/02/2004 61 The Rock Helsby Frodsham Cheshire WA6 9AS **Tel:** (0161) 9294388 w 6345402

H

HALL Emily Katherine 24/12/2002 5 Cullcott Close Yoxford SAXMUNDHAM Suffolk IP17 3GZ w 6279171

HARDCASTLE Sally Annabel 03/01/2008 The Arundel Equine Hospital LLP Tortington Lane Arundel West Sussex BN18 0BG **Tel:** (01903) 883050 w 6378512

HARRIS Donna 20/01/1997 (31/07/2000) The Barn Back Street Modbury Ivybridge Devon PL21 0RF w 6099411

HAYLOCK Sophie Jane 07/04/2006 Hill Farm Hill Road Hempstead Saffron Walden Essex CB10 2PH **Tel:** (01799) 599 238 w 6350913

HEATON Sarah Elizabeth Louise 07/12/2009 31 Hillcrest Avenue Silsden KEIGHLEY West Yorkshire BD20 9NH **Tel:** 07590750312 w 6466347

HOBBINS Kirsty 27/02/2006 Sileby Hall Cossington Road Sileby Loughborough Leicestershire LE12 7RS **Tel:** (01509) 812445/6 w 6354125

HOLMES Katherine Anne 25/09/2008 117 Carter Street Fordham Ely Cambridgeshire CB7 5JU **Tel:** 01638720282 w 6410577

HOPE Heather Madeline 08/07/2008 29 Salkeld Road Penrith Cumbria CA11 8RA **Tel:** 07843209988 w 6416803

HUNT Alexandra Claire 30/09/2008 Sapley Enborne Street Enborne NEWBURY Berkshire RG20 0JS **Tel:** 07920030289 w 6423645

I

IRVING Lynn 30/10/2003 27 Laceys Lane Exning NEWMARKET Suffolk CB8 7HL **Tel:** 07795073635 w 6277400

J

JOHNSON Anna Marie 21/11/2008 Sandcroft Rimington Lane Rimington Clitheroe Lancashire BB7 4DS **Tel:** 01535602988 w 6410621

K

KING Katherine Elizabeth 16/09/2008 The Liphook Equine Hospital Forest Mere Liphook Hampshire GU30 7JG **Tel:** (01428) 723594 w 6433193

KOLBERT Louise Victoria 03/10/2008 The Barn Ratley BANBURY Oxfordshire OX15 6DT w 6404329

L

LAW Anna Elizabeth 30/11/2005 University of Cambridge Madingley Road Cambridge Cambridgeshire CB3 0ES **Tel:** (01223) 337621 w 6350924

LEGG Matthew James 08/08/2008 Bell Equine Veterinary Clinic 104 Butchers Lane Mereworth Maidstone Kent ME18 5GS **Tel:** (01622) 813700 m 6359240

LOWER Helen Amy 07/01/2009 3 Cohort Close CONSETT County Durham DH8 0PG w 6429585

LYONS Natalie Ann 08/10/2008 The Liphook Equine Hospital Forest Mere Liphook Hampshire GU30 7JG **Tel:** (01428) 723594 w 6347811

M

MACASKILL Nicole Gail 19/08/2008 The Liphook Equine Hospital Forest Mere Liphook Hampshire GU30 7JG **Tel:** (01428) 723594 w 6418310

MALYON Terri Ann 15/11/2005 11 Oriole Way Larkfield AYLESFORD Kent ME20 6LN w 6350308

MARNER Katherine Mary 02/06/2004 48a Heath Row Bishop's Stortford Hertfordshire CM23 5DE w 6264618

MARSDEN Katy Anne 14/10/2002 6 Blackfirs Lane Somerford Congleton Cheshire CW12 4QQ **Tel:** (01260) 278914 w 6277246

MARSH Natalie Ann 31/01/2008 7 Greenfields West Grimstead Salisbury Wiltshire SP5 3SH **Tel:** (07980) 838708 w 6410610

MARTIN Joanna Louise 03/09/2008 Sileby Hall Cossington Road Sileby Loughborough Leicestershire LE12 7RS **Tel:** (01509) 812445/6 w 6381504

MARTIN Karen Susan (see SADDLETON, Mrs)

MCHUGH Dawn Patricia DipAVN(Surgical) 01/08/1977 65 High Street Stetchworth Newmarket Suffolk CB8 9TH **Tel:** (01638) 507768 w 6056386

MIDDLECOTE Lucy 15/04/2008 55 The Forge Hempsted GLOUCESTER GL2 5GH **Tel:** (01452) 418249 w 6405561

MILLAR Bonny 15/01/1996 (14/07/1999) Rossdales Equine Hospital Cotton End Road Exning Newmarket Suffolk CB8 7NN **Tel:** (01638) 577 754 w 6097119

MILNE Victoria (nee Cutler) 20/09/1999 (13/12/2001) 48 Parkfield Rank Pucklechurch Bristol Avon BS16 9NP **Tel:** (0117) 9326369 w 6129186

N

NEWMAN Amy Marie 16/07/2009 38 North Street MALDON Essex CM9 5HL **Tel:** 07533111073 w 6347822

NIMMO Gemma Louise 02/11/2004 Coombe Cottage Rake LISS Hampshire GU33 7JD w 6286464

NUTTING Kate Susannah 30/05/2003 Rase Veterinary Centre Gallamore Lane Industrial Estate MARKET RASEN Lincolnshire LN8 3RX **Tel:** (01673) 842448 w 6279347

P

PEROLLS Victoria Zoe 16/01/2009 Flat 4, The Old Diary East End Green Farm East End Green HERTFORD SG14 2PD **Tel:** (07780) 682809 w 6423623

PHILLIPS Catherine Anne 26/01/1994 10 Frome Valley Way ROSS-ON-WYE Herefordshire HR9 5HU w 606722X

POTT Virginia Mabel 09/04/1979 Woodhouse Farm Dalbury Lees Ashbourne Derbyshire DE6 5BS **Tel:** (01332) 824 226 w 6058995

POUCHER Emma 29/08/2008 63 Broad Green Cottages Tortington Lane Tortington Arundel West Sussex BN18 0BQ **Tel:** 01903889811 w 6405572

Q

QUINTON Kathryn Anne 10/05/2007 Redwings Horse Sanctuary Hapton Norwich Norfolk NR15 1SP **Tel:** (01508) 481000 w 6355863

R

RATHBONE Helena Margaret 19/02/2009 97 Carbery Avenue Bournemouth Dorset BH6 3LP **Tel:** 01202428016 w 6405594

REES Emma Louise 02/10/2009 20 Anderson Close Harefield UXBRIDGE Middlesex UB9 6HF w 6492296

RILEY Alison Mary 27/02/2006 Avonvale Veterinary Practice Ltd Ratley Lodge Ratley Banbury Oxfordshire OX15 6DT **Tel:** (01295) 670 501 w 6351661

RIPPINGALE Marie Claire 18/10/2007 184 Woodhouse Road Horsley Woodhouse Ilkeston Derbyshire DE7 6AY w 6401337

ROOKE Carolyn Mair Feirn 01/07/2003 1 Anthony Way Stallingborough GRIMSBY South Humberside DN41 8BD w 6269062

RUSSELL Kelly Jane 27/02/1997 (01/06/2001) Bell Equine Veterinary Clinic 104 Butchers Lane Mereworth Maidstone Kent ME18 5GS **Tel:** (01622) 813700 w 6100258

S

SADDLETON Karen Susan (nee Martin) 25/08/1993 (14/05/1999) 3 Thompsons Meadow Crowfield Ipswich Suffolk IP6 9SU **Tel:** (01449) 760 334 w 6027730

SALT Louise 06/08/2007 Wright & Morten Equine Centre Somerford Park Holmes Chapel Road Somerford Congleton Cheshire CW12 4SW **Tel:** (08458) 330034 w 6384947

SARGENT Michelle Lorraine (see WILSON, Mrs)

SIMPSON Sarah Elizabeth 16/05/2006 Quarteracre 12 Stonehill Road Headley Down Bordon Hampshire GU35 8JJ **Tel:** (01428) 714 056 w 6319640

SLADE Anne-Marie 04/11/2008 Donnington Grove Veterinary Surgery Oxford Road NEWBURY Berkshire RG14 2JB **Tel:** (01635) 47170 w 6387895

SMITH Lucy Rosalind 05/07/2007 Avonvale Veterinary Practice Ltd Ratley Lodge Ratley Banbury Oxfordshire OX15 6DT **Tel:** (01295) 670 501 w 6377896

STEPHENSON Hannah Lynsey 18/02/2008 228 Gresley Wood Road Swadlincote Derbyshire DE11 9QR **Tel:** (01283) 550691 w 6347844

SUTTON Sally Anne 16/07/2007 26 Fletcher Close Tunstead Norwich Norfolk NR12 8RA **Tel:** (01603) 783282 w 6355874

T

TATE Sarah Elizabeth 18/10/2005 Endell Veterinary Group Equine Hospital Southampton Road Clarendon Salisbury Wiltshire SP5 3DG **Tel:** (01722) 710046 w 6348889

THEOBALD Susan Elizabeth 08/09/1998 Taylor & Lees Catley Cross Equine Clinic Halstead Essex CO9 2PE **Tel:** (01787) 269 006 w 6137200

THOMPSON Amy Laura 05/10/2009 3 Dragons Green Sewards End Saffron Walden Essex CB10 2GP **Tel:** (01799) 528293 w 6461342

THROWER Hailey Louise 04/04/2006 Taylor & Lees Catley Cross Equine Clinic Halstead Essex CO9 2PE **Tel:** (01787) 269 006 w 6354136

TIBBETTS Samantha Mary 13/04/2004 Sunnybank 5 Bridgnorth Road Stourton Stourbridge West Midlands DY7 6RP **Tel:** (01384) 873395 w 6271361

V

VOWLES Ruby Mary-Jane 24/09/2009 10 Avenue Road WIMBORNE Dorset BH21 1BT w 6491218

W

WEBBER Joy Marie 16/08/2007 20 Wakedean Gardens Yatton Bristol Avon BS49 4BL **Tel:** (01934) 830122 w 6371857

WICKENS Carina Sarah 13/01/2004 23 Broughton Road Otford SEVENOAKS Kent TN14 5LY w 6291766

WILLIAMS Hannah 19/01/2000 3 Lion Mews Newbury Street Lambourn HUNGERFORD Berkshire RG17 8YY w 6190709

WILSON Michelle Lorraine (nee Wilson, formerly Sargent) 18/02/2000 (09/08/2004) The Horse Clinic and The Pet Clinic at Blackmore Rookery Road Blackmore Ingatestone Essex CM4 OLE **Tel:** (01277) 823858 w 611900X

WOODHEAD Lucy Catherine 22/01/2010 Rainbow Farm Old Malton Malton North Yorkshire YO17 6SG **Tel:** (01653) 695743 w 6491889

WOOLLOFF Sarah Jane 13/10/2009 11 Alpha Street Heavitree EXETER EX1 2SP **Tel:** 01392426054 w 6493407

Y

YOUNG Christine Elizabeth Barnbrook 25/02/2003 Three Counties Equine Hospital Stratford Bridge Ripple Tewkesbury Gloucestershire GL20 6HE **Tel:** (01684) 592099 w 6281195

Section 3

List of Small Animal Veterinary Nurses
List of Equine Veterinary Nurses

The List of Small Animal Veterinary Nurses and Equine Veterinary Nurses is now closed for the addition of the names of newly qualified veterinary nurses

List of Small Animal Veterinary Nurses 2010

Notes:

1. The current Schedule 3 of the Veterinary Surgeons Act 1966 permits those Veterinary Nurses whose names are on the List of Veterinary Nurses, maintained by the Royal College of Veterinary Surgeons, to carry out any medical treatment or minor surgery (not involving entry into a body cavity) to an animal providing the guidance given in Section 4 of this List is complied with.

2. Listed Veterinary Nurses whose names appear in this section are not bound by the *Guide to Professional Conduct for Veterinary Nurses* and the obligations of undertaking compulsory Continuing Professional Development.

3. The first date after a veterinary nurse's name is the date of initial qualification. The date in brackets (if any) is the date of the last restoration to the List, should a nurse's name have lapsed/been removed from the List at any time. These dates are not intended to indicate the periods for which a name has been on the List. Should information be required as to the full period or total periods a name has been on the List, a request should be made to the Registration Department.

4. Small Animal Veterinary Nurses whose names are on the List are entitled to use the post-nominal letters "VN" whilst their name is maintained on the List.

A

ABAZA Jolene (nee Murray) 01/11/1999 (18/05/2005) Inside Pets at Home Unit 1 Didsbury Road STOCKPORT Cheshire SK4 2LQ **Tel:** (0161) 475 5720 w 6152739

ABBISS Elizabeth Mary (nee Williams) 11/02/1998 The Bramleys Pickthorn Lane Chorley Bridgenorth Shropshire WV16 6PU **Tel:** (01746) 718451 w 613172X

ABBOTT Sarah (nee Wilmot) 18/01/1990 58 Udall Gardens Collier Row Romford RM5 2JX **Tel:** 01708-733325 w 6063994

ABLA Melanie (nee Mann) 26/08/1998 1 Dulverton Road Witton Birmingham West Midlands B6 7EQ **Tel:** (0121) 328 1716 w 6102007

ABRAHAM Kay Louise (nee Burgin) 05/02/2001 101 Holly Road Aldershot Hampshire GU12 4SQ **Tel:** (01252) 315007 w 6140596

ADAIR Rebecca Jane 19/10/2001 17 Walton Green Walton-le-Dale Preston PR5 4JL w 6262451

ADAMS Deborah Jean 31/07/1978 14 Gelligaled Road Ystrad PENTRE Mid Glamorgan CF41 7RH **Tel:** (01443) 433431 w 6044450

Sharon Louise (nee Lawrence) 15/01/1996 33 Bridge Close Gillingham Dorset SP8 4LS **Tel:** (01747) 825422 w 6039961

ADAMSON Louise 18/09/2000 (11/11/2008) The Flat Oakham Veterinary Hospital Ashwell Road OAKHAM Rutland LE15 7QH w 6202556

AHEARNE Gillian Anne Patricia (nee Bennett) 03/09/1985 28 Castle View Park Mawnan Smith Falmouth Cornwall TR11 5HB **Tel:** (01326) 251 177 w 6000220

AHERN Imogen 05/05/1999 (01/05/2008) Flat 1 Seaside Pentire Crescent NEWQUAY Cornwall TR7 1PG w 6145324

AIRLIE Karen Anne (see RAMSAY, Mrs)

AKEHURST Emma Jane 04/06/1999 Chichester College Brinsbury Campus North Heath Pulborough West Sussex RH20 1DL **Tel:** (01243) 786 321 w 6145313

AKERS Susan (formerly Swinburne) 12/02/2001 7A Rushen Drive Hertford Heath Hertfordshire SG13 7RB **Tel:** (01992) 420359 w 6204690

Verna Elizabeth 19/08/1992 7a Rushden Drive Hertford Heath Hertford SG13 7RB **Tel:** (01992) 420359 w 604452X

ALDERMAN Anne 03/09/1996 32 Otter Way Wootton Bassett Swindon SN4 7SH **Tel:** (01793) 849972 w 6042690

Charlotte Ann 02/09/1998 (19/04/2005) Greenwood Veterinary Clinic 64 The Greenway Uxbridge Middlesex UB8 2PL **Tel:** (01895) 233095 w 6132563

ALDOUS Emily Anne 20/11/2002 7 South Walsham Road Acle Norwich Norfolk NR13 3EA **Tel:** (01603) 721659 w 6261010

ALEXANDER Catherine (see ARTON, Mrs)

ALEXANDER Heidi (see DOUGLAS, Mrs)

ALEXANDER Maxime Patricia (nee Lines) 30/01/2001 23 Tiffany Gardens East Hunsbury Northampton NN4 0TJ w 6211543

Victoria Ann (nee Freegard) 15/01/1981 Lothian Cottage Lothian Bridge Newtongrange Dalkeith Midlothian EH22 4TS **Tel:** (0131) 663 2495 w 6050770

ALGER Laura Jean DipAVN(Medical) (nee Graham) 08/12/1997 72a Alexandra Road Rochford Essex SS4 3HD **Tel:** (01268) 741636 w 6119870

ALLAN Lesley Elizabeth (see SIMPSON, Mrs)

ALLEN Claire Louise (nee Jones) 15/11/1988 (23/04/2009) 29 St. Leonards Drive Timperley Altrincham Cheshire WA15 7RS **Tel:** (01606) 592557 w 6054141

ALLEN Karen Elizabeth (see OFFORD, Mrs)

Karen Louise (nee Barras) 07/09/1998 8 Tenzing Grove Luton Bedfordshire LU1 5JJ **Tel:** (01582) 483799 w 6128761

ALLEN Marni Jean (see ROGERS, Mrs)

Sarah Joanne (nee Tonks) 09/09/2002 (28/05/2009) 38 Redwood Drive Tividale OLDBURY West Midlands B69 2HY **Tel:** (0121) 522 3706 w 6268281

Tracy Ann 16/09/2002 10 Durnford Street Plymouth PL1 3QL **Tel:** (01752) 266077 w 6266081

ALLIN Margaret Lily (nee Newell) 18/03/1981 (07/04/2005) Bowden Farm Buckland Road Bideford Devon EX39 5EX w 6089196

ALLSOP Karen Heather 22/03/1993 (21/12/2001) 137 Sandy Lane Fair Oak Eastleigh Hampshire SO50 8GF **Tel:** (023) 80693005 w 6014721

ALLUM Beverley Joy (formerly Rigby) 12/09/1995 (26/02/2009) Oakwood House Fuller Road Harleston Norfolk IP20 9EA **Tel:** (01379) 852146 w 6040059

ALSOP Heather Anne (nee Bennett) 01/08/1975 (10/04/2008) 2 Hudnall Lane Little Gaddesden BERKHAMSTED Hertfordshire HP4 1QE **Tel:** (01442) 846824 w 604460X

AMBROSE Lisa Stacey 17/12/2001 215 Wendover Road Aylesbury Buckinghamshire HP21 9PB **Tel:** (01296) 481993 w 6267841

AMIES Mellissa Ann (nee O'Brien) 09/09/2002 (21/12/2005) Eye Veterinary Clinic Marlbrook Leominster Herefordshire HR6 0PH **Tel:** (01568) 616616 w 6262825

AMOS-JONES Sarah Michelle 04/02/2002 Carlton Hall Carlton Lane East Carlton Yeadon Leeds LS19 7BG **Tel:** (0113) 250 9105 w 6260174

ANCELL Paula Jane (see HILL, Mrs)

ANDERSON Caroline Mary 30/01/1995 72 Lewes Road Darlington Durham DL1 4AX **Tel:** (01642) 333395 w 6037035

Claire Louise 04/02/1993 (26/01/2005) Glenbrook Main Road Chillerton Newport Isle of Wight PO30 3ER w 6065608

ANDERSON Jane Sharon (see MAY, Mrs)

Julie Frances 30/01/1998 (31/05/2005) 2 Bradenham Hill Cottage Bradenham HIGH WYCOMBE Buckinghamshire HP14 4HE **Tel:** (07872) 047 189 w 6116814

Kerry 23/01/2003 (15/01/2008) Howletts & Port Lympne Wild Animal Parks Aldington Road Lympne HYTHE Kent CT21 4PD **Tel:** (01303) 234175 w 6281668

Michelle Gillian (nee Linger) 11/10/1993 35 Old Mill Avenue Warboys Huntingdon Cambridgeshire PE28 2TE **Tel:** (01487) 822640 w 6065732

Michelle Joan 26/01/2000 St Mary's House Stamages Lane Painswick Stroud Gloucestershire GL6 6UZ w 6190379

Samantha Jayne (nee Millard) 10/09/1993 (26/01/2004) 3 Westgate Street Southery Downham Market Norfolk PE38 0PA **Tel:** (01366) 377044 w 6026602

Sarah Louise Kaines (formerly Kaines, formerly Anderson) 09/09/1994 (24/01/2008) 39 Hoylake Drive Warmley Bristol BS30 8GS **Tel:** (01179) 608298 w 6027854

ANDERSON Tracy Ann Vera (see TAYLOR, Mrs)

ANDREW Rae Elizabeth 04/04/2001 PDSA Pet Aid Hospital 64 Heyford Road Braunstone Leicester Leicestershire LE3 1SR **Tel:** (0116) 255 8731 w 6204129

ANDREWS Belinda Sally (see ANDREWS-JONES, Mrs)

ANDREWS Denize Eileen Rosina 04/09/1996 29 Lansdowne Road Cardiff CF5 1PQ **Tel:** (029) 20257978 w 6042136

ANDREWS-JONES Belinda Sally DipAVN(Surgical) (nee Andrews) 03/09/1996 42b Benmoor Road POOLE Dorset BH17 7DS **Tel:** (07718) 920932 w 6107683

ANNEAR Penelope Jane 30/07/1987 Rosemullion Veterinary Hospital 66 Melvill Road Falmouth Cornwall TR11 4DD **Tel:** (01326) 313991 w 6044654

ANSCOMB Hazel 30/09/1983 (08/10/1999) 1-5 Hugh Street London SW1V 1QQ **Tel:** (020) 7932 2370 w 6044665

ANTELL Lisa Jane (see BENNETT, Mrs)

ANTHONY Louise Marie (nee Morris) 24/12/2002 189 Station Road Drayton Portsmouth Hampshire PO6 1PY **Tel:** (023) 92 386520 w 6278159

ANTHONY Michelle (see BALDWIN, Mrs)

ANTROBUS Karen Dawn 07/02/2000 Oakmount House Trafalgar Street Burnley Lancashire BB11 1TP **Tel:** (01282) 423640 w 6108166

ANWYL Alexandra Julie 06/09/1999 (24/01/2008) Little Lane Veterinary Clinic 30 Little Lane Wigan WN3 6PX **Tel:** (01942) 231506 w 6146237

APPLEBY Caroline Ruth 24/09/2002 (12/11/2007) 20 Fulmar Road WESTON-SUPER-MARE Avon BS22 6YU **Tel:** (07977) 532213 w 6270459

APPLEYARD Michelle Louise (see BILLARD, Mrs)

ARDREY Gillian Elizabeth 19/08/1992 10 Cherrytree Drive Cambuslang Glasgow Lanarkshire G72 7XZ **Tel:** (0141) 646 0953 w 6008514

ARKLESS Helen Mary 19/01/1996 (24/07/2001) 49 Lilac Road Ormesby Middlesbrough Cleveland TS7 9DE **Tel:** (0161) 7735020 w 6041813

ARNOLD Nadine Deborah 22/07/1993 (12/07/2001) 132 Melton High Street West Melton Rotherham South Yorkshire S63 6RF w 6014936

ARTHUR Michelle Karen 14/10/2002 (17/12/2007) 9 Coombe Shaw Ninfield BATTLE East Sussex TN33 9LQ w 6270954

ARTON Catherine (nee Alexander) 02/08/2001 (22/05/2008) 1 Tern Court Newtonhill STONEHAVEN Kincardineshire AB39 3QF **Tel:** (01569) 739105 w 6190236

ASH Susanne Christina 28/10/1999 Park Veterinary Centre 256 Cassiobury Drive WATFORD Hertfordshire WD17 3PA **Tel:** (01923) 223321 w 6185671

ASHCROFT Rachel Louise (see DUFF, Mrs)

ASHTON Nicola Anne 23/11/2001 83 Devon Street Barrow-in-Furness Cumbria LA13 9PY **Tel:** (01229) 430145 w 6266323

ASHWELL Jennifer 21/07/1993 50 Torrani Way North Wingfield CHESTERFIELD Derbyshire S42 5UU **Tel:** (01246) 853996 w 6066601

ATKINSON Trudie Louise 22/02/1986 37 Tory Bradford-on-Avon Wiltshire BA15 1NN **Tel:** (01225) 864198 w 6044803

ATTRILL Anita Mary (see GARDINER, Mrs)

ATYEO Elizabeth Margaret 21/11/1998 (25/10/2000) Brenmor Cottage Beer Hackett Sherborne Dorset DT9 6QP **Tel:** (01935) 872707 w 6138838

AUTY Caroline Jane (see BUCKLEY, Mrs)

AYLWARD Donna Louise (see BROTHERTON, Mrs)

AYRE Joanne (see JEFFERY, Mrs)

AYRES Sarah (nee Winnett) 04/02/2002 Avenue Cottage Medland Close Wallington Surrey SM6 7BH **Tel:** (0208) 7731849 w 6257160

AYTON Laura Jane 19/03/1999 (08/05/2003) 8 Mostyn View Talwrn Road Coedpoeth Wrexham Clwyd LL11 3PN w 6133192

B

BADCOCK Emma Louise 26/01/1999 (17/12/2009) 39 Le Clos le Breton La Rue de Deloraine St. Saviour JERSEY JE2 7YG **Tel:** (01534) 888409 w 6142731

BADGER Susan Frances 05/08/1976 University of Bristol School of Veterinary Nursing Veterinary Nursing Unit Langford House Langford Somerset BS40 5DU **Tel:** (01179) 289517 w 6000071

BADHAM-MOORE Lisa Megan (formerly Sutherland, nee Sutherland) 20/07/1993 (19/04/2005) 3 Alexandra Road SLEAFORD Lincolnshire NG34 7QW **Tel:** (01529) 419300 w 602756X

BAGGETT Anne Louise (see HAMILTON, Mrs)

BAGGOTT Tracey Jayne (see ISON, Mrs)

BAILES Helen 21/03/2001 6 Long Acre Dairy Lane Estate Houghton le Spring Tyne and Wear DH4 5PZ **Tel:** (0191) 584 2762 w 6214337

BAILEY Angela Claire 25/01/2001 4 Oaks Business Village Revenge Road Chatham Kent ME5 8LF **Tel:** (01634) 671334 w 6203524

BAILEY Anne (see ROBERTS, Mrs)

BAILEY Karen Anne (see BUTT, Mrs)

Laura 24/08/1999 (23/08/2004) 54 Enville Road Kinver STOURBRIDGE West Midlands DY7 6BX **Tel:** (01384) 873660 w 6152466

Michelle Tamzin DipAVN(Surgical) 17/11/1992 PO Box FM676 Famona Bulawayo Zimbabwe w 6044064

BAILEY Ruth (see COX, Mrs)

BAILLIE Philippa Jane (see BLOOMFIELD, Mrs)

BAIN Sandra Olivia 29/07/1977 Blue Cross Animals Hospital Argyle Place London W6 0RQ **Tel:** (020) 8748 5150 w 6044949

BAIRD Deborah Jayne 09/02/1982 (17/01/2003) 1 Farleigh Court Farm Cottages Farleigh Court Road Warlingham Surrey CR6 9PX **Tel:** (01883) 625730 w 604495X

BAKER Rachel Louise (see GOWSHALL, Mrs)

BALCHIN Anna Louise 18/11/2002 8 Cottage Farm Court Stretton on Fosse MORETON-IN-MARSH Gloucestershire GL56 9SR **Tel:** (01608) 664149 w 6263837

BALDOCK Lucy Marguerite Helen (nee Coates) 18/05/1992 49 Langley Grove Sandridge St. Albans Hertfordshire AL4 9DP **Tel:** (01727) 750230 w 6047815

BALDWIN June Editha DipAVN(Surgical) (nee Gray) 01/06/1977 (02/11/1999) The Queens Veterinary School Hospital University of Cambridge Madingley Road Cambridge CB3 0ES w 6051639

Michelle (nee Anthony) 19/10/2001 45 Duxford Grove Faverdale DARLINGTON County Durham DL3 0GH **Tel:** (01325) 365136 w 6270503

Sarah Jeanette 20/02/2001 Alphapet Veterinary Clinic 15 The Precinct West Meads Bognor Regis West Sussex PO21 5SB w 6212544

Sophie Jane 13/08/1991 15 Chestnut Close Tetbury Gloucestershire GL8 8LH **Tel:** (01666) 505997 w 6044982

BALKHAM Fiona Deborah 14/06/2001 12 Beauford Road Horam HEATHFIELD East Sussex TN21 0EB w 611687X

BALL Wendy Joyce 02/08/1993 11 Ontario Close Birmingham B38 9RD **Tel:** (0121) 628 6071 w 6066612

BALMER Josephine Sarah (see BURNFIELD, Ms)

BAMENT Wendy Patricia 29/08/2000 5 Station Road Christchurch Dorset BH23 1QY **Tel:** (077) 112 73716 w 6203810

BANCROFT-LIVINGSTON Philippa Anne (see JACKSON-COX, Mrs)

BANFORD BAKER Kathryn Jane 16/09/1981 28 Fromondes Road Cheam Sutton Surrey SM3 8QR **Tel:** (0208) 6441726 w 6045002

BANHAM Andrea Samantha (nee Lunn) 14/02/1996 14 Burlington Road New Malden Surrey KT3 4NY **Tel:** (020) 8942 2202 w 6025802

BANNISTER Claire Louise (see FLEMING, Mrs)

BANTON Valerie (see TREVALLION, Mrs)

BARBER Catherine Jayne 09/09/1999 26 Mount Street Breaston Derby DE72 3AJ **Tel:** (01332) 873619 w 6184626

Claire Penelope 27/07/1988 (23/04/2009) 61 Long Lane Carlton-in-Lindrick WORKSOP Nottinghamshire S81 9AW **Tel:** (01909) 730912 w 6045024

BARKER Karen Louise (see BYRNE, Mrs)

BARKER Tabitha Lucy Haley (formerly Clarke) 30/01/1995 7 Ryders Langton Green TUNBRIDGE WELLS Kent TN3 0DX **Tel:** (01892) 86820 w 6028304

BARNARD Emma Louise 13/12/2001 1 Colleymore Cottage Coleshill Swindon Wiltshire SN6 7PU **Tel:** (01367) 244070 w 6269293

BARNARD Emma Louise (see DAVIES, Mrs)

Jassy Frances 31/12/1998 (26/10/2000) 74 Mill Lane High Ongar ONGAR Essex CM5 9RL **Tel:** (0208) 5306014 w 609739X

BARNETT Allison Jane 13/09/1999 (27/01/2010) Fairview Farm Wrekin Course Wellington TELFORD Shropshire TF6 5AH **Tel:** (01952) 740374 w 6184824

BARNETT Karen Emily Ann (see CONNELL, Mrs)

BARNETT Vanessa Jayne (see JAYNES, Ms)

BARON Peter 04/11/1998 11 Thistledown Close Eccles Manchester M30 7TD **Tel:** (0161) 278 5797 m 6140610

BARONE Nicola Jamie (nee Boulter) 22/11/2001 De Montfort Veterinary Hospital 44 Merstow Green Evesham Worcestershire WR11 4BH **Tel:** (01386) 446095 w 6264497

BARRACLOUGH Lynne 21/01/1998 28 Dove Road Wombwell Barnsley South Yorkshire S73 0TE w 6115617

BARRAS Karen Louise (see ALLEN, Mrs)

BARRETT Julia Elizabeth (nee Derbridge) 23/08/1999 4 Lark Road Mildenhall BURY ST. EDMUNDS Suffolk IP28 7LA **Tel:** (01268) 566849 w 6117319

BARROW Lesley 01/08/1986 The Glen Elmswell Road Great Ashfield Bury St. Edmunds Suffolk IP31 3HQ **Tel:** (01359) 242633 w 6092959

Sara Louise (nee Trout) 26/01/1994 2 Fox Way Nether Stowey Bridgwater Somerset TA5 1PF **Tel:** (01278) 732942 w 6067285

Valerie Hilda 25/09/2001 P.O Box 52 Hunters Retreat 6017 Eastern Cape South Africa **Tel:** (0027) 766 838 485 w 6228747

BARTLETT Emma Louisa (nee Stringer) 18/01/1999 21 Kenley Avenue Carterton Oxfordshire OX18 3UZ **Tel:** (0161) 437 6831 w 6170711

Susan Louise (nee Burnett, nee Kraatz) 04/03/1999 (17/09/2008) 185 Welland Road Hilton DERBY DE65 5NN **Tel:** (01283) 733628 w 6137255

BARWELL Nicola 05/04/2000 (27/01/2009) Longroyd Farm Cottage Longroyd Road Earby BARNOLDSWICK Lancashire BB18 6NZ w 6134403

BASILE Allison Victoria (see GEORGE, Miss)

BASSINDER Elaine (nee Hudson) 10/09/1973 (18/09/2006) 61 Chudleigh Road Birmingham B23 6HG **Tel:** (0121) 603 8525 w 6084132

BATACANIN Sarah Tracy (see JONES, Mrs)

BATES Kelsey Jane (see STANLEY, Mrs)

BATESON Jennifer Helen 15/03/1989 Flat C, 6 The Avenue Crossgates Leeds West Yorkshire LS15 8JN **Tel:** (01132) 600 970 w 6045192

BATEY Rowena (nee Sneap) 29/09/1999 Ashlea Veterinary Centre Ltd Unit 2B Port Road Business Park Carlisle CA2 7AF **Tel:** (01228) 549177 w 6185462

BAVERSTOCK Elizabeth Ann Lucy (see PARTRIDGE, Mrs)

BAVIN Louise (see WALKER, Mrs)

BAXTER Natasha Leigh (see WATTS, Mrs)

BAYES Charlotte Victoria DipAVN(Surgical) 14/10/2002 Unit A1 Priestley Road Wardley Business Park Worsley Manchester M28 2LY **Tel:** (0161) 794 4999 w 6277224

BAYLIS Sarah DipAVN(Surgical) (nee Cliffe) 16/09/1994 (12/02/2007) 15 Cumbers Drive Ness Neston Merseyside CH64 4AU **Tel:** (0151) 334 2629 w 6031361

BEACH Hilary May 17/05/1988 (03/03/2006) 23 Kings Avenue Highworth Swindon SN6 7AN **Tel:** (01793) 764 511 w 6045239

BEADSWORTH Rachel Clare (nee Looker) 28/01/1994 66 Burnedge Lane Grasscroft OLDHAM OL4 4EB **Tel:** (07941) 226157 w 6066791

BEATT Gillian Margaret 02/02/1998 Parkside Veterinary Group 5 Kings Cross Road Dundee Angus DD2 3PT **Tel:** (01382) 810777 w 6130475

BEATTIE Adele Louisa (nee Williams) 01/09/2000 90 Hadley Grange Church Langley Harlow Essex CM17 9PH **Tel:** (01279) 430449 w 6133625

Lucille Mary Jean (nee Tennant) 27/01/2000 (30/11/2007) 2 Byrehope Road Uphall BROXBURN West Lothian EH52 5SP **Tel:** (01506) 854036 w 6144320

BEAVEN Joanna (see SNOWSILL, Mrs)

BEAZANT Sarah Lesley 15/04/1994 (07/10/1998) 2 Oxhey Avenue Watford Hertfordshire WD19 4HG **Tel:** (01923) 226247 w 6031940

BECK Joanna (nee Nicholson) 25/08/1999 (19/07/2005) Lackham - Wiltshire College Lacock Chippenham Wiltshire SN15 2NY **Tel:** (01249) 466800 w 6132541

BECKETT Joanne Sheila Elizabeth 22/01/1996 (13/02/2002) 47 Kirby Avenue Woodloes Park Warwick CV34 5YY **Tel:** (01926) 497285 w 6037818

BEDDOES Alison Mary 29/07/1974 (15/01/2008) 47 Fairfield Lane Kidderminster Worcestershire DY11 5QJ **Tel:** (01562) 851645 w 604532X

BEDDOWS Margaret Caroline Patricia (see BEDFORD, Mrs)

BEDFORD Margaret Caroline Patricia (nee Beddows) 06/10/1989 (06/07/2000) Sutton Farm Veterinary Surgery Tilstock Crescent Sutton Farm Shrewsbury Shropshire SY2 6HW **Tel:** (01743) 352274 w 6015780

BEEVERS Louise Claire 06/04/2001 37 Stowe Crescent Silvertree Estate Tokai 7945 Cape Town South Africa w 6139310

BELL Deborah Ellen (see GREEN, Miss)

BELL Fiona Jane (see SHEPHERD, Mrs)

BENDIKAS Joanna Lea (nee Quenby) 23/10/2001 26 Finsbury Avenue Derby Derbyshire DE22 4BT w 6205878

BENNELL Susan 10/08/1971 Wildbore Veterinary Group 5 Newcastle Street Worksop Nottinghamshire S80 2AS **Tel:** (01909) 472059 w 6045421

BENNETT Gillian Anne Patricia (see AHEARNE, Mrs)

BENNETT Heather Anne (see ALSOP, Ms)

BENNETT Jayne Linda 26/08/1997 (28/10/2002) Highlands Surgery Ashford Road Tenterden Kent TN30 6LX **Tel:** (01580) 763309 w 6110834

Lisa Jane (nee Antell) 15/08/1990 (21/07/1999) North Park Veterinary Group 64 Fore Street North Tawton Devon EX20 2DT **Tel:** (01837) 82327 w 6044676

BENNETT Rachel Kay (see WILLCOX, Mrs)

BENSKIN Hannah Ruth 17/08/1995 5 Siskin Road Uppingham OAKHAM Rutland LE15 9UL w 6031893

BENSON Julie Marie 01/03/1989 PDSA Hepton Court York Road Leeds LS9 6PW w 6045465

BENTLEY Allison Louise (see BRADBURN, Mrs)

BERESFORD Fiona Jane (see COPELAND, Mrs)

BERKIN Vivien Ann 03/02/2000 C/o Royal College of Veterinary Surgeons 62-64 Horseferry Road LONDON SW1P 2AF w 6191006

BERRIDGE Helen Mary 29/01/2001 (16/03/2007) The Scott Veterinary Clinic 405 Goldington Road Bedford Bedfordshire MK41 0DS **Tel:** (01234) 261 622 w 6211444

BERRY Helen Mary (see WATSON, Mrs)

BERRY Jane (nee Satterley) 21/03/1990 City Vets 101 Buddle Lane St Thomas Exeter EX4 1QS **Tel:** (01392) 250000 w 6045523

Karla Michelle 15/01/1999 (26/10/2000) 46 Surrey Road Dagenham Essex RM10 8ES **Tel:** (0208) 252 0362 w 6137120

BERYCZ Melanie Jane 19/08/1994 31 Wingfield Street Bungay Suffolk NR35 1EZ w 6037308

BESANT Catherine Mary 11/09/1998 224 Winchester Road Shirley Southampton SO16 6TL **Tel:** (023) 8077 9388 w 6139514

BETTS Deborah Louise 22/02/1996 (28/01/2009) 509 New Street Hilcote ALFRETON Derbyshire DE55 5HU w 603660X

BEUKES Christine (see NORRIS, Mrs)

BICHARD Stephanie Jayne 19/04/2002 33 Aintree Drive WATERLOOVILLE Hampshire PO7 8NG w 6268457

BICKNELL Julia (see BRIGGS, Mrs)

BIDWELL Claire Marie 23/08/1999 (26/02/2004) Eastgate Veterinary Group Cotton Lane Bury St. Edmunds Suffolk IP33 1XW **Tel:** (01284) 753961 w 6185264

BIGGS Jacqueline Beryl (see EVANS, Mrs)

BILIK Katherine Louise (see BUTLER, Mrs)

BILLARD Michelle Louise (nee Appleyard) 15/02/2002 5 Westcroft Crescent Westfield Sheffield South Yorkshire S20 8EG w 6205097

BILLING Nancy Elizabeth 10/01/2003 10 Winston Avenue Newton-le-Willows Merseyside WA12 9RW **Tel:** (0797) 632 728 w 6282911

BILLINGTON Angela (nee Hatt) 14/09/1992 (02/11/2009) 30 Nideggen Close THATCHAM Berkshire RG19 4HS w 600670X

BINGHAM Elaine Roma (see O'BRIEN, Mrs)

BIRD Lynda Joan 31/08/2000 34 Southgate Street Bury St. Edmunds Suffolk IP33 2AZ **Tel:** (01284) 701444 w 6202259

BIRKINSHAW Sarah Jane 08/09/1999 Oxton Rakes Farm Oxton Rakes Barlow Dronfield Derbyshire S18 7TH **Tel:** (0114) 2851240 w 6185209

BIRNEY Una Susan 03/05/2001 Hillview Maganey Co Kildare Ireland **Tel:** (059) 863 1498 w 6216999

BIX Elizabeth Anne (formerly Walsh) 16/08/1978 (08/12/2008) 477 Abbey Road Belvedere Kent DA17 5DJ **Tel:** (020) 8306 2325 w 6063076

BLACK Susan Elaine (see LOGAN, Mrs)

BLACKALL Alison Jane (see MACE, Mrs)

BLACKBURN Jane Catherine 02/10/1997 Rowan Heights Grenofen Tavistock Devon PL19 9ER **Tel:** (01579) 346211 w 6116938

BLAGG Karen (nee Lomax) 24/01/1997 76 Main Street Shirebrook MANSFIELD Nottinghamshire NG20 8DL **Tel:** (01623) 744868 w 6098473

BLAIR Tracey Pamela (see DAVIDSON, Mrs)

BLAKE Carly Jayne (see DRAYTON, Mrs)

BLAKE Jennifer Anne 18/01/2001 34 Hillfoot Crescent Pudsey West Yorkshire LS28 7QP **Tel:** (0113) 256 9590 w 6210729

Zoe Louise 15/01/1996 Brelades Veterinary Surgeons 20 Knoll Road Dorking Surrey RH4 3EP **Tel:** (01306) 883086 w 6040230

BLAMIRE Rachel Elizabeth (see MOYLE, Mrs)

BLANDFORD Tracey Anne 27/12/2001 1 Stanton Close Blandford Forum Dorset DT11 7RT **Tel:** (01258) 454786 w 6267302

BLAYER Jane (nee Hampton) 05/08/1980 (23/01/2001) Sherwood Veterinary Group Dudley House 297 Staines Road West Ashford Common Middlesex TW15 1RS **Tel:** (01932) 779979 w 6013932

BLENKIRON Gillian Jane 10/11/1980 (16/01/2001) 10 Institute Street Oakenshaw Crook County Durham DL15 0TB **Tel:** (01388) 747334 w 6045793

BLOOM Candice Anne 05/09/2002 The Hollies Hyde Place Llanhilleth Abertillery Gwent NP13 2RT **Tel:** (077899) 146 98 w 6319090

BLOOMFIELD Philippa Jane (nee Baillie) 13/03/2001 The Ardmore Veterinary Group 57 Cornard Road Sudbury Suffolk CO10 2XB **Tel:** (01787) 372588 w 6203282

BLOSSOM Suzanne Helen (see GLOVER, Mrs)

BLOTT Jodie Elisabeth (see SUMMERS, Mrs)

BLUES Debra DipAVN(Medical) 26/06/1994 76 Carberry Court Whitecraig Musselburgh Midlothian EH21 8PJ **Tel:** (0131) 4680463 w 603214X

BLYTH Alison Marie 14/10/2002 (13/08/2008) 29 Hands Road HEANOR Derbyshire DE75 7HA w 6269051

BLYTHE Sally Ann 25/08/1999 (11/06/2009) Hillview Bromsgrove Road DROITWICH Worcestershire WR9 8LL w 6137528

BODDICE Kathryn Anne (nee Crump) 12/09/2000 6 Dawlish Place LEEDS LS9 9HF w 6203920

BODDISON Lucie Victoria (see HOBDEN, Mrs)

BODIMEAD Jacqueline Bernadette 27/08/1999 13 Beechcroft Brinkley NEWMARKET Suffolk CB8 0SH **Tel:** (01638) 508 011 w 6145663

BOFFEY Ruth Elizabeth (see DEAN, Mrs)

BOGGIS Tracy Jane 12/09/1997 (02/11/2007) 2 Baetty Road Sudbury Suffolk CO10 1PL **Tel:** (01787) 888007 w 6116949

BOLTON Coilla Anne (see DRAKE, Mrs)

BOND Terri Louise (see HORSLEY, Mrs)

BONFIELD Sarah Jane (see CHAPMAN, Mrs)

BONNER Sandra Jane 01/02/1990 (29/01/2002) 100 Colemans Moor Road Woodley Reading Berkshire RG5 4DN w 6045909

BOOKER Lesley Ann (see STILL, Mrs)

BOOKER Sarah (see MCNEELY, Mrs)

BOOTH Emma Louise 14/11/2000 5 Dayhouse Bank Romsley Worcestershire B62 0EU **Tel:** (01562) 710074 w 6203744

Karen Anne 17/01/1997 The Hart Veterinary Centre Browning Drive Kings Meadow Bicester Oxfordshire OX26 2XL **Tel:** (01869) 323 223 w 6097491

Sara 25/10/1989 (22/05/2008) 26 Chelmer Close PLYMOUTH PL7 2YE **Tel:** (01752) 342833 w 6045953

BOOTHROYD Caroline Su 10/12/2002 68 Blackburne Avenue WIDNES Cheshire WA8 8UX **Tel:** (0151) 420 0668 w 6287190

BOSTOCK Claire Isobel 18/02/2000 7 Bolney Court Bewbush Crawley West Sussex RH11 8UB **Tel:** (01293) 553299 w 6191127

BOTHAMLEY Dawn 14/01/2000 Hall Court Veterinary Group 1 St. Leonards Close Dinnington Sheffield S25 2PQ **Tel:** (01909) 562319 w 6149249

BOTT Emma Louise (nee Bott, formerly Watkins) 11/08/1992 C/o Royal College of Veterinary Surgeons 62-64 Horseferry Road LONDON SW1P 2AF w 6008682

BOULTER Nicola Jamie (see BARONE, Mrs)

BOURTON Samantha Elizabeth 11/12/2001 8 St George's Parade Wolverhampton West Midlands WV2 1BD **Tel:** (01902) 425262 w 6270041

BOW Amanda Jane (nee Jenkins, nee Jenkins) 10/12/2002 2 Applegarth Close Snatchill Corby Northamptonshire NN18 8EU **Tel:** (01536) 741105 w 6240649

BOWEN Alison Joan (see WHITELAW, Mrs)

BOWEN Nicola Dawn (nee Davies) 09/02/1998 (29/09/2005) 11 St. Johns Close Burntwood Staffordshire WS7 1QD w 6040503

BOWMAN Anna Marie 02/02/2001 Abbey Veterinary Centre 2 Augusta Street Grimsby Lincolnshire DN34 4TA **Tel:** (01472) 347054 w 6211851

Sharon Wendy 01/10/1991 (30/08/2000) College of Animal Welfare London Road Godmanchester Huntingdon Cambridgeshire PE29 2LJ **Tel:** (01480) 831177 w 6046050

BOWNESS Patricia Anne 09/08/1983 (05/11/2004) Westmorland Veterinary Group Riverside Business Park Natland Road Kendal Cumbria LA9 7SX **Tel:** (01539) 722692 w 6000242

BOXALL Julia Elizabeth (nee Holder) 14/01/1991 (29/12/2000) New Priory Veterinary Practice The Deneway London Rd Brighton East Sussex BN1 8QR **Tel:** (01273) 540430 w 6000945

BOYD Suzannah Jayne Carol (see EASTWOOD, Mrs)

BOYLE Jennifer Forbes 03/02/1986 70 Portland Street Troon Ayrshire KA10 6QU **Tel:** (01292) 311988 w 6000118

BRADBURN Allison Louise (nee Bentley) 25/09/2000 Broom Cottage Veterinary Surgery 28 Chapel Lane Wilmslow Cheshire SK9 5HZ **Tel:** (01625) 525175 w 6204305

BRADBURY Christina 17/08/1995 (21/07/2008) The Flat 31 Bury Road THETFORD Norfolk IP24 3AW **Tel:** (01842) 750609 w 6042282

BRADLEY Andrea Kathleen 27/09/1999 (18/08/2003) 80 Hartford Road HUNTINGDON Cambridgeshire PE29 1XG **Tel:** (01480) 450521 w 6184890

Joanne (nee Underhill) 14/08/1990 64 Coleshill Road Hodge Hill Birmingham B36 8AB **Tel:** (0121) 783 2327 w 6062618

Vanessa Clare 06/09/2000 3 Hawthorne Close Loddon Norwich Norfolk NR14 6UX **Tel:** (01508) 520450 w 6036632

BRADSHAW Deborah (see MILLWARD, Mrs)

BRAID Caroline Ann (nee Fisher-Eames) 25/08/1999 (17/07/2009) The Willows Hare Street BUNTINGFORD Hertfordshire SG9 0AD **Tel:** (01763) 289640 w 6136058

BRANCH Sarah (see MCDIARMID-BRANCH, Mrs)

BRAND Ruth Amy (see ROGERS, Mrs)

BRAND Shona 10/02/1992 1 Gardeners Cottage West Mains Kincaldrum FORFAR Angus DD8 1TU **Tel:** (01307) 820313 w 6046174

BRANDIST Julie 21/01/1980 (23/05/2001) 9 Bladon Close Nuneaton Warwickshire CV11 6DF **Tel:** (024) 76375270 w 6046185

BRAUNTON Heather Patricia 28/07/1978 (12/08/1999) Witten Lodge Heywood Road Northam Bideford Devon EX39 3QB **Tel:** (01237) 473278 w 6046210

BRAY Alison Ruth (see EDWARDS, Ms)

BRAZIER Patricia Jane 11/01/1977 Greenways 240 Bridge Road Sarisbury Green Southampton SO31 7ED **Tel:** (01489) 573442 w 6046232

BREEZE Lindsay Ann (nee Ryan) 18/01/2000 345 St. Annes Hill MIDHURST West Sussex GU29 9NN w 6129288

BRETT Katie 29/08/2000 42 Ashbrook Road Old Windsor Windsor Berkshire SL4 2NB **Tel:** (01753) 841010 w 6203854

BRIDGES Stephanie Louise (see HOBBS, Ms)

BRIERLEY Louise Katy 12/04/2002 1 Duncalfe Drive Four Oaks Sutton Coldfield West Midlands B75 5EX **Tel:** (0121) 3080546 w 6243861

BRIGGS Julia (nee Bicknell) 08/10/1979 (02/11/2007) 11a St Marys Road Cirencester Gloucestershire GL7 1AW **Tel:** (01285) 651056 w 6088079

BRIGGS Suzanne Helen (see IAN, Mrs)

BRIGHT Alison Jane (nee Gear) 05/08/1993 Fern Cottage Veterinary Surgery 233-235 Park Road Sittingbourne Kent ME10 1ER **Tel:** (01795) 476411 w 6066623

BRIGHT Debra Jane (see UPTON, Mrs)

BRIGHTMAN Caroline 28/02/2001 24 Larkway Flitwick Bedfordshire MK45 1NS w 6213369

BRISTOW Tracey Lorraine (nee Sellings) 27/12/2001 75 Ringden Avenue Paddock Wood Tonbridge Kent TN12 6EF **Tel:** (01892) 837144 w 6129594

BRITTAIN Laura Louise (see JEFFERY, Mrs)

BRITTON Sally Joanne (nee Tabor, formerly Waugh) 22/08/1991 (11/04/2008) 72 Fairmile Road CHRISTCHURCH Dorset BH23 2LL **Tel:** (01202) 499270 w 607864X

BROADBRIDGE Jill Louise (see LOWNSBROUGH, Mrs)

BROADHEAD Kate (see GRIFFIN, Mrs)

BROADHURST Claire Mary (nee Stubbs) 12/09/1997 (07/05/2002) Shaw Veterinary Centre Ltd Shaw Village Centre Ramleaze Drive Shaw Swindon Wiltshire SN5 5PY **Tel:** (01793) 881919 w 6118538

BROCKLEHURST Alexandra Claire 08/08/1978 5 Hillside Little Wittenham Abingdon Oxfordshire OX14 4QX **Tel:** (01865) 407348 w 604639X

BROCKWAY Claire DipAVN(Surgical) 20/11/2002 Cedar Veterinary Hospital 69 Christchurch Road Ringwood Hampshire BH24 1DH **Tel:** (01425) 473683 w 6275046

BROOK Jessica Josephine (nee Brook, formerly Carey) 18/09/1997 (08/05/2003) 3 Wren Close Alconbury HUNTINGDON Cambridgeshire PE28 4WG w 6113482

BROOKE Jeanette Marie (see WATSON, Mrs)

BROOKE Laura Ruth 18/09/2000 Willows Hill Farm Northwood Lane Kidderminster DY12 1AT **Tel:** (079) 755 19585 w 6097811

Zoe June (nee Burns) 09/02/1998 Handforth Veterinary Centre 174 Wilmslow Road Handforth Wilmslow Cheshire SK9 3LF **Tel:** (01625) 533654 w 6112059

BROOKS Emma Jennifer 12/09/1996 (25/05/2005) Orchard Dene Newton Thornbury BRISTOL BS35 1LG **Tel:** (01454) 417601 w 6043300

Karoline 23/09/2002 9 Cobham Green Whitnash Leamington Spa Warwickshire CV31 2TH **Tel:** (01926) 470 350 w 6259712

BROTHERTON Donna Louise (nee Aylward) 14/06/2001 (30/01/2003) C/o Royal College of Veterinary Surgeons 62-64 Horseferry Road LONDON SW1P 2AF w 6222147

BROWN Alison Sarah 01/09/1998 C/o Royal College of Veterinary Surgeons 62-64 Horseferry Road LONDON SW1P 2AF w 6116993

BROWN Angela Jayne (see RICHARDSON, Mrs)

Anna-Louise 23/01/2003 (02/11/2007) 111 Canalside REDHILL RH1 2NH w 6184725

BROWN Barbara May (see ELSON, Mrs)

Carol 06/02/1997 20 Walkergate Otley West Yorkshire LS21 1HB **Tel:** (01943) 466676 w 6097833

Caroline Marguerite DipAVN(Surgical) (nee Fraser) 16/08/1982 Moor Cottage Veterinary Hospital London Road Binfield Bracknell Berkshire RG42 4AA **Tel:** (01344) 450345 w 6050759

BROWN Deborah Jane (see PAYNE, Mrs)

Donna Marie 15/09/1997 22 Seggarsdean Park Haddington East Lothian EH41 4NB **Tel:** (01620) 826571 w 6107785

Isla Louise (nee Hargreaves) 06/10/1999 (18/09/2006) 21 Nicol Road BROXBURN West Lothian EH52 6JJ w 6143790

BROWN Jane Margaret (see SALMON, Mrs)

BROWN Karen Anne (see TYLER, Ms)

BROWN Lesley Charlotte (see DOCHERTY, Mrs)

Lesley Sheila 03/08/1978 Alver Veterinary Group 148 Forton Road Gosport Hampshire PO12 3HG **Tel:** (023) 9258 2991/2 w 604655X

Lisa Nicole (nee Tuley) 11/09/1996 Unit 8 Erivan Park Sandbeck Way Wetherby West Yorkshire LS22 7DN **Tel:** (01937) 543860 w 6042566

Marion Elizabeth (nee Nairn) 19/01/1998 McKenzie Bryson & Marshall 21 Hill Street Kilmarnock Ayrshire KA3 1HA **Tel:** (01563) 522701 w 6115548

Nicola Kate 17/01/2000 (19/12/2007) 2 North Cottages Mayes Lane Warnham HORSHAM West Sussex RH12 3SG w 6142775

Tricia Susan 01/11/2000 Les Eturs Veterinary Centre Rue des Eturs Castel Guernsey GY5 7DT **Tel:** (01481) 257708 w 6203557

BROWNRIGG Donna-Marie (nee Smith) 04/02/1992 (04/11/1999) 10 Durnford Street Plymouth PL1 3QL **Tel:** (01752) 266077 w 6060858

BRUCE Claire Jane Gilmour (nee Sadler) 05/09/1990 10 Ranken Drive Hoddlesden Darwen Lancashire BB3 3LT w 6060133

BRUNO Mary Rose 01/05/1980 74 Mansfield Drive Hayes Middlesex UB4 8EB **Tel:** (020) 8848 3964 w 604663X

BRYAN Laura Louise (see HUGHES, Mrs)

BRYANT Clare Elizabeth 18/10/1993 (31/05/2000) The College of Animal Welfare Royal (Dick)School of Veterinary Studies 1 Summerhall Square Edinburgh EH9 1QH **Tel:** (0131) 650 7947 w 6065674

BRYNE Lynn (nee Pearson) 09/09/1987 (16/05/2003) Christon Court Farm Flagstaff Road Christon AXBRIDGE Somerset BS26 2XY **Tel:** (01934) 823328 w 6076234

BRYSON Lindsey (nee Warburton) 17/09/1999 410 Eaton Road West Derby Liverpool L12 3HG **Tel:** (0151) 220 4668 w 6184615

Michelle Ann (nee Thompson) 27/12/2001 11 Silverdale Road St Annes on Sea Lytham St Annes Lancashire FY8 3RE **Tel:** (01253) 722508 w 6268842

BUCHANAN Leanda Nicola (nee Hutchison) 19/02/2001 6 Echline Park SOUTH QUEENSFERRY West Lothian EH30 9XQ **Tel:** (0131) 331 4373 w 6212456

BUCK Jacqueline Mary 07/06/1999 Chestnut Farm House Ludford Road Binbrook Mkt Rasen Lincolnshire LN8 6DR **Tel:** (01472) 398705 w 6170678

BUCKELL Penny 16/11/1990 (28/03/2008) 7 The Borough Brockham BETCHWORTH Surrey RH3 7NB w 6046673

BUCKLEY Caroline Jane (nee Auty) 02/09/1991 (04/02/2009) 10 Lindale Garth Kirkhamgate WAKEFIELD West Yorkshire WF2 0RN **Tel:** (01924) 370112 w 6044825

Nicola Jane (nee Creasey) 02/10/1997 (27/09/2001) Park Veterinary Centre 256 Cassiobury Drive WATFORD Hertfordshire WD17 3PA **Tel:** (01923) 223321 w 6117206

Sherran Ann (nee Fletcher) 22/11/1976 (01/05/2008) 1-3 Hillside Court 498-500 Lickey Road Cofton Hackett Birmingham West Midlands B45 8UU **Tel:** (0844) 800 3475 w 6000082

BUFTON Sarah Elizabeth (see SHONE, Mrs)

BULLARD Jennifer Jane (nee Douglas) 29/07/1975 (18/11/1999) Rosemullion Veterinary Hospital 66 Melvill Road Falmouth Cornwall TR11 4DD **Tel:** (01326) 313991 w 6079654

BULLOCK Annette 02/02/1996 (06/11/2002) 1-5 Hugh Street London SW1V 1QQ **Tel:** (020) 7932 2370 w 6034216

BURCH Marian Eileen (nee Warne) 26/08/1970 (10/04/2002) 3 Denstroude Cottages Denstroude Lane Blean Canterbury Kent CT2 9JX **Tel:** (01227) 472275 w 6082485

BURDEN Ann-Marie Claire 27/01/2000 12 Ratcliffe Road Hedge End SOUTHAMPTON SO30 4HA **Tel:** (01489) 783793 w 6132891

BURGEMAN Lyn Joy 13/08/1973 21 Eagle Close UCKFIELD East Sussex TN22 5WL **Tel:** (01424) 224818 w 6046775

BURGESS Marie Louise (see HARRIS, Miss)

BURGIN Kay Louise (see ABRAHAM, Mrs)

BURKE Carole Anne 01/08/1978 Belmont Veterinary Centre 94 Belmont Road Hereford HR2 7JS **Tel:** (01432) 370155 w 6046786

Elaine Catherine 22/01/1991 (21/06/2001) 7 Warwick Road South Old Trafford Manchester M16 0JW **Tel:** (0161) 8629530 w 6046797

BURLEY Emily Louise (see GAMBLE, Mrs)

BURNETT Julie Louise (see MCNAMARA, Mrs)

BURNETT Ruth Alexandra 05/08/1980 (31/01/2008) 29 Kingsleigh Road STOCKPORT Cheshire SK4 3QF **Tel:** (0161) 442 8014 w 6046866

BURNETT Susan Louise (see BARTLETT, Mrs)

BURNFIELD Josephine Sarah (nee Balmer) 05/08/1980 Hawksdown Veterinary Centre 41 Harestock Road Winchester Hampshire SO22 6NT **Tel:** (01962) 884000 w 6003221

BURNISTON Catherine Anne (nee Hanlon) 26/09/1998 (12/05/2008) 14 Tyne Road OAKHAM Leicestershire LE15 6SJ **Tel:** (07759) 345 861 w 6138918

BURNS Susan Elizabeth 24/02/2000 74 Plasturton Avenue Pontcanna Cardiff CF11 9HJ **Tel:** (029) 20332496 w 6190566

BURNS Zoe June (see BROOKE, Mrs)

BURROW Judith Ann 01/08/1979 Church Walk Veterinary Centre Ltd St Mary's Place Church Walk Ulverston Cumbria LA12 7EN **Tel:** (01229) 583675 w 6046902

BURROWS Nicola (nee Chamberlain) 03/09/1999 (07/11/2005) 2 Buttermere Crescent Rainford St. Helens Merseyside WA11 7LL **Tel:** (01744) 884488 w 6031496

BURT Rachel Marie 16/07/2001 University of Bristol School of Veterinary Nursing Veterinary Nursing Unit Langford House Langford Somerset BS40 5DU **Tel:** (0117) 9289517 w 6226283

BURTON Hannah Yvonne 19/02/2001 (13/11/2007) 24 Atherston Bristol Avon BS30 8YB **Tel:** (0117) 3735575 w 6212390

Janice Irene 30/08/1995 (13/11/2007) 54 Mill Green Warboys HUNTINGDON Cambridgeshire PE28 2SB **Tel:** (01487) 823632 w 6041744

Natalie Lynn 10/10/2000 Cromwell Veterinary Hospital 36-36a St. Johns Street HUNTINGDON Cambridgeshire PE29 3DG **Tel:** (01480) 52601/52222 w 6202292

BUSBY Vanessa Elizabeth 14/09/1995 20 Parkers Circus Chipping Norton Oxfordshire OX7 5LZ **Tel:** (01608) 642 647 w 6024751

Wendy Elizabeth Gravatt 10/08/1984 Fosterton Farmhouse Kirkcaldy Fife KY2 6QZ **Tel:** (01592) 774252 w 6078934

BUSH Joanne Elaine (see YAIR, Mrs)

BUSH Nicola Jayne (nee Bush) 29/09/1992 (20/10/2006) 82 Mokyll Croft Taverham Norwich Norfolk NR8 6UG w 6006754

BUSS Kirsty Anne 11/02/1998 12 A Weyhill Haslemere Surrey GU27 1BX **Tel:** (01428) 645309 w 6097560

BUTLER Katherine Louise (nee Bilik) 30/07/1992 (18/04/2001) Greenhedges 1 Glenwood Ashford Road St Michaels Tenterden Kent TN30 6PR **Tel:** (07931) 436517 w 6005772

BUTLIN Tanya Lisa 17/01/2000 4 Quality Row Cassop DURHAM DH6 4RE **Tel:** (01429) 824011 w 6190786

BUTROID Alison (see SIMPSON, Mrs)

BUTT Karen Anne (nee Bailey) 01/03/1989 (20/06/2007) 3 Ashley Gardens COLCHESTER Essex CO3 3QG **Tel:** (01206) 560760 w 6044916

BUTTIFANT Tracy Ann (see STOKES, Mrs)

BUXTON Tina Angela (nee Buxton, formerly Johns) 29/10/1989 (23/08/2007) Rosemullion Veterinary Practice Isaac House Angel Centre Tyacke Road Helston Cornwall TR13 8RR **Tel:** (01326) 572596 w 6075398

BYLAND Hazel (nee Byland, formerly Davies) 14/01/1982 (06/07/2006) 6 Whitegate Bolton Lancashire BL3 4SU **Tel:** (078) 4086 8197 w 6091434

BYRNE Deena Victoria Dimity 05/09/1997 Andeen Cottage 20 High Street Warmley BRISTOL BS15 4NE w 6117046

Gillian Rose 11/09/1998 35 Iffley Road Oxford OX4 1EA **Tel:** (01865) 242600 w 6021783

Karen Louise (formerly Barker) 12/09/1997 Cedars Llandrinio Llanymynech Powys SY22 6SB w 6036676

BYTHEWAY Cheryl (see SANDS, Mrs)

C

CABLE Deborah Nolene (nee Hamilton) 30/07/2002 29 Albany Road Old Windsor Berkshire SL4 2QD w 6317088

CADMAN Louise Helen 03/02/2000 (07/03/2008) 61 Linley Grove Alsager Stoke-on-Trent ST7 2PR **Tel:** (01270) 884145 w 6191083

CAINE Paula Denise 30/07/1986 48 Napier Crescent Wickford Essex SS12 9NB **Tel:** (01268) 573053 w 6047098

CALEY Tanya Dawn 26/08/1997 Stowe Veterinary Group 54 Bury Road Stowmarket Suffolk IP14 1JF **Tel:** (01449) 613130 w 6097571

CALLAGHAN Coralie Jane (see CAMPAGNA, Mrs)

CALLOW Clare Elizabeth (nee Turbutt) 06/11/1999 Dove House Camp Lane Grimley Worcester Worcestershire WR2 6LX **Tel:** (01562) 777259 w 6185132

CAMPAGNA Coralie Jane (formerly Callaghan) 01/09/1997 (16/03/2004) Downes Veterinary Surgeons Thorpe Bay Surgery 27 Shoebury Road Thorpe Bay Essex SS1 3RP **Tel:** (01702) 584511 w 6043366

CAMPBELL Clare Fiona (nee Woods) 07/01/1986 (31/03/2006) The Wildlife Hospital Trust St. Tiggywinkles Aston Road Haddenham Aylesbury Buckinghamshire HP17 8AF **Tel:** (01844) 292292 w 6047189

CAMPBELL Daun Elizabeth (see FIRTH, Miss)

Hazel Laureen (nee Stark) 05/08/1980 Arwendon 59 Mostyn Avenue Llandudno Conwy LL30 1DZ **Tel:** (01492) 878964 w 604719X

Marian (formerly Stronach) 24/01/1997 (25/10/2006) Ettenbreck Glen Conrie Strathdon Aberdeenshire AB36 8YR **Tel:** (019756) 51257 w 6096523

Serena Julie 27/02/2002 5 Terrace Road Mansfield Nottinghamshire NG18 2BP **Tel:** (01623) 634129 w 6256170

Tracey June (nee Parker) 05/08/1991 6 Tyehurst Crescent COLCHESTER CO4 0NU **Tel:** (01206) 751204 w 6047214

CANNY Michelle (nee Shortt) 31/01/1997 (19/05/2006) The Veterinary Surgery 169 Luton Road Harpenden Hertfordshire AL5 3BN **Tel:** (01582) 462323 w 6040081

CANT Andrew James 14/06/2001 27 Snowshill Drive Bishops Cleeve CHELTENHAM Gloucestershire GL52 8SY **Tel:** (07855) 934196 m 6222169

CANTLON Rachel Larissa 28/04/1992 (27/02/2002) 18 Oldville Avenue Clevedon Avon BS21 6HG **Tel:** (01275) 340196 w 6047258

CAPELL Nikola Claire (see CAPELL-TURNER, Mrs)

CAPELL-TURNER Nikola Claire (nee Capell) 06/09/2000 (16/04/2008) Ash Tree Veterinary Practice 124 Northampton Road Market Harborough Leicestershire LE16 9HF **Tel:** (01858) 462839 w 6204624

CAPEWELL Linda Ann (nee Jones) 29/03/1989 (14/09/1999) 5 Highcliffe Place SHEFFIELD S11 7LW **Tel:** (01142) 301641 w 6047269

CAPON Sarah Louise (see MOSS, Mrs)

CARBERRY Joanne (nee Seed) 17/09/1999 (21/11/2008) 226 Grimsby Road Humberston GRIMSBY South Humberside DN36 4AF **Tel:** (01472) 234670 w 6139434

CARDWELL Tracy Jane 08/09/1998 3 Bridge House Road Marton Blackpool FY4 4XX w 6122125

CAREY Jessica Josephine (see BROOK, Miss)

CARLILE Kelly Lyn (nee Waters) 11/09/1998 (09/04/2009) 7 Willowcroft Road WALLASEY Merseyside CH44 4BR **Tel:** (07941) 916310 w 6133658

CARNEY Sarah Louise (see LINDLEY, Mrs)

CARR Annabel (see DORAN, Mrs)

CARR Donna Michelle 24/08/1990 (22/01/2007) 15 Grangewood East Hunsbury Northampton NN4 0QN w 6047305

Katie Jean (nee Watson) 15/01/1987 220 West 23rd Street North Vancouver British Columbia V7M 2B3 Canada **Tel:** (001) 604 985 0624 w 6063305

CARRICK Jennifer Audrey (nee Carrick-Smailovic) 30/10/2001 3 Main Street Sandhead STRANRAER Wigtownshire DG9 9JF **Tel:** (01776) 830395 w 6259591

CARRICK Joanne Louise (see MERCADO, Mrs)

CARRICK-SMAILOVIC Jennifer Audrey (see CARRICK, Ms)

CARROLL Emma Jane 05/09/1994 Ambleside Farm Ditchley Road Charlbury CHIPPING NORTON Oxfordshire OX7 3QT w 6027140

Janet Helen (nee Mullock) 22/04/2002 385 Leek Road Endon Stoke-on-Trent Staffordshire ST9 9BA **Tel:** (01782) 503166 w 6268699

Verna Patricia 18/01/2000 35 Sandy Lane Taverham Norwich NR8 6JS **Tel:** (01603) 868072 w 6190445

CARTER Donna Jayne 16/01/2002 Fivelands Veterinary Centre 98 Alcester Road BIRMINGHAM B13 8EG **Tel:** (0121) 449 3716 w 6247106

Sarah Jane (nee McGee) 26/09/1988 (19/12/2001) 18 Lawrence Walk Newport Pagnell Buckinghamshire MK16 8RF **Tel:** (01908) 218910 w 6056320

CARTER Sharon Marie (see COTTERELL, Mrs)

CARTMELL Talitha Bryony (nee Haynes) 04/03/1999 Mere Road Veterinary Surgery 24 Mere Road Blackpool Lancashire FY3 9AT **Tel:** (01253) 392 984 w 6116053

CARVER Sharon Louise (nee Pryce) 15/08/1989 (18/11/2009) 11 Woodlands Close Withington SHREWSBURY Shropshire SY4 4PJ **Tel:** (01743) 709365 w 6078140

CASSIDY Claire (nee Williams) 31/01/1996 (10/10/2008) 11 Arran Close HAILSHAM East Sussex BN27 3DZ **Tel:** (01323) 448516 w 6040332

CATTLEY Elizabeth Anne (see TELLWRIGHT, Mrs)

CAUNT Amanda 19/01/2001 17 Teall Court OSSETT West Yorkshire WF5 0PG w 6097924

CAVANAGH Helen Jean (nee Masson) 03/04/1998 1 Fiddlers Yard Woodbush Dunbar East Lothian EH42 1HB **Tel:** (01368) 865280 w 6039553

CAWOOD Marie Ina (see O'CONNOR, Mrs)

CHADWICK Alison Louise (nee Dugdale) 05/02/1998 17 Thames Road Thatcham Berkshire RG18 3DP **Tel:** (01635) 867260 w 6130861

CHALCRAFT Tracy Elizabeth 06/06/1995 (21/02/2001) Grove Lodge Veterinary Group Ltd 18 Upper Brighton Road Worthing West Sussex BN14 9DL **Tel:** (01903) 234866 w 6033041

CHALK Debra Susan 18/08/1982 7 South Way ABBOTS LANGLEY Hertfordshire WD5 0JL **Tel:** (01923) 265814 w 6090747

CHAMBERLAIN Janet Barbara (nee Pink) 06/02/1978 (12/05/1999) Blue Cross 88-92 Merton High St London SW19 1BD **Tel:** (0208) 2541400 w 6047440

CHAMBERLAIN Mary Teresa (see MULLENDER, Mrs)

CHAMBERLAIN Nicola (see BURROWS, Mrs)

CHAMBERLAIN Rhiannon-Lee (see CHAMBERLAIN-DAVIES, Mrs)

CHAMBERLAIN Sharon Teresa 14/09/2001 Fairfield Veterinary Centre 51 Leicester Road Hinckley Leicestershire LE10 1LW **Tel:** (01455) 637642 w 6228175

CHAMBERLAIN-DAVIES Rhiannon-Lee (nee Chamberlain) 27/07/1998 (02/11/2009) 5 Bishopswood Brackla BRIDGEND Mid Glamorgan CF31 2LT w 6112707

CHAMBERS Helen Clare 01/09/2000 331 The Chase (Do not publish) Benfleet Essex SS7 3DN w 6097607

Mary Rose 25/01/1974 (21/07/1998) 3 Sandgate Hill Sandgate Folkestone Kent CT20 2JF **Tel:** (01303) 248501 w 6084289

CHAMBERS Sally Alexandra Brady (see COLLINS, Mrs)

CHANDLER Joanna Elizabeth (see ROSS, Mrs)

CHANDLER Kathleen Ruth 04/10/1999 165 Lower Brook Street Basingstoke Hampshire RG21 7RP **Tel:** (01256) 323 797 w 6138612

CHANT Lyn (nee Phillips, formerly Miles) 18/01/2002 167 Bedwell Crescent STEVENAGE Hertfordshire SG1 1ND w 6275200

CHAPMAN Dawn 18/01/1999 (26/10/2000) Abbey Veterinary Centre 2 Augusta Street Grimsby Lincolnshire DN34 4TA **Tel:** (01472) 347054 w 6108213

Emma Louise 14/10/2002 Macclesfield Veterinary Hospital 26/38 Cumberland Street Macclesfield Cheshire SK10 1BZ **Tel:** (01625) 501500 w 6277235

Sarah Elaine 29/08/1996 (07/02/2007) 44 Vista Way Harrow Middlesex HA3 0SL **Tel:** (0208) 9077061 w 6097618

Sarah Jane (nee Bonfield) 05/08/1980 12 Milford Road West Ealing LONDON W13 9HZ w 6047553

CHARLES Alison Jane (nee Hutchison) 31/07/1987 Daisy Cottage School Road Colkirk FAKENHAM Norfolk NR21 7NW **Tel:** (01485) 600968 w 6053603

CHARLTON Anne Margaret (nee Evans) 27/01/1988 16 Flamingo Close Darlington County Durham DL1 1DW **Tel:** (01325) 355397 w 6013127

Sarah Leigh 04/02/2002 19 Shore Drive Port Sunlight WIRRAL Merseyside CH62 4RN w 6263650

CHEESMUR Georgina Louise (nee Copsey) 21/02/1997 1 Watery Lane Necton Swaffham Norfolk PE37 8EW **Tel:** (01760) 723503 w 6098983

CHEETHAM Audrey Elizabeth Sewell 14/02/1995 Unit A1 Priestley Road Wardley Business Park Worsley Manchester M28 2LY **Tel:** (0161) 794 4999 w 6027344

CHESHAM Shelley Louise 14/04/2000 7 Woodland Way Marlow Buckinghamshire SL7 3LD **Tel:** (01628) 471566 w 6191391

CHEW Sarah Jane 11/02/1994 31 Whitgreave Avenue Low Hill WOLVERHAMPTON WV10 9BS w 6067740

CHILLAS Kim 10/09/1981 82 Bracken Bank Ascot Berkshire SL5 8HR **Tel:** (0207) 3813939 w 6047611

CHRISTIE Eve Odette DipAVN(Surgical) (nee Schalker) 09/09/1999 The Rochford Veterinary Surgery 19 East Street Rochford Essex SS4 1DB **Tel:** (01702) 545558 w 6184912

CHURCHLEY Hannah (see WELMAN, Mrs)

CHURLISH Joan (nee Robson) 09/08/1983 (31/05/2000) 9 Eldon Close Langley Park Durham DH7 9FR **Tel:** (0191) 373 1185 w 6003414

CLARK Caroline (nee Neal) 28/09/1989 (20/01/1999) Luttons House East Lutton Malton North Yorkshire YO17 8TG **Tel:** (01944) 738510 w 6057528

Cathryn Ann 27/09/1999 Bracken Ridge House Ridge Road Aberford Leeds LS25 3DL **Tel:** (0113) 286 6952 w 613498X

CLARK Helen Suzanne (see KING, Mrs)

CLARKE Katie Jane 20/01/1995 273 Dimsdale Parade West NEWCASTLE Staffordshire ST5 8HS **Tel:** (01782) 252852 w 6026158

CLARKE Joanna Lucy Haley (see BARKER, Mrs)

CLARKE Tracy Dawn 23/01/2003 75 Merlin Ave Poplar Farm Nuneaton Warks CV10 9JY **Tel:** (02476) 392406 w 6270052

CLEAVE Tamsyn Anne 23/11/2001 Pelyn Veterinary Group 8 Kings Avenue St. Austell Cornwall PL25 4TT **Tel:** (01726) 68177 w 6267390

CLEGG Aileen Patricia (nee Smith) 10/08/1971 (17/04/2003) The Coneys Galphay Ripon North Yorkshire HG4 3NJ **Tel:** (01765) 658860 w 6047746

CLEMENT Holly Joanne 08/05/2001 2 Broadmead Cottages Green Lane Ashmore SALISBURY SP5 5AJ **Tel:** (01747) 811002 w 6217010

CLIFFE Sarah (see BAYLIS, Mrs)

COATES Lucy Marguerite Helen (see BALDOCK, Mrs)

COBB Helen Patricia 29/07/1986 15 Charlton Grove ROSLIN Midlothian EH25 9NY w 6047826

COCKER Sally Jane (nee Franklin) 02/02/1998 10 Grey Wethers Sandling Maidstone Kent ME14 3DW **Tel:** (01622) 863494 w 6117443

COCKINGS Jennifer Anne (see HARLEY, Mrs)

COCKS Louisa Marie 10/01/2001 Oakmount House Trafalgar Street Burnley Lancashire BB11 1TP **Tel:** (01282) 423640 w 6204734

COE Caroline Jane 28/01/1998 3 Church View Aveley South Ockendon Essex RM15 4LH **Tel:** (01708) 862427 w 613076X

COE Nikki (see WATERS, Mrs)

COE Rebecca Anne 25/09/2000 33 Tregony Way Stenson Fields Derby Derbyshire DE24 3LG w 6203931

COGGINS Philippa Jane 31/01/1977 The Orchard St. Hilary Cowbridge Vale of Glamorgan CF71 7DP **Tel:** (01446) 773811 w 6047859

COLCLOUGH Denise Margaret (nee Turvey, nee Rich) 31/07/1973 Rainbows End 17 Lightwood Road Yoxall Burton-on-Trent Staffordshire DE13 8QD **Tel:** (01543) 472435 (Ex-Directory) w 6014175

COLE Emily Rae 16/08/1995 (18/01/2001) The Manor House Little Tring Tring Hertfordshire HP23 4NR **Tel:** (01442) 823143 w 6035945

COLE Janice Beryl (see TUCKER, Mrs)

COLEMAN Joan Margaret (see MCWHIRTER, Mrs)

COLEMAN Marina (see DAVIS, Mrs)

COLEY Kelly Joy (nee Crook) 16/11/2000 (21/01/2008) 28 Wessex Road DIDCOT Oxfordshire OX11 8BT **Tel:** (01491) 651479 w 6204976

COLLETT Lisa Joanne 22/01/1999 (25/10/2000) 4 Dene Royd Court Stainland Halifax West Yorkshire HX4 9QW **Tel:** (01484) 329930 w 6131719

COLLEY Michelle Kate (nee Parfitt) 14/08/1992 Elmar Ciottage Llantrissent Usk Gwent NP15 1LS **Tel:** 01291-672703 w 6008037

COLLINGS Charlotte Ina May (see MORRISON, Mrs)

COLLINS Rebecca (see PHIPPEN, Mrs)

COLLINS Sally Alexandra Brady (nee Chambers) 13/02/1995 (01/03/2000) RSPCA Norfolk Wildlife Hospital Station Road East Winch Kings Lynn Norfolk PE32 1NR w 6035672

COLLS Kathleen 27/01/1998 93 Newbold Road Chesterfield Derbyshire S41 7PS **Tel:** (01246) 273292 w 6115741

COLMAN Julie Maria (see NEALL, Mrs)

COLVER James Laurence 23/01/2003 Eversleigh Horsell Park Woking Surrey GU21 4LN m 6282724

COMAN Victoria Helen (see SMYTH, Mrs)

COMBEN Jill Caroline (see GIBBINSON, Mrs)

COMBER Zoe Zelda 24/09/1997 (09/11/2009) 36 Burnham Avenue WOLVERHAMPTON WV10 6DX **Tel:** (01902) 448446 w 6039746

CONLONG Sarah Jean 29/01/1998 77 Yarlside Road Barrow-in-Furness Cumbria LA13 0EX **Tel:** (01229) 833107 w 6115752

CONNELL Karen Emily Ann (nee Barnett) 03/09/1997 Richmond Veterinary Clinic 171 Lower Richmond Road Mortlake London SW14 7HX **Tel:** (020) 8878 6080 w 6097403

CONNETT Nadine Le-jette 09/05/2002 White Gate Farm Vicarage Lane Mundon Maldon Essex CM9 6PA **Tel:** (01621) 740302 w 6272945

CONNOR Claire Louise 05/10/2000 Beech House Veterinary Centre Beech House Wilderspool Causeway Warrington WA4 6QP **Tel:** (01925) 445500 w 6203942

CONSTANTINOU Lee-Ann (nee Edwards) 17/08/1995 (18/02/2009) The Hayloft Tyte Farm Ackleton Shropshire WV6 7JH **Tel:** (01746) 783827 w 6040252

CONWAY Amanda Jane (see LEE, Mrs)

COODE Samantha Louise 07/06/2001 Swanspool Veterinary Clinic 1 London Road Wellingborough Northamptonshire NN8 2BT **Tel:** (01933) 222145 w 6221751

COOK Emma Jane 11/09/1997 7 Lewis Grove WIDNES Cheshire WA8 7HH **Tel:** 07775657368 w 6097968

Ruth Anne (nee Watson) 04/09/1989 (11/05/2009) Inside Pets At Home St James Retail Park Edinburgh Way Harlow Essex CM20 2SX **Tel:** (01279) 770104 w 6063327

COOKE Angelique 15/08/1991 Kingsmead Copythorne Crescent Copythorne SOUTHAMPTON SO40 2PE **Tel:** (078843) 86491 w 6048058

COOKSLEY Catherine (formerly Rollitt) 01/09/1988 (11/11/2008) 13 Baden Road Kingswood Bristol Avon BS15 9XD w 6050963

COOPER Amanda Jane (formerly Deakin) 13/12/1984 38 Mossfield Drive Biddulph Stoke-on-Trent Staffordshire ST8 6UL **Tel:** (01782) 510 192 w 6048091

Barbara Claire 09/04/1981 The College of Animal Welfare 6 Eaton Court Road Colmworth Business Park Eaton Socon St Neots Cambridgeshire PE19 8ER **Tel:** (01480) 226180 w 6048105

Charlotte Linsey 18/01/2002 109 Weston Street Walsall WS1 4EF **Tel:** (01922) 720539 w 6265509

COOPER Holly Jane (see FOWLER, Miss)

Julia Margaret (nee Kroner) 29/01/1987 (11/12/2003) Bowbridge Surgery Bowbridge Stroud Gloucestershire GL5 2LA **Tel:** (01453) 762350 w 605471X

Karen Marie (nee Osborn) 28/08/1998 Grove Lodge Veterinary Group Ltd 18 Upper Brighton Road Worthing West Sussex BN14 9DL **Tel:** (01903) 234866 w 6041438

Katherine Elizabeth (nee Harris) 01/02/1994 Donkey Sanctuary Sidmouth Devon EX10 0NU w 6067831

Katie Marie (nee Pell) 25/08/1998 71 Churchill Avenue Bourne Lincolnshire PE10 9QA **Tel:** (01778) 422797 w 6077613

Lesley Rita 21/01/1998 255 Station Road Market Bosworth Nuneaton Warwickshire CV13 0PE **Tel:** (01455) 291784 w 6115763

Lynne Maich 15/01/2001 27 Cairnview Crescent ABERDEEN AB16 5DR w 6205174

Paula Jane (nee Cooper, formerly Peacock) 18/01/1995 (06/06/2006) 28 Vincent Way York North Yorkshire YO24 3HZ w 6023703

COOPER Susan Lynne (see FLANAGAN, Mrs)

COPE Tracey Anne (see COUSINS, Mrs)

COPELAND Fiona Jane (nee Beresford) 29/01/1999 (16/01/2002) C/o RCVS Belgravia House 62-64 Horseferry Road London SW1P 2AF w 6132836

COPPIN Susan Ellen (see MALLUL, Mrs)

COPSEY Georgina Louise (see CHEESMUR, Mrs)

COPUS Michelle Ann (see WALLACE, Mrs)

CORFIELD Philippa Anne (see NEW, Mrs)

CORNOCK Leann Marie (see LAYFIELD, Mrs)

COSGROVE Donna (see HOLLOWAY, Mrs)

COTON Sarah (nee Edge) 24/11/2004 3 Knights Lane Tiddington Stratford-upon-Avon Warwickshire CV37 7BS w 6230606

COTTERELL Sharon Marie (nee Carter) 05/08/1986 (29/08/2000) 34 Kingsbridge Drive Burwood Christchurch 8083 New Zealand w 6048284

COTTINGHAM Sarah 02/09/1998 (10/04/2006) 2 Fossano Court Beacon Road CROWBOROUGH East Sussex TN6 1UQ w 6139401

COULTER Senga Victoria (nee McCormick) 22/09/1999 Cromlyn House Veterinary Hospital 50 Old Coach Road Hillsborough County Down BT26 6PB **Tel:** (02892) 683711 w 6184604

COULTHARD Gillian 30/09/1983 (17/09/2007) The Bridge Veterinary Hospital Victoria Street Middlesbrough Cleveland TS1 5QZ **Tel:** (01642) 242338 w 6048309

COULTON Lisa Victoria 31/08/1995 39 Riverview Street Beckenham Christchurch 8023 New Zealand w 6036392

COUPLAND Chontelle (see VINCENT, Mrs)

COURT Rachel Mary (nee Stokes) 04/09/1991 (12/03/2007) 2 Harwill Grove Churwell Leeds LS27 7QH **Tel:** (0113) 2535409 w 6061341

COUSINS Tracey Anne (nee Cope) 23/10/2001 25 Churchdale Road Frecheville Sheffield South Yorkshire S12 4XW **Tel:** (0114) 2647004 w 6254058

COWAN Samantha Jane Young 06/09/1994 (08/10/2001) C/o Royal College of Veterinary Surgeons 62-64 Horseferry Road LONDON SW1P 2AF w 6022120

COWAP Deborah Louise (see OAKES, Mrs)

COWDEROY Emily Claire 25/02/2002 (10/04/2007) 75 Drury Lane BUCKLEY Clwyd CH7 3DX w 6269403

COWELL Victoria 16/08/1995 (02/11/2009) 15 White Stone Close REDCAR Cleveland TS10 2PS **Tel:** (01642) 494472 w 6042679

COWLEY Natalie Jayne 03/02/1992 (06/11/2000) Veterinary Instrumentation Ltd Broadfield Road SHEFFIELD S8 0XL **Tel:** (0845) 130 9596 w 6048386

COWLEY Terri Louise (see HORSLEY, Mrs)

COX Annalisa 02/02/1995 (12/02/2008) 11 Oxford Street Lambourn Hungerford Berkshire RG17 8XS **Tel:** (01488) 72865 w 6035967

Elizabeth Karen (nee Durbin) 09/05/1991 (14/07/1999) 5 Frenchay Road Weston-super-Mare Somerset BS23 4JL **Tel:** (01934) 624890 w 6049517

Ruth (nee Bailey) 01/10/1997 Southdown View Coneyhurst Billingshurst West Sussex RH14 9DY w 6116869

COZENS Julia Denise (see PARKINSON, Mrs)

CRAINE Sharon Ann (see POLLITT, Mrs)

CRANE Lindsay 03/02/1986 Badmans Cottage 3 The Cottages Stock Lane Langford Bristol BS40 5EW **Tel:** (01934) 852985 w 6048422

CRANMER Sharon (see STOBBS, Mrs)

CRAVEN Samantha (see HANCOCK, Mrs)

CRAWFORD Christina Mary (nee Gardiner) 05/03/2002 Neatham Manor Farmhouse Lower Neatham Mill Lane Neatham ALTON Hampshire GU34 4NP **Tel:** (02392) 454986 w 6268215

CREASE Mary Margaret (nee Murphy) 31/01/1995 Inside Pets at Home Parc Tawe Retail Park Swansea Glamorgan SA1 2AL **Tel:** (01792) 461217 w 6032445

CREASEY Nicola Jane (see BUCKLEY, Mrs)

CRIMES Charlotte Louise 25/08/1998 (13/08/2008) 5 Darwell Avenue Eccles MANCHESTER M30 7AB w 6098010

CRIPPS Victoria (see DAVIES, Mrs)

CRISP Geraldine Ann (see MARRIOTT, Mrs)

CROMEY Barbara Elizabeth (nee Mathews) 21/01/1980 (26/06/2007) RSPCA Wildlife Centre West Hatch Taunton Somerset TA3 5RT **Tel:** (0870) 9061421 w 6088272

CROMPTON Deborah Louise (see HUXLEY, Mrs)

CRONIN Elizabeth Ellen 16/09/2002 (03/11/2009) Kingfisher House Ringwood Road West Totton Southampton Hampshire SO40 7DY **Tel:** (023) 8066 0400 w 6260086

CROOK June Gillian Brenda (see MALTBY, Mrs)

CROOK Kelly Joy (see COLEY, Mrs)

CROSS Lisa Samantha 29/09/1999 (01/06/2009) 11 Kennedy Close Toftwood Dereham Norfolk NR19 1LF w 6145754

CROSSMAN Sarah Jane 02/02/1994 50a Ripon Road BOURNEMOUTH BH9 1RF w 6067401

CROWDER Suzanne Elizabeth (nee Vardey, formerly Harrison) 21/08/1991 (23/10/1998) 93 Newbold Road Chesterfield Derbyshire S41 7PS **Tel:** (01246) 273292 w 6062684

CROWHURST Tracey Jane (nee Daniels) 31/08/1990 (19/11/2007) 10 Oaklea Way UCKFIELD East Sussex TN22 2BL w 6048739

CROWTHER Penelope Ann (see CUSDIN, Mrs)

CRUMP Kathryn Anne (see BODDICE, Mrs)

CRUTTENDEN Christine Joanne (see WOOD, Mrs)

CULLEN Tracy Ruth (nee Davis, nee Fane) 04/08/1987 Hybrid Warren Hill Stud Moulton Road NEWMARKET Suffolk CB8 8QH w 6093351

CULLINANE Bridget Jane 04/02/1988 (23/06/1998) 5 Nothe Parade Weymouth Dorset DT4 8TX **Tel:** (01305) 773835 w 604858X

CUMMINGS Kelly Ann 23/10/2001 11 Annfield Place Dennistoun Glasgow G31 2XQ **Tel:** (0141) 554 1911 w 6261780

CUNNINGHAM Philippa Joanne (nee Liggins) 07/09/1990 (29/06/2001) 16 Station Road Woodford Halse Daventry Northamptonshire NN11 6RB **Tel:** (01327) 262016 w 6055167

Sarah Elizabeth (nee Kidwell) 16/11/2000 21 Sandy Lane Stockton Heath WARRINGTON WA4 2AY w 601817X

CURLING Louise (see PALMER, Mrs)

CURRIE Janice Anne (see HARBISON, Mrs)

CURTIS Sarah Louise (nee Dine) 02/08/1988 (20/05/2009) 15 Leviathan Close FAREHAM Hampshire PO14 2SF **Tel:** (01329) 661460 w 6049211

CUSDIN Penelope Ann (nee Crowther) 23/09/1998 International Zoo Veterinary Group Keighley Business Centre South Street Keighley West Yorkshire BD21 1AG **Tel:** (01535) 692000 w 6135790

CUSS Alison Jane (nee Cuss, formerly Trinder) 20/07/1993 (10/12/2003) Kingfisher Cottage 3 Lechlade Road Highworth Swindon Wiltshire SN6 7HF **Tel:** (01793) 762 031 w 6066543

Sharon Anne (nee Davis) 26/01/1993 (24/10/2000) 14 Sevenfields Highworth Swindon Wiltshire SN6 7NF **Tel:** (01793) 762926 w 606554X

CUTTIFORD Claire Joanne 20/11/2002 Beech House Veterinary Clinic 35 Harrington Road Brighton BN1 6RF **Tel:** (01273) 505071 w 6278335

CUTTING Emma Louise 13/03/2002 30 Coppice Way HARROGATE North Yorkshire HG1 2DQ **Tel:** (01423) 556219 w 6274133

D

DA SILVA Zoe Ann 03/02/2000 (24/03/2004) Guildford College of Further & Higher Education Merrist Wood Campus Worplesdon Guildford Surrey GU3 3PE w 6190313

DAINTY Lorna Joy (nee Flower) 09/02/1996 50 Priory Road Stone Staffordshire ST15 8NT w 6040988

DAINTY Samantha Diane (see LOCKETT, Mrs)

DALE Rachel Elizabeth 13/08/2003 (03/11/2009) 8 Bulls Lane Kings Sutton Banbury Oxfordshire OX17 3RB **Tel:** (01295) 811673 w 6271867

DANIELS Tracey Jane (see CROWHURST, Mrs)

DARBY Nicola Louise 23/09/2002 99 Porthkerry Avenue Welling Kent DA16 2DS w 6254146

DARBYSHIRE Rebecca Noeline (nee Theakston) 28/01/1997 (31/05/2000) Pluckham Farm Fridaythorpe Driffield North Humberside YO25 9SD **Tel:** (01377) 288252 w 6098779

DATHAN Louise Ann (nee Hodgson) 19/10/1992 (24/11/2006) 34 Rosehill Drive Bransgore CHRISTCHURCH Dorset BH23 8NP w 601219X

DAUBNEY Alison Claire (nee Raybould) 10/08/1990 40 Riverdale Seaton Devon EX12 2SL **Tel:** (01297) 22933 w 6059365

DAUNCEY Zoe Anne (see SAGE, Mrs)

DAVEY Helen Louise 12/08/2002 1 Links Close Ewhurst Surrey GU6 7QS **Tel:** (01483) 277871 w 6266851

DAVEY-BRYAN Jane Elizabeth 21/10/1998 Step Cottage 18 High Road Britford Salisbury SP5 4DS w 6138554

DAVID-GRAY Zoe Katherine 30/09/1983 (26/01/2006) 52 Abbeville Road Clapham London SW4 9NF **Tel:** (020) 8772 9922 w 6089924

DAVIDSON Emily Louise 11/10/2000 (20/04/2009) Flat 10 Holm Court 47-49 Westway CATERHAM Surrey CR3 5TQ w 6202831

Kerry Louise 03/02/1997 (13/01/2010) Cedar Cottage Nutwell Road Lympstone EXMOUTH Devon EX8 5AN w 6107912

Tracey Pamela (nee Blair) 21/01/1980 (08/10/1999) Regent Veterinary Group Upper York Street Coventry CV1 3GP **Tel:** (024) 7622 5101 w 6048761

DAVIES Barbara Gail (see SCARROTT, Mrs)

DAVIES Claire (nee Hayman) 22/01/1997 3 Garden Close Staplehurst Tonbridge Kent TN12 0EW **Tel:** (01580) 241892 w 6108563

Emma Louise (nee Barnard) 18/01/1995 Gayton House 40 Hatchlands Road Redhill RH1 6AT **Tel:** (01737) 761475 w 6036938

Erica Jane (nee Williams) 09/08/1991 (29/07/2003) 3 Knowle Lane Drewsteignton EXETER EX6 6QY **Tel:** 01647281145 w 6068358

DAVIES Hazel (see BYLAND, Ms)

Jennifer Lucy 23/01/2003 2 Robertson Road Preston Park Brighton East Sussex BN1 5NL **Tel:** (01273) 566595 w 6284737

Joanne Louise (nee Thornton) 28/08/1998 Sheriffs Highway Veterinary Group 94 Sheriffs Highway Gateshead Tyne and Wear NE9 5SD **Tel:** (0191) 4877319 w 6039338

Karen 05/07/1995 (22/04/2003) 224 Winchester Road Shirley Southampton SO16 6TL **Tel:** (023) 8077 9388 w 6021808

Katharine Anne 18/01/2002 7 Badger Way ALDERSHOT Hampshire GU12 4GA **Tel:** (07971) 403330 w 6268303

Katherine Hamilton 28/01/1998 58 Braithwaite Avenue Romford Essex RM7 0DS **Tel:** (01708) 754335 w 604276X

Katherine Jean 04/04/1996 (12/06/2000) Penmellyn Veterinary Group Station Road St. Columb Major Cornwall TR9 6BX **Tel:** (01637) 880307 w 6038866

Laura Jayne 05/10/2001 (06/10/2008) Sunny Bank 80 Gwscwm Road Pembrey Carms SA16 0YU w 6229616

DAVIES Nicola Dawn (see BOWEN, Mrs)

DAVIES Rebecca Margaret (see WHITE, Mrs)

Victoria (nee Cripps) 07/09/1998 31 Carisbrooke Avenue HIGH WYCOMBE Buckinghamshire HP12 4NL **Tel:** (01494) 443674 w 612962X

DAVIS Elaine (see LODDO, Mrs)

Karen (nee Gregory) 28/01/1994 2 Robertson Road Preston Park Brighton East Sussex BN1 5NL **Tel:** (01273) 566595 w 606781X

Lesa 08/08/1989 (30/01/2001) 100 White Road Quinton Birmingham B32 2TU **Tel:** (0121) 422 5249 w 6048885

Marina (nee Coleman) 21/08/1985 (06/04/2009) 37 Kinsbourne Way Thornhill Southampton SO19 6HB **Tel:** (02380) 464588 w 6048896

DAVIS Nichola Fiona Maria (see GRIFFITHS, Mrs)

Rebecca Susan 01/09/1998 (19/11/2007) 78b Rugeley Road Chase Terrace Burntwood Staffordshire WS7 1AA **Tel:** (01543) 684556 w 6041482

DAVIS Sharon Anne (see CUSS, Mrs)

DAVIS Tracy Ruth (see CULLEN, Mrs)

DAVISON Charlotte Ann 25/02/2003 (24/07/2009) 14/6 Fountainhall Road The Grange EDINBURGH Midlothian EH9 2NN w 6185660

Lynne 20/01/1999 Hall Court Veterinary Group 1 St. Leonards Close Dinnington Sheffield S25 2PQ **Tel:** (01909) 562319 w 6144386

DAVISON Rosamund Kim Penelop (see JAGDHUBER, Mrs)

DAWE Rebecca Maya (formerly Smith) 26/01/1999 (13/02/2002) 88-92 Merton High Street Merton London SW19 1BD **Tel:** (020) 8254 1400 w 6035027

DAWKINS Philippa Jane 17/01/2000 37 Manor Fields Bratton WESTBURY Wiltshire BA13 4ST **Tel:** (01380) 831295 w 6130839

DAWSON Donna Denise 15/11/2001 (19/11/2007) Chapelfield Veterinary Partnership Wellesley Road Tharston Industrial Estate Long Stratton Norfolk NR15 2PD **Tel:** (01508) 530686 w 6263331

DAWSON Lisa (see MARTIN, Mrs)

DAWSON Nicola Joanne (see HAYWARD, Mrs)

DAWSON Sarah Louise (see JORDAN, Mrs)

DAY Alison (see TAYLOR, Mrs)

DAY Sian Elizabeth (nee Thomas) 10/09/1997 53 Bartlett Street Caerphilly Mid Glamorgan CF83 1JT **Tel:** (029) 20861416 w 6043355

DEACON Joy 21/09/1971 3 Springfield Buildings Old Mills Paulton Bristol BS39 7SP **Tel:** (01761) 412898 w 6048987

Kay Patricia 27/09/1999 (02/12/2008) Acorn Veterinary Centre 21 Station Road Studley Warwickshire B80 7HR **Tel:** (01527) 853304 w 6141716

DEAKIN Amanda Jane (see COOPER, Miss)

DEAN Alisa DipAVN(Surgical) 26/01/1996 3 The Birches Neston Merseyside CH64 3SB **Tel:** (0151) 336 5879 w 6041711

Catherine Mary (nee Smith) 09/11/1983 Trentburn St. Bernards Road St. Albans Hertfordshire AL3 5RA w 6048998

Karen Anne 31/03/2003 (18/11/2009) 27 Little Horse Close Earley READING Berkshire RG6 7HL w 6268061

Ruth Elizabeth (nee Boffey) 24/12/2002 The Old Byre Somerford Booths Congleton Cheshire CW12 2JR w 6268633

DEAN Tessa Marjorie Rose (see LESLEY, Mrs)

DEAN Tracey Eleanor 30/10/2001 1 Court Farm Road Longwell Green Bristol BS30 9AA **Tel:** (0117) 932 3660 w 6255191

DEARMAN Sharon Lorraine (see WIGGS, Mrs)

DE'ATH Theresa Louise 05/09/1996 33 Pasture Road Barrowby GRANTHAM Lincolnshire NG32 1BA **Tel:** (07775) 923573 w 6037170

DEEMING Julia Claire (see WEBSTER, Mrs)

DELANEY Toni Alison (see STEVENS, Mrs)

DELLI-BOVI Rebecca Jane 15/01/1988 67 Elm Grove BROMSGROVE Worcestershire B61 0EJ w 6093792

DELMAGE Karenza Daisy (nee Williams) 24/10/1972 (17/08/1999) Mere Road Veterinary Surgery 24 Mere Road Blackpool Lancashire FY3 9AT **Tel:** (01253) 392 984 w 6049051

DEMPSTER Elizabeth Mary (nee Hodgson) 02/02/2001 Grove Veterinary Centre 231-239 Rawlinson Street Barrow-in-Furness Cumbria LA14 1DW **Tel:** (01229) 820402 w 6211928

DENGATE Kerry Lisa 04/02/2002 Northdale Veterinary Surgery 48 Victoria Road Worthing West Sussex BN11 1XE **Tel:** (01903) 202474 w 6263518

DENNISS Anita Lesley DipAVN(Surgical) 19/05/1999 (10/05/2002) Davies Veterinary Specialists Manor Farm Business Park Higham Gobion Hertfordshire SG5 3HR **Tel:** (01582) 883950 w 6170667

DERBRIDGE Julia Elizabeth (see BARRETT, Mrs)

DERBYSHIRE Susan Claire (see VRANCH, Mrs)

DESCOMBES Claire Louise (see WILLIS, Mrs)

DEUS Robyn Karen 04/09/1997 26 Oldfield Lane HECKMONDWIKE West Yorkshire WF16 0JD **Tel:** (01924) 502131 w 611732X

DEW Julie Anne (nee Truman) 16/12/1997 70 Lutterworth Road Pailton Rugby Warwickshire CV23 0QF **Tel:** (01455) 283349 w 6119236

DIAMOND Katherine Elizabeth 22/01/1999 (08/03/2007) Ground Floor Flat 43 Heyford Avenue LONDON SW8 1EA w 612225X

DICK Emma Joanne (see SPEERS, Mrs)

DICKENS Sarah Elizabeth (see EVERARD, Mrs)

DICKIE Angela (see WALLACE, Mrs)

DICKINSON Fiona Jane (nee McCann) 03/02/1992 31 Athol Grove Chorley Lancashire PR6 0LL **Tel:** (01257) 264244 w 6056138

DICKOV Lynne (nee McClure) 29/12/1992 (08/12/2008) 15 Robslee Road Giffnock GLASGOW G46 7AR **Tel:** (0141) 638 9761 w 606642X

DIFFEY Helena Louisa 06/09/1999 (23/04/2008) Vets Now (Telford) 78 Haygate Road Wellington Telford Shropshire TF1 1QN **Tel:** (01952) 253963 w 6184846

DIGGLE Deborah Lorraine 26/08/1999 Elizabeth Smith Veterinary Surgeon Ickwell Road Upper Caldecote Biggleswade Bedfordshire SG18 9BS **Tel:** (01767) 627317 w 6137164

DILLON Jo'ann Ellis (formerly Riches) 08/09/1997 19 Town End Somerby Melton Mowbray Leicestershire LE14 2QQ **Tel:** (01664) 454194 w 6098644

Pauline Margaret (nee Parry) 08/09/1975 (27/10/2000) 278 Lode Lane Solihull West Midlands B91 2HG **Tel:** (0121) 684 5698 w 6058361

DINE Sarah Louise (see CURTIS, Mrs)

DINGLEY Samantha Jane (nee Munn) 21/01/1997 456-458 Hagley Road West Oldbury West Midlands B68 0DL **Tel:** (0121) 422 2902 w 6108428

DINNIN Clare Lucy (see KEENAN, Mrs)

DINSDALE Kelly (see DRYDEN, Mrs)

DIXEY Rachel Emma (nee Shahgaghi) 24/08/1999 Albecq Station Road Wakes Colne COLCHESTER CO6 2DS **Tel:** (07971) 373790 w 6139591

DIXON Charlotte Rosemary 30/08/2000 The Freda Powell Centre 1c Eynsham Drive Thamesmead London SE2 9RQ **Tel:** (020) 8311 6695 w 6202402

DIXON Gemma (see LOVERIDGE, Mrs)

Rachael Louise (formerly Giles) 11/02/1997 (13/12/2004) 9 Cairnsmore Drive Doonfoot Ayrshire KA7 4HW **Tel:** (01292) 443129 w 6038651

Ruth Helen (nee Dixon, formerly Jakeway) 24/01/1996 C/o Royal College of Veterinary Surgeons 62-64 Horseferry Road LONDON SW1P 2AF w 6039688

DOBBS Stephanie Julia 16/06/2000 64 Appin Crescent DUNFERMLINE Fife KY12 7QH w 6186243

DOBNEY Tracey Jayne 14/09/1999 1 Holinshead Place Grange Park Swindon Wiltshire SN5 6DD w 6142888

DOCHERTY Anne Marie (see RITCHIE, Mrs)

DOCHERTY Karen (see NESBITT, Mrs)

DOCHERTY Lesley Charlotte (nee Brown) 19/01/1995 (17/04/2003) Links Veterinary Group 18 High Street MUSSELBURGH Midlothian EH21 7AG **Tel:** (0131) 665 3343 w 603740X

DODD Michelle Louise 16/10/2000 43 Gurney Avenue Tuffley GLOUCESTER GL4 0YB w 6203018

DODDS Joanne (nee Knibb) 09/08/1990 37 Ambleside AYLESBURY Buckinghamshire HP21 9TT w 6054640

Paula Louise 01/09/1998 68 Low Shops Lane Rothwell Leeds LS26 0RH **Tel:** (0113) 282 4123 w 6132745

DOOLEY Christine Elizabeth (nee Waigh) 05/08/1980 203 Castle Way Leybourne West Malling Kent ME19 5HW **Tel:** (01732) 842849 w 6062833

Peter Alexander 12/01/1989 (01/03/2006) 13 Clarkes Drive Uxbridge Middlesex UB8 3UH **Tel:** (01895) 443744 m 6049302

DORAN Annabel (nee Carr) 19/01/1998 50 Chatsworth Road Hazel Grove STOCKPORT Cheshire SK7 6BT **Tel:** (0161) 4836892 w 6110878

DORE Marianne Christine DipAVN(Medical) 23/08/2000 17 Tracey Court Harwell Street Plymouth Devon PL1 5BE **Tel:** (01752) 226455 w 612823X

D'ORIANO Bianca Maria Cristina 23/10/2001 291 Bournemouth Park Road Southend-on-Sea Essex SS2 5LE **Tel:** (01702) 464388 w 6260405

DORMAN Nicola Jayne 22/01/2001 30 Chestnut Avenue Wath-upon-Dearne Rotherham South Yorkshire S63 7PQ **Tel:** (01709) 873844 w 6211433

DOUGALL Shona Kirsteen 03/09/1998 Primrose Cottage Isle of Iona PA76 6SJ **Tel:** (01681) 700359 w 6132304

DOUGLAS Heidi (nee Alexander) 19/01/2001 (21/06/2006) 8 Wildgoose Drive Newnadhar Aberdeenshire AB21 0NG **Tel:** (01651) 869161 w 6210762

DOUGLAS Jennifer Jane (see BULLARD, Mrs)

DOUGLAS Karen Jayne (nee Gallichan) 18/09/1978 (29/12/2000) Burnside of Affleck Udny Ellon Aberdeenshire AB41 6SQ **Tel:** (01651) 842082 w 6000741

DOWNER Stephanie Ann (see ENGLAND, Mrs)

DOWNES Lydia Kate (see SPRIGGS, Mrs)

DOWNS Jennie Louise 10/01/1991 (06/11/2008) 11 The Angel Broad Street LUDLOW Shropshire SY8 1LT w 6049379

DOWSETT Michelle Elizabeth (see LIFELY, Mr)

DOWSON Linda (nee Kitson) 03/08/1993 Widdop Cottage Widdop Road Hebden Bridge West Yorkshire HX7 7AT **Tel:** (01422) 846939 w 6027708

DRAKE Coilla Anne (nee Bolton) 14/01/1999 Cott Westray Orkney KW17 2DA **Tel:** (01857) 677402 w 6170623

DRAYTON Carly Jayne (formerly Blake, nee Wills) 03/09/1996 (30/03/2007) Chicanoa 24 Southwood Avenue Walkford CHRISTCHURCH Dorset BH23 5RN w 6040627

DREW Alison Frances Catherine 06/02/2002 Priory Lodge Veterinary Group 31 Pembury Road TONBRIDGE Kent TN9 2JB **Tel:** (01732) 353668 w 6269601

Susan Jane 19/01/1983 (16/09/2004) Castle Vets Pet Healthcare Centre 1 Tilehurst Road Reading Berkshire RG1 7TW **Tel:** (0118) 957 4488 w 609034X

DRUMMOND Caroline Anne (nee Hughes) 16/08/1982 Ida Cottage Back Lane East Langton Market Harborough Leicestershire LE16 7TB **Tel:** (01858) 545828 w 6049426

DRURY Sonya 10/08/1984 Oathall Veterinary Group 30 Oathall Road Haywards Heath West Sussex RH16 3EQ **Tel:** (01444) 440224 w 6091707

DRYDEN Kelly (nee Dinsdale) 19/01/2000 2 Winston Court Stoney Lane Springwell Village Gateshead Tyne and Wear NE9 7SJ **Tel:** (0191) 431 9011 w 6133931

DU FEU Colette Kim 06/02/1992 (02/11/2009) The Old Coach House Maydencroft Lane Gosmore HITCHIN Hertfordshire SG4 7QA w 6079723

DUFF Rachel Louise (nee Ashcroft) 21/09/2000 12 Drydale Avenue Eastfield Northampton NN3 2RL **Tel:** (01604) 784577 w 6203755

DUFFY Heather 26/04/2002 (08/05/2006) Flat 2 184/2 Main Street Newmills DUNFERMLINE Fife KY12 8SY w 6252793

DUGDALE Alison Louise (see CHADWICK, Mrs)

DUMMER Susan 28/09/1993 (17/04/2003) Merestones Northfields Lane Westergate CHICHESTER West Sussex PO20 3UH **Tel:** (01243) 543545 w 6030878

DUMONT Michelle Lisa (nee Wallace) 17/11/2000 Forest Veterinary Centre Hemnall Street Epping Essex CM16 4LQ **Tel:** (01992) 575790 w 6204470

DUNCAN Clare Louise (see FRAZER, Mrs)

DUNCAN Julie Veronica 30/12/1992 Balkemback Farmhouse Tealing Angus DD4 0RF **Tel:** (01382) 380563 w 6066292

DUNK Sandra Elizabeth 17/01/1996 R S P C A East Winch Wildlife Centre Station Road East Winch King's Lynn Norfolk PE32 1NR w 6041201

DUNLOP Frances Ann 18/11/1970 (20/11/2006) 31 Crockerton Road Tooting London SW17 7HE **Tel:** (0208) 7676767 w 6049481

DUNNE Emma Jane 24/09/2001 (19/03/2003) Handforth Veterinary Centre 174 Wilmslow Road Handforth Wilmslow Cheshire SK9 3LF **Tel:** (01625) 533654 w 6098123

Linda Mary 22/02/2001 Fairfield Veterinary Centre 51 Leicester Road Hinckley Leicestershire LE10 1LW **Tel:** (01455) 637642 w 6202941

DUNSTAN Sara Louise (see RANDALL, Mrs)

DUNSTONE Justine 09/09/1994 Blackthorn Cottage Telscombe LEWES East Sussex BN7 3HY w 6034792

DURANT Kate Joanna (see SMITH, Mrs)

DURBIN Elizabeth Karen (see COX, Mrs)

DURITY Joanna Clare (nee Houldsworth) 06/07/2000 (23/01/2006) Hailey House Duntisbourne Abbotts Cirencester Gloucestershire GL7 7JL w 6184835

DURRANT Janet Louise (nee Lawrence) 09/08/1983 (07/07/2009) Little Orchard The Ridgeway CRANLEIGH Surrey GU6 7HW w 6090113

DUTTON Sarah Jane (nee Keatley) 04/09/1997 11 Warbreck Road Orrell Park Liverpool Merseyside L9 8EE **Tel:** (0151) 525 5064 w 6098371

DYBLE Samantha Georgena (nee Jones) 26/06/1993 5 Clover Way Red Lodge Bury St. Edmunds Suffolk IP28 8TB **Tel:** (01638) 552776 w 6054287

DYER Vanessa Linda 23/08/1994 (23/06/2000) Guildford College of Further & Higher Education Merrist Wood College Worplesdon Guildford Surrey GU3 3PE **Tel:** (01483) 884060 w 6036949

DYSON Caroline Ann 20/09/1994 T/A Dragon Veterinary Centre Prestbury Park New Barn Lane Cheltenham Gloucestershire GL50 4SH **Tel:** (01242) 580 324 w 6027934

E

EASON Diane Elizabeth (nee Laidlow) 03/02/1993 (27/10/2000) 2 Bishops Way Newport Isle of Wight PO30 5WT **Tel:** (01983) 522804 w 6065630

EAST Angela Mary 24/09/2001 Abbey Green Vets Ltd Church Close Broadway Worcestershire WR12 7AH **Tel:** (01386) 852421 w 6138565

EASTWOOD Suzannah Jayne Carol (nee Boyd) 27/09/1999 Woodlands Farm Woodlands Nr Lyndhurst Hampshire SO40 7GL **Tel:** (023) 8029 3556 w 6145630

EATON Cheryl Elizabeth (nee Kay) 11/09/1998 56 Longworth Street Bolton Lancashire BL2 6AR w 6129211

EBECK Liza Kerensa 02/02/2001 (09/04/2009) Small Animal Teaching Hospital University of Liverpool Leahurst Campus Chester High Road Neston Merseyside CH64 7TE **Tel:** (0151) 795 6100 w 6211884

ECCLESTON Victoria Jannine 14/09/1998 29 Leigh Park Lymington Hampshire SO41 9JZ w 6034205

EDDEN Ruth Mary Catherine 20/05/2002 Marches Veterinary Group Ryelands Road Leominster Herefordshire HR6 8PN **Tel:** (01568) 612266 w 6262044

EDEN Dawn Catherine (see PLATTEN, Mrs)

EDGE Sarah (see COTON, Mrs)

EDGE Sarah Margaret 23/01/1992 Three Rivers Veterinary Group Veterinary Clinic London Road Beccles Suffolk NR34 9YU **Tel:** (01502) 712169 w 6049619

EDGERLEY Caroline Elisabeth 28/08/1977 (10/03/2009) 144 Stanley Road Teddington Middlesex TW11 8UA **Tel:** (020) 8973 1599 w 6049630

EDMETT Kelly 25/08/1998 12 Clare Road WELLINGBOROUGH Northamptonshire NN8 3DH **Tel:** (01933) 674822 w 6121802

EDMONDSON Elizabeth (see MOULDING, Mrs)

EDWARDS Alison Ruth (nee Bray) 30/03/1984 Daffodils 16 The Green Winscombe North Somerset BS25 1AH **Tel:** (01934) 843161 w 6089560

Andrea Stacey 28/08/1998 Pinewood Veterinary Practice 23 Crown Street Chorley Lancashire PR7 1DX **Tel:** (01257) 276517 w 6108370

Catherine Juliet (nee Whistler) 05/08/1993 92 Ashingdon Road Rochford Essex SS4 1RE **Tel:** (01702) 547 570 w 6029454

Claire Louise (nee Wright) 09/09/2002 324 Biscot Road Luton Bedfordshire LU3 1AZ **Tel:** (01582) 730105 w 6263507

Gwenan Mai 27/01/2000 LLwyn Bresych Clawddnewydd RUTHIN Clwyd LL15 2NF **Tel:** (01824) 750650 w 6138791

Leah Caroline 05/02/2001 16 Edward Road Fleckney Leicester Leicestershire LE8 8UB **Tel:** (0116) 2404896 w 6099105

EDWARDS Lee-Ann (see CONSTANTINOU, Mrs)

EDWARDS Sarah Louise 10/12/2002 (11/11/2008) 177 Woodside Road Ketley TELFORD Shropshire TF1 5WT **Tel:** (01952) 619007 w 6280876

EGEN Marie (see HURST, Mrs)

EGLEN Sarah Frances Joy 28/08/1998 11-17 The Precinct West Meads Bognor Regis West Sussex PO21 5SB **Tel:** (01243) 842832 w 6136808

EL DABE Helen Margaret (nee Stanners) 16/02/1989 50 The Holme Great Broughton North Yorkshire TS9 7HF **Tel:** (01642) 713599 w 6061192

ELCOCK Holly Elizabeth (nee Fensome) 19/01/1998 (31/10/2005) 3 Nickleby Gardens Totton Southampton Hampshire SO40 8FN **Tel:** (0238) 0860154 w 609915X

ELDRIDGE Natalie Ann 23/10/2001 The Old Barn Shopnoller West Bagborough Taunton Somerset TA4 3ER **Tel:** (01823) 432059 w 6256038

ELIAS Sasha Ann (nee Owen) 02/03/1999 23 Nant yr Efail Glan Conwy Colwyn Bay Conwy LL28 5DR **Tel:** 01492584249 w 6099954

ELLIOTT Sarah Louise (see GREIG, Mrs)

ELLIOTT Victoria Jane 22/01/1998 Tai Wai Small Animal and Exotic Hospital 75 Chik Shun Street Tai Wai Shatin Hong Kong **Tel:** (00) 852 268 71030 w 6099116

ELLIS Amanda Marie 26/01/1998 608 Veterinary Group 608 Warwick Road Solihull West Midlands B91 1AA **Tel:** (0121) 705 3044 w 6041722

Elizabeth Anne 05/10/2000 (02/11/2007) 44 Fountain Place Loanhead Midlothian EH20 9DU **Tel:** (0131) 440 4229 w 6135418

Sarah Elisabeth 22/09/1997 110 Bilton Road Perivale Greenford Middlesex UB6 7BJ **Tel:** (0208) 9985234 w 6117272

ELSON Barbara May (nee Brown) 30/11/1978 (16/11/2004) 4 Manor Farm Cottages Godmanstone Dorchester Dorset DT2 7AH w 6087483

ELSON Juliet Ann (see PEARCE, Mrs)

ELSTON Tamara Margarette Louise (nee Walton) 30/01/2001 Churchfield Veterinary Centre 29 Sackville Street Barnsley South Yorkshire S70 2DB **Tel:** (01226) 733333 w 6211609

EMMERSON Helen Kerry (nee O'Donnell) 12/09/1999 78 Campbell Road IPSWICH IP3 9RE **Tel:** (01473) 254011 w 6185407

EMMERSON Louise Maria (see SMITH, Mrs)

EMMS Danielle Elizabeth (see MEREDITH, Mrs)

ENGLAND Nicola Louise (nee Pummell) 15/02/2002 27 Jones Close Yatton Bristol Avon BS49 4RA **Tel:** (01934) 835 868 w 6263276

Stephanie Ann (nee Downer) 14/08/1986 (23/01/2007) 25 The Ridings Great Baddow Chelmsford Essex CM2 9RR **Tel:** (01245) 494696 w 6049346

ENTWISTLE Joanne Ruth 30/10/2001 West Mount Vet Group Holborow and Tapsfield 41 Burnley Road Todmorden Lancashire OL14 7BU w 6271229

ERRNE Amanda-Jane (nee Rogers) 22/08/1997 (02/11/2009) 36 Beanfield Avenue Green Lane Coventry CV3 6NU **Tel:** (024) 7669 2952 w 6118731

ESSEX Catherine Jane 05/08/1991 (17/10/2008) 47 The Street Kettlestone FAKENHAM Norfolk NR21 0JB **Tel:** (0132888) 822164 w 6049947

ETHERDEN Hazel Elizabeth 24/09/1990 6 Broxell Close Wedgnock Industrial Estate Warwick CV34 5QF **Tel:** (01926) 400255 w 6049958

EVANS Anne Margaret (see CHARLTON, Mrs)

EVANS Claire Elizabeth 17/08/1995 (01/12/2008) 21 Shoemaker Close Astcote Towcester Northamptonshire NN12 8AT **Tel:** (01327) 831056 w 6040004

Denise 22/03/1988 'Llamedos' 11 Sanderling Rise Kingswinford West Midlands DY6 8XN **Tel:** (01384) 296791 w 6049969

EVANS Elaine Marie (see MAIDEN, Mrs)

Gillian Anne 26/07/1993 Alcombe Veterinary Surgery 160 Northfield Avenue London W13 9SB **Tel:** (020) 8567 4597 w 601534X

EVANS Gwenan (see HOWATSON, Mrs)

Jacqueline Beryl (nee Biggs) 14/10/2002 (22/01/2007) Bourne Farm Dingeston Monmouth NP25 4BP **Tel:** (01600) 740637 w 6271999

Jessica Sally 08/09/1999 (25/05/2007) College of Animal Welfare Boltons Park Farm 44 Hawkshead Road POTTERS BAR Hertfordshire EN6 1NB w 6146215

Lauren Elizabeth 19/01/2001 Ground Floor Flat 4 Beacon Road Herne Bay Kent CT6 8SR w 6122373

Tina Marie 27/08/1999 Woodlands Veterinary Hospital Burnett Road Manadon Plymouth Devon PL6 5BH **Tel:** (01752) 700600 w 6040514

EVERARD Sarah Elizabeth (nee Dickens) 20/08/1993 34 Ashwood Gardens West Totton Southampton Hampshire SO40 8SZ **Tel:** (023) 80666340 w 6027479

EVERETT Susan Claire (nee Smith) 27/08/1999 4 Burley Lodge Terrace Leeds LS6 1QA **Tel:** (0113) 226 1520 w 6186089

EVERILL Julie Margaret 30/01/1990 1 Dulverton Road Witton Birmingham West Midlands B6 7EQ **Tel:** (0121) 328 1716 w 6050012

EVERY Jane Louise (see SLEE, Mrs)

EVES Susan Margaret (nee James) 12/09/2000 Banks Farm Barn Manor Road Abridge Romford Essex RM4 1NH **Tel:** (01708) 745 505 w 6202512

EXTON Elizabeth Anne (nee Priestman) 29/07/1975 (22/04/2002) 11 Apperson Court Pocklington YORK YO42 2JD w 6084890

F

FAHEY Wendy (see NASH, Miss)

FAIRFIELD Melissa Kate (see WHITEMAN, Mrs)

FAIRWEATHER Melissa Jane 03/10/1995 4 Douglas Place GLENROTHES Fife KY6 1BA **Tel:** (01592) 756239 w 6027606

Nicola Tracy Michele 05/08/1980 227 Mackenzie Road Beckenham Kent BR3 4SH **Tel:** (020) 8778 4715 w 6088589

FALLON Luisa 15/02/2002 Gateside Cottage Standburn Avonbridge Falkirk FK1 2HN **Tel:** (01324) 861562 w 6267577

FALLOWS Frances (nee Kemp) 01/02/1994 20 Parklands Road Tean STOKE-ON-TRENT ST10 4DT **Tel:** (01538) 722648 w 6067569

FANE Tracy Ruth (see CULLEN, Mrs)

FARMER Alison Emily (see HUGO, Mrs)

FARQUHAR Kim 28/01/2000 10 Maple Drive LARKHALL Lanarkshire ML9 2AR **Tel:** 07747038417 w 6121926

FARQUHARSON Beverly Teresa (nee Parish) 28/01/1992 (22/01/2007) 100 Bury Road Hemel Hempstead Hertfordshire HP1 1HW **Tel:** (01442) 267767 w 6058270

FARR Alice Judith Stephanie (see WYNNE, Mrs)

FARRER Isabel Anna Marie 17/09/1998 Warren House Veterinary Surgery Anchor Road Rochester Kent ME1 2PR **Tel:** (01634) 409988 w 6136025

FARROW Emma Josephine 07/09/1999 (09/01/2006) 3 Clapham Lane Litlington POLEGATE East Sussex BN26 5RQ **Tel:** (079610) 50613 w 6140654

FEARNHEAD Janet Mary Sinclair (see MARDELL, Mrs)

FEAST Patricia Ann 20/02/1981 2 Inglewood Gardens St. Leonards-on-Sea East Sussex TN38 9SA **Tel:** (01424) 852450 w 605017X

FELL Kathryn Anna 24/08/1999 (26/02/2009) Alpha Veterinary Surgery 144 Stanley Road Teddington Middlesex TW11 8UA **Tel:** (020) 8943 2303 w 603484X

FELLOWS Catherine Louise (see GIBBONS, Mrs)

FENSOM Chloe Rebecca 05/09/1996 (06/02/2002) 18 Grundisburgh Road Woodbridge Suffolk IP12 4HG **Tel:** (01394) 380083 w 6099149

FENSOME Holly Elizabeth (see ELCOCK, Mrs)

FENWICK Karen 17/01/1984 6 Orchard Row School Lane Herne Nr Herne Bay Kent CT6 7AW **Tel:** (01227) 375588 w 6050216

FERGUS Colette Rosemary 11/12/2001 19 Creggan Road Cranfield Randalstown Co Antrim BT41 3LN **Tel:** (02894) 472467 w 6237085

FERGUSON Joanna 17/01/1996 136 Lutterworth Road Hinckley Leicestershire LE10 2DW **Tel:** (01455) 449878 w 6077602

FIELD Kathryn Elizabeth 30/09/1983 Windy Ridge Higher Burton East Coker Yeovil Somerset BA22 9LU **Tel:** (01935) 862649 w 605025X

Maxine Ruth 18/01/1996 9 Wyphurst Road Cranleigh Surrey GU6 7AT **Tel:** (01483) 275547 w 6042908

Nicola Marie 09/09/1996 (22/07/2009) Bamber House Springfields Padbury BUCKINGHAM Buckinghamshire MK18 2BS **Tel:** (01280) 813097 w 6033518

FIELD Renay Francis (see RICKARD, Mrs)

FINLAYSON Karen 04/09/1998 61 Parsonage Street Halstead Essex CO9 2JZ **Tel:** (01787) 473637 w 6129561

FINN Cara Jayne 26/10/2000 Warren House Veterinary Surgery Anchor Road Rochester Kent ME1 2PR **Tel:** (01634) 409988 w 6203535

FINNERAL Jane Andrea (see HOLMAN, Mrs)

FIRMIN Sharn Challoner (nee Jones, formerly Higgins) 30/09/1983 (13/02/2002) Writtle College Lordship Road Writtle Chelmsford Essex CM1 3RR **Tel:** (+44) (0) 1245 424200 w 6111372

FIRTH Daun Elizabeth (nee Firth, formerly Campbell) 08/09/1998 (30/05/2003) 19 Braithwaite Street Staincross Barnsley South Yorkshire S75 6BD **Tel:** (01226) 215822 w 6115901

Debra Lynette DipAVN(Surgical) 31/08/1993 4 Manley View Elton Chester Cheshire CH2 4QF **Tel:** (01928) 725696 w 6031077

FISHER Susan Pauline (nee Mayes, formerly Parry) 31/07/1972 16 Ash Close Swanage Dorset BH19 2TF **Tel:** (01929) 425321 w 6013193

FISHER-EAMES Caroline Ann (see BRAID, Mrs)

FISHWICK Janet 10/01/2003 37 Gresford Avenue Sefton Park Liverpool Merseyside L17 2AN **Tel:** (0151) 734 0674 w 6282889

FITZELL Yvonne Elizabeth (see KENNEDY, Mrs)

FITZPATRICK Mary Rose 04/02/2002 (26/04/2005) 52a Abbeville Road Clapham LONDON SW4 9NF **Tel:** (07729) 802883 w 6256379

FLACK Lorraine (nee Johnson) 20/11/2002 (28/01/2009) Briars High Road Laindon BASILDON Essex SS15 6BU **Tel:** (01268) 543700 w 6275299

FLANAGAN Susan Lynne (nee Cooper) 29/08/1995 (15/06/2001) 82 London Road Teynham Sittingbourne Kent ME9 9QH **Tel:** (01795) 520972 w 6019639

Tina Louise 31/08/1989 7 Chamberlain Road Chippenham Wiltshire SN14 0TF w 6050373

FLEMING Amanda Patricia 27/12/2001 (10/03/2004) 6 Copsem Drive Esher Surrey KT10 9HD **Tel:** (01372) 463414 w 6266356

Claire Louise (nee Bannister) 23/07/1993 (08/10/1999) Booval Veterinary Hospital Po Box 33 Booval Queensland 4304 Australia w 6014980

FLETCHER Gillian Mary 09/08/1983 (22/10/2001) 64 Main Street Wentworth Rotherham South Yorkshire S62 7TN **Tel:** (01226) 741657 w 6050420

FLETCHER Sherran Ann (see BUCKLEY, Mrs)

FLETCHER Tammy 02/02/2001 139 James Reckitt Avenue Hull North Humberside HU8 7TJ **Tel:** (01482) 715345 w 6211895

Tamsin Liesel DipAVN(Surgical) 18/09/1998 Lion House Welshampton Ellesmere Shropshire SY12 0PG **Tel:** (01948) 710398 w 6129120

FLINT Yvonne (see GASKIN, Mrs)

FLOWER Barbara Ann 04/08/1981 24 St. Clements Court St Clements Gardens Worcester Worcestershire WR2 5NW **Tel:** (01905) 423382 w 6000694

FLOWER Lorna Joy (see DAINTY, Mrs)

FLOYD Vanessa Beverley Ruth 20/09/1978 40 Bushnell Road London SW17 8QP **Tel:** (020) 8673 8949 w 6050475

FLYNN Louise Violet 22/11/2000 6 Lower Dicker Cottages Lower Dicker Hailsham East Sussex BN27 4BA **Tel:** (01323) 440695 w 6130908

Suzanne 02/02/1994 37 Normandale Road Liverpool L4 8UG **Tel:** (0151) 226 7270 w 6067503

FOGG Alexandra Theresa Ruth 10/12/2002 Argyll Veterinary Clinic 24 Highfield Road Ilfracombe Devon EX34 9LZ **Tel:** (01271) 867711 w 6271207

FOGGON Gayle (nee Jackson) 12/09/2000 (10/11/2009) 80 Oakdene Crescent Portslade BRIGHTON East Sussex BN41 2RN w 6202644

FOLEY Joanne Karen (nee Waller) 24/09/1992 15 London Road Shenley Radlett Hertfordshire WD7 9EW **Tel:** (01923) 856740 w 6006743

FOORD Marie Elaine (nee Matcham) 05/02/1996 (05/11/2004) Ashbrook Veterinary Surgery 212 Battle Road St. Leonards-on-Sea East Sussex TN37 7AL **Tel:** (01424) 754886 w 6028836

FORD Tracy Annette 29/11/2000 (17/12/2008) 15 Bridge Street New Mills HIGH PEAK Derbyshire SK22 4DJ **Tel:** (01663) 743741 w 6040128

FORDHAM Caroline Ellen 29/07/1977 Kinfauns Veterinary Centre Ltd The Street Little Clacton Clacton-on-Sea Essex CO16 9LG **Tel:** (01255) 860555 w 6050577

Nigel James 14/08/1989 (14/06/1999) 24 Middle Touches CHARD Somerset TA20 1NX **Tel:** (01460) 62853 m 6050588

FORNENGO Stephanie Louisa (nee Harris) 28/01/1992 47 Marlborough Park Avenue Sidcup Kent DA15 9DL **Tel:** (0208) 3096587 w 6052381

FORREST Nicola Kristine DipAVN(Surgical) (nee Thixton) 04/10/1993 25a St. Martins Gate HADDINGTON East Lothian EH41 4BA w 6064852

FORSYTH Carrie-Anne (see OTTLEY, Mrs)

FOSS Amanda Clare 28/08/1998 87 Monkwood Road Rawmarsh Rotherham South Yorkshire S62 7JJ **Tel:** (01709) 579491 w 6129437

FOSTER Andrea Elizabeth 12/02/1999 Palma Nova Daws House Launceston Cornwall PL15 7JF **Tel:** (01566) 779181 w 6144364

FOSTER Clare Rebecca (see GITTINGS, Mrs)

FOSTER Deborah Claire (see WILSON, Mrs)

Helen Louise 09/09/1999 45 Bridge Grove DONCASTER South Yorkshire DN5 8HP **Tel:** (01302) 785 356 w 6129029

FOSTER Patricia Angela Jane (see SWAN, Mrs)

FOUNTAIN Gayle Marie 06/02/2002 St Johns Veterinary Surgery 320a High Street Berkhamsted Hertfordshire HP4 1HT **Tel:** (01442) 863101 w 6269623

FOWLER Holly Jane (nee Fowler, formerly Cooper) 05/05/1998 Flat 4 46 Willes Road Leamington Spa Warwickshire CV31 1BY **Tel:** (01926) 420200 w 6130919

Julie May (nee Wood) 28/01/1992 (16/11/2000) 1 Vetch Close Glazebrook Warrington WA3 5BS **Tel:** (0161) 7755093 w 6064160

FOX Caroline Elspeth 09/08/1978 11 Ford View Dudley Cramlington Northumberland NE23 7QD w 6087177

Caroline Jane 25/08/1998 Kirkdean Cottage Blyth Bridge WEST LINTON Peeblesshire EH46 7AJ **Tel:** (01721) 752 758 w 6129222

Lorraine Anne 29/08/1997 1 Glengall Road Bexleyheath Kent DA7 4AW **Tel:** (0208) 3033186 w 6117410

Miranda Jane (nee Green) 10/09/1997 (15/08/2000) Crofton Spearcey Lane Staplehay TAUNTON Somerset TA3 7HJ **Tel:** (01823) 333644 w 6036257

Wendy Julia 18/09/1998 (27/02/2002) 35 Greenways Pagham Bognor Regis West Sussex PO21 4QE **Tel:** (01243) 268783 w 6117421

FOXCROFT Karen Louise 18/09/1998 Mayfield Avenue Walkden Worsley Manchester M28 3JF **Tel:** (0161) 799 5557 w 6076835

FOXELL Kim Elizabeth 01/11/1984 (15/10/2003) Abbotsley Veterinary Group 107 High Street West Malling Kent ME19 6NA **Tel:** (01732) 843080 w 605068X

FOXLEY Patricia Ann 01/11/1984 (28/10/2003) 267 Chester Road Hartford Northwich Cheshire CW8 1LP **Tel:** (01606) 723202 w 6050690

FRANCIS Claire Louise (see WILLIS, Mrs)

FRANCIS Claire Margaret (nee Heffernan, formerly Harris) 28/08/1997 (18/09/2001) 35 Iffley Road Oxford OX4 1EA **Tel:** (01865) 242600 w 6117738

Jennifer Shirley 17/08/1987 653 Devonshire Road BLACKPOOL FY2 0AD **Tel:** (01253) 350 664 w 6050726

FRANKLIN Diana Helen (nee Smith) 06/08/1979 180 St. Ediths Marsh Bromham Chippenham Wiltshire SN15 2DJ **Tel:** (01380) 859881 w 6087891

Helen Louise 01/11/1984 Aqualate Dairy Farm Stafford Road Newport Shropshire TF10 9BZ **Tel:** (01952) 825291 w 6050737

FRANKLIN Sally Jane (see COCKER, Mrs)

FRASER Caroline Marguerite (see BROWN, Mrs)

FRASER-GREEN Heather (see GREEN, Mrs)

FRAZER Clare Louise (nee Duncan) 28/06/2001 Haven Veterinary Practice 35 Holland Road Clacton-on-Sea Essex CO15 6EH **Tel:** (01255) 422150 w 6204426

FREEGARD Victoria Ann (see ALEXANDER, Mrs)

FREELAND Rita Vivienne (see HINTON, Mrs)

FREEMAN Emma Marie 07/04/2000 (22/04/2002) Lodge Farm Barholm Road Tallington STAMFORD Lincolnshire PE9 4RJ w 6190929

Heidi Anne 10/09/1998 219 Witham Road Black Notley BRAINTREE Essex CM77 8NQ **Tel:** (01375) 322028 w 6129197

Joan Mary DipAVN(Surgical) (nee O'Sullivan) 10/01/1991 Northwest Surgeons Delamere House Ashville Point Sutton Weaver Cheshire WA7 3FW **Tel:** (01928) 711400 w 6057958

FREER Susanna Mary Catherine 30/09/1983 C/o RCVS Belgravia House 62-64 Horseferry Road London SW1P 2AF w 6050806

FRENCH Samantha Helen 08/09/1999 (26/03/2001) 43 Page Street Mill Hill London NW7 2EL w 6130930

FRETTER Lee Christian 10/09/1997 16 Church Road Braunston Northants NN11 7HG **Tel:** (01788) 890986 m 6041799

FRIELL Diane Linda (see HAYNES, Mrs)

FROST Debbie 26/04/2002 9 Hayes Walk POTTERS BAR Hertfordshire EN6 2QB **Tel:** (01923) 470022 w 6276487

Melissa Annabel 27/08/1996 Durrell Wildlife Conservation Trust Les Augres Manor La Profonde Rue Trinity JERSEY JE3 5BP **Tel:** (01534) 860000 w 6040150

FRY Helen Clare (nee Rennie) 06/08/1986 (31/12/2002) Quarrington Veterinary Surgery London Road Sleaford Lincolnshire NG34 8NX **Tel:** (01529) 307878 w 6059591

Katie Elizabeth DipAVN(Surgical) (nee Montgomery) 24/08/1998 Totterdale Farm Cottage Tisbury Salisbury wiltshire SP3 6RS **Tel:** (01747) 870624 w 6128295

FULCHER Wendy Joanne DipAVN(Surgical) 26/01/1993 (18/11/2009) 11a Centre Road Soham ELY Cambridgeshire CB7 5AU w 6065550

FURNESS Jane Auld (nee Millar) 21/08/1985 (11/09/2009) 1 Brocket Place Cawston RUGBY Warwickshire CV22 7GX **Tel:** (01788) 819655 w 605084X

FURROKH Ilona Karin Simeen 08/09/1995 Veterinary Department Zoological Society of London Regent's Park London NW1 4RY w 6037330

G

GADHIA Sonya 26/10/2000 25 Grove Hall Road Bushey Watford WD23 2EH **Tel:** (01923) 254631 w 6202699

GAJEWSKI Victoria Louise (nee Seal) 07/09/1998 25 Woodsmoor Lane STOCKPORT Cheshire SK2 7AZ w 6138510

GALBRAITH Kerry Ann 16/11/2001 3/1 305 Glasgow Harbour Terraces Glasgow Lanarkshire G11 6BQ **Tel:** (0141) 357 3706 w 6267170

GALLICHAN Karen Jayne (see DOUGLAS, Mrs)

GALLICHAN Tizane Ila Navarro (see GALLICHAN TREDANT, Mrs)

GALLICHAN TREDANT Tizane Ila Navarro (nee Gallichan) 31/01/2000 Glencraig Cottage South Drive Route Des Genets St Brelade Jersey JE3 8LF w 6190918

GALLIMORE Paula 13/12/2001 (15/04/2004) 41 Dales Green Rookery Stoke-on-Trent ST7 4RH **Tel:** (01782) 511689 w 6123774

GAMBLE Emily Louise (nee Burley) 04/02/2002 259 Bilton Road Rugby Warwickshire CV22 7EQ **Tel:** (01788) 812650 w 6257831

GAMMON Rachel Ann 26/08/1993 (08/10/1999) 238 Bute Street Cardiff CF10 5HT **Tel:** (02920) 494018 w 6019854

GARBUTT Clare Lisa (nee Wilkie) 16/01/1996 (29/09/2005) Castle Vets Pet Healthcare Centre 1 Tilehurst Road Reading Berkshire RG1 7TW **Tel:** (0118) 957 4488 w 6042475

GARDINER Anita Mary (nee Grout, nee Attrill) 19/08/1992 (19/07/1999) 3 Crown Inn Fields Morland Penrith Cumbria CA10 3EB **Tel:** (01931) 714908 w 6007419

GARDINER Anne Margaret (see MUDGE, Mrs)

GARDINER Christina Mary (see CRAWFORD, Mrs)

GARDNER Carol Ann 05/08/1976 17 Sylvan Close Malpas Park Newport Gwent NP20 6JR **Tel:** (01633) 850933 w 6050930

Joanne Ruth 14/02/1997 Amery Veterinary Group Chalet Hill Bordon Hampshire GU35 0DD **Tel:** (01420) 472904 w 6036144

Lynn Marie (nee Hatcher) 21/09/1998 Putlands Veterinary Surgery Maidstone Road Paddock Wood Tonbridge Kent TN12 6DZ **Tel:** (01892) 835456 w 6121755

Margaret Elizabeth 07/09/1999 40 Flying Fields Road Southam Leamington Spa Warwickshire CV47 1GA **Tel:** (01926) 814 593 w 609923X

GARLICK Alexandra Marie (nee Howard) 03/09/1998 37 Littlebrook Avenue SLOUGH SL2 2PD **Tel:** (01628) 664 238 w 6128772

GARRETT Helen Louise 23/01/1996 10 Crindledykes Washington Tyne and Wear NE38 8SA **Tel:** (0191) 4164260 w 604380X

Janine 23/10/2001 (10/04/2007) Northlands Veterinary Hospital 2 Northampton Road Kettering Northamptonshire NN15 7JU **Tel:** (01536) 485 543 w 6259470

GARVEY Julie Siobhan Teresa 26/01/1998 3 Rowan Road TADLEY Hampshire RG26 3RG w 6113008

GASKIN Jenny Louise 23/01/2001 31 St. Peters Avenue Kettering Northamptonshire NN16 0HA **Tel:** (01536) 390708 w 6202281

Yvonne (nee Flint) 24/01/1990 (26/07/2000) 72 St Wilfrids Road West Hallam Ilkeston Derbyshire DE7 6HH **Tel:** (0115) 932 9852 w 6050464

GASSON Debra Ann 13/09/1999 (17/04/2003) The Veterinary Surgery Windmill Court London Road Crawley West Sussex RH10 8NA **Tel:** (01293) 521182 w 6185891

GASTALL Alice Lydia Ireland (see SAGAR, Mrs)

GATLEY Andrea Jane (see HALL, Mrs)

GEAR Alison Jane (see BRIGHT, Mrs)

GEDDIS Heather Lorraine (see LLOYD, Mrs)

GENT Philippa Alison (see MILLARD, Mrs)

GEORGE Allison Victoria (nee George, formerly Basile) 09/08/1989 (11/11/2008) 134-136 Osmaston Road Derby Derbyshire DE1 2RF **Tel:** (01332) 345119 w 6051107

GERMAN Alison Jane 02/09/1999 (04/06/2007) College of Animal Welfare London Road Godmanchester Huntingdon Cambridgeshire PE29 2LJ **Tel:** (01480) 831177 w 6185704

GHIJS Nathalie Maria Lea (see HACK, Mrs)

GIBBINSON Jill Caroline (nee Smith, formerly Comben) 19/01/1996 (19/11/2007) 129 Ashingdon Road Rochford Essex SS4 1RF **Tel:** (01702) 543314 w 6021036

GIBBONS Catherine Louise (nee Fellows) 08/02/2000 132 Buxton Road Disley Stockport Cheshire SK12 2HG **Tel:** (01663) 762 370 w 6135848

GIBBS Emma Jayne (see MATTHEWS, Mrs)

GIBBS Laura Jayne (see HILL, Mrs)

GIBBS Lisa Jane Seton (nee Poole) 24/08/1998 49 Fieldon Close Shirley Solihull West Midlands B90 3EA **Tel:** (0121) 744 1672 w 6135702

GILBERT Nicola Susan 09/08/1989 167 Muirfield Road South Oxhey WATFORD WD19 6JE **Tel:** (07986) 978 822 w 6051195

Rhiannon Elizabeth 06/02/2002 The Bungalow Colchester Road Wivenhoe COLCHESTER CO7 9ET w 6269260

GILES Helen (see KING, Mrs)

GILES Joanne 01/09/2000 (16/05/2003) 60 St. Georges Drive CHELTENHAM Gloucestershire GL51 8NX **Tel:** (07815) 877 006 w 6203084

GILES Rachael Louise (see DIXON, Mrs)

Rebecca (nee Lowry) 02/08/1989 (24/11/2009) Langford Veterinary Services Langford House Langford BRISTOL BS40 5DU **Tel:** (0117) 3319219 w 6055440

GILL Heather Jane (see WOODYATT, Mrs)

GILL Kerrie Layla 29/07/1992 90 Glentrammon Road ORPINGTON Kent BR6 6DH **Tel:** (01689) 858475 w 6051242

GILLAN Pamela Crawford (see MCCOMB, Mrs)

GILLIVER Sarah Katharine 20/11/2000 The Retreat 193 Gardenwood Road East Grinstead West Sussex RH19 1SH **Tel:** (01342) 311331 w 6205482

GILMER Michelle (see MCCONNELL, Mrs)

GILMORE Johanna Teresa 14/03/2000 Elizabeth Street Veterinary Clinic 55 Elizabeth Street London SW1W 9PP **Tel:** (020) 7730 9102 w 6185638

GINGELL Lorraine (see SPENCER, Mrs)

GITTINGS Clare Rebecca (nee Foster) 04/02/2002 (06/12/2006) 17 Mill Way Longdon RUGELEY Staffordshire WS15 4PF **Tel:** (01543) 492070 w 6258172

GLASSON Sara Ann (see HARMAN, Mrs)

GLAZE Ruth Elizabeth (see GOUCHER, Mrs)

GLEN Morag Isabel 03/08/1992 5 Hall Grove Tytherington Macclesfield Cheshire SK10 2HQ **Tel:** (01625) 420405 w 6007805

GLESSING Amy (see WALPOLE, Mrs)

GLESSING Avril Ruth (nee James) 19/10/1999 (19/04/2005) The Veterinary Surgery Inns Park Valley Truckle Camelford Cornwall PL32 9RX **Tel:** (01840) 212229 w 6185011

GLOVER Suzanne Helen (nee Blossom) 12/02/1997 3 Newis Crescent Clifton SHEFFORD Bedfordshire SG17 5HT **Tel:** (01462) 811909 w 6097480

GODDARD Elizabeth Kate (nee Rimell) 16/01/1996 (27/09/2001) 19 Twyniago Pontarddulais Swansea SA4 8HX **Tel:** (01792) 882989 w 6032048

GODDARD Glenda (see KING, Mrs)

GODDEN Melita Dawn (see LLOYD, Mrs)

GODFREY Claire Lesley (nee Struck) 29/08/2000 Pembroke House Millbridge Road MINEHEAD Somerset TA24 8AG **Tel:** (01643) 706471 w 6203040

Janice Elaine 20/01/1987 16 Caernarvon Drive Ilford Essex IG5 0XD **Tel:** (020) 8550 4365 w 6051388

GODFREY Jennifer Leigh (see MOYE, Mrs)

Richard Christian 28/05/1992 (29/04/2002) 120 Ramshead Crescent LEEDS LS14 1PH **Tel:** (01132) 654728 m 6051402

Susan Elizabeth (nee Mead) 06/02/1998 Avonvale Veterinary Centres Ltd 43 Birches Lane Kenilworth Warwickshire CV8 2AB **Tel:** (01926) 854181 w 6116315

GOLDSMITH Melanie 31/08/1999 1 Mafeking Road Wraysbury Staines Middlesex TW19 5AL **Tel:** (01784) 488 299 w 6118458

GOLDWATER Gina Anne 29/08/1997 (31/07/2006) 10 Lincoln Road Hensingham WHITEHAVEN Cumbria CA28 8NP **Tel:** (01946) 691899 w 6107661

GOODFELLOW Joanne Denise (nee Kilner) 23/09/2002 Avonvale Veterinary Centres Ltd 43 Birches Lane Kenilworth Warwickshire CV8 2AB **Tel:** (01926) 854181 w 6249603

GOODWIN Jessica 13/05/1998 50 Channel View Road Eastbourne Sussex BN22 7LN **Tel:** (01323) 731967 w 6130952

Sarah 19/01/1983 R S P C A Stapeley Grange London Road Stapeley Nantwich Cheshire CW5 7JW **Tel:** (01270) 628 755 w 605148X

GORDON Angela (see MCLELLAN, Mrs)

GORDON Fiona Susan 28/02/2001 64 Rayleigh Road Hutton Brentwood Essex CM13 1BH **Tel:** (020) 8599 9949 w 6213413

GORE Nicola Jane 14/08/1991 (05/02/1999) 94 Mount View Road SHEFFIELD S8 8PL **Tel:** (07880) 676162 w 6051490

Nicola Jane 03/09/1998 29 Park Place Brynmill Swansea SA2 0DH **Tel:** (01792) 540493 w 6134946

GORNALL Elizabeth Anne 23/08/1999 14 Riverside Road Hersham Walton-on-Thames Surrey KT12 4PD **Tel:** (01932) 248611 w 603417X

GORSKI Helen Patricia 11/02/1998 (19/08/2002) 5 Hipsmoor Close Kingshurst Birmingham B37 6ND w 6026351

GOTT Lucy Jane (formerly Shaw) 30/09/1998 Small Animal Teaching Hospital University of Liverpool Leahurst Campus Chester High Road Neston Merseyside CH64 7TE **Tel:** (0151) 795 6100 w 6128444

GOUCHER Ruth Elizabeth (nee Glaze) 19/01/1996 8 St George's Parade Wolverhampton West Midlands WV2 1BD **Tel:** (01902) 425262 w 603513X

GOULD Andrea Mary (nee Locke) 27/09/1989 (25/10/2000) 37 Castle Street Aldbourne MARLBOROUGH Wiltshire SN8 2DA **Tel:** (01672) 540153 w 6055305

Helen Marie 08/08/2002 Ballymakeigh Ballymacoda Co Cork Ireland **Tel:** (058) 44476 w 6273011

GOULDING Karen DipAVN(Surgical) 07/08/1989 8 St George's Parade Wolverhampton West Midlands WV2 1BD **Tel:** (01902) 425262 w 6051537

GOWEN Natalie Mary (nee Robinson) 16/01/1996 22 Helmdon Road Trowbridge Wiltshire BA14 9DF **Tel:** (01225) 751786 w 6028698

GOWER Helen Elizabeth (see HARRINGTON, Mrs)

GOWSHALL Rachel Louise DipAVN(Surgical) (nee Baker) 21/08/1984 (14/05/2004) Eastcott Veterinary Hospital 59 Bath Road Swindon Wiltshire SN1 4AU **Tel:** (01793) 528341 w 6051559

GOWTHORPE Rebecca Dawn (see WILD, Mrs)

GRACEY Amanda Louise (see LESIATOI, Mrs)

GRAHAM Anna Georgina 05/10/2001 42 Brook Street Wymeswold Loughborough Leicestershire LE12 6TU w 6229539

GRAHAM Laura Jean (see ALGER, Mrs)

GRAHAM Lisa Carolyn (nee Heyhoe) 18/10/2000 (24/11/2008) 1 Tring Road Halton Aylesbury Buckinghamshire HP22 5PN **Tel:** (01296) 623439 w 6205229

GRAINGER Louise 05/09/2000 4 Melbourne Street Barrow-in-Furness Cumbria LA14 5TU w 6203117

GRANDI Emma Louise 10/09/1998 (17/08/2004) 192 Bolton Road Hawkshaw Bury Lancashire BL8 4JF **Tel:** (07960) 240 692 w 6133840

GRANT Deborah (nee Storey) 24/09/2001 42 Otterburn Way Prudhoe Northumberland NE42 6RD w 6039451

GRASSICK Karyn Michelle 29/08/2000 93 Raeburn Place Ellon Aberdeenshire AB41 9FS **Tel:** (01358) 725882 w 6203161

GRAY Julie Anne (nee Neal) 19/09/1990 High Letham Cottage High Letham Berwick-Upon-Tweed TD15 1UX **Tel:** (01289) 332360 w 605754X

GRAY June Editha (see BALDWIN, Ms)

Karen Gwendoline (nee Rossington) 16/02/1999 (12/05/2008) 30 Brain Close Hatfield Hertfordshire AL10 8BT **Tel:** (01707) 896636 w 6138816

GRAY Karen Lynn (see MARTYNIUK, Mrs)

Suzanne (nee Gray, formerly Wareham) 14/09/2001 2 Cunningham Court Nelson Close NEW MILTON Hampshire BH25 5LF w 611759X

GRAYSHON Michele Anita (see JENKINS, Mrs)

GRAYSMARK Lena Marie 15/01/1998 (18/10/2005) 31 Fitzalan Road Littlehampton West Sussex BN17 5ET **Tel:** (01903) 713806 w 6099295

GREAVES Lisa-Jayne 07/05/1999 The Wylie Veterinary Centre 196 Hall Lane Upminster Essex RM14 1TD **Tel:** (01708) 251200 w 6132450

GREEN Ann Maria 05/09/1996 14 Blackmill Road Chatteris Cambridgeshire PE16 6SR **Tel:** (01354) 693601 w 6099309

Deborah Ellen (nee Green, formerly Bell) 13/01/1988 14 Stalbridge Drive Ferndown Dorset BH22 8HY **Tel:** (01202) 874402 w 6051683

Donna Maria (nee Sadler) 15/02/2002 2 Orchard Close Billinghay LINCOLN LN4 4FJ w 6271570

Heather (formerly Fraser-Green) 21/10/1981 (09/04/2009) Alexander Cottage Norwich Road Hingham Norfolk NR9 4LR **Tel:** (01953) 850343 w 6091514

Lorna 05/09/2000 (22/08/2006) 5 Cornford Road Birchington Kent CT7 0AG **Tel:** (01843) 843055 w 6204789

GREEN Miranda Jane (see FOX, Mrs)

GREEN Rebecca Jane 10/02/1995 (27/05/2008) 2 Dunstan Terrace Cockmount Lane WADHURST East Sussex TN5 6UF **Tel:** (01892) 784716 w 6032128

Rebecca Sara 24/10/2000 Oaklands Farm Sound Lane Sound NANTWICH Cheshire CW5 8BE **Tel:** (01270) 781306 w 6202391

Sarah Jayne 07/08/1990 (29/07/2004) Kingston Maurward College Animal Care Department Dorchester Dorset DT2 8PY **Tel:** (01305) 215179 w 6051730

GREENHALGH Natalie-Jane DipAVN(Surgical) (nee Hinde) 29/03/2000 10 Arrowe Side Greasby WIRRAL Merseyside CH49 2PB **Tel:** (01708) 705679 w 6121722

GREENING Alison Jane (see HYLAND, Mrs)

GREENWOOD Deborah 07/09/1995 Lysdon Farm House Lysdon Farm New Hartley Whitley Bay Tyne and Wear NE26 4PU **Tel:** (0191) 237 0855 w 6031452

Susan Dianne 08/11/1999 (06/12/2005) 49 Lansdowne Road Hayley Green Halesowen West Midlands B63 1BP **Tel:** (0121) 602 1555 w 6149205

GREETHAM Amie Elizabeth 20/02/2001 High House Farm Swineshead Bridge Boston Lincolnshire PE20 3PX **Tel:** (01205) 820519 w 6212566

GREGG Rachael Kay (see HARRIS, Miss)

GREGORY Karen (see DAVIS, Mrs)

GREGSON Christine 28/08/1991 Oakleigh Holmes Lane Winterton Scunthorpe South Humberside DN15 9UF **Tel:** (01724) 734683 w 6051832

GREIG Sarah Louise (nee Elliott) 22/04/2002 56 Bedford Road Great Barford Bedford Bedfordshire MK44 3JF **Tel:** (01234) 871710 w 6253079

GRIERSON Michelle Anne DipAVN(Surgical) 17/08/1993 31 Marley Road WELWYN GARDEN CITY Hertfordshire AL7 4BT **Tel:** (07989) 445884 w 6030459

GRIFFIN Eithne Valerie Elizabeth (see JOHNSTON, Mrs)

GRIFFIN Elizabeth Jane 08/01/1988 (19/11/1998) Berry House Veterinary Practice 41 Nightingale Road Hitchin Hertfordshire SG5 1RE **Tel:** (01462) 432824 w 6051843

Kate (nee Broadhead) 22/11/2001 7 Hill Close Baildon SHIPLEY West Yorkshire BD17 7PB w 6264057

Lucy Victoria 10/12/2002 44 Queen Street East Ardsley WAKEFIELD West Yorkshire WF3 2BE **Tel:** (01924) 871224 w 6279655

GRIFFITHS Claire 14/09/2001 48 Llanfabon Drive Trethomas Caerphilly Mid Glamorgan CF83 8GW **Tel:** (029) 20882445 w 6228197

Nichola Fiona Maria (formerly Davis, nee Davis) 15/08/1995 North Western Laboratories Ltd 23 Mains Lane POULTON-LE-FYLDE Lancashire FY6 7LJ w 6039870

Nicola 23/08/1999 8 Regent Buildings Hall Street Bilston West Midlands WV14 0AB **Tel:** (01902) 493465 w 6135462

GRIMES Helen Kelly Daphine 21/02/1997 (17/03/2006) 2 Whitehall Cottages Whitehall Syderstone KING'S LYNN Norfolk PE31 8SB w 6099331

GRIMSDELL Caroline (see O'CONNOR, Mrs)

GRINSTEAD Tracy Anne (nee Hughes) 15/01/1999 (24/08/2001) Chase Veterinary Group 89-91 Seaside Eastbourne East Sussex BN22 7NL **Tel:** (01323) 639331 w 6099513

GROUT Anita Mary (see GARDINER, Mrs)

GUARD Pauline Anne (nee Hobson) 06/02/2002 Vennaford Swimbridge Barnstaple Devon EX32 0QJ **Tel:** (01271) 830358 w 6266202

GUDGION Letitia 06/11/2000 1 Cowper Avenue Tilbury Essex RM18 8AR **Tel:** (01375) 405588 w 6205207

GUEST Sharon 07/02/2000 120 Coed Celynen Drive Abercarn Newport Gwent NP11 5AT w 6133920

GUINEY Lisa Anne 27/02/1998 (10/04/2008) Mayhew Animal Home Trenmar Gardens LONDON NW10 6BJ **Tel:** (020) 8969 0178 w 6130974

GUITE Deborah Jane 21/08/1995 32 School Lane Irlam Manchester M44 6WF **Tel:** (0161) 776 1136 w 6026238

GUNN Lucy Jane 05/03/2002 (07/10/2009) 17 Edward Street Hinckley Leicestershire LE10 0DH **Tel:** (01827) 897870 w 6271251

GUNTER Nicola Jane 26/03/2002 75 The Fortunes HARLOW Essex CM18 6PH **Tel:** (07799) 268039 w 6270822

GUY Caroline Nicola (nee Sanders) 23/01/2003 23 New Road Ringwood Hampshire BH24 3AU **Tel:** (01425) 474268 w 6276553

GWALCHMAI Emma Jane (formerly Gwalchmai) 08/02/1996 (01/06/2007) 5 Maes Y Llan MEIFOD Powys SY22 6DE **Tel:** (01938) 500139 w 6041675

H

HACK Nathalie Maria Lea DipAVN(Surgical) (nee Ghijs) 08/03/1999 (02/11/2007) 124 Meyrick Avenue LUTON LU1 5JS **Tel:** (01582) 481770 w 6138292

HADDRELL Michelle Elizabeth (nee Pink) 07/04/1994 (31/07/2000) 10 Sir Evelyn Road Borstal Rochester Kent ME1 3NB **Tel:** (01634) 818187 w 6024514

HADGETT Rebecca 03/09/1999 C/o Royal College of Veterinary Surgeons 62-64 Horseferry Road LONDON SW1P 2AF w 6099364

HAINES Heidi Ann (nee Young) 18/01/1999 43 Withies Close Withington HEREFORD HR1 3PS **Tel:** (01432) 851674 w 6119950

Tracy (nee Lynch) 01/09/1997 6 Claremont Court Grundys Lane MALVERN Worcestershire WR14 4HS w 6025777

HALDANE Wendy 19/01/1993 (06/01/2004) 139 Great Meadow Way Aylesbury Buckinghamshire HP19 7GY **Tel:** (01296) 381017 w 6065448

HALFORD Charlotte Anne 04/09/1996 Malin House Woodend Towcester Northamptonshire NN12 8RX **Tel:** (01327) 860456 w 6098258

HALIL Wendy Louise DipAVN(Surgical) 15/02/2001 Spring Lodge Farm Powers Hall End Witham Essex CM8 2HG **Tel:** (01376) 513247 w 6205471

HALL Andrea Jane (nee Gatley) 28/08/1996 8 Aston Street Wem Shrewsbury SY4 5AY **Tel:** (01939) 234227 w 607610X

Emma Jayne 24/05/2002 Acorn Cottage 21 Hazles Cross Road Kingsley STOKE-ON-TRENT ST10 2AX **Tel:** (01538) 750957 w 6262935

Kerry DipAVN(Surgical) 16/09/1998 38 Ipswich Road Stowmarket Suffolk IP14 1BL w 6137018

Merlean Sherlon 02/02/1996 (22/04/2003) Flat 2 10 Cromartie Road London N19 3SJ **Tel:** (0207) 2720984 w 6038822

HALL Wendy Anne (see MORGAN, Mrs)

HALLAS Deborah Ann (nee Slater) 31/08/1994 Hill Top Cottages Top Lane Whatstandwell Matlock Derbyshire DE4 5EN **Tel:** (01773) 857226 w 6034351

HALSE Gemma Louise 21/10/1997 (08/01/2009) 18 Balfour Road Fulwood PRESTON PR2 3BX **Tel:** (01772) 493888 w 6116031

HAMILTON Anne Louise (nee Baggett) 22/07/1993 (27/10/2000) Veterinary Centre 1 Shamrock Street Glasgow G4 9JZ **Tel:** (0141) 332 6944 w 6014947

HAMILTON Deborah Nolene (see CABLE, Mrs)

HAMILTON Tracy Ann (see TIMMS, Mrs)

HAMMERSLEY Jane 21/10/1991 Keepers Barn Kermincham Congleton Cheshire CW12 2LJ **Tel:** (01477) 571774 w 6052144

HAMMERSLEY Zoe Ann (see WARD, Mrs)

HAMMOND Suzannah Michelle 13/12/2001 (03/02/2010) 19 Ullswater Drive Hethersett NORWICH Norfolk NR9 3QD **Tel:** (01603) 813055 w 6273528

HAMPSON Dawn Louise (see SALISBURY, Mrs)

HAMPTON Jane (see BLAYER, Mrs)

HAMPTON Marian Judith (see MOON, Mrs)

HANCOCK Samantha (nee Craven) 04/02/1999 Croft Veterinary Centre 122 Banbury Road Brackley Northamptonshire NN13 6BH **Tel:** (01280) 703451 w 611222X

HANCOX Alison Lesley (see HUNT, Mrs)

HANCOX Eleanor May (nee Johnson) 20/09/1999 Scarsdale Veterinary Hospital 45-47 Kedleston Road Derby DE22 1FN **Tel:** (01332) 345191 w 6138940

HANDS Nicola Clare (see LAST, Mrs)

HANDYSIDE BROWN Fiona Graeme 16/07/2002 43 Rivenhall End WELWYN GARDEN CITY Hertfordshire AL7 2PL **Tel:** (07713) 403 143 w 6266312

HANFORD Sarah Jane 20/08/1999 Emerald Vet Group 5 Heol y Neuadd Tumble LLANELLI Dyfed SA14 6EL **Tel:** (01269) 841242 w 6117647

HANGARTNER Harriet Jane (see NORTH, Mrs)

HANLEY Joanne Elizabeth (see KEOGH, Mrs)

HANLON Catherine Anne (see BURNISTON, Mrs)

HANNAM Wendy Violet Elizabeth (see THOMPSON, Mrs)

HANSON Elizabeth Ann 09/05/2002 (23/01/2006) The Veterinary Hospital Cannock Road Penkridge Stafford ST19 5RY **Tel:** (01785) 712235 w 6272296

Francesca Anna 29/07/2002 Small Animal Teaching Hospital University of Liverpool Leahurst Campus Chester High Road Neston Merseyside CH64 7TE **Tel:** (0151) 795 6100 w 6265916

Kate Simonne 15/02/2002 Oathall Veterinary Group 30 Oathall Road Haywards Heath West Sussex RH16 3EQ **Tel:** (01444) 440224 w 6267445

HANT Samantha Margaret (see TANFIELD, Mrs)

HANYSZYN Kerry Louise (see RUSSELL, Mrs)

HARBISON Janice Anne (nee Currie) 15/11/2001 88 Drumagrove Road Rathkenny Ballymena County Antrim BT43 6QF **Tel:** (0282) 1758214 w 6265113

HARDIE Stacey-Ann 25/01/1993 Flat 2 Maddox Court 11 Stanley Road LONDON E4 7DD **Tel:** (07946) 520 531 w 6066248

HARDING Julie Ann 14/10/2002 21 Acorn Avenue HALSTEAD Essex CO9 1LQ w 6281393

Susan Joy 01/09/1982 32 Isis Avenue Bicester Oxfordshire OX26 2GS **Tel:** (01869) 240761 w 6052279

HARDWICK Suzanne Stephanie (nee Jones) 15/02/1995 (15/01/2007) 165 Ringwood Road Eastbourne East Sussex BN22 8UW **Tel:** (01323) 639361 w 6035242

HARGREAVES Isla Louise (see BROWN, Mrs)

HARGREAVES Jessica 06/02/1997 (12/05/2006) 119 Caxton Road Hoddesdon Hertfordshire EN11 9NX **Tel:** (01992) 447 058 w 6041096

HARLEY Jennifer Anne (formerly Cockings) 22/01/1985 7 Farthing Combe AXBRIDGE Somerset BS26 2DR **Tel:** (01934) 732510 w 6047837

HARMAN Sara Ann (nee Glasson) 01/09/1995 152 Brian Road Chadwell Heath Romford Essex RM6 5BT **Tel:** (0208) 5994481 w 6040354

HARPER Philippa Jane (nee Standley) 12/05/1999 78 The Lane Answorth Nottinghamshire NG16 2QQ **Tel:** (0115) 930 1870 w 6116563

HARRINGTON Helen Elizabeth (nee Gower) 22/11/1988 Spinney Cottage Hamerton Huntingdon Cambridgeshire PE28 5QW **Tel:** (01832) 293341 w 6051548

Jane Rose (nee Musicka) 09/09/1998 (16/12/2008) 66 Dewhurst Road Cheshunt WALTHAM CROSS Hertfordshire EN8 9PE w 6101761

HARRIS Claire Margaret (see FRANCIS, Mrs)

HARRIS Helen Mary 23/09/2002 30 Woodfield Close Exmouth Devon EX8 4HA **Tel:** (01395) 263060 w 6285023

Joanne (nee Wallbank) 21/08/1998 6 St Peters Close Witherley Atherstone CV9 3LY **Tel:** (01827) 713919 w 6024139

HARRIS Katherine Elizabeth (see COOPER, Mrs)

Marie Louise (formerly Burgess) 05/10/2001 94 Main Road Dyke BOURNE Lincolnshire PE10 0AG w 6229528

Nicola Marie (nee Leaney) 06/11/1996 26 Halton Road Grays Essex RM16 4RP w 6031769

Penny 19/01/1987 (29/01/2002) Ashwood Veterinary Clinic 74 Holland Road Sutton Coldfield West Midlands B72 1RE w 605236X

Rachael Kay (nee Harris, formerly Gregg) 02/10/2002 Elms Veterinary Surgery New Dixton Road MONMOUTH Gwent NP25 3SJ **Tel:** (01600) 711511 w 6271801

HARRIS Stacey Victoria (see VAN GENT, Mrs)

HARRIS Stephanie Louisa (see FORNENGO, Mrs)

HARRISON Emma Elizabeth (see SYKES, Mrs)

HARRISON Gloria 17/10/1974 Penllwyn Carmel Caernarfon Gwynedd LL54 7SA **Tel:** (01286) 881134 w 6052392

Jacqueline 22/03/1990 Houghton House 126A Jeffcock Road Wolverhampton West Midlands WV3 7AF **Tel:** (01902) 342775 w 6052406

Matthew David 27/08/1997 The Brook Veterinary Surgery Station Approach Steventon Abingdon Oxfordshire OX13 6RU **Tel:** (01235) 831800 m 6113518

HARRISON Suzanne Elizabeth (see CROWDER, Mrs)

HART Anna Marie 04/08/1988 Avonvale Veterinary Centres Ltd 88 Coventry Street Southam Warwickshire CV47 0EA **Tel:** (01926) 812826 w 6052439

HARTHILL Tracy Susan (nee Lamb) 24/11/1988 (26/02/2001) Sherwood Veterinary Group Dudley House 297 Staines Road West Ashford Common Middlesex TW15 1RS **Tel:** (01932) 779979 w 6003560

HARVEY Debra Louise 01/09/1994 68 Courtlands Close Watford Hertfordshire WD24 5GT **Tel:** (01923) 675821 w 603396X

HASKELL Caroline Clare (nee Hayes) 26/08/1997 Grove Lodge Veterinary Group Ltd 18 Upper Brighton Road Worthing West Sussex BN14 9DL **Tel:** (01903) 234866 w 6099455

HASKINS Sarah Louise 27/02/2002 C/o 3 Marigold Avenue CLACTON-ON-SEA Essex CO16 7DZ w 6269183

HASSALL Marie (nee Williamson) 26/08/1997 (14/01/2008) CVS (UK) Ltd Sandy Lane Diss Norfolk IP22 4HY **Tel:** (01379) 644288 w 6116701

HASSELL Helen Susan (nee Keywood) 07/08/1986 5 Granville Gardens Hall Lane Ullesthorpe LUTTERWORTH Leicestershire LE17 5DD **Tel:** (01455) 202549 w 6092835

HASTIE Christina Louise 23/10/2001 C/o Royal College of Veterinary Surgeons 62-64 Horseferry Road LONDON SW1P 2AF w 6262187

HATCH Marie Claire (nee Whitcher) 04/02/2000 38 Pylewell Road Hythe SOUTHAMPTON Hampshire SO45 6AQ **Tel:** (023) 8084 1000 w 6123457

HATCHER Lynn Marie (see GARDNER, Mrs)

HATT Angela (see BILLINGTON, Mrs)

HATTON Janice Anne 24/08/1995 Church Walk Veterinary Centre Ltd St Mary's Place Church Walk Ulverston Cumbria LA12 7EN **Tel:** (01229) 583675 w 6036188

HAWKER Victoria Clare (see SHERBURN, Mrs)

HAWKES Angela 03/09/1996 Cedar Grove Veterinary Clinic 132 Upper Knockbreda Road Belfast BT6 9QB **Tel:** (028) 9070 5777 w 6096330

HAWKSWORTH Nicola (nee Toye) 31/03/1989 2 The Potlocks Twyford Road Willington Derby DE65 6YA **Tel:** (01283) 703842 w 606239X

HAWLEY Wendy Dawn 05/02/1992 RSPCA Stapeley Grange Wildlife Hospital London Road Stapeley Nantwich Cheshire CW5 7JW **Tel:** (0870) 442 7102 w 6052574

HAYES Caroline Clare (see HASKELL, Mrs)

HAYMAN Claire (see DAVIES, Mrs)

HAYMES Anna Marie 29/11/2000 Ashworth Veterinary Group 60 Bridge Road Cove Farnborough Hampshire GU14 0HP **Tel:** (01252) 542121 w 6203139

Vici Ann Leycester 12/09/1997 (29/09/2004) Rosemullion Veterinary Hospital 66 Melvill Road Falmouth Cornwall TR11 4DD **Tel:** (01326) 313991 w 6110721

HAYNES Diane Linda (nee Friell) 17/01/1984 15 Northern Avenue HENLOW Bedfordshire SG16 6ET w 6052632

HAYNES Talitha Bryony (see CARTMELL, Mrs)

HAYTER Julie Emma 20/11/2002 20 Grace Way Stevenage Hertfordshire SG1 5AA **Tel:** (01438) 360447 w 6277807

HAYTON Catherine Elizabeth (see PRIOR, Mrs)

HAYWARD Nicola Joanne DipAVN(Medical) (nee Dawson) 22/01/1998 10 Deans Close Amersham Buckinghamshire HP6 6LW **Tel:** (01494) 721 456 w 6033165

Zoe Helen 15/01/1998 12 Yates Avenue Aston on Trent Derby Derbyshire DE72 2BG **Tel:** (01332) 792 956 w 613148X

HAZELDEN Charlotte Elizabeth 10/09/1998 (27/01/2010) 33 The Finches SITTINGBOURNE Kent ME10 4PY w 6118491

HEAD Nicola Jane (see JACKSON, Mrs)

HEARD Esther Louise 14/09/2001 Colne Valley Veterinary Practice Off Maudlyn Road Colchester CO1 2GU **Tel:** (01206) 794695 w 6228208

HEATHER Craig Anthony 04/09/1997 (03/04/2002) 47 Kingsmead Road HIGH WYCOMBE Buckinghamshire HP11 1HX **Tel:** (01494) 438234 m 6112004

HEATON Joanna Louise 05/02/1999 (08/05/2006) Park Veterinary Centre 256 Cassiobury Drive WATFORD Hertfordshire WD17 3PA **Tel:** (01923) 223321 w 6129007

Julia Marie 30/07/2002 36 Eavestone Grove HARROGATE North Yorkshire HG3 2XY w 6270261

HEFFERNAN Claire Margaret (see FRANCIS, Mrs)

HELM Maureen 22/11/2001 Zasman Vet 14 Priory Road London N8 7RD **Tel:** (020) 8347 5200 w 6273330

HELME Tricia Joanne (nee Suckling) 17/01/2000 Turvey Hall Wormelow Hereford HR2 8EG **Tel:** (01432) 357222 w 6123322

HEMINSELY Julie (see THOMPSON, Mrs)

HENDERSON Lorna Margaret (see NUTTALL, Mrs)

HENDRIKS Amanda Oliva 29/01/1991 (17/08/2004) 142 Redford Close Feltham Middlesex TW13 4TE w 6052745

HENNESSY Charlotte Emma (nee Tolley) 19/02/2001 178 Chester Road Streetly Sutton Coldfield West Midlands B74 2WS w 6212489

HENRY Melanie Ayrie (nee Timm) 10/06/1994 (24/11/2009) The Cottage 16 Church Lane ELY Cambridgeshire CB7 4JG **Tel:** (01353) 665925 (Work) w 6033347

HENSTRIDGE Angela Helen 15/02/1996 (12/05/2009) 29 Appleshaw Way Perham Down Andover Hampshire SP11 9JU **Tel:** (01980) 601505 w 603521X

HEPPINSTALL Diane 15/01/1999 (27/10/2000) 110 Doncaster Road Hatfield Doncaster South Yorkshire DN7 6AT **Tel:** (01302) 885689 w 6033187

HERMAN Annemieke Nicine 18/09/1998 (10/03/2004) Yarde Gate Bungalow SOUTH MOLTON Devon EX36 3HA w 6034996

HEWITT Tracie Ann Margaret 22/02/2000 (31/10/2002) Veterinary Centre 1 Shamrock Street Glasgow G4 9JZ **Tel:** (0141) 332 6944 w 6108042

HEYHOE Lisa Carolyn (see GRAHAM, Mrs)

HEYNES Charlotte Emily 23/11/1995 (07/02/2002) 10 Middle Lane Cropthorne PERSHORE Worcestershire WR10 3LZ **Tel:** (07974) 202856 w 6038287

HEYS Tracy (see THURSTAN, Mrs)

HEYWOOD Alison Jane (see SANTOS, Mrs)

HIBBLE Hannah Jane (see PARROTT, Mrs)

HICKEY Nadine Isabel 10/12/2002 King Richard Veterinary Centre 29 Glenfield Road East Leicester LE3 5QW **Tel:** (0116) 2517677 w 6276520

HIGGINS Sharn Challoner (see FIRMIN, Mrs)

HIGGINSON Joanna Kenzie Erica DipAVN(Surgical) (nee Streeton) 26/02/1996 49 Blakesware Gardens Edmonton London N9 9HX **Tel:** (0208) 3607117 w 6042883

HILL Fiona Onycha Smithies (nee Mangles) 14/08/1986 (09/11/2009) Dunningworth Barn Tunstall WOODBRIDGE Suffolk IP12 2EQ **Tel:** (01728) 688023 w 605287X

Helen Elizabeth (nee Wilcock) 26/08/1998 (10/02/2005) 17 Prestbury Close Stepping Hill Stockport Cheshire SK2 7HW **Tel:** (0161) 4564463 w 6113041

Helen Louise 08/09/1997 32 Mercia Court Huthwaite SUTTON-IN-ASHFIELD Nottinghamshire NG17 2JX w 6131548

Laura Jayne (nee Gibbs) 23/10/2001 Pines Veterinary Clinic 146a Bath Road Maidenhead Berkshire SL6 4LB **Tel:** (01628) 776699 w 6263133

Paula Jane (nee Ancell) 05/10/2000 12 Avery Close Radgate Warrington Cheshire WA2 0bf w 6146135

Rebecca DipAVN(Surgical) (nee Wilkinson) 23/10/2001 4 Painshawfield Road Stocksfield Northumberland NE43 7EA w 6269271

Sally Jane 24/08/1998 4 Moorside Road Eccleshill BRADFORD West Yorkshire BD2 2EU **Tel:** (01274) 823769 w 6131559

HILLIER Linda Mary 14/08/1968 (10/05/2002) C/o Royal College of Veterinary Surgeons 62-64 Horseferry Road LONDON SW1P 2AF w 6052905

HILLS Nathalie Catherine 10/12/2002 60 Hoblethick Lane Westcliff on Sea Essex SS0 0RH **Tel:** (01702) 342184 w 6281580

HILLYER Rebecca Jane (see READ, Mrs)

HINDE Natalie-Jane (see GREENHALGH, Mrs)

HINES Judith Margaret 24/10/1986 (02/11/2007) Pilgrims Veterinary Clinic London Road West Kingsdown Sevenoaks Kent TN15 6EX **Tel:** (01474) 852661 w 6052949

HINKLY Emma Kate 14/09/1998 161 Kew Road Richmond Surrey TW9 2PN **Tel:** (020) 8940 1090 w 6133884

HINTON Rita Vivienne (nee Freeland) 26/08/1970 The Coppice Knapps Drive Winscombe Avon BS25 1BD **Tel:** (01934) 843184 w 6052960

HIPGRAVE Nicola Claire 15/02/2002 88 Hillyfields Welwyn Garden City Hertfordshire AL7 2EA **Tel:** (01707) 890862 w 6270162

HIRST Leeanne (nee Taylor) 22/04/2002 2 Buttercrambe Road Stamford Bridge York YO41 1AN **Tel:** (01759) 371066 w 6268479

HOAL Sarah Louise 05/09/2000 (10/03/2004) The Veterinary Hospital 118 Victoria Drive Bognor Regis West Sussex PO21 2EJ **Tel:** (01243) 841111 w 6135633

HOARE Laura Ann (nee Stewart) 24/01/1994 9 Longham Copse Downswood Maidstone Kent ME15 8TL **Tel:** (01622) 880184 w 6066215

Tara Jane 22/09/1993 Avenue Veterinary Centre 35 Avenue Road Grantham Lincolnshire NG31 6TJ **Tel:** (01476) 563371/564490 w 6033063

HOBBS Hazel Margaret-Rose (nee Peters) 14/01/1991 Shepherds Cottage 70 Ashcombe Farm Brighton Road Lewes East Sussex BN7 3JP **Tel:** (01273) 476259 w 6058612

Stephanie Louise (nee Hobbs, formerly Bridges) 04/02/2002 Badgers Oak Hastings Road Northiam Rye East Sussex TN31 6NH **Tel:** (01797) 252321 w 6270415

HOBDEN Lucie Victoria (nee Boddison) 27/02/1997 (12/05/2005) Quarry Veterinary Group Brassey Road off Old Potts Way Shrewsbury Shropshire SY3 7FA **Tel:** (01743) 362 556 w 6077497

HOBSON Pauline Anne (see GUARD, Mrs)

HODGES Abigail Caroline 28/08/1998 27 Monument Chase Whitehill Bordon Hampshire GU35 9QS w 6108610

HODGETTS Luan Emily (nee Lucas) 19/02/1998 170 Thornbridge Avenue Birmingham West Midlands B42 2AE **Tel:** (01676) 535033 w 6098484

HODGKINS Vanessa Gail (nee Lindsay) 04/09/1996 (03/08/2005) 3 Dudley Wood Avenue Dudley Wood Dudley West Midlands DY2 0DG w 6098451

HODGKINSON Xanthe Louise 06/02/2002 Colne Valley Veterinary Practice Off Maudlyn Road Colchester CO1 2GU **Tel:** (01206) 794695 w 6267016

HODGSON Elizabeth Mary (see DEMPSTER, Mrs)

HODGSON Louise Ann (see DATHAN, Mrs)

HODGSON Sally (see MORGAN, Mrs)

HODGSON Sally Elizabeth (nee Hodgson) 12/02/2001 3 Dorset Close Great Yarmouth Norfolk NR30 2SB **Tel:** (07973) 404039 w 6204833

HODSON Angela Jane (see SLATTER, Mrs)

HOGARTH Kathryn (nee Robinson) 27/12/2001 (02/12/2008) Beckside Farm Fryup Whitby Yorkshire YO21 2AP **Tel:** (01947) 897259 w 6268897

HOGG Helen Kimberley (see MITCHELL, Mrs)

HOLBROW Sally Elizabeth (nee Richardson) 18/09/1997 1 Tring Road Halton Aylesbury Buckinghamshire HP22 5PN **Tel:** (01296) 623439 w 6118640

HOLDEN Shelley Louise (nee Simmons) 19/01/1998 Small Animal Teaching Hospital University of Liverpool Leahurst Campus Chester High Road Neston Merseyside CH64 7TE **Tel:** (0151) 795 6100 w 6036993

HOLDER Julia Elizabeth (see BOXALL, Mrs)

HOLESWORTH Sarah Anne Louise 04/09/1996 Southwold Thoresby Road Fulstow LOUTH Lincolnshire LN11 0XS w 6023984

HOLLAND Lucy Ann 25/08/1999 (15/11/2005) 34 Flansham Lane Felpham Bognor Regis West Sussex PO22 6AF **Tel:** (01243) 587891 w 6137641

Nicola 18/01/2002 25 Walton Road Mill Park Port Elizabeth 6001 South Africa w 6261516

HOLLAND Rachel Katherine Fishley (see SMALLWOOD, Mrs)

HOLLETT Paula-Louise (nee Lang) 20/07/1993 10 Durnford Street Plymouth PL1 3QL **Tel:** (01752) 266077 w 6015281

HOLLINGTON Natasha Elisabeth (see MULLEY, Ms)

HOLLOWAY Donna (nee Cosgrove) 11/09/1997 Barkham Grove Veterinary Centre 156 Barkham Road Wokingham Berkshire RG41 2RP **Tel:** (0118) 979 0551 w 6107887

HOLMAN Jane Andrea (nee Finneral) 03/09/1997 (19/11/2004) 1 The Chestnuts Main Street Grendon Underwood Aylesbury Buckinghamshire HP18 0UH **Tel:** (01296) 770055 w 6117385

HOLMES Karen Tracey 06/10/1999 Congleton Veterinary Centre West Heath Retail Park Sandbach Road Congleton Cheshire CW12 4NB **Tel:** (01260) 272131 w 6185539

HOLMGAARD PELL Susan Louise (see PELL, Ms)

HOLT Lesley Ann 04/08/1977 110 Chiltern Drive Surbiton Surrey KT5 8LX **Tel:** (020) 8399 6911 w 6053159

Lisa Jane (nee Styles) 20/05/2002 Heath & Reach Veterinary Surgeons Brickhill Road Heath and Reach Leighton Buzzard Bedfordshire LU7 0BA **Tel:** (01525) 237444 w 6262418

HOOK Claire Louise (see STONE, Mrs)

HOOPER Samantha Lynda (formerly Jones, formerly Tayler) 26/08/1997 (14/08/2009) 4 Manor Farm Cottages Rockbourne Fordingbridge Hampshire SP6 3NP **Tel:** (01725) 518797 w 6041416

Theresa Jayne 05/09/1997 Water Meadows Innis Fishery Innis Moor St. Austell Cornwall PL26 8YH **Tel:** (01726) 814626 w 6033697

HOPCROFT Joanne Margaret 16/08/1995 (13/08/2007) Northlands Veterinary Hospital 2 Northampton Road Kettering Northamptonshire NN15 7JU **Tel:** (01536) 485 543 w 6017981

HOPPER Davina Jane 22/03/2004 (04/02/2010) 57 Lilac Crescent Beeston NOTTINGHAM NG9 1PD w 6292162

Janet 26/10/1966 128 Quaker Lane Cleckheaton West Yorkshire BD19 5JG **Tel:** (01274) 874191 w 605324X

HORGAN Clare 27/09/1999 40 Harpesford Avenue Virginia Water Surrey GU25 4RD **Tel:** (01784) 436679 w 6132756

HORLEY Deborah Anne 18/01/1999 Spindlewood White Hill Cresselly Kilgetty Dyfed SA68 0TT **Tel:** (01646) 651489 w 6076052

HORNE Vicki Louise (nee Lamb) 10/09/1997 Pet Doctors Unit 10 Cliffe Industrial Estate South Street Lewes East Sussex BN8 6JL **Tel:** (01273) 474857 w 6033449

HORSLEY Terri Louise (nee Cowley, formerly Bond) 06/02/1997 (08/05/2001) 414-416 Leach Lane Sutton Leach St. Helens Merseyside WA9 4NA **Tel:** (01744) 820505 w 609798X

HORTON Louise 24/09/2002 Warwickshire College Moreton Morrell Centre Moreton Morrell WARWICK Warwickshire CV35 9BL w 6282823

HOSGOOD Sarah Anne 19/10/1990 Apartment 3 131 Maidenwell Avenue LEICESTER Leicestershire LE5 1QD w 6053319

HOUGH Louise Margaret 16/09/1997 (19/07/1999) Macclesfield Veterinary Hospital 26/38 Cumberland Street Macclesfield Cheshire SK10 1BZ **Tel:** (01625) 501500 w 6116075

HOUGHTON Carly Anne 30/10/2001 (07/06/2007) 127 Wennington Road Southport Merseyside PR9 7AH **Tel:** (01704) 214460 w 6261791

HOULDSWORTH Joanna Clare (see DURITY, Mrs)

HOUNSLOW Claire Anne 07/08/1990 9 Creran Walk Linslade Leighton Buzzard Bedfordshire LU7 2YP **Tel:** (01525) 370135 w 6053341

HOWARD Alexandra Marie (see GARLICK, Mrs)

HOWARD Clare (see LANGHAM, Mrs)

HOWARD Tracey Jane 08/09/1997 32 Princes Terrace Brighton Sussex BN2 5JS w 6117862

HOWATSON Gwenan (nee Evans) 21/08/1992 Wern Veterinary Surgery Greenfield Road Ruthin Denbighshire LL15 1EY **Tel:** (01824) 702445 w 6008106

HOWELL Tracey Dawn 06/08/1990 (27/06/2005) 3 Wherry Road Bungay Suffolk NR35 1LG **Tel:** (01986) 892771 w 6058565

HOWELLS Jane Mandy 09/01/1989 17 Hanford Road Aveley South Ockendon Essex RM15 4SS **Tel:** (01708) 862007 w 6053396

HOWES Elizabeth Anne 26/01/1993 (27/04/2005) 17 Church Road Long Hanborough WITNEY Oxfordshire OX29 8JE w 6008445

HOWIE Katherine Jayne (nee Steward) 26/01/2000 Vets Now (Farnham) Leyton House Clinic Hale Road Farnham Surrey GU9 9RB **Tel:** (01252) 737555 w 6129845

HOWLETT Linda Marion 31/07/1972 Broadhouse Bindon Lane East Stoke Wareham Dorset BH20 6AS **Tel:** (01929) 462255 w 6083241

HUBBARD Joanne Sharon (see TAYLOR, Mrs)

HUDSON Elaine (see BASSINDER, Mrs)

HUDSON Jacqueline (nee Taylor, formerly Neal) 15/11/2001 25 Fairfield Close SHOREHAM-BY-SEA West Sussex BN43 6BH **Tel:** (01273) 382434 w 6263804

Kirsty Marie (nee Robson) 24/05/2002 17 Erskines Avenue Aldergrove CRUMLIN County Antrim BT29 4FR **Tel:** (028) 9445 4606 w 6276674

HUGHES Caroline Anne (see DRUMMOND, Mrs)

HUGHES Christine 06/08/1980 1 Glen Craig Terrace Fenwick Kilmarnock Ayrshire KA3 6DE **Tel:** (01560) 600412 w 6053476

Gabrielle Angharad (nee Mitchell) 16/09/2004 (02/11/2009) Grain Barn Mousley House Farm Mousley End Hatton WARWICK CV35 7JG w 6265960

Helen Victoria 04/10/1996 28 Oak Avenue Newport Shropshire TF10 7EF **Tel:** (01952) 419012 w 6098327

Kerisa Jayne 27/08/1999 (19/04/2005) 33 Hawarden Way Mancot Deeside Clwyd CH5 2EL **Tel:** (01244) 533 683 w 613957X

Laura Louise (nee Bryan) 06/02/2002 (18/11/2009) Pruina Petcare St. Georges House Park Lane CROYDON CR9 1NR **Tel:** (0844) 225 5093 w 6260350

Nigel Peter 03/09/1996 (24/06/2003) Church Lane Llanbadarn Fawr Aberystwyth Dyfed SY23 3QU **Tel:** (01970) 612526 m 6077351

HUGHES Tracy Anne (see GRINSTEAD, Mrs)

HUGO Alison Emily (nee Farmer) 12/09/1995 138 Pursey Drive Bradley Stoke Bristol BS32 8DP **Tel:** (0117) 969 3421 w 6027129

HUKE Camilla Kay (see HUKE-JENNER, Mrs)

HUKE-JENNER Camilla Kay (nee Huke) 25/10/1999 The Ark 100 Yarmouth Road Lowestoft Suffolk NR32 4AQ **Tel:** (01502) 517054 w 6185616

HULL Emily Maralyn Maxwell 14/09/2001 (17/03/2006) 6 Kite Lane REDDITCH Worcestershire B97 6TT w 6141545

HUMBLE Jacqueline Elizabeth 31/08/1999 31 The Foxhills Fellside Park Whickham Newcastle upon Tyne NE16 5UU **Tel:** (0191) 488 0145 w 6108326

HUMPHREY Valerie (formerly Verity) 11/09/1972 6 William Ellis Close Old Windsor Windsor Berkshire SL4 2QW **Tel:** (01753) 854843 w 6062731

HUMPHREYS Gail 22/11/1979 Firgrove Veterinary Centre 7 Aylesham Way Yateley Hampshire GU46 6NR **Tel:** (01252) 877799 w 6088170

Sara Louise 16/09/1998 (30/04/2009) Scarsdale Veterinary Hospital 45-47 Kedleston Road Derby DE22 1FN **Tel:** (01332) 345191 w 6131570

HUNT Alison Lesley (nee Hancox) 10/10/1969 Tor View Kennels 41 Ashcott Road Meare Glastonbury Somerset BA6 9SU **Tel:** (01458) 860637 w 6053545

Katie Louise 30/01/1998 (09/08/2004) 39 Queens Road WARE Hertfordshire SG12 7DN **Tel:** (01920) 486234 w 6099546

Melanie (nee Waugh) 15/11/2001 (12/05/2005) Grove Lodge Veterinary Group Ltd 18 Upper Brighton Road Worthing West Sussex BN14 9DL **Tel:** (01903) 234866 w 6264398

Susan Joan 14/01/1982 (24/11/2008) 26 The Lawns FARNBOROUGH Hampshire GU14 0RF **Tel:** (01252) 375771 w 6053556

HUNTER Gail DipAVN(Surgical) 14/09/1989 (04/10/1999) 36 India Drive Inchinnan Renfrew Renfrewshire PA4 9LE **Tel:** (0141) 427 6080 w 6000934

HUNTER Gillian (see LINTON, Mrs)

Heather Kathleen (nee Woore) 28/04/1993 (08/10/1999) 6 Broxell Close Wedgnock Industrial Estate Warwick CV34 5QF **Tel:** (01926) 400255 w 6014845

HUNTER BLAIR Harriet Claire (nee Peck) 31/01/1996 (06/01/2005) Yew Tree Farm Forward Green Stowmarket Suffolk IP14 5HU **Tel:** (01449) 711433 w 604145X

HURST Marie (nee Over, nee Egen) 20/11/2002 Tree View Brigg Road Moortown Lincolnshire LN7 6JA w 6263221

HUTCHINSON Judith Ann (nee Maryindale, formerly Willmott) 15/09/1997 (06/05/2003) 3 Northville Road BRISTOL BS7 0RQ **Tel:** (0117) 9695605 w 6100597

HUTCHISON Alison Jane (see CHARLES, Mrs)

HUTCHISON Leanda Nicola (see BUCHANAN, Mrs)

HUXLEY Deborah Louise (nee Crompton) 08/08/2002 Ashleigh Veterinary Centre 221 Upper Chorlton Road Manchester Greater Manchester M16 0DE **Tel:** (0161) 881 6868 w 6204712

HUXTABLE Claire Louise (nee Sewell) 18/01/2000 12 Donnington Drive CHRISTCHURCH Dorset BH23 4SZ w 6131286

HYAMS Georgina Sarah 27/10/2000 New House Farm Plough Wents Road Chart Sutton Maidstone Kent ME17 3SA **Tel:** (01622) 843445 w 6099557

HYDE Hazel Rebecca (see VERDEN, Mrs)

HYLAND Alison Jane (nee Greening) 16/01/1986 144 Links Way Croxley Green RICKMANSWORTH Hertfordshire WD3 3RN **Tel:** (07875) 582855 w 6000898

I

IAN Suzanne Helen (nee Briggs) 21/08/1998 19 Station Road Edingley NEWARK Nottinghamshire NG22 8BX w 6115650

ILIADIS Shelagh Mary (see NEWTON, Ms)

ILIFFE Zoe Louise (see PAGET, Mrs)

ILLSLEY Julie Mary (nee Matheson) 10/12/2002 3 Bowland Close Herne Bay Kent CT6 7UP **Tel:** (01227) 369298 w 6249493

INDURAIN Sol 24/08/1992 (13/03/2003) 22 Mill Gardens Elmswell Bury St. Edmunds Suffolk IP30 9DQ **Tel:** (01359) 241904 w 6005648

INGLIS Pamela 13/09/1994 3 Dalrymple Court Townhead Kirkintilloch Glasgow G66 3AA **Tel:** (0141) 775 2503 w 6028166

INMAN Karen Louise 12/08/1991 3 Colnbrook Court Hazelhurst Road Tooting London SW17 0TZ **Tel:** (0208) 6727376 w 6053658

INNES Barbara-Ann 02/02/1994 22 Baberton Mains Garden Edinburgh EH14 3BX **Tel:** (0131) 442 2199 w 6067875

IRELAND Deborah Margaret 28/09/1989 Burrows Veterinary Surgery 65 Leigh Road Wimborne Dorset BH21 1AE **Tel:** (01202) 841084 w 605367X

IRVINE Muriel 30/10/1992 (22/12/2009) Alpha Veterinary Surgery 144 Stanley Road Teddington Middlesex TW11 8UA **Tel:** (020) 8943 2303 w 6012098

ISAACS Melissa Jane 16/08/1995 (22/04/2002) 20 Lion Mead HASLEMERE Surrey GU27 1LF **Tel:** (01428) 643726 w 6026668

ISON Tracey Jayne (nee Baggott) 24/08/1989 Feldon Veterinary Centre 257 Coventry Road Hinckley Leicestershire LE10 0NE **Tel:** (01455) 610227 w 6044880

J

JACK Linda 10/09/1998 3 Randolph Crescent Boreland Dysart KIRKCALDY Fife KY1 2YN **Tel:** (01592) 650824 w 6130522

JACKLIN Amy Marie (see WILLIAMSON, Mrs)

JACKSON Caroline Jane 14/09/2001 3 Vermont Street HULL HU5 1NG w 6228219

JACKSON Clare Louise (see SWINDEN, Mrs)

Estelle Norah Marg (nee Riddick) 04/12/2002 (24/11/2009) 5 Lexington Road Chaddesden DERBY DE21 6UW **Tel:** (01332) 608294 w 6018679

JACKSON Gayle (see FOGGON, Mrs)

Judith Ann (nee Langley) 02/04/1969 1 Meadow Court Scruton Northallerton North Yorkshire DL7 0QU **Tel:** (01609) 748438 w 6053727

Lorraine 18/10/1999 University of Glasgow Veterinary School Garscube Estate Glasgow G61 1QH **Tel:** (0141) 330 5848 w 6022153

Nicola Jane (nee Head) 30/08/1990 Downs Farm Yalding Hill Yalding MAIDSTONE Kent ME18 6AL w 6053749

Tina 15/09/1999 Bramley Vets4Pets Limited Old School House Lower Town Street Bramley Leeds Yorkshire LS13 4BN **Tel:** (0113) 255 4466 w 6152488

JACKSON-COX Philippa Anne (nee Bancroft-Livingston) 26/09/1974 Berry House Veterinary Practice 41 Nightingale Road Hitchin Hertfordshire SG5 1RE **Tel:** (01462) 432824 w 6013728

JACOBS Jayne Lindsey 01/12/2000 Talafon St. Davids Road Caernarfon Gwynedd LL55 1EL **Tel:** (01286) 672918 w 6140439

JAGDHUBER Rosamund Kim Penelop (formerly Davison) 11/06/1975 Treanagry Ballinameen Boyle Co Roscomman Ireland **Tel:** (00) 353 71 96 689 49 w 6084835

JAGO Joanne Margaret 23/01/2003 69 Caavendish Road Patchway Bristol BS34 5HJ w 6262913

JAITEH Miranda Kathryn Jane 30/09/1983 (07/10/2009) 101 Glenview LONDON SE2 0SB **Tel:** (020) 8310 6760 w 6063939

JAKEWAY Ruth Helen (see DIXON, Miss)

JAMES Amanda Julie (nee White) 31/01/2000 The Grove Tyndale Road Gossington Slimbridge Gloucestershire GL2 7DL w 6190797

JAMES Avril Ruth (see GLESSING, Mrs)

Jayne Louise (nee Skerten) 15/09/1997 20 Viking Way Winch Wen Industrial Estate Winch Wen Swansea SA1 7DA **Tel:** (01792) 310974 w 6109035

Penelope 17/01/1986 The Bungalow Kingcott Mill Farm Clevedon Road Flax Bourton North Somerset BS48 1LZ **Tel:** (01275) 462452 w 6053807

JAMES Susan Margaret (see EVES, Mrs)

Tracy May 26/02/2000 (22/08/2002) 23 Bafford Lane Charlton Kings Cheltenham Gloucestershire GL53 8DN w 6110812

JAYNES Vanessa (nee Plested, formerly Barnett) 25/03/2002 77-79 Bournemouth Road Chandlers Ford Eastleigh Hampshire SO53 3AP **Tel:** (02380) 255565 w 6264926

JEFFERY Joanne (nee Ayre) 27/08/1999 2 Dolphin Court Railway Street HERTFORD SG14 1RP **Tel:** (01992) 501502 w 6184923

Laura Louise (nee Brittain) 25/03/2002 1 Plover Close Edenbridge Kent TN8 6BQ w 6274760

JEFFERYS Emma Elizabeth 22/08/1994 119 Spruce Drive BICESTER Oxfordshire OX26 3YF **Tel:** (01869) 325474 w 6032274

JEFFREY Jane Patricia (nee Temple) 26/08/1976 (30/03/2001) 29 Polwarth Crescent Brunton Park Newcastle upon Tyne NE3 2EE **Tel:** (0191) 2170502 w 6003378

JENKINS Amanda Jane (see BOW, Mrs)

JENKINS Jennifer Anne 25/02/2004 (02/11/2009) 12 The Moorings COWES Isle of Wight PO31 7FB w 6288488

Michele Anita (nee Grayshon) 25/11/1992 Green Hollow School Road Ruyton XI Towns Shrewsbury SY4 1JT **Tel:** (01939) 261216 w 6044235

JENNER Estelle (nee Wall) 28/07/1992 (04/11/2008) 12 Church Road Kessingland LOWESTOFT Suffolk NR33 7TQ **Tel:** (01502) 7442291 w 6008285

JEPHCOTT Sandra 18/09/1997 Waverley Cottage 9 East Street Colne Nr. Huntingdon Cambridgeshire PE28 3LZ **Tel:** (01487) 840710 w 6117909

JINKS Elizabeth Louise 06/09/1999 140 Harborne Road Oldbury West Midlands B68 9JG **Tel:** (0121) 501 1828 w 6112831

JOHNS Joanna Margaret (nee Lamphee) 06/08/1990 68 Canefields Avenue Plympton Plymouth Devon PL7 1XH **Tel:** (01752) 342183 w 6054797

JOHNS Tina Angela (see BUXTON, Ms)

JOHNSON Eleanor May (see HANCOX, Mrs)

JOHNSON Helen Ruth 16/09/1991 37 Finchley Crescent Whelley Wigan Lancashire WN2 1AZ **Tel:** (01942) 825985 w 6053986

JOHNSON Julie Clare (see MCMORRAN, Mrs)

JOHNSON Lorraine (see FLACK, Mrs)

Lynne (nee Owens) 11/05/1983 (04/08/2004) 3 Meadowdale Close High Clarence Middlesbrough Cleveland TS2 1TJ **Tel:** (01642) 562149 w 6054039

Marion Euphemia Morrison 28/07/1975 Oban Veterinary Surgeons 14 Tweeddale Street Oban Argyll PA34 5DD **Tel:** (01631) 562876 w 6054050

JOHNSON Marion Patricia (see LINES, Miss)

Michael Paul 14/10/2002 (21/01/2008) 33 Fenton Road BIRMINGHAM B27 6HY m 6259888

Rita Caroline DipAVN(Surgical) (nee Williams) 30/07/1979 Newnham Court Veterinary Group Bearsted Road Weavering Maidstone Kent ME14 5EL **Tel:** (01622) 734555 w 6054061

Victoria 29/09/1999 (17/03/2006) 61 Hawthorne Avenue SOUTH SHIELDS Tyne and Wear NE34 8BD w 6184714

JOHNSTON Eithne Valerie Elizabeth (nee Griffin) 19/12/1977 Bank Farm Holyhead Road Kingswood Albrighton Wolverhampton West Midlands WV7 3AP **Tel:** (01902) 374517 w 6054072

JOLLEY Lisa Elaine (nee Waterson) 01/11/2000 University of Cambridge Madingley Road Cambridge Cambridgeshire CB3 0ES **Tel:** (01223) 337621 w 6203128

JONAS Samantha Lian 15/02/2002 Silva House Veterinary Clinic Silver Street Midsomer Norton Radstock Somerset BA3 2ET **Tel:** (01761) 412223 w 6257457

JONES Claire Louise (see ALLEN, Mrs)

JONES Diane Pamela 12/02/1996 The Green Tranch Road PONTYPOOL Gwent NP4 6BG **Tel:** (07855) 125535 w 6077340

Helen 19/12/1988 Orchard Veterinary Centre 21 Church Street Oldbury West Midlands B69 3AF **Tel:** (0121) 544 8951 w 6054163

JONES Helen Louise (see REEVE, Miss)

Karen Elizabeth 16/02/1999 26 Cambridge Road Milton Cambridge Cambridgeshire CB24 6AW **Tel:** (01223) 426600 w 6140279

JONES Linda Ann (see CAPEWELL, Mrs)

Lucy-Ann 14/10/2002 C/o Royal College of Veterinary Surgeons 62-64 Horseferry Road LONDON SW1P 2AF w 6275695

Nicola Jane (nee Morse) 27/02/2002 (10/04/2008) 65 Albion Road PONTYPOOL Gwent NP4 6LE **Tel:** (07967) 706913 w 6254432

Nicola Mary 29/10/1998 (30/05/2008) 1 Bransdale Close Great Sankey WARRINGTON WA5 3FW w 6140665

JONES Patricia Muriel Farquhar (see SHAW, Mrs)

JONES Paula (see SMITH, Mrs)

JONES Samantha Georgena (see DYBLE, Mrs)

JONES Samantha Lynda (see HOOPER, Mrs)

Sarah Tracy (nee Batacanin) 15/01/1998 30 Brewer Mead Chippenham Wiltshire SN15 3FB **Tel:** (01249) 661542 w 6130668

JONES Sharn Challoner (see FIRMIN, Mrs)

JONES Suzanne Stephanie (see HARDWICK, Mrs)

Victoria Ann Carruthers 04/02/2002 Kennel Farm Southampton Road Clarendon SALISBURY SP5 3DG **Tel:** (01722) 710844 w 6274177

JORDAN Melanie 24/01/2000 Easton College Easton Norwich Norfolk NR9 5DX w 6191072

Sarah Louise (nee Dawson) 15/11/2001 (10/11/2009) 17 Oxford Street Long Eaton Nottingham Nottinghamshire NG10 1JR w 6253794

Sharon Wendy 10/09/1998 (29/06/2007) 9 Newfields WELWYN GARDEN CITY Hertfordshire AL8 6YS **Tel:** (01707) 331939 w 6118695

JOYES Lynne Catherine 15/11/2001 55 Axbridge Forest Park Bracknell Berkshire RG12 0XB **Tel:** (01344) 481 085 w 6256445

K

KADDU Celine 25/02/1992 (16/05/2003) 30 Hurst Road Northumberland Heath Erith Kent DA8 3EN w 6054323

KAINES Sarah Louise (see ANDERSON, Ms)

KAY Cheryl Elizabeth (see EATON, Mrs)

KEALEY Kim 14/10/2002 (05/02/2010) 12 Shortlands Close EASTBOURNE East Sussex BN22 0JE **Tel:** (01323) 504516 w 6261670

KEATLEY Sarah Jane (see DUTTON, Mrs)

KEELEY Anne Roberta 17/11/1965 121 Cedar Road Croydon CR0 6UJ **Tel:** (020) 86863013 w 6054367

KEENAN Clare Lucy (nee Dinnin) 24/08/1995 Veterinary Centre 41 Peartree Lane Welwyn Garden City Hertfordshire AL7 3UA **Tel:** (01707) 336919 w 6036654

KEEP Rachael Michelle (nee Marner) 10/09/1999 15 Stoneage Close North Bersted Bognor Regis West Sussex PO22 9QN **Tel:** (01243) 863 423 w 6136819

KELLY Alison Jane (see MCGRATH, Mrs)

KELLY Amanda Jane 20/01/2000 (12/03/2004) New Era Veterinary Hospital Victoria Road St Saviour Jersey JE2 7QG **Tel:** (01534) 730521 w 6185176

Emma Jane (nee Quinn) 20/11/2002 15-17 Acacia Grove West Kirby WIRRAL Merseyside CH48 4DD **Tel:** (0151) 625 9916 w 6265993

Julie Anne 20/05/2002 31 Glenalmond Road HARROW Middlesex HA3 9JY **Tel:** (020) 8204 9004 w 6274694

Sarah Jane 23/07/1993 Broad Lane Vets Ltd 255 Broad Lane Coventry West Midlands CV5 7AQ **Tel:** (024) 7646 4789 w 601526X

Sharon Louise 10/09/1996 (16/05/2005) Church view 11 Bede Close Higham Ferrers Northamptonshire NN10 8LT **Tel:** (01933) 412021 w 6037421

KEMP Barbara 25/01/1993 35 Parkhead Drive Sighthill Edinburgh EH11 4SP **Tel:** (0131) 539 1704 w 6065583

KEMP Frances (see FALLOWS, Mrs)

Laura (nee McKenzie) 10/02/1992 (31/05/2000) 211 Hawkhill Dundee DD1 5LA **Tel:** (01382) 660384 w 6056444

KEMP Michelle Arthurina Crawford (see KERR, Mrs)

Tina Ann 23/01/2001 25 Heath Road Alresford Colchester Essex CO7 8DT **Tel:** (01206) 825319 w 6205504

KENDALL Nina Louise (see MACLEAN, Mrs)

KENNEDY Yvonne Elizabeth (nee Fitzell) 20/01/2000 Cathermone Midleton Co Cork Ireland **Tel:** (0035321) 4639114 w 6121937

KENT Michaela Louise 10/04/1997 13 Rosewood Drive Higher Walton Preston PR5 4ER w 6098393

KEOGH Joanne Elizabeth (nee Hanley) 03/09/1996 Veterinary Centre 41 Peartree Lane Welwyn Garden City Hertfordshire AL7 3UA **Tel:** (01707) 336919 w 6099397

KERR Michelle Arthurina Crawford (formerly Kemp) 04/09/1991 West Lodge Balmuto Kirkcaldy Fife KY2 5XA **Tel:** (01592) 870472 w 6054505

KEYWOOD Helen Susan (see HASSELL, Mrs)

KIDWELL Sarah Elizabeth (see CUNNINGHAM, Mrs)

KIENTZEL Celia Mary (nee Whiting) 30/07/1975 Betussou Cazes-Mondenard 82110 France w 6063699

KILLINGBACK Nadia Rachel Marie (see RODGERS, Miss)

KILNER Joanne Denise (see GOODFELLOW, Mrs)

KINCHIN Lynda Erica 22/08/1967 Norsted Kennels Cromer Road North Walsham Norfolk NR28 0NB **Tel:** (01692) 402469 w 6054549

KIND Tracy Jane 04/02/2002 18 Stourton Place Horncastle Lincolnshire LN9 5AZ **Tel:** (01507) 522952 w 6268083

KING Frances Mary 16/08/1982 3 Bell Hill Hook Norton Banbury Oxfordshire OX15 5NG w 605455X

Glenda (nee Goddard) 18/09/1998 (04/05/2007) 123 Exeter Street Salisbury Wiltshire SP1 2SG **Tel:** (01722) 337117 w 6129379

Helen (nee Giles) 21/07/1993 (14/05/2007) Chestnut Veterinary Group 1 Hoe Lane Ware Hertfordshire SG12 9LS **Tel:** (01920) 468874 w 6066576

Helen Suzanne (nee Clark) 19/01/1998 21 East Close STEVENAGE Hertfordshire SG1 1PP **Tel:** (01438) 244843 w 6112762

Samantha Alison 29/01/1999 (07/11/2005) 7 Higher Church Street HAYLE Cornwall TR27 4LR w 6134174

KING Sarah Jane (see KOSTUK, Mrs)

KING Sylvia Ann 13/08/1965 9 Abbey Court Cerne Abbas Dorchester Dorset DT2 7JH **Tel:** (01300) 341195 w 6054571

KINREAD Kathryn Ellen (nee Price) 14/09/1998 26 Ffordd-Y-Rhos Treuddyn Mold Flintshire CH7 4NJ **Tel:** (01352) 770184 w 6098622

KIRBY Donna Iris (nee Sharman) 29/08/1995 (15/09/2009) 37 Edinburgh Close Market Harborough Leicestershire LE16 7QQ **Tel:** (01858) 419224 w 603230X

KIRBYSHIRE Claire Emma (nee Miles) 06/02/2002 34 St. Johns Avenue BURGESS HILL RH15 8HH w 6267885

KIRK Josephine 02/09/1997 1-5 Hugh Street London SW1V 1QQ **Tel:** (020) 7932 2370 w 6099615

Lorna Sadie 05/09/1996 (16/06/2004) Fieldside Cottage Padnal Littleport ELY Cambridgeshire CB6 1NS **Tel:** (01353) 860296 w 6042191

KIRRANE Joanne 19/01/2000 Cornerstones The Leys Whiston Stoke-on-Trent ST10 2JE **Tel:** (01538) 266727 w 6190401

KITCHEN Abby Louise (see WATTS, Mrs)

KITCHING Anne Elizabeth (see WRIGHT, Mrs)

KITSON Emma Louise 16/01/2002 (07/08/2008) Flat 6 Glenpatrick Buildings Glenpatrick Road Elderslie JOHNSTONE Renfrewshire PA5 9UH **Tel:** (01505) 323709 w 6274221

KITSON Linda (see DOWSON, Mrs)

KNAPTON Lucy Alice (see WIGG, Mrs)

KNIBB Joanne (see DODDS, Mrs)

KNIGHT Gemma Louise 04/02/2000 (01/02/2002) 41 Falcon Close Rayleigh Essex SS6 9BH **Tel:** (01268) 781 496 w 6131049

Helen Victoria 09/12/1991 (05/08/1999) Castle Vets Pet Healthcare Centre 1 Tilehurst Road Reading Berkshire RG1 7TW **Tel:** (0118) 957 4488 w 6054651

KNIGHT Justine (see SPIVEY, Mrs)

KNIGHTON Karen 14/09/2001 Rusthall Veterinary Surgery 20 Ashley Gardens Rusthall Tunbridge Wells Kent TN4 8TU **Tel:** (01892) 511715 w 6228230

KNOTT Nicola McCall (formerly Reeder) 04/02/1993 (08/02/2002) 20 Brunswick Avenue Waterloo Street Hull HU2 9AY **Tel:** (01482) 224452 w 6054662

KNOX Helen 30/01/2001 16 Stryd Hywel Harris Ystrad Mynach Hengoed Mid Glamorgan CF82 7DN **Tel:** (01443) 815982 w 6211532

Natasha 15/10/1999 25 Larch Way Southwood FARNBOROUGH Hampshire GU14 0QN **Tel:** (01252) 664643 w 6140406

KOHLER Kathryn Jane 02/11/2000 27 Daryl Road Heswall Wirral Merseyside CH60 5RD **Tel:** (0151) 342 7646 w 6204646

KOMOROCZY Joanna (nee Lyon) 20/01/1999 195 Kingston Crescent Chatham Kent ME5 8YZ **Tel:** (01634) 301822 w 609974X

KOSTUK Sarah Jane (nee King) 03/08/1992 The Veterinary Centre Queen Annes Road GREAT YARMOUTH Norfolk NR31 0LE **Tel:** (01493) 416700 w 600793X

KRAATZ Susan Louise (see BARTLETT, Mrs)

KRONER Julia Margaret (see COOPER, Mrs)

L

LAAR Janine (see RAWLES, Mrs)

LAIDLOW Diane Elizabeth (see EASON, Mrs)

LAIN Susan Jane 11/10/1973 (20/01/2010) PO BOX 311 Nottingham Road 3280 Kwazulu Natal South Africa **Tel:** (002733) 2666934 w 6084187

LAINTON Janet (nee Vickers) 10/09/1998 27 Morning Field Road Inverness Inverness-Shire IV2 6AU w 6134538

LAITHWAITE Carolyn Gail 13/10/2000 107 Raithby Drive Wigan Lancashire WN3 5PZ **Tel:** (01942) 321711 w 6204910

LAKE Alison Jane 14/09/1995 (23/06/2009) 4 Hall Farm Church Road Teversham Cambridgeshire CB1 9AP **Tel:** (01223) 292170 w 6033653

LAMB Elaine (nee Willoughby) 27/01/1994 (23/10/2001) 62 Little Brook Road Sale Cheshire M33 4WG **Tel:** (0161) 962 8418 w 6066780

LAMB Tracy Susan (see HARTHILL, Mrs)

LAMB Vicki Louise (see HORNE, Mrs)

LAMBERT Kerry Susan (nee Price) 04/10/1999 (10/02/2009) 17 Friesian Close Fleet Hampshire GU51 2TP **Tel:** (01252) 624315 w 6118560

Natasha 16/09/1998 7 Hurst Road Croydon CR0 1JT **Tel:** (020) 8686 3972 w 6099659

LAMERTON Ann Marie (see ORMAN, Mrs)

LAMPHEE Joanna Margaret (see JOHNS, Mrs)

LAMPING Vanessa Laura (nee Lightfoot) 15/11/2001 11 Blackthorn Close Portslade East Sussex BN41 2EU **Tel:** 01903-234-866 w 6249339

LANE Sharon (see MORRIS, Mrs)

LANG Cathryn Suzanne (see VILLARS, Mrs)

LANG Paula-Louise (see HOLLETT, Mrs)

LANGDALE Heather Lesley (nee Roberts) 03/09/1996 14 Well Close Great Preston LEEDS LS26 8BG **Tel:** (01924) 501597 w 6100189

LANGHAM Clare (nee Howard) 21/01/1994 (19/11/2001) Southbourne Veterinary 254 Main Road EMSWORTH Hampshire PO10 8JJ w 6066102

LANGLEY Judith Ann (see JACKSON, Mrs)

LANGLEY Sarah Lacey (nee Tucker) 29/07/1992 (03/09/2008) 2 Hillview Moat Lane Taynton GLOUCESTER GL19 3AR **Tel:** (01452) 790787 w 6008252

LARRINGTON Nicola 12/10/2000 28a Harold Road Dartford Kent DA2 7SA w 6152422

LAST Nicola Clare (nee Hands) 20/11/2002 (06/11/2008) 643 Bramford Road IPSWICH Suffolk IP1 5BD **Tel:** (01473) 742652 w 6265971

LAURIE Margaret 29/01/1999 1 Derwent View Park Head Estate Winlaton Tyne and Wear NE21 6LW **Tel:** (0191) 4144252 w 6138543

LAVELLE Roseanne 09/08/1983 32 Houstonfield Quadrant Houston Johnston Renfrewshire PA6 7EX **Tel:** (01505) 610181 w 6001086

LAWES Victoria Ann 04/09/1997 (24/08/2009) 60 Coastguard Cottages Beach Road Sea Palling Norwich NR12 0UH **Tel:** (01692) 598481 w 6041234

LAWRENCE Janet Louise (see DURRANT, Mrs)

LAWRENCE Marlies Ald (nee May) 03/09/1998 556 Bath Road Brislington Bristol Somerset BS4 3JZ **Tel:** (01179) 775911 w 6112478

LAWRENCE Sharon Louise (see ADAMS, Mrs)

LAWRIE Denise Elizabeth 23/09/2002 (09/01/2006) 297 Sandycombe Road Kew Richmond Surrey TW9 3LU **Tel:** (020) 8940 0014 w 6275717

LAWTON Sally Louisa (nee Shepherd) 03/09/1998 (22/02/2005) Barnsley Vets4Pets Limited 161 Wilthorpe Road Barnsley South Yorkshire S75 1JQ **Tel:** (01226) 289000 w 6128309

LAYFIELD Leann Marie (nee Cornock) 16/02/2000 (07/11/2005) 61 Primmers Place WESTBURY Wiltshire BA13 4QZ w 6190984

LAZENBY Gayl-Marie (see LAZENBY TRUBY, Mrs)

LAZENBY TRUBY Gayl-Marie (nee Lazenby) 19/01/1996 88 Garthdee Road ABERDEEN AB10 7AR **Tel:** (079) 899 65551 w 6033926

LE GUEN Brigitte Claire 15/02/2002 17 Windmill Rise Hundon Sudbury Suffolk CO10 8EQ **Tel:** (01440) 786270 w 6265124

LEACH Jessica Lucy 15/02/1999 (13/08/2007) Hope Manor Farmhouse Cutts Heath Road Milbury Heath Wotton under Edge Gloucestershire GL12 8PS **Tel:** (01454) 269339 w 6145776

Laura Suzanne Katherine 03/02/1999 Inside Pets at Home Colne View Retail Park Cowdray Avenue Colchester Essex CO1 1YN **Tel:** (01206) 771984 w 6139423

LEANEY Jane Nanette 01/04/2003 (20/11/2009) Garden Flat 17 St Andrews Rd Portslade East Sussex BN41 1DB **Tel:** (01273) 439320 w 6277719

LEANEY Nicola Marie (see HARRIS, Mrs)

LEANING Helen 21/08/1995 Southfield Veterinary Centre South Walks DORCHESTER Dorset DT1 1DU **Tel:** (01305) 262913 w 6033700

LEARY Sarah Jane 04/02/2002 9 Oak Drive Tewkesbury Gloucestershire GL20 8QN **Tel:** (01684) 295976 w 6264112

LEATHERBARROW Janet (see WOODCRAFT, Mrs)

LEATHERDALE Sandra Fay 31/07/1986 11-17 The Precinct West Meads Bognor Regis West Sussex PO21 5SB **Tel:** (01243) 842832 w 6054968

LEDGER David Jonathan 24/08/1999 Springfield Veterinary Group 39 Moorgate Road Rotherham South Yorkshire S60 2AD **Tel:** (01709) 377241 m 6026715

LEE Amanda Jane (nee Conway, formerly McBride) 06/02/1997 6 Hillside Mount Pudsey West Yorkshire LS28 9DQ **Tel:** (0113) 2577725 w 6026781

LEE Philippa Jane (see MCFARLING, Mrs)

Samantha Jayne 26/10/1999 124 Blackpool Old Road Poulton-le-Fylde Lancashire FY6 7RJ **Tel:** (01253) 885522 w 6030040

LEEDHAM Susan (see SHEPHERD, Mrs)

LEEDHAM-PAGE Susan (see SHEPHERD, Mrs)

LEETE Jayne Louise 06/09/1990 (05/10/2001) First Vets 39 Leighswood Road Walsall West Midlands WS9 8AH **Tel:** (01922) 451158 w 6055098

LEIVESLEY Rosalind Elaine 22/10/1977 (30/07/2007) Seafield Veterinary Group 144 Land Street Keith Banffshire AB55 5DL **Tel:** (01542) 882209 w 6055101

LENNOX Vanessa Dawn (nee Lennox, formerly Withers) 20/02/1996 (03/05/2007) 5 The Pantiles Queens Park Billericay Essex CM12 0UA **Tel:** (01277) 651009 w 6042894

LESIATOI Amanda Louise (nee Gracey) 20/02/1992 (06/01/2005) 36 Alpine Road Bristol Avon BS5 6BD w 605156X

LESLEY Tessa Marjorie Rose (nee Dean) 18/03/1981 (06/12/2004) Les Hautgard Les Hautgard Vale Guernsey Channel Islands GY3 5HZ w 6089174

LETCHFORD Vicki Jane 16/03/2001 (15/05/2008) 2 Hardknott Row WORCESTER WR4 0TD w 6202897

LETT Joanne Victoria 24/09/1999 32 Newmarket Road Fordham Ely Cambridgeshire CB7 5LL w 6186045

LEWIS Lisa Bronwen Fleur 17/01/2000 43 Clare Avenue DARLINGTON County Durham DL3 8SJ **Tel:** (01325) 362101 w 6190698

Pamela Jayne 01/03/2001 339 Upholland Road Billinge Wigan Lancashire WN5 7AJ **Tel:** (01695) 623165 w 6213424

Sandra Jayne 16/08/1982 184 Marley Fields Leighton Buzzard Bedfordshire LU7 4WN **Tel:** (01525) 385508 w 6055156

LIFELY Michelle Elizabeth (nee Dowsett) 28/10/1996 (13/07/2000) Passey Veterinary Surgery 24 Passey Place Eltham London SE9 5DQ **Tel:** (020) 8850 3206 w 6099080

LIGGINS Philippa Joanne (see CUNNINGHAM, Mrs)

LIGHTFOOT Vanessa Laura (see LAMPING, Mrs)

LILWALL Claire Ann 14/08/2002 (17/02/2009) 9 Leigh Street HEREFORD HR4 9PD **Tel:** (01432) 379498 w 6271218

LINDLEY Melissa Jane (see STUBBS, Mrs)

LINDLEY Sarah Louise DipAVN(Medical) (nee Carney) 26/03/2002 Unit A1 Priestley Road Wardley Business Park Worsley Manchester M28 2LY **Tel:** (0161) 794 4999 w 6249680

LINDSAY Vanessa Gail (see HODGKINS, Mrs)

LINE Kerry Jane (formerly Putnam) 14/01/1986 (25/09/2006) 10 Halsetown St. Ives Cornwall TR26 3NA **Tel:** (01736) 797569 w 6059208

LINES Marion Patricia DipAVN(Surgical) (formerly Johnson) 24/11/1997 99 Montpelier Gardens East Ham London E6 3JE w 6116122

LINES Maxime Patricia (see ALEXANDER, Mrs)

LING Edwina Margaret (see NORBURY, Mrs)

LING Vikki Louise 22/11/2000 Street Grove Farm Bruisyard Road Peasenhall Saxmundham Suffolk IP17 2HG **Tel:** (01728) 660209 w 6203216

LINGER Michelle Gillian (see ANDERSON, Mrs)

LINTON Gillian (nee Hunter) 22/02/2000 4 Station Court Pittenweem Fife KY10 2QY **Tel:** (01333) 312811 w 6144502

LISTER Sally Jane 23/08/1995 8 All Saints Walk Worlington Bury St. Edmunds Suffolk IP28 8SP **Tel:** (01638) 715 083 w 6030732

LITHGOW-MACLEAN Angela 03/02/1998 (14/05/2007) Weighbridge Referral Centre Kemys Way Swansea Enterprise Park Morriston Swansea SA6 8QF **Tel:** (01792) 796660 w 6024718

LITTLER Paula Jane 25/03/2002 9 Moor Royd Honley Holmfirth West Yorkshire HD9 6ES w 6277587

LIVETT Carol Charlotte 01/08/1989 40 Lon Conwy Benllech Tyn-y-Gongl Gwynedd LL74 8RP **Tel:** (01248) 853067 w 6055258

LLOYD Christine (see LOUGHRAN, Mrs)

LLOYD Heather Lorraine (formerly Geddis) 05/08/1980 108 Norton Road Stotfold Hitchin Hertfordshire SG5 4PG **Tel:** (01462) 733782 w 6051071

LLOYD Katie Louise (see MOORCROFT, Mrs)

Melita Dawn (formerly Godden) 28/07/1992 (30/01/2007) 19 Bryn Terrace Cwmdare Aberdare Mid Glamorgan CF44 8RB **Tel:** (01685) 883883 w 6002206

LLOYD-DAVIES Clare Alexandria 18/01/1999 68 St. Andrews Road COLWYN BAY Clwyd LL29 6DL **Tel:** (01492) 875634 w 6098462

LOACH Sally Ann (see WORTHING, Mrs)

LOADES Janet 23/08/2000 Parkside Veterinary Group 5 Kings Cross Road Dundee Angus DD2 3PT **Tel:** (01382) 810777 w 6202721

LOCKE Andrea Mary (see GOULD, Mrs)

LOCKE Tracey 02/02/2001 Kohat New Row Gonerby Hill Foot Grantham Lincolnshire NG31 8HJ w 6211939

LOCKETT Samantha Diane (nee Lowe, formerly Dainty) 29/09/1999 Shires Veterinary Practice Eccleshall Road Stone Staffordshire ST15 0HJ **Tel:** (01785) 813955 w 6133079

LODDO Elaine (nee Davis) 06/02/1991 Chestnut House Veterinary Centre Sutton Grange Saltshouse Road Hull HU8 9HL **Tel:** (01482) 787366 w 6048863

LODING Clair Anne 05/03/2002 79 Cranston Park Avenue Upminster Essex RM14 3XD **Tel:** (01708) 220890 w 6273231

LOFTUS Alison Ita 13/08/1987 (17/04/2003) Garden Flat 59 Talbot Road London N6 4QX **Tel:** (020) 77942612 w 6055316

LOGAN Clare Alison 05/09/1994 (04/01/2000) 130 Pyrles Lane Loughton Essex IG10 2NW w 6025256

Sharon 04/09/1979 (13/07/1999) Mole End 1 Marshalls Cottages Chappel Road Great Tey Colchester CO6 1JL **Tel:** (01206) 210652 w 6055327

Susan Elaine (formerly Black) 03/08/1989 (07/08/2008) 7 Maes Ffyddion Rhuddlan RHYL Clwyd LL18 2YE **Tel:** (01745) 591205 w 6000264

LOMAX Karen (see BLAGG, Mrs)

LONG Natalie Jane 26/01/2000 15 Craiglands Jersey Farm St. Albans Hertfordshire AL4 9AH **Tel:** (01727) 759 283 w 6190940

LONGDON Caroline 04/09/1997 34 Keswick Drive Lake View Northampton NN3 6NZ **Tel:** (01604) 462926 w 6118083

LONGHURST Kim Lorraine (nee White) 05/10/1992 (11/09/2008) 56 Attlee Drive Dartford KENT DA1 5DE **Tel:** (01322) 221397 w 601200X

LONGTHORPE Julie Lesley (nee Smith) 27/08/1996 PDSA Hepton Court York Road Leeds West Yorkshire LS9 6PW **Tel:** (0113) 240 8818 w 6098702

LONSDALE Sarah Jane 17/09/1996 (28/01/2004) 21 Goldings Road LOUGHTON Essex IG10 2QR w 6099739

LOOKER Rachel Clare (see BEADSWORTH, Mrs)

LOUGHRAN Christine (nee Lloyd) 24/08/1994 345 Aigburth Road Liverpool Merseyside L17 0BL **Tel:** (0151) 728 7676 w 6037090

LOVERIDGE Gemma (nee Dixon) 23/01/2003 The Veterinary Hospital Colwill Road Estover Plymouth Devon PL6 8RP **Tel:** (01752) 702646 w 6267225

LOWE Samantha Diane (see LOCKETT, Mrs)

LOWE Sarah Louise (see WEST, Mrs)

LOWNSBROUGH Jill Louise (formerly Broadbridge) 19/02/1996 (07/10/1998) 4 Harlea Avenue Hindley Green Wigan Lancashire WN2 4SL **Tel:** (01942) 256280 w 6036610

LOWRY Rebecca (see GILES, Mrs)

LUCAS Luan Emily (see HODGETTS, Mrs)

LUCK Miranda Ann Nicola 20/09/1995 (07/07/2008) Hale Cottage Cricketers Close Ockley DORKING Surrey RH5 5BA **Tel:** (01306) 627855 w 6030131

LUMBRERAS Maria Carmen 01/09/1999 (14/01/2010) 24 Homefield Park SUTTON Surrey SM1 2AN w 6185594

LUMLEY Alison Claire 24/02/2000 The Ardmore Veterinary Group 57 Cornard Road Sudbury Suffolk CO10 2XB **Tel:** (01787) 372588 w 6191193

LUNN Andrea Samantha (see BANHAM, Mrs)

LUPTON Melloney Jane (see NICHOLLS, Miss)

LYNCH Gemma Anne (see STUCKEY, Mrs)

LYNCH Tracy (see HAINES, Mrs)

LYON Joanna (see KOMOROCZY, Mrs)

LYONS Dianne Patricia 26/08/1969 69 Lower Anchor Street Chelmsford CM2 0AU **Tel:** (01245) 350012 w 6055520

Jane Margaret 14/01/1982 (21/06/2006) 12 Chapel Hay Lane Churchdown Gloucester Gloucestershire GL3 2ET **Tel:** (01452) 854 458 w 606319X

M

MACDONALD Diane DipAVN(Medical) 01/11/1984 31 Fifth Street Newtongrange DALKEITH Midlothian EH22 4PH **Tel:** (0131) 650 7650 w 6055553

Helen Jane 16/01/1994 Clockhouse Veterinary Hospital Wallbridge Stroud Gloucestershire GL5 3JD **Tel:** (01453) 752555 w 6067208

MACE Alison Jane (nee Blackall) 18/01/1995 (24/07/2000) 10 Pavenham Close Lower Earley Reading Berkshire RG6 4DX **Tel:** (0118) 9861715 w 6034737

MACEY Michelle Marie (see MACEY-RICHARDSON, Mrs)

MACEY-RICHARDSON Michelle Marie (nee Macey) 01/03/2001 Cliffe Veterinary Group 21 Cliffe High Street Lewes East Sussex BN7 2AH **Tel:** (01273) 473232 w 6213435

MACFADYEN Carol (see SELLARS, Mrs)

MACFADYEN Elizabeth Christine Mary 07/03/1973 25 High Street Roade Northampton NN7 2NW **Tel:** (01604) 863672 w 6055586

MACGILLIVRAY Janice Elizabeth DipAVN(Surgical) 01/02/1972 The Aviaries Alyth Road Old Rattray Blairgowrie Perthshire PH10 7DY **Tel:** (01250) 876051 w 6055597

MACGILLIVRAY Kirsty (see YOUNG, Mrs)

MACINTOSH Heather Anne 24/12/2002 2 Castleblair Mews Dunfermline Fife KY12 9DZ w 6282251

MACKENZIE Caroline 04/09/1997 (19/01/2010) c/o Mr C Mackenzie 6 Langlands Terrace Kyle of Lochalsh Ross-Shire IV40 8AW **Tel:** (01599) 530259 w 6043570

MACLEAN Nina Louise (nee Kendall) 31/08/1994 16 Keysland Thundersley Essex SS7 3TW **Tel:** (01268) 771857 w 6024773

MACLEOD Allison (see SMITH, Miss)

MACNEE Lorna Ruth 30/08/2001 (06/04/2009) Heureux Ville Au Roi St. Peter Port GUERNSEY GY1 1NZ **Tel:** (01481) 722545 w 6205130

MACWILLIAMS Fiona (see WILSON, Mrs)

MAFFITT Tracy Lynn (formerly Vance) 14/01/1982 34 Eastbourne Road Aintree Liverpool L9 0JF **Tel:** (0151) 474 5655 w 6062673

MAGO Anjali 13/12/2002 Flat 29, Roberts Court 45 Barkston Gardens LONDON SW5 0ES **Tel:** (020) 73706822 w 6327153

MAIDEN Elaine Marie (nee Evans) 03/09/1993 (26/01/2004) 13 Pearsons Terrace HEXHAM Northumberland NE46 3DZ w 6026726

MAINWARING Lynne Marie (see PARKINSON, Mrs)

MALE Lisa Corinne (nee Webb) 10/08/1984 164 Rugby Road Binley Woods Coventry WARWICKSHIRE CV3 2AZ **Tel:** (02476) 545503 w 6063382

MALLUL Susan Ellen (nee Coppin) 31/01/1992 46 Fairby Road LONDON SE12 8JR **Tel:** (0208) 8525721 w 6048193

MALTBY June Gillian (nee Crook) 22/12/1976 (15/03/2007) 47 Yapton Road Barnham Bognor Regis West Sussex PO22 0AX **Tel:** (01243) 555656 w 6055713

MALTWOOD Bonnie Jayne (see SIMMONS, Mrs)

MANGLES Fiona Onycha Smithies (see HILL, Mrs)

MANN Alia-Dawn Svanhvit 24/01/2000 14 Hilfield Yateley Hampshire GU46 6XP **Tel:** (01252) 877741 w 6184670

Alison 01/10/1999 94 Southroyd Park Pudsey West Yorkshire LS28 8AX **Tel:** (0113) 2109473 w 6116268

Lisa Marie 10/05/2001 (23/05/2003) 11 Noden Drive Lea Ross-on-Wye Herefordshire HR9 7NB **Tel:** (01989) 750542 w 6202468

MANN Melanie (see ABLA, Mrs)

MANNING Amelia Jane 15/11/2001 (01/06/2009) 29 Burnside Street Allaston DERBY Derbyshire DE24 8QT w 6204503

MANT Sonia Dawn 24/02/1995 Greengates Lyng Easthaugh Lyng Norwich NORFOLK NR9 5LN **Tel:** 01603879483 w 603193X

MARCHANT Angela (see STAFFORD, Mrs)

MARCHANT Cherie Louise 24/09/2001 33 Tower Road South, Warmley Bristol Avon BS30 8BL **Tel:** (07971) 804217 w 6228615

MARDELL Janet Mary Sinclair (nee Fearnhead) 13/12/2001 (16/12/2009) Little Frogmore Farm Warninglid Lane Plummers Plain HORSHAM West Sussex RH13 6NY **Tel:** (01403) 891172 w 6256962

MARINER Lia Jean 13/09/2000 (05/11/2004) 21 Hillfield Road Selsey Chichester West Sussex PO20 0LB **Tel:** (01243) 602635 w 6203579

MARLEY Daniel Joseph 24/01/1997 Forge House Llangattock Crickhowell Powys NP8 1LD m 6108756

MARMO Maria Letitia Christine 01/03/1994 (02/11/2009) 19 Swan Cottages Wittersham TENTERDEN Kent TN30 7PA **Tel:** (01797) 270568 w 6026023

MARMOT Helen Jayne 15/11/2001 49 Whittington Close Hythe Southampton SO45 5EZ **Tel:** (023) 80847781 w 6262121

MARNER Rachael Michelle (see KEEP, Mrs)

MARRIOTT Geraldine Ann (nee Crisp) 07/09/1978 (29/07/2003) Three Ways Mansfield Road Blidworth Mansfield Nottinghamshire NG21 0LR **Tel:** (01623) 796778 w 6055804

MARRISON Marina Lesley 25/08/1995 (21/02/2001) Grove Lodge Veterinary Group Ltd 18 Upper Brighton Road Worthing West Sussex BN14 9DL **Tel:** (01903) 234866 w 6034453

MARRON Sheelagh 14/01/1988 58 Winnock Road Colchester CO1 2BJ **Tel:** (01206) 797739 w 6002975

MARSAN Jennifer Kate (see MARSAN-STOTT, Mrs)

MARSAN-STOTT Jennifer Kate (nee Marsan) 24/12/2002 (10/12/2009) 60 Broadmeadow View TEIGNMOUTH Devon TQ14 9BS **Tel:** (01626) 774454 w 6269777

MARSDEN Penelope Jane 04/02/1994 8 Warton Avenue Bierley BRADFORD West Yorkshire BD4 6JG w 6067580

Sarah Jane Elizabeth 24/01/2000 4 The Hawthorns Bluntisham HUNTINGDON Cambridgeshire PE28 3XL **Tel:** (01487) 843393 w 6148904

MARSH Gay Davina 11/11/1994 149 West End March Cambridgeshire PE15 8DE **Tel:** (01354) 651875 w 6037498

MARSHALL Kelly Diane 24/01/2001 15 Bridle Road Bromborough Wirral Merseyside CH62 6AP **Tel:** (0151) 2001599 w 6205779

Rosina Mary 04/08/1981 30 Hall Carr Lane Longton Preston Lancashire PR4 5JJ **Tel:** (01772) 616676 w 6055870

MARTIN Joanna Frances 04/08/1989 33 Broadley Green Windlesham Surrey GU20 6AJ **Tel:** (01276) 472618 w 605594X

Lisa (nee Dawson) 07/08/1991 5 Hawfield Grove Sutton Coldfield West Midlands B72 1YD **Tel:** (0121) 373 3299 w 6048921

Rebecca Joanne (nee Tuffs) 24/09/1999 North Lindsey College Kingsway SCUNTHORPE South Humberside DN17 1AJ **Tel:** (01724) 294197 w 6186419

Tina Paulette 01/09/1995 7 Mount Gardens St. Davids Haverfordwest Pembrokeshire SA62 6BS **Tel:** (01437) 720465 w 6031871

MARTYNIUK Karen Lynn (nee Gray) 10/09/1999 50 Makbrar Road Dumfries Dumfriesshire DG1 4BA **Tel:** (01387) 248226 w 6185363

MARYINDALE Judith Ann (see HUTCHINSON, Mrs)

MASON Donna Marie (see MASON-NEWMAN, Mrs)

MASON Elizabeth Sophie 18/09/1998 (13/03/2003) 9 Northfield Road Blaby LEICESTER LE8 4GU **Tel:** (0116) 2771602 w 6131093

MASON-NEWMAN Donna Marie (nee Mason) 01/11/2000 31 Foxes Rake CANNOCK Staffordshire WS11 5UD w 6204723

MASSON Helen Jean (see CAVANAGH, Mrs)

MASTERS Alison Jayne 29/12/1983 The Valley Veterinary Group Tutts Clump Bradfield READING RG7 6JU **Tel:** (0118) 9744352 w 6089764

Sharon Ann DipAVN(Surgical) 01/03/1984 89 Willow Street Romford ESSEX RM7 7JH **Tel:** (01708) 721554 w 6013615

MATCHAM Marie Elaine (see FOORD, Mrs)

MATHESON Julie Mary (see ILLSLEY, Mrs)

MATHEW Catherine Melanie 03/11/2000 67 Main Street Wheldrake YORK YO19 6AB w 6205614

MATHEWS Barbara Elizabeth (see CROMEY, Mrs)

MATOS Pamela Ellen 13/02/1985 (06/04/2009) 35 Alexander Street Bayswater London W2 5NU **Tel:** (020) 7229 2040 w 6001213

MATTHEWS Emma Jayne (nee Gibbs) 03/09/1998 Walton Lodge Veterinary Group 101 North Road Poole Dorset BH14 0LT **Tel:** (01202) 747678 w 610799X

Joanna 18/12/1986 (10/11/2003) 9 Elm Tree Lane Leavenheath Colchester Essex CO6 4UL **Tel:** (01206) 262991 w 6056036

MATTHIAS Amanda Jayne (see MOYLE, Mrs)

MAY Brian Kieron 22/08/2000 11 St. Clements Crescent Wallyford Musselburgh Midlothian EH21 8BB **Tel:** (0131) 6533705 m 6203865

Jane Sharon (nee Anderson) 09/01/1989 33 Norries Drive Wallingford Oxfordshire OX10 8JT **Tel:** (01491) 839970 w 6000038

Karen Sheila 27/07/1979 Hill House Cottage Hillhouse Lane Sadberge Darlington County Durham DL2 1SL **Tel:** (01325) 332226 w 6056080

Katharine Patricia 05/04/2005 (23/06/2009) 21 Bourne Road Godalming Surrey GU7 3NL **Tel:** (01483) 417647 w 6329760

MAY Marlies Ald (see LAWRENCE, Mrs)

MAYES Susan Pauline (see FISHER, Mrs)

MAYNARD Sally (nee Paremain) 16/02/2000 54 Claydon Road Horsell Surrey GU21 4XE **Tel:** (07769) 710537 w 6134775

MCADAM Christine Ann (see WRIGHT, Mrs)

MCALLISTER Lucy Jane DipAVN(Surgical) 17/08/1995 64a Hampton Road TWICKENHAM TW2 5QB w 6037749

MCBETH Kathleen Caroline Lindsay 01/10/1971 Aigaiou Pelagous 46 15341 Ag. Paraskeui Attikis Greece **Tel:** (00302) 06082830 w 601278X

MCBRIDE Amanda Jane (see LEE, Mrs)

Sarah Elizabeth 21/08/1998 (08/12/2008) 11 Low Row North Bitchburn CROOK County Durham DL15 8AJ w 612217X

MCCABE Helen Rosalind 09/08/1983 (27/02/2002) Moor Cottage Veterinary Hospital London Road Binfield Bracknell Berkshire RG42 4AA **Tel:** (01344) 450345 w 6056116

MCCANN Fiona Jane (see DICKINSON, Mrs)

MCCARTNEY Zoe Justine 28/06/2002 (13/04/2007) 15 North Way Hyde Cheshire SK14 1RU **Tel:** (0161) 3511509 w 6140632

MCCLURE Karen Louisa 24/08/1990 (15/01/2008) 30 Main Street New Abbey DUMFRIES DG2 8BY **Tel:** (01387) 850544 w 6001304

MCCLURE Lynne (see DICKOV, Mrs)

MCCOLGAN Rosemary Patricia 31/08/2000 23 Carricklynn Avenue Strabane County Tyrone BT82 9BF **Tel:** (02871) 886038 w 6032886

MCCOMB Pamela Crawford DipAVN(Surgical) (nee Gillan) 19/01/1987 University of Glasgow Veterinary School Garscube Estate Glasgow G61 1QH **Tel:** (0141) 330 5848 w 6051275

MCCONNELL Michelle (nee Gilmer) 09/08/1991 (22/02/2007) 47 Loughries Road Newtownards Co Down BT23 8RW **Tel:** (02891) 811568 w 6051300

MCCORMICK Senga Victoria (see COULTER, Mrs)

MCCULLEY Judith Lesley 22/07/1993 (26/11/2008) 35 Northfield Duffus Elgin Morayshire IV30 5RW w 6015328

MCDIARMID-BRANCH Sarah (formerly Talbott, nee Branch) 23/12/1992 51 Main Road Dyke Bourne Lincolnshire PE10 0AF **Tel:** (01778) 393640 w 606511X

MCDONALD Helen Patricia 31/01/1995 (05/11/2004) 85 Cross Road MALDON Essex CM9 5ED **Tel:** (01621) 855069 w 6037159

Lyn Sharon 29/08/1995 (29/01/2002) Weipers Centre Equine Hospital University of Glasgow Faculty of Veterinary Medicine 464 Bearsden Road Bearsden Glasgow G61 1QH **Tel:** (0141) 330 5999 w 6035548

Susan Anne 26/07/1988 (20/05/2009) 'Karibu' 6 Chippenham Road Corston Malmesbury Wiltshire SN16 0HQ **Tel:** (01666) 826618 w 6056251

MCDOWELL Elaine Anne (formerly Pearson) 17/08/1990 35 St. Martins Green Trimley St. Martin FELIXSTOWE Suffolk IP11 0UW w 605850X

Marie Louise 05/11/1982 The Shed Pickering Forest Celbridge Co Kildare Ireland w 6056284

MCELREA Alison Grierson (nee Nicol) 01/03/2001 Back Rogerton Farm Auchinleck Cumnock Ayrshire KA18 2ND **Tel:** (01290) 420310 w 6133432

MCFADYEN Fiona Anne DipAVN(Surgical) 26/01/1998 PDSA PetAid Hospital Stoneygate Lane Felling Gateshead Tyne & Wear NE10 0LX **Tel:** (0191) 4382881 w 6108723

MCFARLING Philippa Jane (nee Lee) 01/08/1986 (03/03/2006) Fish Farm House Main Road Itchen Abbas Winchester Hampshire SO21 1BQ **Tel:** (01962) 779 248 w 6055010

MCGAW Kristina 18/07/2002 (03/06/2009) 131a Frimley Road CAMBERLEY Surrey GU15 2PS **Tel:** (01276) 22414 w 6316637

MCGEE Sarah Jane (see CARTER, Mrs)

MCGINN Diane (see MCKAY, Mrs)

MCGOWAN Agata 11/09/1997 27 Skeaping Close NEWMARKET Suffolk CB8 0GP w 611812X

MCGRAND Elizabeth Anita (see MORGAN, Mrs)

MCGRATH Alison Jane (formerly Kelly) 12/01/2001 T A Grinter 61 Molesworth Road Stoke Plymouth PL1 5PF **Tel:** (01752) 562575 w 6204888

MCGUIGAN Eliza Sarah Rhiannon 02/07/2001 Park Veterinary Centre 256 Cassiobury Drive WATFORD Hertfordshire WD17 3PA **Tel:** (01923) 223321 w 6205284

MCGUINNESS Jayne Elizabeth 15/02/2002 Lancaster Farm Burned House Lane Preesall Poulton-le-Fylde Lancashire FY6 0PQ **Tel:** (0773) 441 3336 w 6270723

MCHALE Lara Mary (nee Prince) 30/01/1998 Calder Veterinary Group/Calder Vets Savile Road Dewsbury West Yorkshire WF12 9LN **Tel:** (01924) 465592 w 6116461

MCINTOSH Sheila 19/03/1980 (06/04/2009) Easter Bush Veterinary Centre University of Edinburgh Easter Bush Roslin Midlothian EH25 9RG **Tel:** (0131) 650 7650 w 6056397

MCKAY Diane (nee McGinn) 03/09/1996 66 Ribadoo Road Leitrim Castlewellan County Down BT31 9SY **Tel:** (0284) 377 8749 w 6042704

MCKEAG Nicola Louise (nee Swan) 30/08/1994 Cromlyn House Veterinary Hospital 50 Old Coach Road Hillsborough County Down BT26 6PB **Tel:** (02892) 683711 w 602975X

MCKEANE Amanda Jane DipAVN(Surgical) 24/09/2001 (05/05/2004) 11 Cloverfield Drive Soham Ely Cambridgeshire CB7 5FT **Tel:** (01353) 725180 w 6228626

MCKENZIE Laura (see KEMP, Mrs)

MCKENZIE Susan Claire 13/01/1999 25 Hailey Place Cranleigh Surrey GU6 7EG **Tel:** (01483) 277956 w 613471X

MCKNIGHT Yvonne 15/02/2002 24 St. Margaret Street Dunfermline Fife KY12 7PE **Tel:** (01383) 732897 w 6253464

MCLAUGHLIN Elaine 30/01/1996 (23/03/2009) 5 Chatham Road Gorton MANCHESTER M18 7JG **Tel:** (0161) 371 2954 w 603054X

MCLEAN Susan Alison (nee Young) 21/08/1991 (19/03/2002) 1478 Pollokshaws Road Glasgow G43 1RN **Tel:** (0141) 649 5471 w 6064455

MCLELLAN Angela (nee Gordon) 31/08/1999 13 Bughtknowes Drive Bathgate West Lothian EH48 4DP **Tel:** (01501) 740958 w 610801X

MCMANN Claire June (see MILLINGTON, Mrs)

MCMORRAN Julie Clare (formerly Johnson) 16/08/1989 77 Moffat Road Dumfries Dumfriesshire DG1 1PB **Tel:** (01387) 279510 w 6054006

MCMULDROW Kim Annette 30/03/1976 (18/07/2007) 301 York Road SHREWSBURY SY1 3QA **Tel:** (01743) 367586 w 6056488

MCNAMARA Elaine Bridget Ann DipAVN(Surgical) 09/09/1996 (30/01/2002) 3 Moat Lane Abbots Ripton Huntingdon Cambridgeshire PE28 2PD **Tel:** (01487) 773201 w 6108745

Julie Louise (nee Burnett) 23/10/2000 38 Parsons Close PLYMOUTH PL9 9UY w 6190467

MCNAY Helen Fiona 05/02/1992 Hamilton House Throughgate Dunscore DUMFRIES DG2 0UG **Tel:** (07718) 020230 w 6056524

MCNEELY Sarah (nee Booker) 17/09/1998 (17/04/2003) 5 St. Johns Road Kirkheaton Huddersfield West Yorkshire HD5 0NE **Tel:** (01484) 306850 w 6128910

MCNICOL Bonnie (see THOMAS, Mrs)

MCPHERSON Valerie Nancy 28/10/1977 (02/02/2000) Clovelly Brookfield Drive Hoveringham Nottingham NG14 7JW **Tel:** (01159) 664130 w 6056535

MCTAGGART Leann Jane 12/04/2001 256 New Road Croxley Green RICKMANSWORTH Hertfordshire WD3 3HH **Tel:** (01923) 721417 w 6202413

MCVICAR Sarah Jayne 13/10/2000 Lower Place Veterinary Centre 455 Oldham Road Rochdale Lancashire OL16 4TD **Tel:** (01706) 713380 w 6134141

MCWHIRTER Joan Margaret (nee Coleman) 19/08/1968 (30/11/2000) 28 Ivy Road Leicester LE3 0DF **Tel:** (0116) 2541505 w 6056579

MEAD Susan Elizabeth (see GODFREY, Mrs)

MEE Kay 20/08/1999 16 Fleming Close ROCHDALE Lancashire OL12 9RL **Tel:** (01706) 373268 w 6041405

Marie Paula (nee Theaker) 09/01/1989 Ambivet Veterinary Group 24 Mundy Street HEANOR Derbyshire DE75 7EB **Tel:** (01773) 717780 w 6061920

MEIGH Sharron Elizabeth 12/05/1971 (20/11/2003) 2 The Buckleys Alvechurch Birmingham B48 7NF **Tel:** (0121) 445 3487 w 6056659

MEMBRY Kelly Irene 15/11/2001 (23/05/2003) 27 Adhurst Road Havant Hampshire PO9 2HP **Tel:** (01243) 841111 w 6270195

MEPHAM Claire Louise 23/01/1998 18 Winterbourne Close Lewes East Sussex BN7 1JY w 6131140

MERCADO Joanne Louise DipAVN(Medical) (nee Carrick) 17/01/2000 The Oxford Cat Clinic 78a West Way OXFORD OX2 9JU w 612938X

MEREDITH Danielle Elizabeth (nee Emms) 27/01/1992 (13/11/2007) 14 Exon Street Walworth LONDON SE17 2JW w 6049889

MERRIN Samantha Louise 14/01/2000 15 Ashby Court READING Berkshire RG2 8PG w 6030776

MERRITT Karin Anne 06/08/1991 Cambridge Veterinary Group Ltd 89a Cherryhinton Road Cambridge Cambridgeshire CB1 7BS **Tel:** (01223) 249331 w 6056692

MESSENGER Kate Victoria 31/01/2000 (14/10/2005) The Flat Amery Hill Veterinary Hospital Amery Hill ALTON Hampshire GU34 1HS **Tel:** (01420) 489777 w 6128455

MICKLEBURGH Suzanne Mary 23/01/1991 (06/11/2008) Tall Trees Hartwith Bank Summerbridge Harrogate North Yorkshire HG3 4HY **Tel:** (01423) 781105 w 6056717

MIDDLETON Angela Jane (nee Prime) 29/08/1986 21 The Limes Sawston Cambridge CB2 4DH **Tel:** (01223) 562265 w 6056739

Angela Sheila 18/01/2000 Petmedics Memorial Road Walkden Manchester M28 3DS **Tel:** (0161) 799 2299 w 6134516

Joyce Daphne 15/09/1972 114 Dulwich Road Holland-on-Sea Clacton-on-Sea Essex CO15 5LU **Tel:** (01255) 812397 w 6061090

MILBURN Deborah Anne (see PAISLEY, Mrs)

MILES Annabel Clare 21/09/1984 Rickney Farm Rickney Hailsham East Sussex BN27 1SF **Tel:** (01323) 763063 w 6056783

MILES Claire Emma (see KIRBYSHIRE, Mrs)

MILES Lyn (see CHANT, Mrs)

MILLAR Jane Auld (see FURNESS, Mrs)

MILLARD Philippa Alison (nee Gent) 09/09/1996 (29/05/2001) Woodlands Veterinary Clinic Salisbury Avenue Warden Hill Cheltenham Gloucestershire GL51 3GA **Tel:** (01242) 255133 w 6034624

MILLARD Samantha Jayne (see ANDERSON, Mrs)

MILLER Helen Louise 08/09/2005 (25/06/2009) 30 Burgundy Gardens BASILDON Essex SS13 1NP **Tel:** (01268) 449171 w 6321004

MILLETT Claire Marie (see PERKINS, Mrs)

MILLIGAN Nicola 10/03/1994 (17/01/2003) Manor Veterinary Centre 113-119 Kent Road Halesowen West Midlands B62 8PB **Tel:** (0121) 422 5411 w 6018442

MILLINGTON Claire June (nee McMann) 15/01/1998 20 Brunswick Avenue Waterloo Street Hull HU2 9AY **Tel:** (01482) 224452 w 6112274

Clare Harriet 08/08/1991 (21/01/2008) 11 Snelgate Cottages Epsom Road East Clandon Guildford Surrey GU4 7RL **Tel:** (01483) 211082 w 6001337

MILLS Claire Joanne (see WALKER, Mrs)

MILLS Connie Borre (nee Rasmussen) 01/02/1994 Blacksmith Cottage Blacksmith Road Fiskerton LINCOLN LN3 4HE **Tel:** (01522) 754180 w 6067616

Lisa 07/08/1987 (13/01/2003) 9 The Crescent Dunscroft Doncaster South Yorkshire DN7 4ER **Tel:** (01302) 843209 w 605682X

Sandra Jane 28/08/1991 (20/05/2002) Belmont Veterinary Centre 94 Belmont Road Hereford HR2 7JS **Tel:** (01432) 370155 w 6056830

MILLWARD Deborah (nee Bradshaw) 09/11/1983 42 Main Road Asfordby Valley Melton Mowbray Leicestershire LE14 3SW **Tel:** (01664) 812882 w 6046119

MILSOM Jasmine 21/09/1971 Milton Keynes Veterinary Group Fyfield Barrow Walnut Tree Milton Keynes MK7 7AN w 6056852

MINARDS Mary Elizabeth 28/08/1980 The Flat 10 Peverell Park Road Plymouth Devon PL3 4NA **Tel:** (01752) 662312 w 6056863

MINOR Deborah (nee Wardrobe) 01/09/1998 Bridgefield Veterinary Surgery Central Carpark Wem Shropshire SY4 5AA **Tel:** (01939) 232291 w 6137743

MINSHALL Amanda 02/08/1978 Springfield Veterinary Group 39 Moorgate Road Rotherham South Yorkshire S60 2AD **Tel:** (01709) 377241 w 6056874

MITCHARD Louisa Kate 28/08/1996 (05/11/2004) University of Bristol School of Veterinary Nursing Veterinary Nursing Unit Langford House Langford Somerset BS40 5DU **Tel:** (0117) 928 9517 w 6039859

MITCHELL Gabrielle Angharad (see HUGHES, Mrs)

MITCHELL Helen Kimberley (nee Hogg) 03/02/1997 23 Birkdale Drive The Fair Ways Shiney Row Houghton le Spring Tyne and Wear DH4 4QH **Tel:** (0191) 385 6661 w 6035537

MITCHINSON Jill Frances 03/08/1988 (12/02/2008) Value Vets 304 Vicarage Road Kings Heath Birmingham B14 7NH **Tel:** (0121) 444 4154 w 6056943

Joanne 03/02/1992 (12/03/2004) 2 Picton Grove Liverpool Merseyside L15 1HL **Tel:** (0151) 7345939 w 6056932

MITTENS Heidi Maria 06/03/2001 615 Wells Road Whitchurch Bristol BS14 9BE **Tel:** (01275) 832410 w 6122169

MITTON Desiree Theodora 10/01/2001 1-5 Hugh Street London SW1V 1QQ **Tel:** (020) 7932 2370 w 6204195

MIZON Katie Emma 06/02/1998 (15/08/2007) Helston Edward Road Devizes Wiltshire SN10 5AR w 6118163

MOAR Sharon Ann (see SCOTT, Mrs)

MOIZER Clare Louise 26/02/1997 Ashleigh Veterinary Centre 221 Upper Chorlton Road Manchester Greater Manchester M16 0DE **Tel:** (0161) 881 6868 w 609851X

MOLLOY Helena Louise 26/01/2000 7 Lodge Farm Elvetham HOOK Hampshire RG27 8AS w 6190412

MOLONEY Elaine 06/01/1989 34 Commercial Street Crook County Durham DL15 9HR **Tel:** (01388) 763743 w 6050624

MONSEY Louise Margaret 02/03/2001 Arbury Road Veterinary Surgery 32 Arbury Road Cambridge CB4 2JE **Tel:** (01223) 361911 w 6213589

MONTGOMERY Katie Elizabeth (see FRY, Mrs)

MOODY Joanne Roma 10/01/2003 (16/01/2009) 8 Chapel Street Adlington Chorley Lancashire PR7 4JL **Tel:** (01257) 475276 w 6261043

MOODY Laura-Anne (see WEBB, Mrs)

MOODY Susan Carole 05/03/1999 St Johns Veterinary Surgery 320a High Street Berkhamsted Hertfordshire HP4 1HT **Tel:** (01442) 863101 w 6134571

MOON Marian Judith (nee Hampton) 06/08/1991 Cobblestone Mews Broomhill Road Speldhurst Tunbridge Wells Kent TN3 0TD **Tel:** (01892) 864963 w 6052202

MOORCROFT Katie Louise (nee Lloyd) 19/01/1998 (23/06/2006) Vets Now (Coventry) 34 Barker Butts Lane Coundon Coventry West Midlands CV6 1DT **Tel:** (02476) 595354 w 604364X

MOORE Alison Clare (see TURNER, Mrs)

MOORE Denise Lynne 17/08/1979 156 Moorings Way SOUTHSEA Hampshire PO4 8YN w 605703X

Karen Elizabeth 11/01/2001 (17/04/2003) Rontgen Avdeling bygg 11 Norges Veterinaerhogskole Ullevalsveien 72 Pb 8146, Dep 0033 0454 Oslo Norway w 6205801

Lynette Clair 20/09/1999 (29/12/2004) 1 Speedwell Close LUTON LU3 4AF w 6134414

Margaret Clare 04/08/1977 Yewgate Cottage Remenham Hill Remenham Henley-on-Thames Oxfordshire RG9 3ES **Tel:** (01491) 414113 w 6002308

Michelle 17/08/1979 26 Market Place Bridlington East Yorkshire YO16 4QL **Tel:** (01262) 679278 w 6057084

MORAN Avril Adele 25/09/2000 68 Maple Avenue Talke STOKE-ON-TRENT ST7 1JW **Tel:** (01782) 774987 w 6203458

MORBEY Lucy Helen 22/08/1994 De Montfort Veterinary Hospital 44 Merstow Green Evesham Worcestershire WR11 4BH **Tel:** (01386) 446095 w 602940X

MORGAN Elizabeth Anita (formerly McGrand, formerly Winkworth) 20/04/1999 (11/09/2006) Gardeners Cottage Kimmeridge Wareham Dorset BH20 5PD **Tel:** (01929) 480 715 w 6144499

Sally (nee Hodgson) 06/09/1999 Hillview 4 The College Marsh Gibbon Bicester Oxfordshire OX27 0HW **Tel:** (01869) 278 208 w 6185396

Sally Ann 15/09/1997 38 Chilwell Gardens South Oxhey Watford Hertfordshire WD19 6NA **Tel:** (0208) 4284326 w 6099863

Wendy Anne (nee Hall) 20/02/1981 18 Overstone Drive Coldham Wisbech Cambridgeshire PE14 0NG **Tel:** (01945) 860587 w 6052100

MORGANS Jacqueline 11/02/1998 The Animal Hospital Stinchcombe Dursley Gloucestershire GL11 6AJ **Tel:** (01453) 542092 w 6041460

MORRIS Caroline Anne (see RICHARDSON, Mrs)

MORRIS Eleanor Jane (nee Morris) 12/08/1991 1 Roman Way Stretton Sugwas Hereford Herefordshire HR4 7AG **Tel:** (01432) 760767 w 6057200

Imogen Elizabeth 10/09/1999 (12/12/2002) Fir Trees Beechfield Lane Frilsham Hermitage THATCHAM Berkshire RG18 9XD w 613746X

MORRIS Louise Marie (see ANTHONY, Mrs)

Sharon (nee Lane) 18/01/1999 33 Ffordd Allt-wen Gowerton SWANSEA SA4 3HG w 6134935

MORRISON Charlotte Ina May (nee Collings) 09/09/1996 Christchurch Veterinary Surgery 49 Christchurch Street Ipswich Suffolk IP4 2DF **Tel:** (01473) 255789 w 603978X

Leanne 30/03/2001 (06/01/2005) 5 Oakbank Crescent Perth PH1 1DD w 6214623

Victoria Louise (nee Prince) 24/01/1994 (21/04/2009) 87 Watford Road Cotteridge Birmingham B30 1NP **Tel:** (0121) 459 4333 w 6066179

MORSE Nicola Jane (see JONES, Mrs)

MOSS Sarah Louise DipAVN(Surgical) (nee Capon) 03/08/1988 (27/03/2001) Christchurch Veterinary Surgery 49 Christchurch Street Ipswich Suffolk IP4 2DF **Tel:** (01473) 255789 w 604727X

MOTTRAM Joanne (see TELFORD, Mrs)

MOULDING Elizabeth (nee Edmondson) 27/07/1979 (19/02/2001) 5 Hambledon Terrace Higham Burnley Lancashire BB12 9BN **Tel:** (01282) 866005 w 6014346

MOYE Jennifer Leigh (nee Godfrey) 08/09/1995 (18/09/2006) Rosemullion Veterinary Hospital 66 Melvill Road Falmouth Cornwall TR11 4DD **Tel:** (01326) 313991 w 6039065

MOYLE Amanda Jayne (nee Matthias) 17/01/1996 (12/05/2005) 23 Highertown Highertown Truro Cornwall TR1 3QE **Tel:** (01872) 273408 w 6035559

Rachel Elizabeth (nee Blamire) 25/08/1999 The Lodge 42 High Seaton Workington Cumbria CA14 1LJ w 6145346

MUDGE Anne Margaret (nee Gardiner) 06/01/1993 7 Church Lane Kingston Lewes East Sussex BN7 3LN w 6066441

MULHOLLAND Caroline (see RUSTAGE, Mrs)

MULLEN Jennifer (nee Wason) 05/03/2002 29 Hannahston Avenue Drongan Ayr Ayrshire KA6 7AX **Tel:** (01292) 591950 w 6264343

MULLENDER Mary Teresa (formerly Chamberlain) 12/12/1991 456-458 Hagley Road West Oldbury West Midlands B68 0DL **Tel:** (0121) 422 2902 w 6047462

MULLEY Natasha Elisabeth (nee Mulley, formerly Hollington) 20/01/1997 11 Victory Close Bury St. Edmunds Suffolk IP33 2DB **Tel:** (01284) 764170 w 6036075

MULLOCK Janet Helen (see CARROLL, Mrs)

MUNDAY Sharon Trina 24/09/1998 81 Whitley Wood Road READING Berkshire RG2 8HY w 6119972

MUNDY Emma Jane (nee Weisberg) 11/09/1997 113 Mirfield Road Witney Oxfordshire OX28 5BH **Tel:** (01993) 891521 w 6028676

MUNN Samantha Jane (see DINGLEY, Mrs)

MUNNS Faye-Marie 29/08/2000 7 Tall Trees Colnbrook SLOUGH SL3 0JS **Tel:** (01753) 682511 w 6152320

MURPHY Helen Elizabeth 14/02/1995 (17/04/2003) 116 Wareham Road Corfe Mullen Wimborne Dorset BH21 3LH **Tel:** (01202) 698899 w 6033019

Lynsey Melanie (nee Potter) 01/09/1997 Meadow Cottage Carter Lane Warsop Vale MANSFIELD Nottinghamshire NG20 8XF w 6043876

MURPHY Mary Margaret (see CREASE, Mrs)

MURRAY Janice Elizabeth DipAVN(Surgical) 21/02/1980 131 Greenrock Road Bishopton PA7 5AT **Tel:** (01505) 863688 w 6001290

MURRAY Jolene (see ABAZA, Mrs)

MURRAY-LESLIE Catherine Arbella 25/09/2000 (19/05/2006) 7 Holyoake Drive Heather Coalville Leicestershire LE67 2QD w 6202776

MURTAGH Sharon Marie 10/01/2003 P D S A Woolfall Heath Avenue LIVERPOOL L36 3YD **Tel:** (0151) 4803226 w 6282900

MUSGRAVE Janet 03/09/1997 Willows Veterinary Group Middlewich Veterinary Surgery 39 Newton Heath Middlewich Cheshire CW10 9HL **Tel:** (01606) 833731 w 603759X

MUSICKA Jane Rose (see HARRINGTON, Mrs)

MUSTOE Julie Suzanne (see SHIPPEY, Mrs)

MYATT Julie Winifred 11/10/1989 Park House Farm Ellenhall Stafford ST21 6HT **Tel:** (01785) 850381 w 6057470

MYERS Elizabeth Anne 06/02/2002 266 Harrogate Road Eccleshill Bradford Yorkshire BD2 3RH **Tel:** (01274) 400500 w 6270558

Lyndsey Jane 02/03/2001 33 Upper Way Farnham Surrey GU9 8RG w 6213600

N

NAIRN Marion Elizabeth (see BROWN, Mrs)

NASH Sarah Louise (see PEARCE, Mrs)

NASH Wendy (formerly Fahey) 16/09/1981 3 Greenaway Close Great Barr Birmingham B43 7HT **Tel:** (0121) 366 6540 w 6050045

NATHAN Mary-Ann (nee Valler, formerly Nathan) 27/08/1999 (01/08/2001) 39 Button Lane Bearsted Maidstone Kent ME15 8DW **Tel:** (01622) 734 546 w 6135167

NATYNCZUK Theresa Anne 11/11/1992 57 Coverdale Luton Bedfordshire LU4 9JP **Tel:** (01582) 583179 w 6057481

NAYLOR Amanda 24/06/1987 (13/04/2000) Orchard Cottage Coombes Moor PRESTEIGNE Powys LD8 2HY **Tel:** 01544262862 w 6057492

Vikki 28/08/1998 (08/02/2005) Companion Care Unit 5 Wessex Gate Retail Park Broodstone Way Poole Dorset BH15 3TE w 6118254

NEAL Andrea Ruth 21/09/1989 8 Bookham Grove Great Bookham Leatherhead Surrey KT23 4NS **Tel:** (01372) 451338 w 6057506

Barbara Ann 24/08/1977 (26/11/2007) 'Evergreens' 49 Main Road North Dagnall Berkhamsted Hertfordshire HP4 1QZ w 6057517

NEAL Caroline (see CLARK, Mrs)

NEAL Jacqueline (see HUDSON, Mrs)

NEAL Julie Anne (see GRAY, Mrs)

NEALL Julie Maria (nee Colman, nee Neall) 07/09/1995 (15/01/2008) 55 Keene Way Galleywood Chelmsford CM2 8NT **Tel:** (01245) 258617 w 6042861

NEIL Laura Elizabeth Livingstone 10/02/1999 52 Thomson Drive Airdrie Lanarkshire ML6 9DG **Tel:** (01236) 761387 w 6130544

NEILSON-TOY Georgiana Bianca Amarylis 23/08/1994 (23/01/2006) 17 Glebelands Nunney Frome Somerset BA11 4NQ **Tel:** (01373) 836800 w 6032106

NELSON Adele Louise (see ROGERS, Mrs)

NELSON Michelle Louise 15/01/1999 C/o Royal College of Veterinary Surgeons 62-64 Horseferry Road LONDON SW1P 2AF w 6133953

NESBITT Karen (nee Docherty) 17/01/1996 343 Gladsmuir Road Hillington Glasgow G52 2JY **Tel:** (0141) 882 8783 w 6041609

NEVILLE Katherine Anne 23/01/2003 4 Gardeners Close CHEDDAR Somerset BS27 3EG **Tel:** (01934) 742949 w 6267940

NEW Philippa Anne (nee Corfield) 03/09/1996 Elms Veterinary Surgery 30 Gloucester Street Faringdon Oxfordshire SN7 7HY **Tel:** (01367) 242416 w 6039699

NEWCOMBE Emma Louise 02/10/2000 87 Watford Road Cotteridge Birmingham B30 1NP **Tel:** (0121) 459 4333 w 6129164

NEWELL Margaret Lily (see ALLIN, Mrs)

NEWEY Emma Louise Rosemary (nee Wilton) 26/08/1999 25 Stanford Road Liberty Gardens Thetford Norfolk IP24 1FH **Tel:** (01366) 727219 w 6184802

NEWNHAM Nicole Mary (nee Ward) 27/02/2002 Northdale Veterinary Surgery 48 Victoria Road Worthing West Sussex BN11 1XE **Tel:** (01903) 202474 w 6263749

NEWPORT Katie Victoria (nee Newport) 13/03/2002 36 Pennymoor Drive ALTRINCHAM Cheshire WA14 4UT **Tel:** (0161) 929 1887 w 6254542

NEWTON Jack Anthony Dudgeon 07/05/2002 The Old Forge Hurcott Somerton Wiltshire TA11 6AA m 6261879

NEWTON Sandra (see STRONG, Miss)

Shelagh Mary (nee Newton, formerly Iliadis) 29/07/1992 2 Arlen Way HEYWOOD Lancashire OL10 4PY w 6004790

NICHOLLS Melloney Jane (formerly Lupton) 10/10/1994 Pines Veterinary Clinic 146a Bath Road Maidenhead Berkshire SL6 4LB **Tel:** (01628) 776699 w 6035140

NICHOLS Samantha Arunkumar (nee Shah) 02/09/1999 (26/11/2008) 88 Cressing Road Braintree Essex CM7 3PW **Tel:** (01376) 324569 w 6185231

NICHOLSON Joanna (see BECK, Mrs)

NICHOLSON Ruth (see WATERS, Mrs)

NICKERSON Joanne Noele 03/03/2000 27 Oldbutt Road SHIPSTON-ON-STOUR Warwickshire CV36 4EG **Tel:** (01608) 662411 w 6190643

NICKLESS Sarah 08/02/1985 (09/07/2007) Linhay Veterinary Rehabilitation Jubilee Barn Dawlish Devon EX7 0QW **Tel:** (01626) 867614 w 6057710

NICOL Alison Grierson (see MCELREA, Mrs)

NICOL-SMITH Elizabeth Helen 10/08/1984 (28/04/2006) 35 Alexander Street Bayswater London W2 5NU **Tel:** (020) 7229 2040 w 6057721

NOAKES Anne Kathleen 18/08/1995 Holly Cottage Hempnall Road Woodton Bungay Suffolk NR35 2LS **Tel:** (01508) 482764 w 6026136

NOBLE Vicky 22/09/1999 (02/11/2007) Coomara Veterinary Practice Coomara Carleton Carlisle Cumbria CA4 0BU **Tel:** (01228) 524740 w 6143961

NORBURY Edwina Margaret (nee Ling) 26/08/1976 (01/11/1984) Feldon Veterinary Centre 257 Coventry Road Hinckley Leicestershire LE10 0NE **Tel:** (01455) 610227 w 6085770

NORCOP Susan Jane 14/01/1982 13 Croft Crescent Penkhull Stoke-on-Trent Staffordshire ST4 5EP **Tel:** (01782) 846226 w 6091423

NORCROSS Catharine Hilary (see PUCKNELL, Mrs)

NORMAN Alexandra DipAVN(Surgical) 20/11/1986 Anchor Lane AYLESBURY Buckinghamshire HP20 1AJ **Tel:** (01296) 745377 w 6057754

NORRIS Christine (nee Beukes) 15/10/2003 PO Box 22053 Fish Hoek Cape Town 7974 South Africa w 6348020

NORTH Harriet Jane (nee Hangartner) 31/07/1987 10 Chequers Lane Glemsford SUDBURY Suffolk CO10 7PW **Tel:** (01787) 282661 w 6061228

Janet 31/07/1989 DBARC Nelsons Lane Hurst Berkshire RG10 0RR **Tel:** (0118) 934 1122 w 6001392

NORTHALL Andrea Jayne (nee Pearce) 10/03/1994 27 Lundy View Smiths Wood Birmingham B36 0LY **Tel:** (0121) 770 4020 w 6025686

NURSEY Zoe Amanda (see SHUTE, Mrs)

NUTTALL Lorna Margaret (nee Henderson) 06/08/1992 Colne Valley Veterinary Practice Off Maudlyn Road Colchester CO1 2GU **Tel:** (01206) 794695 w 6007860

O

OAKES Deborah Louise (nee Cowap) 23/01/1998 86 Orford Avenue Warrington Cheshire WA2 7QQ **Tel:** (01925) 232221 w 6024536

OBEROI Kulwinder Singh 30/08/1994 59 Beauchamp Road Sutton Surrey SM1 2PY **Tel:** (020) 8643 2409 m 6041493

O'BRIEN Elaine Roma (nee Bingham) 18/08/1987 (12/05/2008) 7 Dunstone Road Plymstock Plymouth Devon PL9 8RG **Tel:** (01752) 406182 w 6057867

Maria (nee Robinson) 06/08/1992 (26/01/2004) Fivelands Veterinary Centre 98 Alcester Road BIRMINGHAM B13 8EG **Tel:** (0121) 449 3716 w 6014834

OBRIEN Mellissa Ann (see AMIES, Mrs)

O'CALLAGHAN Abigail Lucy 20/09/1999 309a Liverpool Road SOUTHPORT Merseyside PR8 3DE **Tel:** (01704) 572 592 w 6185143

O'CONNOR Caroline (nee Grimsdell, formerly Wilson) 09/01/1991 38 Deanfield Road Henley-on-Thames Oxfordshire RG9 1UG **Tel:** (01491) 579922 w 6051901

Marie Ina (nee Cawood) 28/06/2002 544 Old Chester Road Rock Ferry Birkenhead Merseyside CH42 4PF **Tel:** (0151) 6459270 w 6274386

Michelle Patricia 15/09/1997 3 Thistledown Close Rhostyllen WREXHAM Clwyd LL14 4EZ **Tel:** (01978) 366978 w 6043162

ODDELL Susan Jane 29/06/1989 (08/10/1999) 10 Westcroft North Newbald York YO43 4TX **Tel:** (01430) 827710 w 6058011

O'DONNELL Anne Marie 27/01/1997 (02/11/2009) 32 Foxland Avenue Rednal BIRMINGHAM B45 9QE w 6036563

ODONNELL Helen Kerry (see EMMERSON, Mrs)

OFFORD Karen Elizabeth (nee Allen) 23/09/1998 Stowe Veterinary Group 54 Bury Road Stowmarket Suffolk IP14 1JF **Tel:** (01449) 613130 w 6135779

OLIVER Alison Jane 16/08/1993 Windlebrook Veterinary Clinic 46 High Street Bagshot Surrey GU19 5AW **Tel:** (01276) 73516 w 6015951

Amanda Lillian 09/09/1996 (17/02/2004) 35 Furnace Hill Halesowen West Midlands B63 3LY **Tel:** (0121) 585 7013 w 6022346

Anne Denise 12/02/2001 63 Norwich Road Wroxham Norwich Norfolk NR12 8RX **Tel:** (01603) 783 920 w 6204866

Gwen DipAVN(Surgical), DipAVN(Medical) 07/08/1989 73 New Road Bedfont Feltham Middlesex TW14 8HR w 6058044

Tracey Karen 09/02/1996 Flat 44 St. Leonards Court House Lane Sandridge St. Albans Hertfordshire AL4 9UZ **Tel:** (01727) 843139 w 6042453

OLIVIER Jennifer Marie 26/03/2002 8 Yardley Road Grendon NORTHAMPTON NN7 1JH **Tel:** (07871) 898 020 w 6273209

OLLIVER Maria Jayne 28/08/1997 10 Durnford Street Plymouth PL1 3QL **Tel:** (01752) 266077 w 610887X

OLSEN Judith Ann (nee Spoors) 29/01/1992 16 Ludlow Drive West Monkseaton Whitley Bay Tyne and Wear NE25 9QG w 6061137

O'NEILL Patricia 28/07/1992 (19/12/2001) 29 Roakes Avenue Addlestone Surrey KT15 2HF **Tel:** (01932) 564191 w 6004826

O'REILLY Melanie Jane 06/12/1990 (08/05/2001) 48 Harvest Hill EAST GRINSTEAD West Sussex RH19 4BT w 606263X

ORGAN Celine Geraldine Marie (see SANDERS, Mrs)

ORMAN Ann Marie (nee Lamerton) 05/08/1980 22 Hollybrook Close Shipley Southampton Hampshire SO16 6SY **Tel:** (023) 80784096 w 6054786

OSBORN Karen Marie (see COOPER, Mrs)

OSBORNE Michaela Ann (see ROSE, Mrs)

OSBORNE Sarah Carol 21/08/1998 PDSA 1c Eynsham Drive London SE2 9RQ w 6108880

OSHEA Stacey Marie (see WILLIAMS, Mrs)

OSULLIVAN Joan Mary (see FREEMAN, Mrs)

O'SULLIVAN Marie 10/09/1981 (29/10/2002) Culleen Tubber Co. Clare Ireland **Tel:** (091) 633344 w 6091591

OTTLEY Carrie-Anne (nee Forsyth) 28/02/2001 27 Haygarth Knebworth Hertfordshire SG3 6HE **Tel:** (01438) 216801 w 6134731

OVER Marie (see HURST, Mrs)

OWEN Donna Marie 16/07/2002 Parkside Hotel 11 Clarence Road North WESTON-SUPER-MARE Avon BS23 4AT **Tel:** (01934) 626354 w 6275167

Michelle Louise 07/08/2002 Maindee House Veterinary Surgeon Mount Pleasant Road Pontnewydd Cwmbran Gwent NP44 1AN **Tel:** (01633) 483208 w 6263540

OWEN Sasha Ann (see ELIAS, Mrs)

OWENS Lynne (see JOHNSON, Mrs)

OXLADE Tracy Ann 07/09/1998 49 College Road College Town SANDHURST Berkshire GU47 0RA **Tel:** (0208) 9421931 w 6122216

OXLEY Julie 10/09/1996 161 Oregon Way Chaddesden Derby DE21 6UP **Tel:** (01332) 345191 w 6077442

OXLEY Linda Ann (see SLATER, Mrs)

P

PAGE Verity Ann 26/03/2002 (29/11/2005) 130 The Lakes Larkfield AYLESFORD Kent ME20 6SL w 6265839

PAGET Zoe Louise (nee Iliffe) 10/12/2002 4 Old Road Bishops Itchington Southam Warwickshire CV47 2RS w 6271471

PAGGI Catherine Jane 10/02/2000 27 Wood Street Chelmsford CM2 9AU **Tel:** (01245) 609084 w 6190555

PAISLEY Deborah Anne (nee Milburn) 19/08/1991 6 Wavell Drive Rosehill Industrial Estate Carlisle CA1 2ST **Tel:** (01228) 521393 w 6056772

PALLIER Susan Juliet 03/09/2002 428 Buxton Road Great Moor Stockport Cheshire SK2 7JQ **Tel:** (0161) 456 6570 w 6266015

PALMER Louise (nee Curling) 05/10/1990 (22/06/1999) 13 Draycote Road Waterlooville Hampshire PO8 0NE **Tel:** (01730) 300350 w 6048637

Michelle Louise (nee Stokes) 21/02/1997 (24/06/2002) 20 Farrow Road Whaplode Drove SPALDING Lincolnshire PE12 0TS **Tel:** (01406) 330907 w 6100393

Rachael Louise (nee Palmer) 01/09/1997 (27/07/1999) 45 Lock Hill Thorne DONCASTER South Yorkshire DN8 5EP w 6112037

PANES Leanne Zoe 27/01/2000 6 Bellevue Road Minster on Sea Sheerness Kent ME12 2RH w 6099976

PAPE Deborah Patricia 23/09/1999 (06/03/2008) 199 Grange Road Darlington County Durham DL1 5NT **Tel:** (01325) 351111 w 6040219

PAREMAIN Sally (see MAYNARD, Mrs)

PARFITT Michelle Kate (see COLLEY, Mrs)

PARISH Beverly Teresa (see FARQUHARSON, Mrs)

PARKER Alison DipAVN(Surgical) 05/08/1980 Tyddyn Du Llanfairtalhaiarn Abergele Clwyd LL22 8YY **Tel:** (0191) 5672098 w 6058281

Ann Frances 05/09/1996 13 Queens Crescent Glasgow G4 9BL **Tel:** (0141) 332 1934 w 6025697

Julie Marie 30/09/1997 Lebry House 3 Throughgate Dunscore Dumfries Dumfriesshire DG2 0UG **Tel:** (01387) 820202 w 6033198

PARKER Tracey June (see CAMPBELL, Mrs)

Victoria Samantha 15/09/1999 Bryn Eithin Caergeiliog HOLYHEAD Anglesey LL65 3EQ w 6134527

PARKINSON Julia Denise (nee Cozens) 21/06/1983 Rushwood Boarding Kennels and cattery Shab Hill Birdlip Gloucestershire GL4 8JX w 6090168

Lynne Marie (nee Mainwaring) 12/02/1996 (31/12/2002) 13 Millfield Close Wilberfoss YORK YO41 5PP **Tel:** (01759) 388408 w 6032514

PARNWELL Claire Elizabeth 26/08/1998 (08/07/2009) 44 Mill Road Whittlesey PETERBOROUGH PE7 1SN w 6129426

PARRINDER Anne-Marie (nee Parrinder, formerly Thorne) 26/01/1994 (12/12/2005) 47 Victoria Street Staple Hill Bristol BS16 5JP **Tel:** (01179) 566880 w 6067263

PARRIS Heather Jane 23/10/2001 Hayne Farm Howley Chard Somerset TA20 3DX **Tel:** (01460) 62502 w 6267566

PARROTT Hannah Jane (nee Hibble) 05/09/1996 (07/11/2000) 1 Cornwall Road Stamford Lincolnshire PE9 1LQ **Tel:** 01780764991 w 604049X

PARRY Debbie 16/01/1991 8 Regent Buildings Hall Street Bilston West Midlands WV14 0AB **Tel:** (01902) 493465 w 6058350

PARRY Pauline Margaret (see DILLON, Mrs)

PARRY Susan Pauline (see FISHER, Mrs)

PARSONS Jo-Anne 23/01/1995 Fourwinds Pennsylvania Lane Tiptree COLCHESTER Essex CO5 0UE w 6033992

PARTISS Jill Barbara (nee Reade) 16/08/1982 (31/05/2000) Bicton College East Budleigh Budleigh Salterton Devon EX9 7BY **Tel:** (01395) 562327 w 6059401

PARTRIDGE Elizabeth Ann Lucy (nee Baverstock) 05/03/1997 (31/07/2009) Leightor Farm Poundsgate NEWTON ABBOT Devon TQ13 7PB **Tel:** (01364) 631550 w 6097436

PATEL Mena Kumari (nee Rao) 19/08/1993 (28/11/2000) 8 St George's Parade Wolverhampton West Midlands WV2 1BD **Tel:** (01902) 425262 w 6015962

PATRICK Janet Patricia (nee Southwell) 29/01/1996 (13/03/2003) Pennington House Veterinary Centre Newlands Road LEIGH Lancashire WN7 4HA **Tel:** (01942) 673777 w 6037975

PATTERSON Susan (see RICHARDSON, Mrs)

PAUL Joanne Helen 21/08/1998 77 Gillshill Road Hull HU8 0JJ **Tel:** (01482) 787996 w 6138827

PAULSDOTTIR Steinunn Johanna (see PAULSDOTTIR-JENKINS, Mrs)

PAULSDOTTIR-JENKINS Steinunn Johanna (formerly Paulsdottir) 18/08/1983 (06/07/2006) Hawthorne Lodge Veterinary Practice Ltd 1 Old Parr Road Banbury Oxfordshire OX16 5HT **Tel:** (01295) 259446 w 608998X

PAVEY Wendy Michelle 20/02/1987 66 Avalanche Road Portland Dorset DT5 2DL w 6001508

PAYNE Deborah Jane (nee Brown) 05/02/2001 Banstead Village Veterinary Surgery 170A High Street Banstead Surrey SM7 2NZ **Tel:** (01737) 210011 w 6203183

Juliet 05/09/1997 (07/03/2001) 9 Carson Close Stretton on Fosse Moreton-in-Marsh Gloucestershire GL56 9SJ **Tel:** (01608) 662397 w 6043854

PAYTON Sally Joanne 11/12/2001 152 Elliott Street Tyldesley MANCHESTER M29 8FJ **Tel:** (01942) 886174 w 6253156

PEACOCK Paula Jane (see COOPER, Mrs)

PEARCE Andrea Jayne (see NORTHALL, Mrs)

PEARCE Juliet Ann (nee Elson) 21/09/1992 (11/02/2009) 17 Warres Road Taunton Somerset TA2 8QF **Tel:** (01823) 252385 w 6049867

Sarah Louise (nee Nash) 30/06/2003 27 Portland Road East Grinstead West Sussex RH19 4EB **Tel:** (01342) 327799 w 6269381

PEARSALL Deborah Louise 09/09/1997 12 Manscroft Road HEMEL HEMPSTEAD Hertfordshire HP1 3HU **Tel:** (01442) 211 319 w 611847X

PEARSON Elaine Anne (see MCDOWELL, Mrs)

PEARSON Lynn (see BRYNE, Mrs)

PEARSON Vanessa (see STOKES, Mrs)

PECK Harriet Claire (see HUNTER BLAIR, Mrs)

PECK Kerry Joanne 31/10/1988 (16/02/2007) 8 Bury Court Stone Street Cambridge CB1 2RX **Tel:** (01223) 67419 w 6058510

PEERS Susan Helen 03/09/1991 Sunny House Farm 8 Draycott Road Upper Tean Stoke-on-Trent Staffordshire ST10 4JF **Tel:** (01538) 722332 w 6058521

PEGG Rebecca Louise 29/01/1996 134-136 Osmaston Road Derby Derbyshire DE1 2RF **Tel:** (01332) 345119 w 6043526

Victoria Jayne 06/04/2001 (13/08/2007) 14 Taylor Drive Woodsetts WORKSOP Nottinghamshire S81 8SH **Tel:** (01909) 565375 w 6144375

PELL Katie Marie (see COOPER, Mrs)

PELL Susan Louise (nee Pell, formerly Holmgaard Pell) 11/03/1994 (26/09/2003) 7 Holden Road Southborough Tunbridge Wells Kent TN4 0QG w 6024900

PEMBERTON Judith Emma (nee Rodmell) 27/08/1997 (10/04/2002) The Scott Veterinary Clinic 405 Goldington Road Bedford Bedfordshire MK41 0DS **Tel:** (01234) 261 622 w 6030710

PENGELLY Julia Gail (see SAMPSON, Mrs)

PENN Christina Black 29/08/2000 Hillhead Farm Limerigg Slamannan FALKIRK FK1 3BY **Tel:** (01324) 851337 w 6031703

Emma Jane 17/01/1996 (02/02/1999) 59 Lodge Drive Moulton Northwich Cheshire CW9 8RG **Tel:** (01606) 556685 w 6039848

PENNELL Alison 19/01/2000 Nantglas Fach Llangybi Lampeter Dyfed SA48 8NW **Tel:** (01570) 493493 w 6190324

PEPPER Christine Louise 20/08/1991 8 Gresham Road Derby DE24 8AW **Tel:** (07932) 656161 w 6058554

PERCIVAL Sharon Lynne 17/11/2000 Oakdene Capenhurst Lane Great Sutton Ellesmere Port Cheshire CH66 2NT **Tel:** (0151) 339 3801 w 6205251

PERKINS Claire Marie (nee Millett) 08/02/1999 18 Roseville Avenue Longwell Green Bristol Avon BS30 9UD **Tel:** (0117) 960 9937 w 6121824

Megan Moira 30/04/2001 12 The Street Oare Faversham Kent ME13 0PY **Tel:** (01795) 591651 w 6216504

Valerie Ann 01/03/1979 14 Knightswick Road Canvey Island Essex SS8 9PA **Tel:** (01268) 510506 w 6058576

PERRETT Catherine Fiona 01/09/1998 (29/04/2002) 266 Harrogate Road Eccleshill Bradford Yorkshire BD2 3RH **Tel:** (01274) 400500 w 6118505

PERRY Emma Kate 01/12/2000 (07/09/2005) 1 Vineyard Close Lytchett Matravers Poole Dorset BH16 6DD **Tel:** (01202) 625504 w 6204217

PETERS Hazel Margaret-Rose (see HOBBS, Mrs)

PETRIE Gillian Shirley 20/05/2002 (21/01/2010) 42 Claremount View Coatbridge Lanarkshire ML5 4GA **Tel:** (01234) 422952 w 6263353

PHILLIPS Clare Helen (see PITTAWAY, Mrs)

Heidi Ann (nee Rodda) 10/12/2002 13 Meeres Court Lane SITTINGBOURNE Kent ME10 3PZ **Tel:** (07971) 948459 w 6249229

PHILLIPS Lyn (see CHANT, Mrs)

PHILP Caroline Teresa (nee Philp, formerly Wannell) 30/08/1994 (14/05/1998) 31 Nightingale Close Rowland's Castle Hampshire PO9 6EU **Tel:** (023) 92413584 w 6032296

PHILP Debbie Jane (see QUENBY, Mrs)

PHILPOTT Elaine 05/08/1976 4 Scarborough Way Coventry West Midlands CV4 8DE **Tel:** (02476) 470750 w 6058747

PHIPPEN Rebecca (nee Collins) 21/06/2002 (11/11/2008) 12 Alamein Avenue WATCHET Somerset TA23 0TY **Tel:** (01643) 707857 w 6264739

PIGGOTT Judith Karen 17/08/1981 34 Rosebery Crescent Kingfield Woking Surrey GU22 9BL **Tel:** (01483) 714 191 w 6089469

PILE Anita Ruth (see SCOTT, Mrs)

PILLAR Claire Elizabeth 18/01/1995 16 Valley Drive Wembury PLYMOUTH Devon PL9 0EZ w 6029057

PINFOLD Anna Christine 04/02/2002 19 Hayes Way BECKENHAM Kent BR3 6RJ **Tel:** (020) 8650 0861 w 6257303

PINK Jane Carolyn (see CHAMBERLAIN, Miss)

PINK Michelle Elizabeth (see HADDRELL, Mrs)

PINNINGTON Jill 29/08/2000 63 London Road South Poynton Stockport Cheshire SK12 1LA **Tel:** (01625) 859019 w 6152728

PITTAWAY Clare Helen (nee Phillips) 16/07/2002 65 Golf Links Road Hull North Humberside HU6 8RD **Tel:** (01482) 343571 w 6266730

PITTS Elaine Anne (see ROBERTS, Mrs)

PITTS Natasha Claire DipAVN(Surgical) 04/09/1998 26 Sandpiper Way LEIGHTON BUZZARD Bedfordshire LU7 4SS w 6133818

Sarah Louise 02/09/1998 410 Eaton Road West Derby Liverpool L12 3HG **Tel:** (0151) 220 4668 w 6098611

PLATTEN Dawn Catherine (nee Eden) 24/01/1989 Yewgate Cottage Remenham Hill Remenham Henley-on-Thames Oxfordshire RG9 3ES **Tel:** (01491) 414113 w 6049608

PLESTED Vanessa Jayne (see JAYNES, Ms)

PLUMB Gillian Dawn (see WASHINGTON, Mrs)

POLLARD Caroline Ann 01/11/1984 (23/06/2000) 1A Monks Pond Street Northampton NN1 2LF **Tel:** (01604) 637175 w 6058893

Deborah Jane DipAVN(Surgical) (nee Reeve) 10/08/1990 (01/03/2002) 5 Russet Road Maidenhead Berkshire SL6 3HL **Tel:** (01628) 671556 w 605949X

Tina Rebecca 30/08/1990 (11/12/2003) 69 Kinver Close Great Woodley Romsey Hampshire SO51 7JW **Tel:** (01794) 511441 w 6058918

Valerie Anne DipAVN(Surgical) (nee Smith) 30/01/1996 36 The Glades East Grinstead West Sussex RH19 3XW **Tel:** (01342) 410116 w 6038232

POLLITT Sharon Ann (nee Craine) 19/02/2001 (03/12/2009) 10 Burton Avenue Rainhill Merseyside L35 9JN **Tel:** (0151) 430 7033 w 6212412

POOLE Lisa Jane Seton (see GIBBS, Mrs)

PORTER Samantha Clair 17/09/1998 49a High Street WALTON-ON-THAMES Surrey KT12 1DH w 6135087

POSTINGS Victoria 24/07/2000 205 Mount Pleasant Kingswinford West Midlands DY6 9SP **Tel:** (01384) 277689 w 6146113

POTTER Claire Elizabeth (see TAYLOR, Mrs)

POTTER Lynsey Melanie (see MURPHY, Mrs)

POTTS Clare Andrea 27/12/2001 Veterinary Instrumentation Ltd Broadfield Road SHEFFIELD S8 0XL w 6205361

POWELL Joanne Elizabeth 14/01/1982 13 Hawkins Road Neston Cheshire CH64 9TD **Tel:** (0151) 336 6260 w 6059048

Nancy Jane 19/01/1998 28 Brook Road Rubery Birmingham B45 9UH **Tel:** (0121) 6802513 w 6113620

Natasha 19/09/1997 (04/01/2010) Woodlands Veterinary Hospital Burnett Road Manadon Plymouth Devon PL6 5BH **Tel:** (01752) 700600 w 6108949

POWLEY Caroline Fraser 24/01/2000 24 Birchwood Avenue Sidcup Kent DA14 4LF **Tel:** (0208) 3001660 w 6190247

PRICE Kathryn Elizabeth Anne 17/09/1998 (16/11/2003) R S P C A East Winch Wildlife Centre Station Road East Winch King's Lynn PE32 1NR w 6123719

PRICE Kathryn Ellen (see KINREAD, Mrs)

PRICE Kerry Susan (see LAMBERT, Mrs)

Sarah Kate DipAVN(Medical) 08/08/2002 Wey Referrals 125-129 Chertsey Road Woking Surrey GU21 5BP **Tel:** (01483) 729194 w 6190896

Tanya Theresa 25/08/1999 (12/12/2005) 1 The Drive Kingsley Park Northampton NN1 4RY **Tel:** (01604) 710411 w 6142797

PRIESTMAN Elizabeth Anne (see EXTON, Mrs)

PRIME Angela Jane (see MIDDLETON, Mrs)

PRIMMER Kate Joanna (see SMITH, Mrs)

PRINCE Lara Mary (see MCHALE, Mrs)

PRINCE Victoria Louise (see MORRISON, Mrs)

PRIOR Catherine Elizabeth (nee Hayton) 05/08/1980 (22/07/1999) The Hart Veterinary Centre Browning Drive Kings Meadow Bicester Oxfordshire OX26 2XL **Tel:** (01869) 323 223 w 6088512

Elizabeth 15/11/2001 59 Bucklebury Bracknell Berkshire RG12 7YJ **Tel:** (01252) 876782 w 6257259

PRITCHARD Karen Julie 15/11/2001 27 Greenacres Shoreham-by-Sea West Sussex BN43 5WY **Tel:** (01273) 446 455 w 6258282

Verity Kathryn 24/08/1999 6 Harding Close Redbourn ST. ALBANS Hertfordshire AL3 7NT **Tel:** (07793) 358208 w 6118571

PRYCE Sharon Louise (see CARVER, Mrs)

PUCKNELL Catharine Hilary DipAVN(Surgical) (nee Norcross) 25/02/1991 The Chevin Calcraft Road Corfe Castle WAREHAM Dorset BH20 5EL w 6001494

PULLAN Claire Victoria (nee Wicks) 09/05/2005 (01/06/2009) Breaks Fold Farm West End Summerbridge Harrogate North Yorkshire HG3 4BB **Tel:** (01943) 880277 w 6299675

PULMAN Joanna Jane 02/10/1978 Firgrove Veterinary Centre 7 Aylesham Way Yateley Hampshire GU46 6NR **Tel:** (01252) 877799 w 6059194

PUMMELL Nicola Louise (see ENGLAND, Mrs)

PURCHASE Lucy (nee Saunders) 31/08/1999 18 Wood Avenue Coven Wolverhampton West Midlands WV9 5DP **Tel:** (01902) 798749 w 6185110

PUTNAM Kerry Jane (see LINE, Miss)

PYALL Carol 22/01/1987 (21/07/1999) Binniehill Cottage Binniehill Road Slamannan FALKIRK FK1 3BG w 6059219

Q

QUENBY Debbie Jane (nee Philp) 06/09/1999 5 Dial Close Little Paxton ST. NEOTS Cambridgeshire PE19 6QN w 6128750

QUENBY Joanna Lea (see BENDIKAS, Mrs)

QUICK Tracey Marie 09/09/1998 30 The Crescent Hadleigh Benfleet Essex SS7 2HF **Tel:** (01702) 551802 w 6100098

QUINN Emma Jane (see KELLY, Mrs)

QUINN Laura Grant (see ROBERTSON, Mrs)

QUINN Susan Avril 05/11/2001 (23/05/2005) St Clair Veterinary Group 2 Pottery Street Kirkcaldy Fife KY1 3ET **Tel:** (01592) 599500 w 6035129

QUITMAN Janelle Dawn 19/01/1983 3 Coolers Farm Horsebridge Road Broughton Stockbridge Hampshire SO20 8BN **Tel:** (01794) 301754 w 6059241

R

RACE Anne Elizabeth 01/11/1984 58 Bramble Lane MANSFIELD Nottinghamshire NG18 3NX w 6059263

RADECKA Susan 30/03/1984 (03/03/2006) 8 Hampden Road Ashford Kent TN23 6JL **Tel:** (01233) 633841 w 6076948

RADWELL Rachel 16/02/1998 (08/01/2009) 47 Upper George Street Higham Ferrers Rushed Northamptonshire NN10 8JN w 6113438

RAFFERTY Carole Louise 21/08/1985 (08/01/1999) 191 Gorsemoor Road Heath Hayes Cannock Staffordshire WS12 3HR **Tel:** (01543) 458424 w 6059274

RAINE Joanna Kate 10/01/2001 Grove Lodge Veterinary Group Ltd 18 Upper Brighton Road Worthing West Sussex BN14 9DL **Tel:** (01903) 234866 w 6204756

RALLEY Janet Maureen 08/09/1997 50 New Village Dudley West Midlands DY2 0DP **Tel:** (01384) 633570 w 6108960

RAMSAY Karen Anne (nee Airlie) 08/09/1994 2075 Paisley Road West Cardonald Glasgow G52 3JH **Tel:** (0141) 883 8118 w 6032092

Nicolette Amanda 06/01/1993 15 Greythorne Road Woking Surrey GU21 3PG **Tel:** (01483) 756811 w 6066474

RAMSDEN Emma Clare 02/10/2001 A-Z Animal Care Greenways Garden Centre Ashford Road Bethersden Ashford Kent TN26 3LF **Tel:** (01233) 822411 w 6229341

RANDALL Annette Elizabeth 10/11/1971 Davies Veterinary Specialists Manor Farm Business Park Higham Gobion Hertfordshire SG5 3HR **Tel:** (01582) 883950 w 605930X

Sara Louise (nee Dunstan) 09/01/1990 145 Pasley Street Stoke Plymouth PL2 1DT **Tel:** (01752) 318609 w 6049492

Shelly 21/08/1998 Mrs P Darling 254 Main Road Emsworth Hampshire PO10 8JJ **Tel:** (01428) 729838 w 6118607

RAO Mena Kumari (see PATEL, Mrs)

RASMUSSEN Connie Borre (see MILLS, Mrs)

RAWLES Janine (nee Laar) 07/02/1983 20 Shortlands Gardens Shortlands Village Bromley Kent BR2 0EA **Tel:** (0208) 2893671 w 6054742

RAWLINS Kirsty Marie (nee Smith) 06/09/1999 20 Church Close Drayton Bassett Nr Tamworth

Staffordshire B78 3UJ **Tel:** (01827) 285883 w 6186012

RAYBOULD Alison Claire (see DAUBNEY, Mrs)

READ Michelle 28/09/1995 (15/05/2000) Fernlea Veterinary Clinic Blackhorse Road Kingswood Bristol BS15 8DZ **Tel:** (0117) 960 6145 w 6035016

Rebecca Jane (nee Hillyer) 03/02/1994 (03/03/1999) 14 Otter Street Hilton DERBY DE65 5NS **Tel:** (01332) 727190 w 6067842

READ Sarah Jane (see SPARK, Mrs)

READE Helen Elizabeth (nee Young) 11/08/1986 (25/04/2007) Ashwood Farm Ashwood Lane Ash Parva WHITCHURCH Shropshire SY13 4DX w 6064433

READE Jill Barbara (see PARTISS, Mrs)

REAY Dianne 21/10/1981 101 Aycliffe Avenue Springwell Gateshead Tyne and Wear NE9 7BX **Tel:** (0191) 4821054 w 6059423

REECE Linda May 14/08/1981 (16/01/2002) 259 Bilton Road Rugby Warwickshire CV22 7EQ **Tel:** (01788) 812650 w 6059445

REEDER Nicola McCall (see KNOTT, Mrs)

REEVE Deborah Jane (see POLLARD, Mrs)

REEVE Helen Louise (nee Reeve, formerly Jones) 30/01/2001 1 Caldecott Place Rugby Warwickshire CV21 3TT **Tel:** (01788) 540706 w 6211576

REEVES Anna Lisa 20/11/2002 37 Victoria Park Colwyn Bay Conwy LL29 7AJ **Tel:** (01492) 534755 w 6269722

Joanne 07/09/1990 (11/11/2003) Connaught House Veterinary Hospital 38 Broad Street Kingswinford West Midlands DY6 9LP **Tel:** (01384) 295949 w 6059514

REGAN Laura Jane (nee Robinson) 26/08/1997 (06/03/2008) Bank House Red Lane Light Oaks STOKE-ON-TRENT ST2 7LT w 6131672

REID Emma Jane 25/02/2003 31 Charles Street Sileby Loughborough Leicestershire LE12 7RH **Tel:** (01509) 812889 w 6254806

Linda Anne 10/08/1978 (23/12/2009) 118 Dumbuck Road Silverton DUMBARTON G82 3LZ w 6059558

Sharon Louise 25/08/1999 Veterinary School University of Glasgow 464 Bearsden Road Bearsden Glasgow G61 1QH w 6130566

RENDLE Matthew Edwin 02/09/1992 (16/05/2005) 2 Oxhey Avenue Watford WD19 4HG **Tel:** (01923) 240961 m 600646X

RENNIE Helen Clare (see FRY, Mrs)

REYNOLDS Vikki-Luan 04/02/2002 Station Farm London Road Six Mile Bottom Newmarket Suffolk CB8 0UH **Tel:** (01638) 572012 w 6270096

REYNOLDS-WARNES Suzanne Mary 12/09/1996 (26/06/2001) 94 Dawes Road Fulham London SW6 7EJ **Tel:** (020) 7381 3939 w 6033212

RICH Denise Margaret (see COLCLOUGH, Mrs)

RICH Gillian Barbara (nee Scott) 27/08/1999 (15/01/2007) The Mayhew Animal Home Trenmar Gardens Kensal Green London NW10 6BJ **Tel:** (020) 8969 0178 w 6184659

RICHARDS Hannah Marie 25/08/1998 147 Rooker Avenue WOLVERHAMPTON WV2 2DS w 6128331

Jane 20/03/1974 Godalming Veterinary Surgery The Old Auction Mart Station Approach Godalming Surrey GU7 1EU **Tel:** (01483) 422644 w 6059627

Mary Joy Rose DipAVN(Medical) 14/11/2000 42 Wilmington Gardens Barking Essex IG11 9TP **Tel:** (020) 8594 1299 w 6203733

Sarah Louise 19/01/1998 Broad Lane Vets Ltd 255 Broad Lane Coventry West Midlands CV5 7AQ **Tel:** (024) 7646 4789 w 6100167

RICHARDSON Angela Jayne (nee Brown) 25/01/1995 (15/08/2005) 9 Roper Street Workington Cumbria CA14 3BZ **Tel:** (01900) 61517 w 6034486

Caroline Anne (nee Morris) 16/11/2000 10 Newbury Drive Urmston MANCHESTER M41 7FA **Tel:** (0161) 748 3525 w 6202688

Caroline Jane 22/08/1986 9 Station Road Hopton-On-Sea Great Yarmouth Norfolk NR31 9BE **Tel:** (01502) 731854 w 6059638

Karen Mary (nee Wallis) 17/01/1996 (27/03/2002) 20 Medway Turners Hill CRAWLEY West Sussex RH10 4NR **Tel:** (01342) 715897 w 6038640

Kenneth Earnest 23/08/1999 5 Bramley Court Hatton Derby Derbyshire DE65 5QT **Tel:** (01283) 520938 m 6137776

Kerry Samantha 26/08/1999 (20/01/2010) Kerry Lee 2 Westwood Clipstone Drive Forest Town MANSFIELD Nottinghamshire NG19 0JH w 6152295

RICHARDSON Sally Elizabeth (see HOLBROW, Mrs)

RICHARDSON Susan (nee Patterson) 29/09/1992 (12/08/1999) South Lodge Elvingston Estate TRANENT East Lothian EH33 1EH **Tel:** (01875) 852826 w 6006776

RICHES Jo'ann Ellis (see DILLON, Mrs)

RICHES Katherine 24/11/2000 5 Blacksmith Lane Thorpe on the Hill Lincoln LN6 9BQ **Tel:** (01522) 684874 w 6203403

RICHMOND Kathryn Jane (nee Rushworth) 24/08/1999 Lodge Cottage Langley Lane Goosnargh PRESTON PR3 2JT **Tel:** (01995) 643457 w 6108483

RICKARD Renay Francis (nee Field) 15/03/1990 (17/08/1999) Pelyn Veterinary Group Nomansland Edgcumbe Road Lostwithiel Cornwall PL22 0DZ **Tel:** (01208) 872254 w 6050260

RICKETTS Emma Jane 03/09/2001 (14/05/2007) Mainstone Veterinary Clinic Mainstone Romsey Hampshire SO51 6BA **Tel:** (01794) 513157 w 6204998

RIDDICK Estelle Norah Marg (see JACKSON, Mrs)

RIDSDALE Hazel 20/11/2002 Heath & Reach Veterinary Surgery Kingswood Farm Brickhill Road Leighton Buzzard LU7 0BA w 6273495

RIGBY Beverley Joy (see ALLUM, Miss)

RIGHELATO Kathleen Margaret 13/03/1977 71 Chatsworth Drive Bush Hill Park Enfield Middlesex EN1 1EU **Tel:** (0208) 3636500 w 6059682

RIMELL Elizabeth Kate (see GODDARD, Mrs)

RITCHIE Anne Marie (nee Docherty) 22/11/2001 (01/12/2008) 69 Glaive Road GLASGOW G13 2HT **Tel:** (0141) 954 2527 w 6252111

ROBBINS Angela Mary 15/02/2001 17 Nutclough Hebden Bridge West Yorkshire HX7 8HA **Tel:** (01422) 842696 w 6205020

ROBERTS Anne (nee Bailey) 09/09/1996 21 Lawrence Grove Kingshill Dursley Gloucestershire GL11 4EY **Tel:** (01453) 548860 w 6097389

Elaine Anne (nee Pitts) 24/08/1989 (04/01/2005) Northcott Farm Yeoford Crediton Devon EX17 5HD **Tel:** (01647) 24598 w 6058816

ROBERTS Heather Lesley (see LANGDALE, Mrs)

Jane (nee Turner) 26/03/2002 3 Bryn Road Bryn WIGAN WN4 0AA **Tel:** (01942) 721562 w 6271295

Kylie Rebecca 06/10/1999 114 The Chantrys FARNHAM Surrey GU9 7AN **Tel:** (01252) 737220 w 6134979

Lynn Marie 21/09/1984 Chy Kerenza Parc Morrep Praa Sands Penzance Cornwall TR20 9TE **Tel:** (01736) 763251 w 6091864

Sarah Marie 10/01/2003 5 Hoathly Mews Kents Hill MILTON KEYNES MK7 6JH w 6280458

ROBERTSON Laura Grant (nee Quinn) 29/08/1996 18 Kilmore Road Kilmore Drumnadrochit Inverness Inverness-Shire IV63 6TS **Tel:** (01456) 459080 w 6038800

Lucy Teresa 19/01/1989 55 Havenfield Road HIGH WYCOMBE Buckinghamshire HP12 4SY **Tel:** (07958) 768077 w 6059784

ROBEY Lorraine Marie (see SOUTTER, Mrs)

ROBINSON Kathryn (see HOGARTH, Mrs)

ROBINSON Laura Jane (see REGAN, Mrs)

ROBINSON Maria (see O'BRIEN, Mrs)

ROBINSON Natalie Mary (see GOWEN, Mrs)

ROBSON Joan (see CHURLISH, Mrs)

ROBSON Kirsty Marie (see HUDSON, Mrs)

ROBSON Sandra Lindsay Christina 26/08/1970 Clevedon Crest Hill Peaslake Guildford Surrey GU5 9PE **Tel:** (01306) 730448 w 6001585

Shelagh Lyndsay 07/05/1969 (25/01/2002) 608 Veterinary Group 608 Warwick Road Solihull West Midlands B91 1AA **Tel:** (0121) 705 3044 w 6059831

RODDA Heidi Ann (see PHILLIPS, Mrs)

RODGERS Nadia Rachel Marie (nee Rodgers, formerly Killingback) 10/09/1999 (27/02/2003) 26 Tolverne Road LONDON SW20 8RA **Tel:** (07971) 068854 w 6152692

Rachael Louise (nee Williams) 21/03/2001 39 Holifast Road Wylde Green Sutton Coldfield West Midlands B72 1AP **Tel:** (0121) 682 2398 w 6098881

RODHAM Rachel Mary 21/01/1980 (28/06/2000) 104 Thorpe House Avenue SHEFFIELD S8 9NJ **Tel:** (0114) 2810221 w 6059853

RODMELL Judith Emma (see PEMBERTON, Mrs)

RODWELL Carolyn Emma 01/02/1995 (18/12/2003) Chevening House Station Road Henbury Bristol BS10 7QQ **Tel:** (0117) 950 5888 w 602692X

ROGERS Adele Louise (nee Nelson) 11/09/1996 (26/01/2005) 49 Henley House The Spinnakers Aigborth LIVERPOOL L19 3RZ **Tel:** (07801) 565241 w 6041777

ROGERS Amanda-Jane (see ERRNE, Mrs)

Barbara Jean (nee Williams) 28/10/1986 (04/10/2002) Wyatts Crawley End Chrishall Royston Hertfordshire SG8 8QL **Tel:** (01763) 838 264 w 6063870

Marni Jean (nee Allen) 15/02/1994 (15/10/2001) 7b Ballyblack Road Portaferry NEWTOWNARDS County Down BT22 1PY **Tel:** (0284) 2729621 w 6068460

Ruth Amy (nee Brand) 20/05/2002 42 Hallcroft Road Whittlesey Peterborough Cambridgeshire PE7 1JW **Tel:** (01235) 550934 w 6255983

ROLFE Lisa Joanne (see WOOLDRIDGE, Mrs)

ROLLITT Catherine (see COOKSLEY, Mrs)

ROONEY Amanda Yvonne 16/09/1998 (03/09/2001) 215d Stoke Newington Church Street LONDON N16 9ET **Tel:** (0208) 8081376 w 6100225

ROPE Beverly Jane (see SHINGLETON, Mrs)

ROSE Michaela Ann (nee Osborne) 22/09/1988 (16/11/2006) 7 Paxcroft Way Trowbridge Wiltshire BA14 7DG **Tel:** (01225) 340683 w 6001417

ROSS Debbie Lee 08/04/2003 Ardmohr Stirling Road Milnathort Kinross KY13 9XR **Tel:** (01577) 863494 w 6257512

Jane 14/09/1998 Cornerways Station Road East Preston Littlehampton West Sussex BN16 3AJ **Tel:** (01903) 770795 w 6135291

Joanna Elizabeth (nee Chandler) 25/08/1994 East Ongley Farmhouse Beech Lane Biddenden ASHFORD Kent TN27 8HF **Tel:** (01580) 291503 w 6031088

Katrina Louise 17/01/1996 The Annex Hill Barn Bourton Hill Bourton-on-the-Water Gloucestershire GL54 2LF w 6027275

ROSSINGTON Karen Gwendoline (see GRAY, Mrs)

ROUZEL Amy Elizabeth 09/09/1996 105 Hunters Oak Hemel Hempstead Hertfordshire HP2 7SZ **Tel:** (01442) 401 282 w 6043774

ROWE Michelle Amanda (see SHIELDS, Mrs)

ROWLAND Dawn Louise 13/03/2002 16 Sapphire Gate Copsewood Coventry CV2 5JQ **Tel:** (02476) 441 639 w 6264871

ROWLANDS Margaret Kate 31/01/1994 (05/11/2004) Upton Garth Upton Bude Cornwall EX23 0LY **Tel:** (01288) 325724 w 6067660

Valerie Anne 09/08/1983 Rosemount Veterinary Centre 24 Old Woking Road West Byfleet Surrey KT14 6HP **Tel:** (01932) 341058 w 606001X

ROWLEY Amanda (see ROWLEY-EVANS, Mrs)

ROWLEY Emma Jane 01/02/1996 11 Delft Gardens Waterlooville Hampshire PO8 8SP **Tel:** (02392) 241825 w 6035581

ROWLEY-EVANS Amanda (nee Rowley) 30/10/2001 (29/06/2009) 2 Marron Close Leyland Lancashire PR25 1RX **Tel:** (01772) 465264 w 6252749

ROWSE Paula 14/10/2002 Pencarrow Fore Street Probus Truro Cornwall TR2 4LQ **Tel:** (01726) 882073 w 613412X

RUNDLE Leanne 14/12/2000 19 Chapel Lane Spondon Derby DE21 7JS **Tel:** (01332) 666078 w 6204822

RUSHWORTH Kathryn Jane (see RICHMOND, Mrs)

RUSSELL Janet Ann 11/11/1994 (29/05/2001) Bardyke Bank Upwell Wisbech Cambridgeshire PE14 9HH **Tel:** (01945) 772245 w 6037501

Kerry Louise (nee Hanyszyn) 10/09/1998 176 London Road Clacton-on-Sea Essex CO15 4DU **Tel:** (01255) 812365 w 6128706

RUSTAGE Caroline (nee Mulholland) 30/01/1997 4 Hawthorne Grove Paddington Warrington Cheshire WA1 3EQ **Tel:** (01925) 838786 w 6039258

RYAN Lindsay Ann (see BREEZE, Mrs)

RYCROFT Alison Clare 08/08/1991 (28/04/2004) Southfield Veterinary Centre South Walks DORCHESTER Dorset DT1 1DU **Tel:** (01305) 262913 w 6095610

RYLEY Kirsty Louise 23/06/1999 154 Worcester Road Malvern Worcestershire WR14 1AA **Tel:** (01684) 573333 w 6036406

RYMER Rachel 14/02/1994 Elcombe Farm Uley Dursley Gloucestershire GL11 5BP **Tel:** (01453) 860 265 w 6068201

S

SABERI Sophie 24/03/1998 (05/06/2006) Newdigate Veterinary Surgery George Horley Place Church Road Newdigate DORKING Surrey RH5 5DW **Tel:** (01306) 632863 w 6118786

SADLER Claire Jane Gilmour (see BRUCE, Mrs)

SADLER Donna Maria (see GREEN, Mrs)

Jane Elizabeth 01/10/1982 Hill Farm Church Hill Kinver STOURBRIDGE West Midlands DY7 6HX w 609069X

SADLER Kate Louise (see SCOTT, Mrs)

SAGAR Alice Lydia Ireland (nee Gastall) 05/08/1987 (07/08/2003) 321 Blackburn Road West End Oswalotwistle Lancs BB5 4NQ **Tel:** (01254) 889595 w 6014233

SAGE Zoe Anne (nee Dauncey) 17/01/1995 24 Caudledown Lane Stenalees St. Austell Cornwall PL26 8TG **Tel:** (01726) 850 995 w 6030346

SAGGARS Katie Louise 04/02/2002 Larkmead Veterinary Group Ilges Lane Cholsey Wallingford Oxfordshire OX10 9PA **Tel:** (01491) 651379 w 6254080

SALISBURY Dawn Louise (nee Hampson) 06/02/1995 20 Ryecroft Avenue Tottington Bury Lancashire BL8 3LX **Tel:** (01204) 886465 w 6034511

Rachael Mary 18/09/1995 (26/01/2004) 22 Mitton Gardens Stourport-on-Severn Worcestershire DY13 9AE **Tel:** (01299) 879847 w 6032208

SALMON Charlotte Agnes 17/11/2000 Meon Crescent High Street Soberton Southampton Hampshire SO32 3PN w 6203007

Jane Margaret (nee Brown) 05/09/1988 Cumberland House Colchester Road Ardleigh Colchester Essex CO7 7NS w 6046505

SAMPSON Julia Gail (nee Pengelly) 12/02/1993 (18/07/2001) The Castle Veterinary Group Limited Pennygillam Way Launceston Cornwall PL15 7ED **Tel:** (01566) 772371 w 6058532

SANBAR Claire 28/06/2002 RSPCA Putney Animal Hospital 6 Clarendon Drive London SW15 1AA **Tel:** (0300) 123 0716 w 6269744

SANDERS Caroline Nicola (see GUY, Mrs)

SANDERS Celine Geraldine Marie (nee Organ) 19/09/1991 (18/11/2008) Westerly 9 Station Road Kimberley Norwich Norfolk NR18 9HB **Tel:** (010603) 759502 w 6058088

SANDS Cheryl (nee Bytheway) 25/02/2003 The Animal Health Centre Ltd Parkway Centre Coulby Newham Middlesbrough Cleveland TS8 0TJ **Tel:** (01642) 576333 w 6272659

SAN-MIGUEL Anna (see TANKARD, Mrs)

SANSOM Jackie Mellissa 23/03/2001 Country Cottage Mill Road Walpole Highway Wisbech Cambridgeshire PE15 0HU **Tel:** (01945) 781198 w 6202963

Naomi 25/01/1994 (28/08/2007) The Old School Station Road Clutton BRISTOL BS39 5RA **Tel:** (0117) 962 8706 w 606618X

SANTOS Alison Jane (nee Heywood, formerly Thomas) 04/09/1997 (02/11/2000) 11 Robert Avenue Somersham Cambridgeshire PE28 3EX w 6117749

SASIN Anne-Marie 02/08/2002 Unit 10 Berkshire House County Park Business Park Shrivenham Road Swindon Wiltshire SN1 2NR w 6276124

SATCHELL Louise 04/09/1997 64 Hatch Ride Crowthorne Berkshire RG45 6LB **Tel:** (01344) 420431 w 6113198

SATTERLEY Jane (see BERRY, Mrs)

SAUNDERS Lucy (see PURCHASE, Mrs)

SAVILL Carolyn Hilda DipAVN(Surgical) (nee Sudding) 09/11/1990 58 Albemarle Road Churchdown Gloucester Gloucestershire GL3 2HE **Tel:** (01452) 712194 w 6061487

SCARLETT Erin Michelle (see SCARLETT-MCNAIR, Mrs)

SCARLETT-MCNAIR Erin Michelle (nee Scarlett) 16/08/1995 9 Shearwater Crescent DUNFERMLINE Fife KY11 8JX **Tel:** (01383) 724456 w 602844X

SCARROTT Barbara Gail (nee Davies) 23/08/1990 55 St. Kenelms Avenue Hayley Green HALESOWEN West Midlands B63 1DN **Tel:** (0121) 550 3643 w 6048772

SCHALKER Eve Odette (see CHRISTIE, Mrs)

SCHOLES Elizabeth Helen 25/03/2002 19 Kiln Court Salendine Nook HUDDERSFIELD HD3 3GH w 6275959

SCHUMANN Anna Maria 20/12/2000 (27/02/2004) 212 Caswell Close Farnborough Hampshire GU14 8TQ **Tel:** (01252) 376809 w 6026963

SCOTT Aimee-Louise Teresa (formerly Woodward) 19/12/1991 (22/10/2003) Downsview 5 Cootham Brow Storrington Pulborough West Sussex RH20 4JP **Tel:** (01903) 745190 w 6050340

Anita Ruth (nee Pile) 30/07/2002 (24/03/2006) Shaw Veterinary Centre Ltd Shaw Village Centre Ramleaze Drive Shaw Swindon Wiltshire SN5 5PY **Tel:** (01793) 881919 w 6241958

Clare 28/06/2002 3 Hollyhocks Lane Barkston Ash Tadcaster North Yorkshire LS24 9TT **Tel:** (01937) 557753 w 6271097

SCOTT Gemma Marianne (see WILSON, Mrs)

SCOTT Gillian Barbara (see RICH, Mrs)

Helen Rowena 19/01/2000 39 Hassop Way Beaufront Park Bedlington Northumberland NE22 7LE **Tel:** (01670) 829351 w 6148981

Johanne Elizabeth 19/08/2002 The Old Police Station 4 High Street Barton upon Humber North Lincolnshire DN18 5PA **Tel:** (01652) 636359 w 6264387

Karen DipAVN(Surgical) 21/01/1998 181 Craigmillar Castle Avenue EDINBURGH EH16 4DN w 611919X

Kate Louise (nee Sadler) 14/09/1999 91 Ascot Walk Newcastle upon Tyne Tyne and Wear NE3 2UZ **Tel:** (0191) 2715472 w 6138758

Lorraine Ellen 09/08/1983 (22/06/2004) Hill Park Veterinary Group 1 Lindfield Road Romford RM3 9BJ **Tel:** (01708) 344455/386046 w 6060370

Natalie Louise 27/02/2002 (07/11/2005) Priory Veterinary Ltd Gwalia Gardens Pwllhai CARDIGAN Dyfed SA43 1DB **Tel:** (01239) 612479 w 6255114

Sharon Ann (nee Moar) 22/08/1994 (24/11/1998) Westside Veterinary Surgery West Side Bixter SHETLAND ZE2 9NA **Tel:** (01595) 810456 w 6036370

SCOTT-WILL Tessa Belle 26/01/1994 (13/11/2008) 34 Beacon Gate LONDON SE14 5UB w 6067241

SCRASE Karin Vivecca (nee Southern, nee Scrase) 10/08/1978 (24/03/2006) 7 St. Johns Terrace Pendeen Penzance Cornwall TR19 7DP **Tel:** (01736) 787430 w 6061068

SCRIMSHAW Fiona Ann 06/09/1995 (04/10/2002) 17 Hereford Close WALSALL WS9 8HX **Tel:** (01922) 745063 w 603847X

SCRYMINGER Laura Marie 22/11/2001 Grove House Holt Road Fakenham Norfolk NR21 8JG **Tel:** (01328) 862137 w 6261747

SEAL Victoria Louise (see GAJEWSKI, Mrs)

SEATON Alison Mary 19/04/1993 (17/09/2004) 7 Brackley Lane Calvert Buckingham Buckinghamshire MK18 2HF **Tel:** (01296) 733504 w 6014798

SEED Joanne (see CARBERRY, Mrs)

SEIERSEN Lise Jane 08/08/1991 7 Roedeer Cottages Raskelf York YO61 3UY **Tel:** (01347) 823446 w 6060494

SELLARS Carol (nee Macfadyen) 10/12/2002 (23/06/2009) 48 Selworthy Drive Crewe CW1 3RR **Tel:** 01270-258538 w 6263584

SELLARS Helen Barbara (see THORNTON, Mrs)

SELLINGS Tracey Lorraine (see BRISTOW, Mrs)

SEWELL Claire Louise (see HUXTABLE, Mrs)

SEYMOUR Jennifer Susan 15/01/1981 19 Wheatcroft Close Penkridge Stafford ST19 5JS **Tel:** (01785) 714182 w 6068711

SHACKLETON Nicholas Andrew 22/11/2001 Flat 3 42 Tatton Road South Heaton Moor STOCKPORT Cheshire SK4 4LU **Tel:** (07807) 928254 m 6264277

SHADBOLT Naomi Rebecca 09/09/1999 122 Fosseway Avenue Moreton-in-Marsh Gloucestershire GL56 0EA **Tel:** (01608) 650097 w 6186023

SHAH Samantha Arunkumar (see NICHOLS, Mrs)

SHAHGAGHI Rachel Emma (see DIXEY, Mrs)

SHANNON Amy 23/01/2003 52 Maker Rd Torpoint Cornwall PL11 2HZ **Tel:** (01752) 562575 w 6276168

SHARMAN Donna Iris (see KIRBY, Mrs)

SHARP Clare Elizabeth 27/09/1999 Hykeham Green Lincoln Road North Hykeham Lincoln Lincolnshire LN6 8NH **Tel:** (01522) 683300 w 6147707

Diana 11/10/1965 45 Graemesdyke Avenue LONDON SW14 7BH **Tel:** (020) 88762966 w 6060519

Sarah Jane Fergusson 20/04/2001 (09/10/2008) RSPCA Putney Animal Hospital 6 Clarendon Drive London SW15 1AA **Tel:** (0300) 123 0716 w 6113664

SHARRY Fiona Caroline 30/09/1999 (10/04/2008) 1-5 Hugh Street London SW1V 1QQ **Tel:** (020) 7932 2370 w 6185649

SHAW Joanne 05/09/1997 (17/02/2000) 17 The Crest Hillcrest WHITEHAVEN Cumbria CA28 6TJ **Tel:** (07779) 339938 w 6108133

SHAW Lucy Jane (see GOTT, Ms)

Patricia Muriel Farquhar (nee Jones) 03/09/1996 Woodside Felon's Oak Rodhuish Minehead Somerset TA24 6QT **Tel:** (01984) 641461 w 6076030

SHEARING Virginia Victoria 28/09/2000 79 Priory Road Shirehampton Bristol Avon BS11 9TF w 6204327

SHEPHERD Fiona Jane (formerly Bell) 05/02/1996 (11/06/2002) The Dog House Easter Craigs Craighall Blairgowrie Perthshire PH10 7JB **Tel:** (01250) 876483 w 6041915

Hannah 22/08/1995 (03/08/2007) The Avenue Veterinary Clinic 33 St. Peters Avenue Kettering Northamptonshire NN16 0HB **Tel:** (01536) 512200 w 6036858

Julie Dawn 27/08/1999 63 Norwich Road Wroxham Norwich Norfolk NR12 8RX **Tel:** (01603) 783 920 w 6185429

SHEPHERD Sally Louisa (see LAWTON, Mrs)

Sandra Dawn 13/02/1989 13 St. Thomas Drive Hatch End Middlesex HA5 4SX **Tel:** (0208) 4202055 w 6059296

Sarah 23/03/2000 Oundle Veterinary Surgery 92 South Road Oundle Peterborough PE8 4BP **Tel:** (01832) 273521 w 6123628

Susan (nee Leedham, formerly Leedham-Page) 07/08/1987 (17/02/2000) 267 Bristnall Hall Road Oldbury Warley West Midlands B68 9NF **Tel:** (0121) 544 4327 w 6055054

SHERBURN Victoria Clare (nee Hawker) 15/01/1999 (17/10/2006) The Avenue Veterinary Group 31 Park Road Bingley West Yorkshire BD16 4BL **Tel:** (01274) 510868 w 6138452

SHERIFF Kate Louise 08/08/2002 (04/04/2008) Town & Country Veterinary Group 40 King Street Blackburn Lancashire BB2 2DH **Tel:** (01254) 681455 w 6143735

SHERLOCK Allison Dianne 18/01/1999 The Veterinary Surgery Tetts Farm West Street Hinton St. George Somerset TA17 8SB **Tel:** (01460) 73398 w 613949X

SHIELDS Michelle Amanda (nee Rowe) 10/09/1996 21 The Terrace Finchfield Wolverhampton West Midlands WV3 9EW **Tel:** (01902) 342775 w 6098655

SHILLINGFORD Clair Lorraine 06/09/1999 The Addiscombe Road Veterinary Centre 263 Addiscombe Road Croydon CR0 7HX **Tel:** (020) 8654 0151 w 6145200

SHINGLETON Beverly Jane (nee Rope) 13/12/1984 61 Greenoaks Lancing West Sussex BN15 0HE **Tel:** (01273) 890454 w 6059911

SHIPLEY Dawn (see WARD, Mrs)

SHIPPEY Julie Suzanne (nee Mustoe) 06/08/1990 (07/09/2005) 14 Halsey Drive Hemel Hempstead Hertfordshire HP1 3SF **Tel:** (01442) 269099 w 605746X

SHIPPEY Lisa Jane (see WILLIAMS, Mrs)

SHOEMARK Nadean Ann 10/01/2003 8 Balmoral Close Penycoedcae PONTYPRIDD Mid Glamorgan CF37 1XE **Tel:** (01656) 766353 w 6259932

SHONE Sarah Elizabeth (nee Bufton) 18/09/2000 Averley House Farm Hinckley Road Sapcote Leicester LE9 4LH **Tel:** (01455) 271277 w 6202765

SHORTT Michelle (see CANNY, Mrs)

SHUFFLEBOTHAM Debra 11/01/1988 (26/07/1999) Weighbridge Referral Centre Kemys Way Swansea Enterprise Park Morriston Swansea SA6 8QF **Tel:** (01792) 796660 w 6093861

SHUTE Elizabeth Joanne 09/09/2002 7 Jubilee Close Syston Leicester Leicestershire LE7 1JB w 6275211

Zoe Amanda (nee Nursey) 24/08/1993 1 Seaview Road Drayton Portsmouth Hampshire PO6 1EN **Tel:** (02392) 371679 w 6015995

SIBLEY Amanda Grace 29/01/1998 The Freda Powell Centre 1c Eynsham Drive Thamesmead London SE2 9RQ **Tel:** (020) 8311 6695 w 6018817

SIDAOUI Pamela Joy 01/08/1978 (22/04/2002) 51 Sunbury Lane Walton-on-Thames Surrey KT12 2HX **Tel:** (01932) 225168 w 6060632

SIMM Joanne DipAVN(Surgical) 18/09/1995 Carisbrooke House Middridge Road Rushyford Ferryhill County Durham DL17 0NH **Tel:** (01388) 722234 w 6028745

SIMMONS Bonnie Jayne (nee Maltwood) 10/09/1990 (18/11/2005) 11 Larch Close Ruskington Sleaford Lincolnshire NG34 9GB **Tel:** (01526) 830433 w 6055724

SIMMONS Clare Deborah (see WOODS, Mrs)

SIMMONS Shelley Louise (see HOLDEN, Mrs)

SIMPSON Alison (nee Butroid) 21/01/1994 Nottingham Trent University Brackenhurst SOUTHWELL Nottinghamshire NG25 0QF **Tel:** (0115) 848 8046 w 6065812

Lesley Elizabeth (nee Allan) 09/09/1997 Moray Coast Veterinary Group West Road Greshop Estate Forres Morayshire IV36 2GW **Tel:** (01309) 672243 w 6107628

SIMS Claire Helen 02/03/2001 Cornerways Stone Road Yaxham Dereham Norfolk NR19 1RR **Tel:** (01362) 692850 w 6213545

SINCLAIR Sandra Louise (nee Wilkins) 27/09/1991 (18/03/2004) PDSA Pet Aid Hospital 64 Heyford Road Braunstone Leicester Leicestershire LE3 1SR **Tel:** (0116) 255 8731 w 6095869

SKEEL Eleanor Clare 28/06/2002 Cecil Avenue Veterinary Centre 1 Cecil Avenue Sale Cheshire M33 5BW **Tel:** (0161) 973 0375 w 6275816

SKERTEN Jayne Louise (see JAMES, Mrs)

SKINNER Sharon Susan 31/01/1997 Arden House Animal Hospital 56 Pembroke Road Ruislip Middlesex HA4 8NF **Tel:** (01895) 633600 w 6077318

SLADE Brenda Josephine 01/10/1971 Priory Veterinary Ltd Gwalia Gardens Pwllhai CARDIGAN Dyfed SA43 1DB **Tel:** (01239) 612479 w 6060734

Elizabeth Henrietta Leoni 27/07/2000 (04/06/2004) 6 Cabin Moss Bracknell Berkshire RG12 0WB **Tel:** (01344) 303961 w 6190863

SLATER Deborah Ann (see HALLAS, Mrs)

SLATER Gail Sharron 17/06/1993 (07/10/2003) 17-19 Church Road Leyland Lancashire PR25 3EJ **Tel:** (01772) 432039 w 6014404

Linda Ann DipAVN(Surgical) (nee Oxley) 28/07/1992 16 Norman Court Potters Bar Hertfordshire EN6 1HY **Tel:** (01707) 664987 w 6004837

SLATTER Angela Jane (nee Hodson) 19/02/1996 (11/05/2005) East Hamptonne La Rue De La Hague St. Peter Jersey JE3 7DB **Tel:** (01534) 744641 w 6036621

SLEE Jane Louise (nee Every) 07/03/1991 (24/06/2003) Clay House Abbotsham BIDEFORD Devon EX39 5AS **Tel:** (01271) 327256 w 6060767

SLOW Jean May 10/10/1972 46 Barnet Road London Colney St. Albans Hertfordshire AL2 1AU **Tel:** (01727) 825966 w 6060778

SMALL Tracy (see THURSTAN, Mrs)

SMALLWOOD Rachel Katherine Fishley (nee Holland) 28/08/1998 128 Woodlands Road Charfield WOTTON-UNDER-EDGE Gloucestershire GL12 8LU **Tel:** (01454) 260337 w 6131005

SMART Rebecca Louise (see WATERS, Mrs)

SMEDLEY Ann Marie 30/10/1998 (28/04/2008) 32 Pool Street Macclesfield Cheshire SK11 7NX **Tel:** (01625) 612434 w 6141443

SMITH Aileen Patricia (see CLEGG, Mrs)

SMITH Alison Hazel 08/11/1991 (26/02/2004) University of Cambridge Deptof Clinical Veterinary Medicine Madingley Cambridge CB3 0ES **Tel:** (01223) 337647 w 6060814

Allison (formerly MacLeod) 23/01/2003 123 Burte Court BELLSHILL Lanarkshire ML4 3GB **Tel:** (01698) 344 377 w 6282372

Angela 27/02/2002 1 Dulverton Road Witton Birmingham West Midlands B6 7EQ **Tel:** (0121) 328 1716 w 6257281

Antonia Helen Mary 08/09/1993 (31/10/2003) 15 Dean Close Nottingham Nottinghamshire NG8 2BX **Tel:** (07967) 764162 w 6026894

Catherine Anne 04/02/2000 28 Primrose Close Purley on Thames Reading Berkshire RG8 8DG w 6145721

SMITH Catherine Mary (see DEAN, Mrs)

Claire Elizabeth 09/02/1998 (13/04/2006) 1 Southview Cottages Magdalen Laver Ongar Essex CM5 0ER **Tel:** (01279) 426 027 w 6118323

Claire Marie 18/08/1992 (13/03/2003) 7 Albert Street Chadsmoor Cannock Staffordshire WS11 5JA **Tel:** (01543) 502392 w 600881X

David Alexander 27/11/2000 (20/01/2005) Scarsdale Veterinary Hospital 45-47 Kedleston Road Derby DE22 1FN **Tel:** (01332) 345191 m 6202743

SMITH Diana Helen (see FRANKLIN, Mrs)

Donna Louise 04/11/1997 12 Aspen Court SHILDON County Durham DL4 2RQ w 6118334

SMITH Donna-Marie (see BROWNRIGG, Mrs)

SMITH Jill Caroline (see GIBBINSON, Mrs)

SMITH Joanna Claire (see YOUNG, Ms)

Joanna Louise 17/11/2000 (17/02/2009) 15 Marley Avenue NEW MILTON Hampshire BH25 5LQ w 6202435

Judith Mary 06/09/2001 Pelyn Veterinary Group 8 Kings Avenue St. Austell Cornwall PL25 4TT **Tel:** (01726) 68177 w 6227867

SMITH Julie Lesley (see LONGTHORPE, Mrs)

Kate Joanna (nee Durant, formerly Primmer) 03/08/1992 Keele House 30 Sea Lane East Preston West Sussex BN16 1NE **Tel:** (01903) 775227 w 6005422

Kathryn Elizabeth (nee Willis) 17/01/1995 2 New Farm Moor End Lane Rodwell Bedford Bedfordshire MK43 7HZ **Tel:** (01234) 782534 w 603652X

Kim Josephine 21/01/1998 Equipet Veterinary Hospital 24 Nicol Street Kirkcaldy Fife KY1 1NY **Tel:** (01592) 641333 w 6036315

SMITH Kirsty Marie (see RAWLINS, Mrs)

Lisa Ann (nee Wilson) 06/02/2002 (15/12/2006) 10 Rowletts View BIGGLESWADE Bedfordshire SG18 0FD w 6273264

Lisa Michelle EVN 04/09/1997 (02/11/2009) 200 St. Ediths Marsh Bromham CHIPPENHAM Wiltshire SN15 2DJ w 6100349

Louise Maria DipAVN(Surgical) (formerly Emmerson) 21/08/1995 (17/02/2009) Keepers Cottage Bragbury Lane Datchworth KNEBWORTH Hertfordshire SG3 6QZ w 6037137

Melanie Jane 07/09/1992 (05/10/2001) 17 Butterworth Path Luton Bedfordshire LU2 0TP **Tel:** (01582) 617533 w 6006459

SMITH Nicola (see WELDON, Mrs)

Paula (nee Jones) 14/09/1998 Weighbridge Referral Centre Kemys Way Swansea Enterprise Park Morriston Swansea SA6 8QF **Tel:** (01792) 796660 w 6030506

Penny Ann 25/08/1999 6 Hamilton Road South Willesborough Ashford Kent TN24 0DJ **Tel:** (01233) 634 793 w 6043457

SMITH Rebecca Maya (see DAWE, Miss)

Rosalind Helen 28/08/1968 C/o Hangzhou Yusei Industrial Co Ltd No 335 Hongxing Road Xiaoshan Hangzhou Zhejiang 311231 China w 606095X

SMITH Susan Claire (see EVERETT, Mrs)

Tessa Frances 09/08/1983 (02/11/1999) 119 Guisborough Road Nunthorpe Middlesbrough Cleveland TS7 0JD **Tel:** (01642) 316748 w 6060971

SMITH Valerie Anne (see POLLARD, Mrs)

SMYTH Victoria Helen (nee Coman) 18/09/1998 38 Wilfred Owen Drive Birkenhead Merseyside CH41 0HA w 6135101

SNEAP Rowena (see BATEY, Mrs)

SNELLING Lisa Alison (nee Swallow) 09/10/1989 (02/11/2007) The Old Bakehouse High Street Partridge Green Horsham West Sussex RH13 8HU **Tel:** (01403) 710332 w 6061589

SNOWSILL Joanna (nee Beaven) 15/01/1993 Hannam House Lamberts Lane Midhurst West Sussex GU29 9EA **Tel:** (01730) 816833 w 6065211

SNUTCH Allison Jayne 06/09/1990 Northlands Veterinary Hospital 2 Northampton Road Kettering Northamptonshire NN15 7JU **Tel:** (01536) 485 543 w 6061024

SOMERVILLE Isobel Jean 24/01/1995 (17/12/2009) Dragons Lair Killanley Ballina Co Mayo Ireland **Tel:** (00353) 9637702 w 6032616

SOPP Kathryn Margaret (see WESTCOTT, Mrs)

SOUTHERN Karin Vivecca (see SCRASE, Mrs)

SOUTHERNWOOD Teresa 08/09/1997 (18/11/2005) Easton College Easton Norwich Norfolk NR9 5DX w 6031598

SOUTHWELL Janet Patricia (see PATRICK, Mrs)

SOUTTER Lorraine Marie (nee Robey) 16/03/2001 (11/02/2009) 25 New Church Road HOVE East Sussex BN3 4AD **Tel:** (01273) 727433 w 6214161

SPALDING Jodi Rae 15/11/2001 6 Fitzroy Close Bracknell Berkshire RG12 7GP **Tel:** 01344868761 w 6250945

SPARK Sarah Jane (nee Read) 08/09/1997 27 Pyes Meadow Elmswell BURY ST EDMUNDS Suffolk IP30 9UF w 6118618

SPARKE Claudine Helen 23/08/1990 481 Carlton Road WORKSOP Nottinghamshire S81 7PL **Tel:** (07876) 438990 w 6053975

SPARROW Caroline Heather (see WHYBROW, Mrs)

SPEERS Emma Joanne (nee Dick) 01/09/2000 (15/12/2006) Balla-Noo-Martyn 9 St. Martins Park Owston Ferry DONCASTER South Yorkshire DN9 1FE **Tel:** (01427) 728359 w 6203425

SPENCER Lorraine (nee Gingell) 17/08/1992 Wick Farm Keevil Trowbridge Wiltshire BA14 6NH **Tel:** (01380) 828875 w 6005477

SPIVEY Justine (nee Knight) 31/07/1992 (10/12/2003) Sunnytop 1A The Park Mayfield Ashbourne Derbyshire DE6 2HT **Tel:** (01335) 342375 w 6008489

SPOORS Judith Ann (see OLSEN, Mrs)

SPRIGGS Lydia Kate (nee Downes) 25/10/2000 74 Lady Margarets Avenue Deeping St. James PETERBOROUGH PE6 8TQ **Tel:** (01778) 341503 w 6204008

SPRINGALL Kelly 12/04/2002 The Wylie Veterinary Centre 196 Hall Lane Upminster Essex RM14 1TD **Tel:** (01708) 251200 w 6276773

STABLER Linda Margaret 23/10/2000 Park Veterinary Centre 256 Cassiobury Drive WATFORD Hertfordshire WD17 3PA **Tel:** (01923) 223321 w 6203700

STAFFORD Angela (nee Marchant) 21/01/1994 (23/06/2006) 39 Buxton Road Congleton Cheshire CW12 2DU **Tel:** (01260) 290 191 w 6067219

STAGG Helen Frances 12/09/2000 9 Manor Close Crayford Dartford Kent DA1 4EX **Tel:** (01322) 523153 w 6204118

Malcolm 19/08/1994 (15/01/2008) 7 Scotney Way Pontprennau Cardiff CF23 8PJ **Tel:** (029) 2054 9380 m 6018883

STALKER Christine 19/12/1974 (03/01/2001) 8 Old School Close Barnton NORTHWICH Cheshire CW8 4GR **Tel:** (01606) 754 524 w 6061170

STANDLEY Philippa Jane (see HARPER, Mrs)

STANIER Rebecca Wilson 22/08/2000 926 Walsall Road Great Barr Birmingham West Midlands B42 1TG **Tel:** (0121) 357 4286 w 6152590

STANLEY Kelsey Jane (nee Bates) 18/10/1999 (25/08/2009) 20 Palmer Close Stansted Mountfitchet Stansted Essex CM24 8FB **Tel:** (01279) 815975 w 6152615

STANNERS Helen Margaret (see EL DABE, Mrs)

STANSFIELD Diana May (see STANTON, Mrs)

STANTON Diana May DipAVN(Surgical) (nee Stansfield) 11/10/1993 2 Buttercrambe Road Stamford Bridge York YO41 1AN **Tel:** (01759) 371066 w 6064819

STARK Hazel Laureen (see CAMPBELL, Mrs)

STEPHENS Helen Jane DipAVN(Surgical) 18/01/2002 104 Greenacres Kirkby-in-Ashfield Nottingham Nottinghamshire NG17 7GF **Tel:** 07939454828 w 6266708

STEPHENSON Catherine Mary DipAVN(Surgical) 28/09/1999 12 Everard Lane Caterham Surrey CR3 6QS **Tel:** (01883) 381187 w 6152794

STEPTOWE Fiona Kimberly 14/09/1998 The Wylie Veterinary Centre 196 Hall Lane Upminster Essex RM14 1TD **Tel:** (01708) 251200 w 6128998

STEVENS Toni Alison (nee Delaney) 25/08/1998 16 Willow Lea Tonbridge Kent TN10 3RF **Tel:** (0207) 5648520 w 6117294

STEWARD Katherine Jayne (see HOWIE, Mrs)

STEWART Laura Ann (see HOARE, Mrs)

STEWART Phillipa 28/01/1998 28 Riverside Close Whitley Coventry CV3 4AU **Tel:** (024) 76223232 w 6022663

Suzanne Helen 22/11/2001 Lincvet 43 Friars Lane Lincoln Lincolnshire LN2 5AL **Tel:** (01522) 534842 w 6268787

STICKINGS Michelle Anne 31/07/1992 (27/02/2002) Priory Lodge Veterinary Group 31 Pembury Road TONBRIDGE Kent TN9 2JB **Tel:** (01732) 353668 w 600830X

STILES Karen 04/02/2002 Melrose Farm Reigate Road Hookwood Surrey RH6 0AP **Tel:** (01293) 773282 w 6269238

STILL Lesley Ann (nee Booker) 23/08/1990 (03/09/2008) 5 Mid-Kent Shopping Centre Castle Road Allington Maidstone Kent ME16 0PU **Tel:** (01622) 663166 w 6045920

STOBBS Sharon (nee Cranmer) 21/03/2001 26 Earlswood Drive Alderholt FORDINGBRIDGE Hampshire SP6 3EN **Tel:** (01425) 654139 w 6214359

STOKES Michelle Louise (see PALMER, Mrs)

STOKES Nicola Jayne 16/03/2001 (14/01/2009) 24 The chesters Westlea SWINDON SN5 7DB **Tel:** (01793) 872 938 w 6214150

STOKES Rachel Mary (see COURT, Mrs)

Tracy Ann (nee Buttifant) 25/08/1995 (18/11/1999) 48 Kennedy Avenue East Grinstead West Sussex RH19 2DG **Tel:** (01342) 327 941 w 6027989

Vanessa (nee Pearson) 11/02/1998 456-458 Hagley Road West Oldbury West Midlands B68 0DL **Tel:** (0121) 422 2902 w 6131195

STONE Claire Louise (nee Hook) 03/08/1990 Animed Veterinary Centre 24 Oxford Street Whitstable Kent CT5 1DD **Tel:** (01227) 273005 w 6053181

STOOKS Rachael Elizabeth 10/12/2002 Kingsnorth Veterinary Centre Ashford Road Kingsnorth Ashford Kent TN23 3EA **Tel:** (01233) 640022 w 6285331

STOREY Angela Elizabeth 24/01/1995 (11/11/2008) 1 High Chibburn Farm Widdrington MORPETH Northumberland NE61 5EF w 6035311

STOREY Deborah (see GRANT, Mrs)

STREETON Joanna Kenzie Erica (see HIGGINSON, Mrs)

STRICKLAND Lisa 20/01/1999 (27/10/2000) Chevening House Station Road Henbury Bristol BS10 7QQ **Tel:** (0117) 950 5888 w 6140326

Paula Danielle 17/01/1984 1 Handel Avenue St. George Bristol BS5 8DS w 6001698

STRIKE Christine Mowbray DipAVN(Surgical) 05/02/1970 2 The Old Byre Dove Bank Kirby-In-Furness Cumbria LA17 7XD w 6061432

STRINGER Emma Louisa (see BARTLETT, Mrs)

STRONACH Marian (see CAMPBELL, Miss)

STRONG Sandra (formerly Newton) 07/02/1985 (11/11/2002) 22 Thornton Road LONDON SW12 0LF **Tel:** (0207) 2289606 w 6015554

STRUCK Claire Lesley (see GODFREY, Mrs)

STUBBS Claire Mary (see BROADHURST, Mrs)

STUBBS Melissa Jane (nee Lindley) 31/07/1992 (08/05/2009) Warren Farm Uttoxeter Road Hollywood STONE Staffordshire ST15 8RB **Tel:** (01889) 505336 w 6008354

Victoria 29/03/2000 (05/11/2004) 57-59 Broadleys Clay Cross Chesterfield Derbyshire S45 9JN **Tel:** (01246) 862266 w 6027796

STUCKEY Gemma Anne (nee Lynch) 10/12/2002 1-2 Park Street Anlaby Road Hull HU3 2JF **Tel:** (01482) 223688 w 6279215

STURDY Charlotte Louise 10/11/1999 Top Cat Veterinary Centre 146 Mackie Avenue Patcham Brighton BN1 8SB **Tel:** (01273) 504800 w 6185792

STURGESS Melanie Jane 03/08/1989 The Farm Coldharbour Lane Carrington Boston Lincolnshire PE22 7JG **Tel:** (01205) 480205 w 6001268

STYLES Jemma Elizabeth 27/02/1998 (07/03/2002) 5a Heather Way Rise Park ROMFORD RM1 4SX **Tel:** (01708) 724005 w 6100407

STYLES Lisa Jane (see HOLT, Mrs)

SUCKLING Tricia Joanne (see HELME, Mrs)

SUDDING Carolyn Hilda (see SAVILL, Mrs)

SULLIVAN Alison 30/07/1979 30 Lochaber Road Bearsden Glasgow G61 2JU **Tel:** (0141) 942 0422 w 6061498

Joanne Valerie 02/02/1996 30 Grosvenor Road Romford Essex RM7 0QT **Tel:** (01708) 723974 w 603070X

Katrina Susannah (nee Walker) 15/10/1992 29 Hillcroft Crescent RUISLIP Middlesex HA4 9HL **Tel:** (0208) 8424430 w 6011990

SUMMERFIELD Tracy Jane 01/02/1999 The Wylie Veterinary Centre 196 Hall Lane Upminster Essex RM14 1TD **Tel:** (01708) 251200 w 6137175

SUMMERS Debra Jayne 23/02/1994 Hollycroft 66 Roston Drive Hinckley Leicestershire LE10 0XP **Tel:** (01455) 616012 w 6068380

Jodie Elisabeth (nee Blott) 14/02/2002 59 Great Brockeridge Westbury-onTrym BRISTOL BS9 3UA **Tel:** (0117) 962 2828 w 6264002

SUMNER Deborah Ann 15/09/1998 (21/06/2005) 57 Churchill Avenue Cheddleton LEEK Staffordshire ST13 7EJ w 6133228

SUTHERLAND Lisa Megan (see BADHAM-MOORE, Mrs)

SUTTON Charlotte Louise Gwillim 08/11/2000 (22/09/2003) Brickworks Cottage Monk Sherborne Road Ramsdell Tadley Hampshire RG26 5PR **Tel:** (01256) 850101 w 6141589

Karen Louise 08/09/1997 Pool Farm Veterinary Surgery Main Road Betley Crewe Cheshire CW3 9AB **Tel:** (01270) 820007 w 6112638

SWALLOW Lisa Alison (see SNELLING, Mrs)

SWALLOW Lucy Victoria 18/01/2002 Shires Veterinary Practice Eccleshall Road Stone Staffordshire ST15 0HJ **Tel:** (01785) 813955 w 6265707

SWAN Nicola Louise (see MCKEAG, Mrs)

SWAN Patricia Angela Jane (nee Foster) 06/02/1989 28 Glenhome Walk Dyce Aberdeen AB21 7FJ **Tel:** (01224) 723166 w 6002873

SWARBRICK Anne Patricia 07/09/1995 (03/10/2003) 2 Chancel Terrace Barnwell Peterborough PE8 5PY **Tel:** (01832) 274512 w 6039101

SWINBURNE Susan (see AKERS, Ms)

SWINDEN Clare Louise (nee Jackson) 05/03/2002 MacQueen Veterinary Surgery 1 Hopton Park London Road Devizes Wiltshire SN10 2EY **Tel:** (01380) 728505 w 6253596

SYDENHAM Nadina Gay 26/08/1976 Mount Veterinary Hospital 21 High Street Wellington Somerset TA21 8QS **Tel:** (01823) 662286 w 6061603

SYKES Emma Elizabeth (nee Harrison) 09/09/1998 2 Leicester Lane Desford LEICESTER LE9 9JJ w 6170634

T

TABERNER Cala 02/11/1990 (07/10/2005) 8 Humber Crescent Sutton Leach ST HELENS Merseyside WA9 4HD **Tel:** (01744) 609957 w 6060610

TABOR Sally Joanne (see BRITTON, Mrs)

TAI Lisa Wynne (nee Woolls) 10/02/1999 (13/08/2008) 201 Treffry Road TRURO Cornwall TR1 1UF **Tel:** (07793) 206097 w 6021706

TALBOTT Sarah (see MCDIARMID-BRANCH, Mrs)

TANFIELD Samantha Margaret (nee Hant) 23/09/1998 2 Archibald Close Pocklington YORK YO42 2DJ **Tel:** (01759) 304714 w 613586X

TANKARD Anna (nee San-Miguel) 26/02/1998 Kingston House 83-85 Main Street Pembroke Pembrokeshire SA71 4DB **Tel:** (01646) 622943 w 6113416

TARLING Jane Lesley 22/01/1985 (15/05/2000) Fernlea Veterinary Clinic Blackhorse Road Kingswood Bristol BS15 8DZ **Tel:** (0117) 960 6145 w 6061680

TATE Clare 23/10/2001 (29/06/2009) 33 Woodmancote DURSLEY Gloucestershire GL11 4AF w 6122001

TAYLER Samantha Lynda (see HOOPER, Mrs)

TAYLOR Alison (nee Day) 07/02/1989 (26/01/2004) Orchard Veterinary Group Wirrall Park Road Glastonbury Somerset BA6 9XE **Tel:** (01458) 832972 w 6013739

Claire Elizabeth (nee Potter) 23/11/2001 2 Ivy Cottages Blaxhall Church Road Tunstall Nr Woodbridge Suffolk IP12 2DB **Tel:** (01728) 668908 w 6257380

Clare Louise DipAVN(Surgical) 19/08/1994 1 Willow Drive Devizes Wiltshire SN10 2SN w 6029115

Fiona Susan 29/08/2000 The Blue Cross Animal Hospital Nelson Street Grimsby South Humberside DN32 7SH **Tel:** (01472) 343278 w 6203546

Francis Aaran 30/01/1997 7 Bramble End Alconbury Huntingdon Cambridgeshire PE28 4EZ **Tel:** (01480) 896533 m 6100429

Hazel Julia Dakin 27/07/1993 Madgewicks Brook Lane Albury Guildford Surrey GU5 9DH **Tel:** (01483) 202154 w 6044359

TAYLOR Jacqueline (see HUDSON, Mrs)

Jenny Margaret 07/05/2002 Walnut Tree House Watercress Lane Off Mill Road Mattishall Norfolk NR20 3RJ **Tel:** (01362) 850223 w 6269447

Joanne Sharon (nee Hubbard) 25/01/1994 33 Southwell Estate Eccleshall Stafford Staffordshire ST21 6EB **Tel:** (01785) 859 193 w 6066135

Judith Sharon 18/01/1991 53 Brownhill Lane Holmbridge Holmfirth HD9 2QW **Tel:** (01484) 687214 w 606175X

TAYLOR Leeanne (see HIRST, Mrs)

Nicholas 27/07/1988 10 Bishopsfield Cricklade SWINDON SN6 6BS **Tel:** (01793) 752543 m 6061807

Nicola C 17/08/1987 Glendale Cotehill Carlisle Cumbria CA4 0AZ **Tel:** (01228) 561561 w 6061818

Tracy Ann Vera (nee Anderson) 10/04/1996 (12/09/2002) 33 Hareburn Road Blackdog Bridge of Don ABERDEEN AB23 8AR **Tel:** (01224) 708285 w 6043209

TAYLOR Vicki Anne (see TURNER, Mrs)

TEANBY Elizabeth Jane 20/01/1997 Eastfield Veterinary Clinic Ltd Station Road North Thoresby GRIMSBY Lincolnshire DN36 5QU **Tel:** (01472) 840209 w 6037545

TELFORD Joanne (nee Mottram) 10/09/1996 (12/05/2005) Quarry Veterinary Group Brassey Road off Old Potts Way Shrewsbury Shropshire SY3 7FA **Tel:** (01743) 362 556 w 6099885

TELLWRIGHT Elizabeth Anne (nee Cattley) 15/09/1998 (24/11/2009) 41 Ford Road Newport Shropshire TF10 7TU **Tel:** (01952) 405261 w 6131490

TEMPLE Jane Patricia (see JEFFREY, Mrs)

TENNANT Lucille Mary Jean (see BEATTIE, Mrs)

TENNANT Susan Elizabeth 21/02/1997 68 Jones Green LIVINGSTON West Lothian EH54 8QD **Tel:** (01506) 412134 w 6108144

TERRY Sharon 30/01/2001 53 Combwell Crescent Abbey Wood London SE2 9LZ **Tel:** (020) 8310 7900 w 6109090

Wendy Jane 14/01/1977 Orchard Veterinary Centre 21 Church Street Oldbury West Midlands B69 3AF **Tel:** (0121) 544 8951 w 6001825

TETHER Carolyn Jayne 18/12/1989 (23/01/2006) 8 Bartletts Row Somerton Somerset TA11 6QW **Tel:** (01458) 274 395 w 606191X

THEAKER Marie Paula (see MEE, Mrs)

THEAKSTON Rebecca Noeline (see DARBYSHIRE, Mrs)

THEOBALD Caron Jane 20/11/1989 (13/11/2007) Newnham Court Veterinary Group Bearsted Road Weavering Maidstone Kent ME14 5EL **Tel:** (01622) 734555 w 6001836

THIXTON Nicola Kristine (see FORREST, Mrs)

THOMAS Alison Jane (see SANTOS, Mrs)

THOMAS Bonnie (nee McNicol) 09/09/2002 Bond Street Veterinary Clinic 1 Ryles Park Road Macclesfield Cheshire SK11 8AH **Tel:** (01625) 425637 w 6243377

Catherine Tracy 18/09/1990 Ty Arc Brackla Park BRIDGEND Mid Glamorgan CF31 2BF **Tel:** (01656) 653918 w 6061942

Julie 02/02/2001 3 Cambron Two Mile Ash Milton Keynes MK8 8BZ **Tel:** 01908669111 w 6211840

Kelly Jane 05/10/2001 29 Warwick Road Wellesbourne Warwickshire CV35 9NA **Tel:** (01789) 841072 w 6229572

Samantha Jayne 03/09/2002 17 Masefield Way Pontypridd Mid Glamorgan CF37 5HD **Tel:** (01443) 406484 w 6257765

THOMAS Sian Elizabeth (see DAY, Mrs)

THOMLINSON Margaret Ann 09/08/1972 (14/01/1999) 43 St Nicholas Street Norton Malton North Yorkshire YO17 9AQ **Tel:** (01653) 697299 w 6083423

THOMPSON Christina 13/09/1989 (22/08/2005) 341 Bramhall Lane Stockport Cheshire SK3 8TP **Tel:** (0161) 456 2030 w 6062017

Helen 01/09/1997 Gunnerside 65 Salters Lane Tamworth Staffordshire B79 8BH **Tel:** (07971) 467890 w 609878X

Julie (nee Heminsely) 04/08/1981 The Old Vicarage Bewholme Driffield North Humberside YO25 8EB **Tel:** (01964) 537009 w 6052734

THOMPSON Michelle Ann (see BRYSON, Mrs)

THOMPSON Susan Patricia (see WEATHERLEY, Ms)

Tara Jeana Annamatilda 27/01/1995 Ebony House Linenhall Street Dundalk Co Louth Ireland **Tel:** (08723) 60883 w 6037680

Wendy Violet Elizabeth (nee Hannam) 27/08/1997 The Surgery The Square GILLINGHAM Dorset SP8 4NA **Tel:** (01747) 822428 w 6108541

THOMSON Gary John 15/08/1990 (21/07/1999) Teignview Veterinary Group Hospital Hill Dawlish Devon EX7 9NS **Tel:** (01626) 862020 m 6062072

Jean Seton 01/09/2000 Dundas Veterinary Group 99 Dundas Street Edinburgh EH3 6SD **Tel:** (0131) 557 1819 w 6202842

Margaret 05/08/1976 (29/11/2005) 33 Junction Road Kirkwall Orkney KW15 1AG **Tel:** (01856) 873403 w 6062119

THORNE Anne-Marie (see PARRINDER, Ms)

THORNTON Helen Barbara (nee Sellars) 22/01/1998 (16/03/2001) North View Mill Road West Chiltington West Sussex RH20 2PY **Tel:** (01798) 815638 w 6118866

THORNTON Joanne Louise (see DAVIES, Mrs)

THOROGOOD Michelle Louise 12/04/1999 149 Old Folkestone Road Aycliffe DOVER Kent CT17 9HD **Tel:** (01304) 206487 w 610043X

THURSTAN Tracy (formerly Small, nee Heys) 30/01/1995 (16/05/2003) 362 Gisburn Road Blacko NELSON Lancashire BB9 6LS **Tel:** (01282) 690884 w 6036155

TILLING Samantha Tracy 12/09/1996 Skinners Hill Barn Eyford Park Upper Slaughter CHELTENHAM Gloucestershire GL54 2JN w 6100440

TIMM Melanie Ayrie (see HENRY, Mrs)

TIMMS Tracy Ann (nee Hamilton) 01/09/1997 Castle Vets Pet Healthcare Centre 1 Tilehurst Road Reading Berkshire RG1 7TW **Tel:** (0118) 957 4488 w 6035366

TIMPERLEY Debra Ann (nee Whitford) 13/05/2003 (16/11/2009) 10 Lomond Close Euxton CHORLEY Lancashire PR7 6FU **Tel:** (01257) 272777 w 6275585

TITHERINGTON Linda Kay 14/09/1998 3 Saleswood Avenue Eccleston St. Helens Merseyside WA10 5NG **Tel:** (01744) 631 347 w 6138226

TODD Dafni Josephine 12/01/1989 (29/01/2004) Park Veterinary Centre 256 Cassiobury Drive WATFORD Hertfordshire WD17 3PA **Tel:** (01923) 223321 w 6062287

TOLLEY Charlotte Emma (see HENNESSY, Mrs)

TONER Emma Jane 24/08/1998 The Old School Grizebeck KIRKBY-IN-FURNESS Cumbria LA17 7XH **Tel:** (01229) 889 786 w 6131708

TONKS Sarah Joanne (see ALLEN, Mrs)

TORRES Josefa Miguela 07/10/1998 (23/10/2000) Davies Veterinary Specialists Manor Farm Business Park Higham Gobion Hertfordshire SG5 3HR **Tel:** (01582) 883950 w 6137652

TOSH Jessica Victoria Davison 01/03/1996 Curlew Cottage Red House Lane Elstead GODALMING Surrey GU8 6DR **Tel:** (01252) 703300 w 6039203

TOTTEY Helen Wendy 19/01/1996 (28/06/2000) 18 Warnford Walk Merryhill Wolverhampton WV4 4YR **Tel:** (01902) 659111 w 6042646

TOWLER Sarah Jane 04/08/1986 The Bungalow Low Mill Dalston Carlisle Cumbria CA5 7JU **Tel:** (01228) 711 945 w 6062378

TOYE Nicola (see HAWKSWORTH, Mrs)

TRASK Hayley Clare 07/12/1990 42 Langdons Way Tatworth CHARD Somerset TA20 2TF **Tel:** (01460) 220663 w 6062403

TRAWFORD Diana Lee Hampden 18/08/1997 Paccombe House Harcombe Sidmouth Devon EX10 0PR **Tel:** (01395) 597356 w 6109115

TREMAIN Charlotte Frances 09/09/1975 (06/11/2002) Tremain Veterinary Practice Ltd 1 Farm Mill Lane WITNEY Oxfordshire OX28 4BJ **Tel:** (01993) 703146 w 6062436

TREVALLION Valerie (nee Banton) 23/04/1971 Ash Veterinary Surgery Aberdare Road Georgetown Merthyr Tydfil Mid Glamorgan CF48 1AT **Tel:** (01685) 385117 w 6082769

TRIGG Melanie Anna (see WHITLING, Mrs)

TRILL Claire Anna 06/09/2000 27 Marchants Drive Camber East Sussex TN31 7RF **Tel:** (01797) 225720 w 6205691

TRINDER Alison Jane (see CUSS, Ms)

TROUT Sara Louise (see BARROW, Mrs)

TRUEMAN Pearl Michelle 01/08/1988 (06/07/2000) 19 Low Street Tingley Wakefield West Yorkshire WF3 1RL **Tel:** (0113) 259 7310 w 606247X

TRUMAN Julie Anne (see DEW, Mrs)

TUCKER Janice Beryl (nee Cole) 06/08/1986 24 Churchill Road Whitchurch Tavistock Devon PL19 9BU **Tel:** (01822) 613971 w 6047870

Katie Jayne (nee Webber) 04/08/1993 37 Broadoak Road Langford Bristol Avon BS40 5HD **Tel:** (01934) 852210 w 6008296

TUCKER Sarah Lacey (see LANGLEY, Mrs)

TUFFS Rebecca Joanne (see MARTIN, Mrs)

TULEY Lisa Nicole (see BROWN, Mrs)

TURBUTT Clare Elizabeth (see CALLOW, Mrs)

TURNER Alison Clare (nee Moore) 28/08/1997 56 Eldorado Close Studley Warwickshire B80 7LB **Tel:** (01527) 458226 w 6116326

Cindy Louise 15/01/1987 (12/05/1999) 21 High Street Highworth Swindon SN6 7AG **Tel:** (01793) 765335 w 6062549

Emma Jane 23/10/2000 The Veterinary Practice Millennium Way Braintree Essex CM7 3GX **Tel:** (01376) 325511 w 6135655

TURNER Geraldine Theresa (see WILLIAMS, Mrs)

Jacqueline Elaine 23/09/1999 41 Barkstone Drive SHREWSBURY Shropshire SY1 3XT w 6142913

TURNER Jane (see ROBERTS, Mrs)

Vicki Anne (nee Taylor, nee Taylor) 02/09/1998 Oathall Veterinary Group 30 Oathall Road Haywards Heath West Sussex RH16 3EQ **Tel:** (01444) 440224 w 6131355

TURVEY Denise Margaret (see COLCLOUGH, Mrs)

TWISS Helen Claire (see WRIGHT, Mrs)

TYLER Karen Anne (formerly Brown) 14/09/1998 64 Randsfield Avenue Brough East Yorkshire HU15 1BG w 613535X

TYRRELL Mandy 10/12/1992 (22/02/2008) 10 Pondtail Close HORSHAM West Sussex RH12 5HS w 6008423

U

UDDIN Rebecca Jayne 04/02/2002 6 Chycornick Terrace Gulval PENZANCE Cornwall TR18 3BU **Tel:** (01736) 367226 w 6259206

UNDERHILL Joanne (see BRADLEY, Mrs)

UPSHALL Tracy Claire 02/02/1996 (10/12/2003) Lynwood Veterinary Group Station Road Wimborne Dorset BH21 1RQ **Tel:** (01202) 882101 w 6039054

UPTON Debra Jane (nee Bright) 29/07/1986 (24/10/2003) 371/373 Hagley Road Edgbaston Birmingham West Midlands B17 8DL **Tel:** (0121) 429 3833 w 6000231

V

VALLER Mary Ann (see NATHAN, Mrs)

VAN GENT Stacey Victoria (nee Harris) 18/01/1999 2 Reedland Crescent Faversham Kent ME13 7HR w 6108552

VANCE Tracy Lynn (see MAFFITT, Ms)

VARDEY Suzanne Elizabeth (see CROWDER, Mrs)

VERDEN Hazel Rebecca (nee Hyde) 08/02/1996 (28/07/2008) 26 Taylors Crescent CRANLEIGH Surrey GU6 7EL **Tel:** (01483) 267076 w 6036552

VERITY Valerie (see HUMPHREY, Mrs)

VERNON Kathryn Ann 23/01/1998 86 Orford Avenue Warrington Cheshire WA2 7QQ **Tel:** (01925) 232221 w 6030958

VICKERS Janet (see LAINTON, Mrs)

VICKERS Shelley Belinda 01/10/1999 The Veterinary Hospital Colwill Road Estover Plymouth Devon PL6 8RP **Tel:** (01752) 702646 w 6185990

VILLARS Cathryn Suzanne (nee Lang) 19/09/1994 (09/04/1998) 23 Dale Lane Blidworth Mansfield Nottingham NG21 0SA w 6030120

Ruth Morag 30/08/1989 (19/05/1999) 28 Dorset Street Lincoiln LN2 5NS **Tel:** (01522) 821682 w 6062775

VINCE Mark Brendon 10/03/1999 4 Ringstead Buildings Ringstead Road Catford London SE6 2BN **Tel:** (020) 8697 0857 m 6137051

VINCENT Chontelle (nee Coupland) 18/08/1995 (30/07/2007) 160 Lanchester Way Castle Bromwich Birmingham B36 9LE **Tel:** (0121) 749 7841 w 6032489

VINCENT Kathryn Emma (see WARR, Mrs)

VINING Annette Marguerite 09/02/1982 (30/10/2000) 224 Winchester Road Shirley Southampton SO16 6TL **Tel:** (023) 8077 9388 w 6062800

VIRGO Lynne 17/01/1991 (16/07/2009) The Young Veterinary Partnership 57 Lampton Road Hounslow TW3 4DH **Tel:** (020) 8570 0489 w 6062811

Yvonne June 18/01/2002 6 Lacca Close Longlevens Gloucester GL2 0XB **Tel:** (01452) 506907 w 6253959

VRANCH Susan Claire (nee Derbyshire, nee Vrnach) 06/09/1996 c/o Dr. Cecilia Gorrel 17 Burnt House Lane Pilley LYMINGTON SO41 5QN **Tel:** (01590) 678715 w 6036836

VRNACH Susan Claire (see VRANCH, Mrs)

W

WAIGH Christine Elizabeth (see DOOLEY, Mrs)

WAKEHAM Rebecca Jane 25/08/1998 3 Park Row New Road Aylburton Lydney Gloucestershire GL15 6DT **Tel:** (01594) 841889 w 6122136

WALKER Anna Ruth 15/08/1995 (15/05/2008) Trinity House Church Street Eckington PERSHORE Worcestershire WR10 3AN **Tel:** (01386) 751936 w 6039134

Claire Joanne (formerly Mills) 15/11/2001 2 Sherwin Farm Cottages Abbots Wick Lane Great Wigborough Colchester Essex CO5 7RT w 6239813

Hayzellle Balnave 04/12/2000 (08/02/2005) 5 Irvine Crescent Bathgate West Lothian EH48 2QS **Tel:** (01506) 655922 w 6205372

Jane Elisabeth 27/07/1978 (12/11/2007) 59 Salcombe Road Lipson Plymouth PL4 7NF **Tel:** (01752) 266159 w 6062913

Jean Margaret 25/11/1974 20 Delvin Road Bristol BS10 5EJ **Tel:** (01179) 755965 w 6062924

WALKER Katrina Susannah (see SULLIVAN, Mrs)

Louise (nee Bavin) 23/08/2000 Craigpark Veterinary Centre 3 Ralston Road Barrhead Glasgow G78 2QQ **Tel:** (0141) 881 9499 w 6140337

WALL Anna-Lisa 15/09/2000 (12/11/2007) 16 Camden Terrace BRIGHTON East Sussex BN1 3LR **Tel:** (01273) 454040 w 6141308

WALL Estelle (see JENNER, Mrs)

Joanne Avril 23/08/2000 Eye Veterinary Clinic Marlbrook Leominster Herefordshire HR6 0PH **Tel:** (01568) 616616 w 6202545

Kerry Rae 26/09/2000 Connaught House Veterinary Hospital 38 Broad Street Kingswinford West Midlands DY6 9LP **Tel:** (01384) 295949 w 6204030

WALLACE Alice Anne 26/08/1969 Little Witty Whitgift Goole East Yorkshire DN14 8HL **Tel:** (01405) 704855 w 6062990

Angela DipAVN(Surgical) (nee Dickie) 18/01/1995 18 Westray Drive Kilmarnock Ayrshire KA3 2GR **Tel:** (01563) 520989 w 6035388

Michelle Ann (nee Copus) 23/09/2002 41 The Smithy Bramley Tadley Hampshire RG26 5AY **Tel:** (01256) 883272 w 6264695

WALLACE Michelle Lisa (see DUMONT, Mrs)

WALLBANK Joanne (see HARRIS, Mrs)

WALLER Joanne Karen (see FOLEY, Mrs)

WALLINGTON Linda 05/09/1974 (27/05/2004) Somerville Leckford Stockbridge Hampshire SO20 6JQ **Tel:** (01264) 810479 w 6063043

WALLIS Karen Mary (see RICHARDSON, Mrs)

WALLMAN Catherine Vanessa 23/08/1999 (17/04/2003) 4 Penstock Mews Godalming Surrey GU7 1NB **Tel:** (01483) 853880 w 614554X

WALMSLEY Helen Louise 18/01/1999 2 Albert Street Lytham Lytham St. Annes Lancashire FY8 5EB **Tel:** (01253) 737187 w 6098837

WALPOLE Amy (nee Glessing) 31/08/2000 (12/11/2008) 26 Boleyn Way Boreham CHELMSFORD CM3 3JL **Tel:** (07802) 638335 w 6202996

WALSH Elizabeth Anne (see BIX, Mrs)

WALSH Kerry Michelle 06/04/1996 (02/02/2000) 17 All Saints Road BURTON-ON-TRENT Staffordshire DE14 3LS **Tel:** (01283) 515 679 w 6028428

Niamh Carol 21/03/2000 5 College Green Dunshaughlin Co. Meath Ireland w 6191017

WALTERS Alison Claire 05/02/1996 24 Natalie Close Bedfont Middlesex TW14 8PJ **Tel:** (0208) 8909575 w 6032398

Katie Elizabeth 05/09/2000 Flat 5 24 Wilbury Road HOVE East Sussex BN3 3JP w 6203898

WALTON Tamara Margarette Louise (see ELSTON, Mrs)

WANNELL Caroline Teresa (see PHILP, Miss)

WARBURTON Lindsey (see BRYSON, Mrs)

WARD Dawn DipAVN(Medical) (nee Shipley) 01/09/1999 1 Ryedale Cottage Great Habton Malton North Yorkshire YO17 6TU **Tel:** (01653) 668432 w 6145368

Jenny Helen 27/08/1996 12B York Road Weybridge Surrey KT13 9DT **Tel:** (01932) 855856 w 6077522

WARD Nicole Mary (see NEWNHAM, Mrs)

Zoe Ann (nee Hammersley) 14/08/2002 1 Garrow Drive Lymington Hampshire SO41 9LP **Tel:** (01590) 677541 w 6140428

WARDLE Anna 19/01/1998 Vale Cottage Vale Road Chalfont St Peter GERRARDS CROSS Buckinghamshire SL9 9SD **Tel:** (0411) 041227 w 6101739

WARDROBE Deborah (see MINOR, Mrs)

WARE Nancy 13/12/2001 (05/01/2006) Gatehouse Veterinary Centre Chester Road Lavister Rossett Wrexham Clwyd LL12 0DF **Tel:** (01244) 570364 w 6138601

WAREHAM Suzanne (see GRAY, Miss)

WARNE Marian Eileen (see BURCH, Mrs)

WARNE Racheal Ann Louise (see YOUNGSON, Mrs)

WARR Kathryn Emma (nee Vincent) 06/11/2003 (15/01/2010) R S P C A Stapeley Grange London Road Stapeley NANTWICH Cheshire CW5 7JW w 6262242

WARREN Charlene 20/11/2002 (02/11/2009) Renwar House Taverham Lane Norwich Norfolk NR8 5BE **Tel:** (01603) 748363 w 6280161

Elizabeth Jane 09/09/1996 Sir Harold Harmsworth Memorial Hospital 22 Sonderburg Road London N7 7QD **Tel:** (0870) 753 8081 w 6099648

Nicola Jane 04/02/2002 17 Foxcroft Close Burntwood Staffordshire WS7 4ST **Tel:** (01543) 317322 w 6268424

Vanessa Lorna 21/07/1993 Higher Pilehayes Farm Woodbury Salterton Exeter EX5 1PN **Tel:** (01395) 232659 w 6066237

WASHINGTON Gillian Dawn (nee Plumb) 20/09/1999 28a High Street South Stewkley LEIGHTON BUZZARD Bedfordshire LU7 0HR w 6185319

WASON Jennifer (see MULLEN, Mrs)

WATERS Kelly Lyn (see CARLILE, Mrs)

WATERS Nikki (nee Coe) 15/09/2000 6 Nicholson Grove Wickford Essex SS12 9PL w 6202666

Rebecca Louise (nee Smart) 29/08/2000 (31/10/2005) MacQueen Veterinary Surgery 1 Hopton Park London Road Devizes Wiltshire SN10 2EY **Tel:** (01380) 728505 w 6204459

Ruth (nee Nicholson) 09/09/1996 (10/12/2003) 14a Kit Lane Owermoigne DORCHESTER Dorset DT2 8HP **Tel:** (01420) 487461 w 6099932

WATERSON Lisa Elaine (see JOLLEY, Mrs)

WATKINS Emma Louise (see BOTT, Miss)

WATSON Helen Mary (nee Berry) 01/02/1994 35 St Olaves Close Staines Middlesex TW18 2LH **Tel:** (01784) 257212 w 6067332

Jeanette Marie (nee Brooke) 30/03/2001 90 Westbourne Road Selby North Yorkshire YO8 9DA **Tel:** (01757) 701146 w 6214535

Jill Margrethe 10/08/1984 Eaton Veterinary Practice Ltd 30-32 Eaton Street NORWICH Norfolk NR4 7LD **Tel:** (01603) 455196 w 6063291

WATSON Katie Jean (see CARR, Mrs)

WATSON Ruth Anne (see COOK, Mrs)

Shane Alan 26/02/2000 (31/01/2002) Rosewyn Church Lane Lelant ST. IVES Cornwall TR26 3HY **Tel:** (01736) 753140 m 6131388

WATT Jacqueline Ann 16/09/1981 (06/01/2005) 18 Bridle Lane Streetly Sutton Coldfield West Midlands B74 3HB **Tel:** (0121) 352 1023 w 6063338

Kathryn Marie 15/02/2002 Christchurch Veterinary Surgery 49 Christchurch Street Ipswich Suffolk IP4 2DF **Tel:** (01473) 255789 w 6268369

Rebecca Jane 04/02/2002 3 Wiltshire Road Wyton on the Hill Huntingdon Cambridgeshire PE28 2EX **Tel:** (01733) 246 328 w 6262506

WATTS Abby Louise (nee Kitchen) 23/01/1998 (08/05/2002) 139 Hazleton Way Waterlooville Hampshire PO8 9DR w 6117997

Natasha Leigh (nee Baxter) 03/05/2000 (09/06/2004) 615 Wells Road Whitchurch Bristol BS14 9BE **Tel:** (01275) 832410 w 6190676

WAUGH Melanie (see HUNT, Mrs)

WAUGH Sally Joanne (see BRITTON, Mrs)

WEATHERLEY Susan Patricia (formerly Thompson) 29/07/1974 (08/05/2003) 7 South Parade Horley Row Horley Surrey RH6 8BH **Tel:** (01293) 771560 w 6084507

WEAVER Fay Ella 05/03/2002 (02/11/2007) 69 Duchess Way Bristol Avon BS16 1EX **Tel:** (0117) 939 0686 w 6272516

Michelle 15/02/2002 171 Manchester New Road Middleton Manchester M24 1DE **Tel:** (0161) 643 3097 w 6266719

WEBB Clare Margaret 26/01/2000 96 Parsons Way Wootton Bassett Swindon SN4 8DJ **Tel:** (01793) 853560 w 6190511

Laura-Anne (nee Moody) 11/12/2001 Beggars Roost 41 Chalk Hill West End Southampton Hampshire SO18 3BY **Tel:** (02380) 464506 w 6262869

WEBB Lisa Corinne (see MALE, Mrs)

WEBB Lorraine (see WHITE, Mrs)

WEBBER Katie Jayne (see TUCKER, Mrs)

WEBER Niamh Geraldine 05/03/2002 2 Finglen Gardens Milngavie Glasgow G62 7RW **Tel:** (0141) 563 8730 w 6264981

WEBSTER Amanda Marie DipAVN(Medical) 28/09/2000 28 Melford Bridge Road Thetford Norfolk IP24 2HH **Tel:** (01842) 762349 w 6203909

Joanna Marie (nee Wright) 07/02/1996 (02/08/1999) Stowe Veterinary Group 54 Bury Road Stowmarket Suffolk IP14 1JF **Tel:** (01449) 613130 w 6032591

Julia Claire (nee Deeming) 01/08/1983 Anchor Farm Anchor Newcastle Craven Arms Shropshire SY7 8PR **Tel:** (01686) 670932 w 604903X

Julie Anne 18/01/2000 86 Orford Avenue Warrington Cheshire WA2 7QQ **Tel:** (01925) 232221 w 6134108

WEDGE Anita Diane 27/08/1987 (17/10/2003) 1 Hartland Avenue Coseley Bilston West Midlands WV14 9AN w 6002024

WEISBERG Emma Jane (see MUNDY, Mrs)

WEISS Jane Louise 06/09/1999 54 Heath Drive Ware Hertfordshire SG12 0RJ **Tel:** (01920) 465 994 w 6185044

WELDON Nicola (nee Smith) 17/10/2000 31 Sandstone Drive Whiston Prescot Merseyside L35 7LS **Tel:** (0151) 431 0545 w 6191380

WELLS Amanda Jane 16/01/2002 (13/08/2008) The Freda Powell Centre 1c Eynsham Drive Thamesmead London SE2 9RQ **Tel:** (020) 8311 6695 w 6270569

Clare Hardy 27/01/1994 (20/07/2001) The Gables 17 Avenue Road Malvern Worcestershire WR14 3AY **Tel:** (01684) 572420 w 6067310

WELLSTEAD Claire Louise 18/01/1995 (21/07/1999) 7 Tudor Close Ashford Middlesex TW15 3HZ **Tel:** (01784) 243775 w 6030856

WELMAN Hannah (nee Churchley) 13/03/2002 The Veterinary Hospital 118 Victoria Drive Bognor Regis West Sussex PO21 2EJ **Tel:** (01243) 841111 w 6270382

WELSMAN Hannah 02/09/1998 (10/04/2008) 23 High Street EBBW VALE Gwent NP23 6BU **Tel:** (01495) 308778 w 6122147

WEST Karen 17/09/1999 (03/03/2009) Inside Pets at Home Rom Valley Way Retail Park Rom Valley Way ROMFORD Essex RM7 0AN **Tel:** (01708) 720920 w 6152626

Sarah Louise (nee Lowe) 02/10/2001 (06/08/2009) The Avenues Veterinary Clinic 22 Garston Lane WATFORD Hertfordshire WD25 9QJ **Tel:** (01923) 894274 w 6229308

WESTCOTT Kathryn Margaret (nee Sopp) 24/08/1994 4 Second Avenue Stanford-le-Hope Essex SS17 8DP **Tel:** (01375) 643565 w 6032321

WESTON Donna June (nee Wiltshire) 22/05/2001 Medivet Veterinary Group 237 St Albans Road WATFORD WD24 5BP **Tel:** (01923) 243429 w 6218264

WHEAT Tracey Jane DipAVN(Surgical) 20/05/1993 70 Deyncourt Road Fallings Park Wolverhampton WV10 0SY **Tel:** (01902) 683889 w 6014914

WHELAN Aine Martina 20/04/2001 (02/11/2009) 28 Park Lane Avenue Abbeyside Dungarvan Co Waterford Ireland w 6141410

Edel Mary 04/10/2001 (02/11/2009) 20 Riverview Villierstown Co. Waterford Ireland **Tel:** 058-42314 w 6229429

WHISTLER Catherine Juliet (see EDWARDS, Mrs)

WHITCHER Marie Claire (see HATCH, Mrs)

WHITE Amanda Julie (see JAMES, Mrs)

WHITE Gina Elizabeth 01/09/1994 (27/01/2010) 5 Grape Vine Close High Wycombe Buckinghamshire HP11 1RT **Tel:** (01494) 438 183 w 6033438

Jacqueline Anne 03/09/1990 (01/09/2006) 3 Beechlands Bishop's Stortford Hertfordshire CM23 3PL **Tel:** (01279) 834 293 w 6095166

Janet Lesley 21/01/1980 (01/03/2006) 33 Gladstone Road KINGSTON UPON THAMES Surrey KT1 3HD **Tel:** (0208) 288 2692 w 6063622

Jennifer Mary (nee Wintersgill) 01/12/2000 Warwickshire College Moreton Morrell Warwick Warwickshire CV35 9BL **Tel:** (01926) 318000 w 6204382

WHITE Kim Lorraine (see LONGHURST, Mrs)

Lisa Ann 26/01/1998 (16/07/2003) Cogges Veterinary Surgery Cogges Hill Road Witney Oxfordshire OX28 3XY **Tel:** (01993) 772 627 w 6113562

Lisa Jane 30/01/2001 17 Embassy Close Blacon Chester CH1 5AN **Tel:** (01244) 383791 w 6211631

Lorraine (nee Webb) 11/09/1997 54 Enville Road Kinver STOURBRIDGE West Midlands DY7 6BX **Tel:** (01384) 873660 w 6043005

Natalie Dawn 26/03/2002 4 Calartha Terrace Boscaswell Downs Pendeen PENZANCE Cornwall TR19 7DX w 6272131

Rebecca Margaret (nee Davies) 16/02/1994 87 Walsh Avenue BRISTOL BS14 9SQ **Tel:** (01275) 790 115 w 6068278

Ross Devereux DipAVN(Surgical) 23/01/1995 Warwickshire College Moreton Morrell Warwick Warwickshire CV35 9BL **Tel:** (01926) 318000 m 6033711

Tammy 08/02/1994 33 West View Rough Close Stoke-on-Trent Staffordshire ST3 7PH **Tel:** (01782) 388665 w 6068256

WHITEHEAD Sarah 29/08/1997 (09/11/2009) 261 Wigan Road Euxton CHORLEY Lancashire PR7 6HZ w 6116665

WHITEHOUSE Lisa Roma 28/08/1997 2 Temple Street Lower Cornal Dudley West Midlands DY3 2PE **Tel:** (01384) 837397 w 6098870

WHITEHURST Lisa Marie (see WILLIAMS, Mrs)

WHITELAW Alison Joan (nee Bowen) 27/07/1992 (08/02/2008) 32 Purcell Avenue Lichfield Staffordshire WS13 7PJ w 6005783

WHITELEY Susan Janette 25/08/1999 Ingholme Sedbergh Cumbria LA10 5HR **Tel:** (05396) 21946 w 614271X

WHITEMAN Melissa Kate (nee Fairfield) 06/09/1999 (20/01/2005) 151 Milton Road Nunsthorpe Grimsby North East Lincolnshire DN33 1DN **Tel:** (01472) 593 581 w 6185528

WHITFORD Debra Ann (see TIMPERLEY, Mrs)

WHITING Celia Mary (see KIENTZEL, Mrs)

WHITLING Melanie Anna (nee Trigg) 17/11/2000 9 Wenlock Close Padgate Warrington Cheshire WA1 4JX **Tel:** (01925) 251259 w 6204184

WHITTAKER Karen 26/04/2002 (08/02/2008) 22 Oval Road North Dagenham Essex RM10 9EL **Tel:** (020) 8252 7149 w 6205273

Sarah Louise DipAVN(Surgical) 23/08/1990 The Veterinary Centre 271 Reading Road Henley-on-Thames Oxfordshire RG9 1EL **Tel:** (01491) 574490 w 6063713

WHYBROW Caroline Heather (nee Sparrow) 23/11/2001 16 Avon Close Lee-on-the-Solent Hampshire PO13 8JQ **Tel:** (02392) 367 562 w 6258117

WICKS Claire Victoria (see PULLAN, Mrs)

WIGG Lucy Alice (nee Knapton) 07/02/2005 (20/05/2009) 5 Medley Way St Lawrence Bay Southminster Essex CMO 7JZ **Tel:** (01621) 779976 w 6296276

WIGGS Sharon Lorraine (nee Dearman) 30/10/2001 1 Trumper Road STEVENAGE Hertfordshire SG1 5JZ w 6272923

WILCOCK Helen Elizabeth (see HILL, Mrs)

WILD Rebecca Dawn (nee Gowthorpe) 01/09/1997 (23/12/2009) 1 Prospect Villas Barlow Common Road Barlow Selby North Yorkshire YO8 8JF **Tel:** (01757) 617466 w 6119054

WILDGOOSE Julia 24/04/1981 (29/01/2003) 1 Fitzgerald Road Wanstead London E11 2ST **Tel:** (020) 89892666 w 6063779

WILDMAN Jenifer Louise 26/03/2002 15 Heritage Way LLANYMYNECH Powys SY22 6LL **Tel:** (01691) 830671 w 6258238

WILKES Lisa Jane 31/01/1996 21 Keeble Close Tiptree Colchester CO5 0NU **Tel:** (01621) 816612 w 6040944

WILKIE Clare Lisa (see GARBUTT, Mrs)

WILKINS Kerry 15/08/1989 31 Maypole Road Maidenhead Berkshire SL6 0NA **Tel:** (01628) 668244 w 6063815

WILKINS Sandra Louise (see SINCLAIR, Mrs)

WILKINSON Margaret Denise 22/06/2001 West Mount Vets Ltd 41 Burnley Road Todmorden Lancashire OL14 7BU **Tel:** (01706) 814110/812568 w 6223533

WILKINSON Rebecca (see HILL, Mrs)

WILLCOX Rachel Kay (nee Bennett) 09/09/1998 Fulford House Torbay Road Castle Cary Somerset BA7 7DT **Tel:** (01963) 350307 w 6038312

WILLIAMS Adele Caroline 18/01/2002 Orchard Veterinary Surgery 121a The Hundred Romsey Hampshire SO51 8BZ **Tel:** (01794) 830288 w 6273869

WILLIAMS Adele Louisa (see BEATTIE, Mrs)

WILLIAMS Barbara Jean (see ROGERS, Mrs)

WILLIAMS Claire (see CASSIDY, Mrs)

Elizabeth Mary 29/01/1979 3 Cae Haf Northop Hall Mold Flintshire CH7 6GB **Tel:** (01244) 821504 w 6063892

WILLIAMS Elizabeth Mary (see ABBISS, Mrs)

WILLIAMS Erica Jane (see DAVIES, Mrs)

Fiona Mary 18/09/1998 (28/01/2010) Southill Veterinary Group Balsam Fields Wincanton Somerset BA9 9HE **Tel:** (01963) 33226 w 603986X

Geraldine Theresa (nee Turner) 26/03/2002 9 Waynefleet Grove Millfield Lane York North Yorkshire YO10 3AR **Tel:** (01904) 411127 w 6268490

WILLIAMS Karenza Daisy (see DELMAGE, Mrs)

Lisa Jane (nee Shippey) 26/01/1999 (28/04/2004) 2 Redcar Road Guisborough Cleveland TS14 6DB **Tel:** (01287) 633255 w 6123581

Lisa Marie 12/10/2000 (24/11/2006) 52 Dunscore Road Wigan Lancashire WN3 6TH **Tel:** (01942) 200046 w 6204701

Lisa Marie (nee Whitehurst) 02/02/1990 456-458 Hagley Road West Oldbury West Midlands B68 0DL **Tel:** (0121) 422 1312 w 6063666

Lynsey Marie 01/11/1999 Colne Valley Veterinary Practice Off Maudlyn Road Colchester CO1 2GU **Tel:** (01206) 794695 w 6185858

WILLIAMS Rachael Louise (see RODGERS, Mrs)

WILLIAMS Rita Caroline (see JOHNSON, Mrs)

Stacey Marie (nee O'Shea) 26/03/2002 4 Jubilee Terrace CAMBORNE Cornwall TR14 7AN **Tel:** 01209-613457 w 6277884

WILLIAMSON Amy Marie (nee Jacklin) 03/11/2000 (18/11/2008) 3 Acthorpe Cottages Acthorpe South Elkington Louth Lincolnshire LN11 0SD w 6205185

WILLIAMSON Marie (see HASSALL, Mrs)

WILLIS Claire Louise (nee Francis, formerly Descombes) 26/02/1996 Celia Hammond Veterinary Hospital 233-235 Lewisham Way London SE4 1UY **Tel:** (0208) 691 2100 w 6034238

WILLIS Kathryn Elizabeth (see SMITH, Mrs)

WILLMOTT Judith Ann (see HUTCHINSON, Mrs)

WILLOUGHBY Elaine (see LAMB, Mrs)

WILLS Carly Jayne (see DRAYTON, Mrs)

WILLSMORE Charlotte Louise 08/05/2002 76 Fairmead Avenue Daws Heath Benfleet Essex SS7 2UJ **Tel:** (01702) 553501 w 6261461

WILLSON Carol 29/07/1974 Campston Cottage Campston Hill Pandy Abergavenny Gwent NP7 8EE **Tel:** (01843) 890696 w 6063983

WILMOT Sarah (see ABBOTT, Mrs)

WILSON Beth Jaime 23/08/2000 26 Ramsden Avenue Langold Worksop Nottinghamshire S81 9PB w 6203997

Caroline 14/09/1976 (01/11/2006) Three Sisters 9 Thame Road Long Crendon Aylesbury Buckinghamshire HP18 9AS **Tel:** (01844) 208688 w 6068755

WILSON Caroline (see O'CONNOR, Mrs)

Deborah Claire (nee Foster) 20/11/2002 4 Sentinel Close Waterlooville Hampshire PO7 8LX **Tel:** (023) 92 426450 w 6278830

Elaine Marguerite 18/09/1998 (03/03/2006) 22a Carrydarragh Road Moneymore Magherafelt County Londonderry BT45 7YX **Tel:** (028) 867 47666 w 6100600

Fiona (nee MacWilliams) 27/07/1987 7 Fir Road Sutton Surrey SM3 9JY **Tel:** (020) 8644 7329 w 6055633

Gemma Marianne (nee Scott) 05/09/2000 32 Leighton Avenue Meols WIRRAL Merseyside CH47 0LZ w 6137186

Georgina Margaret 21/09/1984 43 Alma Court Alma Vale Road Clifton Bristol BS8 2HJ **Tel:** (0117) 9238764 w 6002807

Helen Louise 30/03/2001 The Mews Veterinary Centre Preseland Road LIVERPOOL Merseyside L23 5TE **Tel:** (0151) 924 2025 w 6214634

WILSON Lisa Ann (see SMITH, Mrs)

Melanie Jane 07/08/1990 Maes Glas Veterinary Group Church Acre Brackla Bridgend Mid Glamorgan CF31 2JT **Tel:** (01656) 652 751 w 6064025

WILTON Emma Louise Rosemary (see NEWEY, Mrs)

WILTSHIRE Donna June (see WESTON, Mrs)

WINCOTT Emma 27/02/2002 26 Buckstone Wood Edinburgh EH10 6QW **Tel:** (0131) 445 7954 w 6271702

WINKWORTH Elizabeth Anita (see MORGAN, Mrs)

Mary Catherine 06/04/2001 Veterinary Centre 41 Peartree Lane Welwyn Garden City Hertfordshire AL7 3UA **Tel:** (01707) 336919 w 6215140

WINNETT Sarah (see AYRES, Mrs)

WINTERSGILL Jennifer Mary (see WHITE, Mrs)

WISHART Alison Margaret 19/08/1992 16 Melbury Court Sunderland Tyne and Wear SR6 9HZ **Tel:** (07769) 702619 w 6005615

WITHERS Vanessa Dawn (see LENNOX, Miss)

WITTS Claire Elizabeth 15/02/2002 29 Stonebridge Close MARLBOROUGH Wiltshire SN8 2AE **Tel:** (01672) 513451 w 6131446

WITTY Winifred Margaret Lindsay 12/10/1978 Wareham 160 Caterham Drive Coulsdon Surrey CR5 1JL **Tel:** (0208) 668 1558 w 6064091

WOOD Christine Joanne (nee Cruttenden) 18/08/1987 (20/05/1999) Oakside Goldbridge Road Newick Lewes East Sussex BN8 4QP w 6064138

Davinia Clare 13/03/2002 Christchurch Veterinary Surgery 49 Christchurch Street Ipswich Suffolk IP4 2DF **Tel:** (01473) 255789 w 6267654

Diane 22/01/1987 Shearbridge Veterinary Group 2 Legrams Lane Bradford West Yorkshire BD7 1ND **Tel:** (01274) 731299 w 6064149

WOOD Julie May (see FOWLER, Mrs)

WOODBRIDGE Hannah Clair 31/08/2000 (30/11/2007) 1 Clifton Terrace Portscatho TRURO Cornwall TR2 5HR **Tel:** (01872) 580263 w 6113686

WOODCRAFT Janet (nee Leatherbarrow) 08/01/1979 7 Drake Hall Westhoughton BOLTON BL5 2RA **Tel:** (01942) 814181 w 6087610

WOODHALL Carolyn 09/09/2002 11 Addison Road Toronto Bishop Auckland Co Durham DL14 7RN **Tel:** (01388) 604381 w 6286134

WOODS Clare Deborah (nee Simmons) 02/09/1994 (16/11/1998) 4 Denshire Court Baston PETERBOROUGH PE6 9QL **Tel:** (01778) 560772 w 6027832

WOODS Clare Fiona (see CAMPBELL, Mrs)

Colleen Lesley 06/09/1995 105 Prestwood Road West Wednesfield Wolverhampton WV11 1HY **Tel:** (01902) 863600 w 6028552

Lorna Marie 24/12/2002 70 Castle Lane West Moordown Bournemouth Dorset BH9 3JU **Tel:** (01202) 533630 w 6271856

WOODWARD Aimee-Louise Teresa (see SCOTT, Mrs)

WOODWARD Kim Lesley 19/09/1999 42 Danesby Rise Denby Ripley Derbyshire DE5 8RG w 6186078

WOODYATT Heather Jane (nee Gill) 06/09/1999 Trinity Cottage New Church Lane Ulverston Cumbria LA12 7AF w 6146306

WOOLDRIDGE Lisa Joanne (nee Rolfe) 11/01/1993 4 Gainsborough Avenue Kintbury HUNGERFORD Berkshire RG17 9XN **Tel:** (01488) 658130 w 6065302

WOOLLS Lisa Wynne (see TAI, Mrs)

WOORE Heather Kathleen (see HUNTER, Mrs)

WORTHING Sally Ann DipAVN(Surgical) (nee Loach) 26/07/1993 Belle Vue Lodge Bartestree Hereford Herefordshire HR1 4BB **Tel:** (01432) 851871 w 6015292

WREN Susan Elizabeth 10/10/1974 (02/11/2000) Brook House Veterinary Hospital 12 Landguard Road Southampton Hampshire SO15 5DJ **Tel:** (02380) 228570 w 6064295

WRIGHT Anne Elizabeth (nee Kitching) 19/01/1995 Thorndale Calton Skipton North Yorkshire BD23 4AD **Tel:** (01729) 830713 w 603708X

Christine Ann (nee McAdam) 12/09/2000 (06/11/2008) Sundean Veterinary Clinic 11 High Street LYDNEY Gloucestershire GL15 5DP **Tel:** (01594) 840404 w 6024230

WRIGHT Claire Louise (see EDWARDS, Mrs)

Helen Claire (nee Twiss) 04/12/1998 16 Holders Close Billingshurst West Sussex RH14 9HL **Tel:** (01403) 783742 w 6139558

Helen Elizabeth 03/03/1997 38 Molyneux Road Waterloo Liverpool L22 4QZ **Tel:** (0151) 9490626 w 6098917

WRIGHT Joanna Marie (see WEBSTER, Mrs)

Lorraine Agnes 09/09/1999 "The Perch" 98a Mottram Road Broadbottom HYDE Cheshire SK14 6BB w 614933X

WYATT Joanne Alison 22/08/1994 CVS (UK) Ltd Animed Veterinary Hospital & Equine Unit Botley Road Shedfield Southampton Hampshire SO32 2JG **Tel:** (01329) 833112 w 603687X

WYLE Jessica Rose 30/01/2001 42 Belmont Road Reading RG30 2UU **Tel:** (01189) 674303 w 6211642

WYNNE Alice Judith Stephanie (nee Farr) 10/11/2000 12 The Paddock Cross Lanes Wrexham Clwyd LL13 0TX **Tel:** (01978) 780241 w 6203689

Y

YAIR Joanne Elaine (nee Bush) 30/07/1992 (05/11/2004) 19 Blundies Lane Enville Stourbridge West Midlands DY7 5HU **Tel:** (01384) 877063 w 6005794

YATES Victoria Clare 13/03/1997 (28/07/2008) 40 Barrington Road Altrincham Cheshire WA14 1HJ **Tel:** (0161) 928 8367 w 6098928

YOCKNEY Alexandra Louise 06/01/1999 The Veterinary Centre 271 Reading Road Henley-on-Thames Oxfordshire RG9 1EL **Tel:** (01491) 574490 w 613965X

YOUNG Christine Linda 21/08/1990 The Freda Powell Centre 1c Eynsham Drive Thamesmead London SE2 9RQ **Tel:** (020) 8311 6695 w 6064411

YOUNG Heidi Ann (see HAINES, Mrs)

YOUNG Helen Elizabeth (see READE, Mrs)

Joanna Claire DipAVN(Surgical) (nee Young, formerly Smith) 28/10/1991 (17/10/2006) 11 Northampton Road Lavendon OLNEY Buckinghamshire MK46 4EY w 6064444

Kirsty (nee MacGillivray) 15/03/1999 (21/06/2006) Barony College Parkgate Dumfries DG1 3NE **Tel:** (01387) 860251 w 6139569

Lee Victoria 13/05/2002 54 Stempe Close Hawkinge Folkestone Kent CT18 7PQ **Tel:** (0136) 886 4145 w 6264156

YOUNG Susan Alison (see MCLEAN, Mrs)

Teresa 14/11/1967 2 Offini Close West Bromwich West Midlands B70 6TA **Tel:** (0121) 553 1547 w 6064466

YOUNGSON Racheal Ann Louise (nee Warne) 06/08/1992 (01/04/2004) 2 Marsh Lane Worlingham Beccles Suffolk NR34 7PE **Tel:** (07941) 422313 w 600558X

Z

ZIEBART Darlene 05/09/1994 (13/03/2003) 6 Hillside Close Woodford Green Essex IG8 7QP **Tel:** (0208) 5052482 w 6037192

List of Equine Veterinary Nurses 2010

Notes:

1. The current Schedule 3 of the Veterinary Surgeons Act 1966 permits those Veterinary Nurses whose names are on the List of Veterinary Nurses, maintained by the Royal College of Veterinary Surgeons, to carry out any medical treatment or minor surgery (not involving entry into a body cavity) to an animal providing the guidance given in Section 4 of this List is complied with.
2. Listed Veterinary Nurses whose names appear in this section are not bound by the *Guide to Professional Conduct for Veterinary Nurses* and the obligations of undertaking compulsory Continuing Professional Development.
3. The first date after a veterinary nurse's name is the date of initial qualification. The date in brackets (if any) is the date of the last restoration to the List should a nurse's name have lapsed/been removed from the List at any time. These dates are not intended to indicate the periods for which a name has been on the List. Should information be required as to the full period or total periods a name has been on the List, a request should be made to the Registration Department.
4. Equine Veterinary Nurses whose names are on the List are entitled to use the postnominal letters "EVN" whilst their name is maintained on the List.

B

BONNER Sandra Jane 01/02/1990 (29/01/2002) 100 Colemans Moor Road Woodley Reading Berkshire RG5 4DN w 6045909

BUFTON Sarah Elizabeth (see SHONE, Mrs)

H

HAINES Tracy (nee Lynch) 01/09/1997 6 Claremont Court Grundys Lane MALVERN Worcestershire WR14 4HS w 6025777

HEYNES Charlotte Emily 23/11/1995 (07/02/2002) 10 Middle Lane Cropthorne PERSHORE Worcestershire WR10 3LZ **Tel:** (07974) 202856 w 6038287

HOUGH Louise Margaret 16/09/1997 (19/07/1999) Macclesfield Veterinary Hospital 26/38 Cumberland Street Macclesfield Cheshire SK10 1BZ **Tel:** (01625) 501500 w 6116075

I

ISAACS Melissa Jane 16/08/1995 (22/04/2002) 20 Lion Mead HASLEMERE Surrey GU27 1LF **Tel:** (01428) 643726 w 6026668

J

JONES Victoria Ann Carruthers 04/02/2002 Kennel Farm Southampton Road Clarendon SALISBURY SP5 3DG **Tel:** (01722) 710844 w 6274177

L

LYNCH Tracy (see HAINES, Mrs)

M

MORAN Avril Adele 25/09/2000 68 Maple Avenue Talke STOKE-ON-TRENT ST7 1JW **Tel:** (01782) 774987 w 6203458

S

SHONE Sarah Elizabeth (nee Bufton) 18/09/2000 Averley House Farm Hinckley Road Sapcote Leicester LE9 4LH **Tel:** (01455) 271277 w 6202765

SMITH Alison Hazel 08/11/1991 (26/02/2004) University of Cambridge Deptof Clinical Veterinary Medicine Madingley Cambridge CB3 OES **Tel:** (01223) 337647 w 6060814

Lisa Michelle EVN 04/09/1997 (02/11/2009) 200 St. Ediths Marsh Bromham CHIPPENHAM Wiltshire SN15 2DJ w 6100349

T

TRIGG Melanie Anna (see WHITLING, Mrs)

W

WHITLING Melanie Anna (nee Trigg) 17/11/2000 9 Wenlock Close Padgate Warrington Cheshire WA1 4JX **Tel:** (01925) 251259 w 6204184

Section 4

Veterinary Nurses and the Veterinary Surgeons Act 1966

Veterinary Nurses and the Veterinary Surgeons Act 1966

Introduction

1. Under the Veterinary Surgeons Act 1966 the general rule is that only a veterinary surgeon may practise veterinary surgery. There are, however, a number of exceptions to this rule, and two of them concern veterinary nurses. This note explains the law as it applies to them.

Definition of veterinary surgery

2. Veterinary surgery as defined in the Act means the art and science of veterinary surgery and medicine and, without prejudice to the generality of the foregoing, shall be taken to include

   (a) the diagnosis of diseases in, and injuries to, animals including tests performed on animals for diagnostic purposes;

   (b) the giving of advice based upon such diagnosis;

   (c) the medical or surgical treatment of animals; and

   (d) the performance of surgical operations on animals.

What can be done by people other than veterinary surgeons

3. Schedule 3 to the Act allows anyone to give first aid in an emergency for the purpose of saving life and relieving suffering. The owner of an animal, or a member of the owner's household or employee of the owner, may also give it minor medical treatment. There are a number of other exceptions to the general rule, mainly relating to farm animals, in addition to the exceptions which apply to veterinary nurses. The rules on veterinary nurses are explained below.

What can be done by veterinary nurses

4. Veterinary nurses, like anyone else, may give first aid and look after animals in ways which do not involve the practice of veterinary surgery. In addition, veterinary nurses may do the things specified in paragraphs 6 and 7 of Schedule 3 to the Veterinary Surgeons Act 1966 as amended by the Veterinary Surgeons Act 1966 (Schedule 3 Amendment) Order 2002, SI 2002/1479. The text of these paragraphs is set out in the annex below.

Qualified veterinary nurses

5. Paragraph 6 of the Schedule applies to veterinary nurses whose names are entered on the list maintained by RCVS. Listed veterinary nurses include Registered Veterinary Nurses for this purpose.

6. Listed veterinary nurses may administer any medical treatment or any minor surgery (not involving entry into a body cavity) under veterinary direction. The Schedule does not, however, authorise a veterinary nurse

to carry out any of a number of procedures which are specified in Part II of the Schedule. These excluded procedures are the castration of a horse, pony, ass or mule, the castration or spaying of a cat or dog, and a number of other procedures relating to farm animals.

7. The animal must be under the care of a veterinary surgeon and the treatment must be carried out at the veterinary surgeon's direction. The veterinary surgeon must be the employer of the veterinary nurse or be acting on behalf of the nurse's employer. The directing veterinary surgeon must be satisfied that the veterinary nurse is qualified to carry out the treatment or surgery.

Student veterinary nurses

8. Paragraph 7 of the Schedule applies to student veterinary nurses. A student veterinary nurse is someone enrolled for the purpose of training as a veterinary nurse at an approved training and assessment centre or a veterinary practice approved by such a centre.

9. A student veterinary nurse may administer any medical treatment or any minor surgery (not involving entry into a body cavity) under veterinary direction. Schedule 3 does not, however, allow the nurse to castrate a horse, pony, ass or mule, castrate or spay a cat or dog, or carry out certain procedures relating to farm animals.

10. The animal must be under the care of a veterinary surgeon and the treatment must be carried out at the veterinary surgeon's direction. The veterinary surgeon must be the employer of the veterinary nurse or be acting on behalf of the nurse's employer.

11. The treatment or minor surgery must be carried out in the course of the student veterinary nurse's training.

12. The treatment or surgery must be supervised by a veterinary surgeon or a listed veterinary nurse. In the case of surgery the supervision must be direct, continuous and personal.

Medical treatment and minor surgery

13. The Act does not define any medical treatment or any minor surgery (not involving entry into a body cavity). Ultimately it would be for the courts to decide what these words mean.

Guidance

14. Veterinary nurses should only carry out medical treatment or minor surgery after considering in each individual case whether they are competent to do so, taking into account their training and experience, the nature of the treatment or procedure and the condition of the patient. The directing veterinary surgeon should take the same matters into account in deciding whether the nurse is qualified to carry out the treatment.

Anaesthesia

15. There is separate guidance at RCVSonline on the role of veterinary nurses in the maintenance and monitoring of anaesthesia (www.rcvs.org.uk/advicenotes).

RCVS

March 2009

EXTRACTS FROM SCHEDULE 3 TO THE VETERINARY SURGEONS ACT 1966

Note: section 19(4)(b) of the Act allows a person who is not a veterinary surgeon to do anything specified in Part 1 of Schedule 3 to this Act and not excluded by Part II of that Schedule.

Extract from Part I of the Schedule

6. Any medical treatment or any minor surgery (not involving entry into a body cavity) to any animal by a veterinary nurse if the following conditions are complied with, that is to say

    (a) the animal is, for the time being, under the care of a registered veterinary surgeon or veterinary practitioner and the medical treatment or minor surgery is carried out by the veterinary nurse at his direction;

    (b) the registered veterinary surgeon or veterinary practitioner is the employer or is acting on behalf of the employer of the veterinary nurse; and

    (c) the registered veterinary surgeon or veterinary practitioner directing the medical treatment or minor surgery is satisfied that the veterinary nurse is qualified to carry out the treatment or surgery.

    In this paragraph and in paragraph 7 below

    veterinary nurse means a nurse whose name is entered in the list of veterinary nurses maintained by the College.

7. Any medical treatment or any minor surgery (not involving entry into a body cavity) to any animal by a student veterinary nurse if the following conditions are complied with, that is to say

    (a) the animal is, for the time being, under the care of a registered veterinary surgeon or veterinary practitioner and the medical treatment or minor surgery is carried out by the student veterinary nurse at his direction and in the course of the student veterinary nurse's training;

    (b) the treatment or surgery is supervised by a registered veterinary surgeon, veterinary practitioner or veterinary nurse and, in the case of surgery, the supervision is direct, continuous and personal; and

    (c) the registered veterinary surgeon or veterinary practitioner is the employer or is acting on behalf of the employer of the student veterinary nurse.

    In this paragraph

student veterinary nurse means a person enrolled under bye-laws made by the Council for the purpose of undergoing training as a veterinary nurse at an approved training and assessment centre or a veterinary practice approved by such a centre;

approved training and assessment centre means a centre approved by the Council for the purpose of training and assessing student veterinary nurses.

Part II of the Schedule

Nothing in section 19(4)(b) of this Act shall authorise—

(a) the castration of a male animal being—

  (i) a horse, pony, ass or mule,

  (ii) a bull, boar or goat which has reached the age of two months,

  (iii) a ram which has reached the age of three months, or

  (iv) a cat or dog;

(b) the spaying of a cat or dog;

(c) the removal (otherwise than in an emergency for the purpose of saving life or relieving pain or suffering) of any part of the antlers of a deer before the velvet of the antlers is frayed and the greater part of it has been shed;

(d) the desnooding of a turkey which has reached the age of 21 days;

(e) the removal of the combs of any poultry which have reached the age of 72 hours;

(f) the cutting of the toes of a domestic fowl or turkey which has reached the age of 72 hours;

(g) the performance of a vasectomy or the carrying out of electro-ejaculation on any animal or bird kept for the production of food, wool, skin or fur or for use in the farming of land;

(h) the removal of the supernumerary teats of a calf which has reached the age of 3 months; or

(i) the dehorning or disbudding of a sheep or goat, except the trimming of the insensitive tip of an ingrowing horn which, if left untreated, could cause pain or distress.

Section 5

Holders of the Diploma in Advanced Veterinary Nursing (Surgical)

Holders of the Diploma in Advanced Veterinary Nursing (Medical)

Listed and Registered Veterinary Nurses who are holders of the Diploma in Advanced Veterinary Nursing (Surgical)

Name	Year
Andrews, Victoria Joyce	2001
Andrews-jones, Belinda Sally	2004
Archer, Emma	2006
Armstrong, Sarah Jane	2008
Armstrong, Sarah Jane	2009
Attwater, Fiona Jane	2002
Bailey, Michelle Tamzin	1998
Baldwin, June Editha	1992
Barnett, Wendy Jane	1999
Barton, Sarah-Gay	2006
Bayes, Charlotte Victoria	2008
Baylis, Sarah	1999
Bealey, Joanna Ruth	2006
Bevan, Rebecca Louise	2004
Birch, Nicola	1997
Boswell, Victoria Louise	2007
Bowcott, Amy	2006
Bowman, Verity Jane	1993
Branscombe, Elizabeth Ann	1994
Brennand, Kerry Louise	2009
Brewer, Julie Ann	1995
Brockway, Claire	2008
Brown, Caroline Marguerite	1992
Burke, Julia Ann	2001
Burnett, Janet	1992
Carver, Donna	1998
Challis, Katherine Jane	2002
Chandler, Sharon	1993
Chaplin, Helen Judith	2006
Charlesworth, Linda Anne	2007
Chivers, Elaine Ann	2008
Christie, Eve Odette	2007
Cockburn, Cheryl Anne	2002
Coles, Geraldine Elaine	2000
Cosgrove, Michelle Marie	1996
Cottrell, Jane	1996
Cox, Donna Alison	1998
Creighton, Dorothy Elizabeth	1997
Cullum-hanshaw, Kathryn Sarah	1999

Name	Year
Cummins, Wendy Jane	1998
Daniels, Lois	1995
Darby, Lynn	1994
Davey, Marie	2007
Dean, Alisa	2005
Denniss, Anita Lesley	2003
Dingle, Katie Jane	2001
Duggan, Shenade Lucinda	2005
Elliott, Julii	2000
Firth, Debra Lynette	2005
Fletcher, Tamsin Liesel	2003
Forrest, Nicola Kristine	1998
Freeman, Joan Mary	1995
Fry, Katie Elizabeth	2003
Fulcher, Wendy Joanne	1996
Gaskin, Sharon Theresa	1992
George, Caroline Sally-Jane	1993
Glenwright, Gail Ann	1998
Goddard, Lucy Ann	2004
Gordon, Karen	2002
Goulding, Catherine Tracey	1996
Goulding, Karen	1996
Gowshall, Rachel Louise	1992
Greenhalgh, Natalie-Jane	2006
Grierson, Michelle Anne	1998
Guinan, Diane Elizabeth	1997
Hack, Nathalie Maria Lea	2003
Halil, Wendy Louise	2005
Hall, Kerry	2004
Hamilton, Janis Christine	1995
Harris, Janet Lois	1997
Hayes, Laura	2003
Hemingway, Elaine	2002
Higginson, Joanna Kenzie Erica	2000
Hill, Nichole Anita Teresa	2004
Hill, Rebecca	2006
Hodgson, Verity	2009
Holder, Abigail Ruth	1997
Hollis, Caroline Mary	1994

Name	Year
Hollyoak, Ursula	2001
Holmes, Paula	2007
Hopkins, Sian Elizabeth	1992
Hopley, Lorraine Margaret	2003
Howarth, Susan Dianne	2000
Howell, Joy Sarah Helen	1992
Hughes, Helen	2003
Hunter, Gail	1994
Jackson, Nadine Emily	2008
Jeffery, Andrea Karen	1995
Johnson, Julie Ann	2007
Johnson, Rita Caroline	1998
Kelly, Audrey	1999
Kilbane, Hayley Jayne	2005
Killner, Josephine	2001
King, Emily Jane	2008
Knight, Leigh Patricia	2005
Lear, Tracey Elizabeth	2001
Leworthy, Katie May	2009
Lines, Marion Patricia	2002
Lutwyche, Tracy Anne	2008
Macdonald, Jill Mary Fiona	2006
Macgillivray, Janice Elizabeth	1994
Magee, Annaliese Helen	2003
Marshall, Catherine Mary	2003
Martin, Carole	1993
Masters, Sharon Ann	1992
Matthews, Joanna	2000
Maxwell, Nina	1992
Mcallister, Lucy Jane	1998
Mccomb, Pamela Crawford	1993
Mcfadyen, Fiona Anne	2003
Mchugh, Dawn Patricia	1992
Mckeane, Amanda Jane	2005
Mcnamara, Elaine Bridget Ann	2002
Mcnellan, Angela Mary	2002
Milne, Louise	1998
Moon, Louise Mary	1999
Morgan, Samantha Francis	2008
Moss, Sarah Louise	1994
Mothersdale, Susan	1997
Murray, Cheryl Linda	2006
Murray, Janice Elizabeth	1992
Nartey, Gertrude Dede-Ofoley	2004
Nichols, Katy Ann	2004
Norman, Alexandra	1995

Name	Year
Nuttall, Linzi Angela	2002
O'dwyer, Louise Mary	2004
Oliver, Gwen	1995
Orpet, Hilary Anne	1993
Osborne, Davina Elizabeth	2007
Parker, Alison	1992
Parry, Josephine Jeanette	2001
Passingham, Caroline Michelle	2007
Pitts, Natasha Claire	2005
Pollard, Deborah Jane	1998
Pollard, Valerie Anne	2003
Pollock, Jacqueline Ann	2007
Prisk, Denise Margaret	2006
Pucknell, Catharine Hilary	1999
Rankin, Rachel Louise	2006
Read, Tracey Joy	1994
Rees, Michelle Melanie	2004
Richmond, Michelle Linda	2005
Roberts, Deborah	2006
Robinson, Alison Clare	2003
Robinson, Susan Jane	2005
Russell, Tracey Jane	2003
Rutland, Gary Alan	2007
Sample, Kerry Anne	2007
Savill, Carolyn Hilda	1994
Scott, Karen	2003
Shellim, Claire Vanessa	2006
Sheppard, Angela Louise	2007
Shield, Kirstie May	2006
Silver, Sarah Helen	2005
Simm, Joanne	2000
Simpson, Shirley	2003
Skelton, Alison Jean	1992
Skinner, Kerry Marie	2007
Slater, Linda Ann	1999
Smith, Holly Suzanne	1998
Smith, Jennifer	1992
Smith, Louise Maria	2004
Smith, Wendy Louise	1997
Stanton, Diana May	1999
Stephens, Helen Jane	2006
Stephenson, Catherine Mary	2005
Stone, Kelly Louise	2008
Stoner, Belinda Jane	2001
Strike, Christine Mowbray	2000
Taylor, Clare Louise	2007

Name	Year
Thomas, Jane Alison	2006
Thompson, Carol	1996
Thompson, Jennifer	2007
Thompson, Jennifer	2008
Thompson, Kathryn Alison	2007
Thompson, Lisa Michelle	2006
Tomlinson, Sarah Louise	2001
Varlow, Margaret Hilary	2001
Wallace, Angela	2000
Ward, Anne Marie	2000
Weekes, Clare Joanne	2007
Welsh, Perdita	1994
Wheat, Tracey Jane	1998

Name	Year
White, Ross Devereux	1999
Whiting, Sandra Samantha	2003
Whittaker, Sarah Louise	2000
Wilde, Simone Sharon	2002
Williams, Stephanie	1997
Withers, Julia Margaret	2001
Woodley, Rachael Lucy	2006
Woods, Sara Dee	2006
Worthing, Sally Ann	1998
Yates, Josephine Margaret	1993
Young, Alison Sarah	2005
Young, Joanna Claire	1999

Listed and Registered Veterinary Nurses who are holders of the Diploma in Advanced Veterinary Nursing (Medical)

Name	Year
Adams, Alice Elizabeth	2007
Alger, Laura Jean	2005
Birch, Nicola	2004
Blues, Debra	2002
Brudenell, Natalie Anne	2008
Burke, Julia Ann	2006
Campbell, Susan Mary	2009
Chandler, Sharon	2003
Chapman, Kara Marie	2008
Collins, Sarah Michelle	2005
Cory, Julie	2002
Crook, Sarah Rachel	2007
Cummins, Wendy Jane	2002
Defries, Claire Ilana Natalie	2007
Donovan, Michelle Rowena Simone	2009
Dore, Marianne Christine	2008
Drummond, Juliet Christina	2003
Dyer, Rachel Elizabeth	2008
Fletcher, Virginia	2007
Fontaine, Samantha Joanna	2007
Gallagher, Kerrie-Ann	2008
Garrod, Rachel Elizabeth Clare	2003
Goddard, Lucy Ann	2007
Gordon, Karen	2007
Hayes, Laura	2006
Hayward, Nicola Joanne	2005
Hill, Nichole Anita Teresa	2009
Howarth, Susan Dianne	2003
Jameson, Katherine Jane	2004
Jermey, Victoria Jayne	2007
Johnson, Emma Jeanne	2009
Jones, Marie	2002
Killner, Josephine	2006
Lindley, Sarah Louise	2005
Macalister, Gemma Irene	2008
Macdonald, Diane	2002
Mcmillan, Samantha Jane	2006
Mercado, Joanne Louise	2008
Mogridge, Gemma Catherine	2006
Morgan, Samantha Francis	2003
O'byrne, Evelyn	2004
O'dwyer, Louise Mary	2007
Oliver, Gwen	2005
Parry, Judith Elizabeth	2006
Patten, Melanie Rachel	2005
Price, Sarah Kate	2008
Rendell, Michelle	2005
Richards, Mary Joy Rose	2004
Riches-tomei, Julie Louise	2003
Richmond, Michelle Linda	2002
Roberts, Linda Jane	2006
Rooney, Helen Elizabeth	2005
Rudd, Suzanne	2004
Tindall, Lynsey Anne	2008
Wakefield, Karen	2006
Ward, Dawn	2003
Ward, Rebecca Julia	2007
Webster, Amanda Marie	2007
Wedd, Cindy Ann	2006
Wilde, Simone Sharon	2005
Wood, Gemma Enid	2008